HIV Infection in Primary Care

HIV Infection in Primary Care

Editors

R. MICHAEL BUCKLEY, MD

Clinical Professor of Medicine,
Department of Medicine,
University of Pennsylvania;
Chairman, Department of Medicine,
The Pennsylvania Hospital,
Philadelphia, Pennsylvania

STEPHEN J. GLUCKMAN, MD

Professor of Medicine,
Department of Medicine,
University of Pennsylvania;
Chief, Infectious Diseases Clinical Services,
Hospital of the University of Pennsylvania,
Philadelphia, Pennsylvania

with 41 illustrations

W.B. SAUNDERS COMPANY
An Imprint of Elsevier Science
Philadelphia   London   New York   St. Louis   Sydney   Toronto

W.B. Saunders Company
An Imprint of Elsevier Sciences

The Curtis Center
Independence Square West
Philadelphia, Pennsylvania 19106

Publishing Director: Steven Merahn
Acquisitions Editor: Elizabeth Fathman
Editorial Assistant: Paige Mosher Wilke
Publishing Services Manager: Pat Joiner
Project Manager: David Stein
Designer: Mark Oberkrom

Library of Congress Cataloging-in-Publication Data

HIV infection in primary care / editors, R. Michael Buckley, Stephen J. Gluckman.
   p. ; cm.
  Includes bibliographical references and index.
  ISBN 0-7216-8601-X
   1. AIDS (Disease) 2. Primary care (Medicine) I. Buckley, R. Michael. II. Gluckman, Stephen J., M.D.
   [DNLM: 1. HIV Infections—complications. 2. HIV Infections—diagnosis. 3. AIDS-Related Opportunistic Infections—diagnosis. 4. AIDS-Related Opportunistic Infections—therapy. 5. Primary Health Care. WC 503.1 H676 2002]
  RC606.6 .H586 2002
  616.97′92—dc21

                                                2002017603

HIV INFECTION IN PRIMARY CARE   ISBN 0-7216-8601-X

Copyright © 2002, Elsevier Science (USA). All rights reserved.

All rights reserved. No part of this publication may be reproduced, stored in a retrieval system, or transmitted, in any form or by any means, electronic, mechanical, photocopying, recording, or otherwise, without written permission of the publisher.

Printed in the United States of America

02 03 04 05/ 9 8 7 6 5 4 3 2 1

CONTRIBUTORS

JENNIFER L. ALDRICH, MD
Adjunct Assistant Professor,
Department of Medicine,
Division of Infectious Diseases,
Hospital of the University of Pennsylvania;
Director of Clinical HIV Services,
Department of Ambulatory Health Services,
Philadelphia Department of Public Health,
Philadelphia, Pennsylvania

YVETTE E. APPIAH, MD
Housestaff PGY-IV,
Department of Dermatology,
Hospital of the University of Pennsylvania,
Philadelphia, Pennsylvania

TODD D. BARTON, MD
Fellow, Section of Infectious Diseases,
University of Pennsylvania,
Philadelphia, Pennsylvania

PETER BERTHOLD, LDS, PhD, DMD
Professor and Chair,
Department of Dental Care Systems,
University of Pennsylvania,
School of Dental Medicine,
Philadelphia, Pennsylvania

KATHLEEN BRADY, MD
Instructor in Medicine,
Department of Medicine,
Division of Infectious Disease,
University of Pennsylvania,
Philadelphia, Pennsylvania

MICHAEL N. BRAFFMAN, MD
Clinical Associate Professor of Medicine,
Department of Medicine,
University of Pennsylvania;
Chief, Infectious Diseases Section,
Pennsylvania Hospital,
Philadelphia, Pennsylvania

R. MICHAEL BUCKLEY, MD
Clinical Professor of Medicine,
Department of Medicine,
University of Pennsylvania;
Chairman, Department of Medicine,
The Pennsylvania Hospital,
Philadelphia, Pennsylvania

CHARLES R. CANTOR, MD
Clinical Assistant Professor of Neurology,
Department of Neurology,
University of Pennsylvania School of Medicine,
Pennsylvania Hospital,
Philadelphia, Pennsylvania

ELIZABETH M. COLSTON, MD, PhD
Fellow, Department of Medicine,
Division of Infectious Diseases,
University of Pennsylvania,
Hospital of the University of Pennsylvania,
Philadelphia, Pennsylvania

KEVIN J. CROSS
Medical Student,
University of Pennsylvania School of Medicine,
Philadelphia, Pennsylvania

NEIL O. FISHMAN, MD
Assistant Professor of Medicine,
Division of Infectious Diseases,
University of Pennsylvania;
Director, Department of Healthcare Epidemiology
    and Infection Control,
Director, Antimicrobial Management Program,
University of Pennsylvania Medical Center,
Philadelphia, Pennsylvania

IAN FRANK, MD
Associate Professor,
Department of Medicine,
University of Pennsylvania,
Philadelphia, Pennsylvania

MICHAEL GLICK, DMD
Professor, Department of Diagnostic Sciences,
University of Medicine and Dentistry
    of New Jersey/New Jersey Dental School,
Newark, New Jersey

STEPHEN J. GLUCKMAN, MD
Professor of Medicine,
Department of Medicine,
University of Pennsylvania;
Chief, Infectious Diseases Clinical Services,
Hospital of the University of Pennsylvania,
Philadelphia, Pennsylvania

STEPHEN M. GOLDMAN, MD
Clinical Assistant Professor of Ophthalmology,
University of Pennsylvania;
Chief, Section of Ophthalmology,
Assistant Surgeon,
Department of Surgery,
The Pennsylvania Hospital,
Philadelphia, Pennsylvania

AMY L. GRAZIANI, PharmD
Associate Professor, Adjunct Faculty,
Department of Pharmacy Practice,
University of the Sciences in Philadelphia,
Philadelphia College of Pharmacy and Science;
Clinical Pharmacist Specialist,
HIV and Anti-Infectives,
Department of Pharmacy Services,
University of Pennsylvania Medical Center,
Philadelphia, Pennsylvania

PAUL R. GROSS, MD
Clinical Professor,
Department of Dermatology,
University of Pennsylvania;
Head, Section of Dermatology,
The Pennsylvania Hospital,
Philadelphia, Pennsylvania

ROBERT GROSS, MD, MSCE
Assistant Professor of Medicine and Epidemiology,
Department of Medicine,
Division of Infectious Disease,
Department of Biostatistics and Epidemiology,
University of Pennsylvania School of Medicine,
Philadelphia, Pennsylvania

ROBERT M. GROSSBERG, MD
Instructor, Department of Medicine,
Division of Infectious Diseases,
University of Pennsylvania School of Medicine;
Instructor, Department of Medicine,
Division of Infectious Diseases,
Philadelphia Veterans Administration Medical Center,
Philadelphia, Pennsylvania

JOSEPH HASSEY, MD
Clinical Assistant Professor of Medicine,
Temple University School of Medicine,
Division of Infectious Diseases,
Abington Memorial Hospital,
Abington, Pennsylvania

KELLY J. HENNING, MD
Clinical Assistant Professor of Medicine,
University of Pennsylvania;
Department of Medicine,
Division of Infectious Diseases,
The Pennsylvania Hospital,
Philadelphia, Pennsylvania

DAVID H. HENRY, MD
Clinical Associate Professor of Medicine,
University of Pennsylvania;
Hematology-Oncology Section,
The Pennsylvania Hospital;
Director, HIV Malignancy Program,
University of Pennsylvania Health System,
Philadelphia, Pennsylvania

JANET M. HINES, MD
Assistant Professor of Medicine,
Department of Internal Medicine,
Division of Infectious Diseases,
University of Pennsylvania School of Medicine;
Associate Director, Immunodeficiency Program,
Department of Medicine,
Division of Infectious Diseases,
University of Pennsylvania Medical Center,
Philadelphia, Pennsylvania

STUART N. ISAACS, MD
Assistant Professor,
Department of Medicine,
Division of Infectious Diseases,
University of Pennsylvania;
Department of Medicine/Infectious Diseases,
Hospital of the University of Pennsylvania;
Philadelphia Veterans Administration Medical Center,
Philadelphia, Pennsylvania

KARA JUDSON, MD
Division of Infectious Diseases,
University of Pennsylvania Medical Center,
Philadelphia, Pennsylvania

JAY R. KOSTMAN, MD
Clinical Associate Professor of Medicine,
Division of Infectious Diseases, Department of Medicine,
University of Pennsylvania School of Medicine;
Head, Division of Infectious Diseases,
Presbyterian Medical Center,
University of Pennsylvania Health System,
Philadelphia, Pennsylvania

EBBING LAUTENBACH, MD, MPH
Assistant Professor of Medicine and Epidemiology,
Senior Scholar,
Center for Clinical Epidemiology and Biostatisics,
Department of Medicine, Division of Infectious Diseases,
University of Pennsylvania School of Medicine;
Hospital Epidemiologist,
Department of Medicine,
Division of Infectious Diseases,
Presbyterian Medical Center,
Philadelphia, Pennsylvania

ROB ROY MacGREGOR, MD
Professor, Department of Medicine,
Division of Infectious Diseases,
University of Pennsylvania School of Medicine;
Attending Physician,
Department of Medicine,
Hospital of the University of Pennsylvania,
Philadelphia, Pennsylvania

LEO McCLUSKEY, MD
Assistant Professor of Neurology,
Department of Neurology,
University of Pennsylvania School of Medicine,
Philadelphia, Pennsylvania

DANIEL K. MEYER, MD
Assistant Professor of Medicine,
Division of Infectious Diseases,
Cooper Hospital—University Medical Center,
University of Medicine and Dentistry of New Jersey,
Robert Wood Johnson Medical School at Camden,
Camden, New Jersey

ANNE H. NORRIS, MD
Instructor in Medicine,
University of Pennsylvania,
Philadelphia, Pennsylvania

K. ADU NTOSO, MD
Clinical Associate Professor of Medicine,
University of Pennsylvania School of Medicine;
Section of Renal Disease and Hypertension,
The Pennsylvania Hospital,
Philadelphia, Pennsylvania

BRET J. RUDY, MD
Assistant Professor of Pediatrics,
Craig Dalsmer Division of Adolescent Medicine,
University of Pennsylvania School of Medicine;
Medical Director,
Adolescent HIV Infection,
Children's Hospital of Philadelphia,
Philadelphia, Pennsylvania

RICHARD M. RUTSTEIN, MD
Associate Professor of Pediatrics,
University of Pennsylvania School of Medicine;
Medical Director, Special Immunology Service,
Division of General Pediatrics,
Children's Hospital of Philadelphia,
Philadelphia, Pennsylvania

MINDY SCHUSTER, MD
Assistant Professor of Medicine/Infectious Diseases,
Department of Medicine/Infectious Diseases,
University of Pennsylvania,
Philadelphia, Pennsylvania

JOHN J. STERN, MD
Clinical Associate Professor of Medicine,
Department of Medicine,
University of Pennsylvania School of Medicine;
Division of Infectious Diseases,
Department of Medicine,
The Pennsylvania Hospital,
Philadelphia, Pennsylvania

JAMES TANG, MD
PGY 1 in the Transitional Year Program,
Lemuel Shattuck Hospital,
Jamaica Plain, Massachusetts

ROGER E. WEISS, MD
Clinical Associate,
Department of Psychiatry,
University of Pennsylvania Health System;
Active Staff, Department of Psychiatry,
The Pennsylvania Hospital,
Philadelphia, Pennsylvania

To our patients

PREFACE

In the two decades that we have been treating individuals infected with the human immunodeficiency virus (HIV) much has changed. In the early 1980s, we learned how to recognize and treat opportunistic infections (OIs) that even the most experienced infectious disease clinicians had rarely seen. Despite our best efforts, patients died, often within weeks of the appearance of these infections. As antiretrovirals were introduced and as we became more experienced at preventing OIs, there appeared a glimmer of hope that we might someday begin to control this most clever and deadly virus. Further progress toward this goal has been made with the introduction of combination therapy and highly active antiretroviral therapy (HAART).

These new therapies, however, have changed the way that health professionals care for people with HIV, and have shifted treatment strategies to the outpatient setting. As patients are living longer and as fewer are being hospitalized, the clinical burden of care is actually increasing. It is likely that primary care practitioners will continue to see more of these patients in their offices and clinics. This book is designed to give primary care providers concise and practical information on the diagnosis and management of patients infected with HIV. Part I, *Early Infection,* focuses on evaluating and testing patients at risk for HIV infection. These chapters discuss how to evaluate and counsel newly diagnosed patients, how to monitor their immune system, when and how to treat them before they are severely immunosuppressed, and ultimately how to keep them well for as long as possible. Part II, *Symptomatic Progressive Infection,* focuses on the diagnosis and treatment of OIs and other manifestations of progressive infection. Part III, *Late Infections,* discusses some special aspects of HIV infection, and the differential diagnosis of common syndromes in full-blown AIDS.

The care of the HIV-infected patient is occasionally complex and at times requires careful consultation and clear communication among the patient, the primary health care provider, and an AIDS specialist. We have collaborated with our primary care colleagues in the care of many HIV-positive patients, and we have learned much from one another. It is in that spirit that this book is written.

You, in primary care, will be providing the continuity of care for many of these patients, care that is both difficult and highly rewarding. We believe that you will find this text useful as you face this challenge.

R. MICHAEL BUCKLEY
STEPHEN J. GLUCKMAN

ACKNOWLEDGMENTS

We are indebted to the many colleagues who authored the chapters in this book. They are a group of highly skilled clinicians, researchers, and teachers, dedicated to contributing new knowledge to the field, to taking excellent care of patients with HIV, and to teaching others to do so as well. Each has contributed his or her valuable time and expertise to share considerable experience and knowledge with others. We acknowledge their efforts and thank them.

We are also grateful to David Stein and Paige Mosher Wilke for their professional and patient advice and editorial assistance.

R. MICHAEL BUCKLEY
STEPHEN J. GLUCKMAN

CONTENTS

PART I EARLY INFECTION, 1

1. **The Virus, Its Epidemiology, and the Natural History of Infection**, 3
   KELLY J. HENNING

2. **Acute HIV-1 Infection**, 14
   ELIZABETH M. COLSTON, R. MICHAEL BUCKLEY

3. **Testing for the Virus**, 20
   JAY R. KOSTMAN

4. **Initial Management of HIV Infection**, 24
   STEPHEN J. GLUCKMAN

5. **Antiretroviral Therapy**, 30
   IAN FRANK, AMY L. GRAZIANI

6. **Prevention of Opportunistic Infections**, 44
   KARA JUDSON, NEIL O. FISHMAN

PART II SYMPTOMATIC PROGRESSIVE INFECTION, 55
Section One: *Opportunistic Infections*, 57

7. ***Pneumocystis Carinii* Pneumonia**, 57
   JAMES TANG, JOHN J. STERN

8. **Mycobacterial Infections**, 68
   ROB ROY MacGREGOR

9. **Fungal Infections**, 79
   DANIEL K. MEYER, MINDY SCHUSTER

10. **Cytomegalovirus and Other Herpes Family Viral Infections**, 85
    KATHLEEN BRADY

11. **Toxoplasmosis and Other Protozoal Infections**, 96
    EBBING LAUTENBACH, STUART N. ISAACS

12. **Bacterial Infections in HIV**, 108
    ROBERT M. GROSSBERG

Section Two: *Symptoms and Signs Indicative of Progressive Infection*, 118

13. **Skin Manifestations of HIV Infection**, 118
    YVETTE E. APPIAH, PAUL R. GROSS

14. **Oral Manifestations of HIV Infection**, 132
    MICHAEL GLICK, PETER BERTHOLD

15. **Ocular Complications of AIDS**, 141
    STEPHEN M. GOLDMAN

16. **Renal Disease in HIV**, 154
    K. ADU NTOSO

17. **Central Nervous System Complications**, 166
    CHARLES R. CANTOR, LEO McCLUSKEY

18. **Neuropsychiatric Complications of HIV Infection**, 177
    ROGER E. WEISS

19. **Gastrointestinal Disease**, 193
    ROBERT GROSS

PART III LATE INFECTION, 203
Section One: *Differential Diagnosis of Common Syndromes*, 205

20. **Pneumonia**, 205
    MICHAEL N. BRAFFMAN

21. **HIV and Diarrhea**, 216
    TODD D. BARTON, ANNE H. NORRIS

22. **Wasting**, 223
    JENNIFER L. ALDRICH, JOSEPH HASSEY

23. **Fever of Unknown Origin**, 229
    KEVIN J. CROSS, JANET M. HINES, STEPHEN J. GLUCKMAN

Section Two: *Special Aspects*, 236

24. **Malignancy in HIV-Infected Patients**, 236
    DAVID H. HENRY

25. **HIV Infection in Children and Adolescents**, 249
    RICHARD M. RUTSTEIN, BRET J. RUDY

Part I

EARLY INFECTION

1 The Virus, Its Epidemiology, and the Natural History of Infection

KELLY J. HENNING

The Virus

The acquired immunodeficiency syndrome (AIDS) is caused by human immunodeficiency virus type 1 (HIV-1), an association that was not discovered until 1983-1984. HIV-1 is a human retrovirus, an RNA virus that is somewhat unique in that it replicates via a DNA intermediate.

Retroviruses are enveloped and contain two identical single-stranded RNA molecules, allowing for frequent genetic change through a mechanism called recombination. Retroviruses integrate their RNA genomes as a DNA provirus in the chromosomes of cells that they infect, and the provirus is replicated along with the cell's genes.

The classification of retroviruses is based on nucleotide and amino acid sequence comparisons. HIV-1 is a member of the lentivirus group, as is the HIV-2 virus, the simian immunodeficiency virus, the feline immunodeficiency virus, and the ovine/equine/bovine lentiviruses. There are two human lentiviruses: HIV-1, the most common HIV type found throughout the world, and HIV-2, principally found in persons from West Africa. These two human lentiviruses have the most complex genome structure and expression strategy of any of the retroviruses. HIV-1 and HIV-2 are thus prone to frequent mutations of their genomes.

There are at least eight distinct steps in the HIV-1 replication cycle: virus attachment, entry, reverse transcription of the viral genome, integration, gene expression, assembly, budding, and maturation (Fig. 1-1). In the first step the viral envelope attaches to the specific host-cell receptors. The host cell receptor is the CD4 molecule that CD4 lymphocytes and some macrophages express on their surfaces. However, the CD4 molecule alone is not sufficient to permit HIV-1 entry into cells. Other human-specific accessory factors, such as fusin and CC-CKR-5, have recently been identified that work with the CD4 molecule. Fusin is a co-receptor for T-trophic HIV-1 strains. CC-CKR-5 is a co-receptor for macrophage-trophic HIV-1 strains, the strains that are believed to be the key pathogenic strains in vivo. CC-CKR-5 is a receptor for the β-chemokines regulated on activation, normal T cell expressed and secreted (RANTES), macrophage inhibitory protein (MIP)-1 α, and MIP-1 β. These chemokines are small chemotactic cytokines that attract leukocytes to sites of inflammation. α-Chemokines activate neutrophils, whereas β-chemokines activate T lymphocytes, basophils, eosinophils, and macrophages. Exciting new work in this area has opened up new avenues of possible therapy and prevention of HIV-1 infection.

Following attachment and cell entry, viral nucleoprotein complexes enter the target cell cytoplasm. Within these complexes, reverse transcriptase (RT) directs the synthesis of a DNA copy of the viral RNA genome. The viral DNA–containing complexes then migrate to the nucleus and integrate into the cell's chromosomal DNA under the direction of the viral integrase protein. The integrated viral DNA forms a provirus. Expression of the provirus produces spliced and unspliced viral messenger RNA (mRNA) that encodes for the regulatory and structural *(gag* and *gag-pol)* viral proteins. The *gag* and *gag-pol* viral polyprotein precursors and genomic-length viral RNA are assembled into new virus particles at the cell surface. As HIV-1 particles bud through the cell membrane, they acquire a lipid bilayer that contains the envelope proteins. During or slightly after budding, the viral protease cleaves *gag* and *gag-pol* precursor polyproteins to the mature individual proteins, which generates infectious virus.

HIV is composed of three basic components: the envelope, the RNA genome, and structural proteins (Table 1-1). The envelope of all retroviruses is composed of a lipid bilayer that is derived from the cell membrane. The HIV envelope contains viral surface (gp 120) and transmembrane envelope proteins (gp 41). The HIV genome consists of a dimer of identical single-stranded RNA molecules. In contrast to the simple retroviruses that contain only the *gag* (capsid proteins), *pol* (protease, RT, integrase, and RNase), and *env* (envelope) genes, HIV-1 and HIV-2 are complex retroviruses because they also possess regulatory genes that can enhance or perhaps depress viral expression. The regulatory proteins of HIV-1 are *tat, rev, vpu, vpr, vif,* and *nef* (Table 1-2). All of the regulatory proteins have a positive effect, to stimulate or enhance the production of HIV-1 particles in infected cells.

There is substantial genetic variation of HIV because of the extremely high replication rate in infected individuals, the poor fidelity of the viral RT system, and the substantial viral load. A swarm of quasispecies of HIV develops in different people or even within an individual. The quasispecies are related but distinct HIV variants that diverge increasingly over time. The greatest variation occurs in the *env* gene, with lesser variations in the *gag* and *pol* genes. In the V3 region of the *env* gene, this hypervariability is associated with the immune response against the virus. The more variability, the less chance for a single vaccine prototype. Nine subtypes, clades, or genotypes of HIV-1 have been characterized based on *env* sequences (Fig. 1-2 and Table 1-3). Subtypes A through H constitute the major group for HIV-1, group M. An additional ninth subtype I has been described. Divergent or outlying strains of HIV-1, outside group M, have been described and categorized as group O.

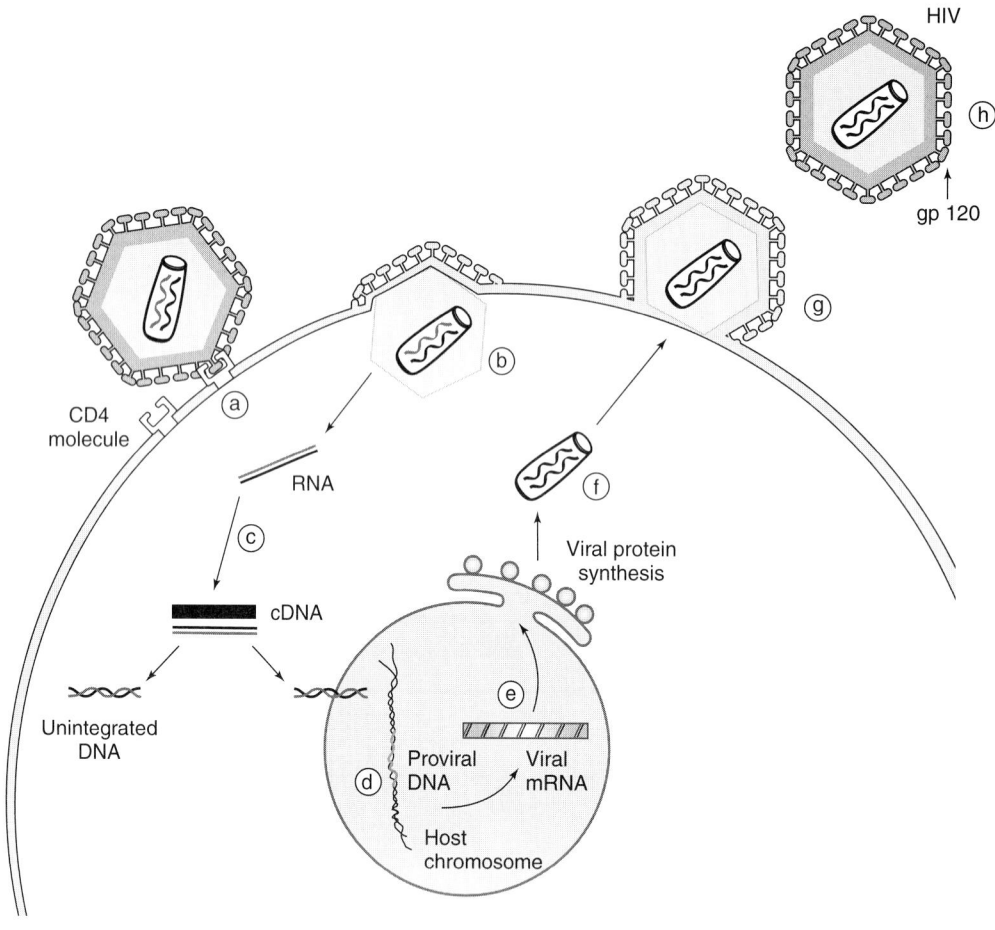

FIG. 1-1 The HIV replication cycle. The 8 principal steps are represented as: (a) attachment, (b) entry, (c) reverse transcriptase, (d) integration, (e) gene expression, (f) assembly, (g) budding, (h) maturation. (Modified from Hardy WD: The human immunodeficiency virus, *Med Clin North Am* 80:1244, 1996.)

TABLE 1-1
HIV-1 Structural Proteins

Retroviral gene	Current protein name	HIV proteins	Polyprotein precursor
gag	Matrix (MA)	p17	
gag	?	p6	
gag	Capsid (CA)	p24	pr 55gag
gag	Nucleocapsid (NC)	p9	
pol	Protease (PR)	p10	p190gag-pol
pol	Reverse transcriptase (RT)	p50	
pol	RNase H (RN)	p15	
pol	Integrase (IN)	p32	
env	Surface (SU)	gp 120	9p 160env
env	Transmembrane (TM)	gp 41	

Modified from Hardy WD: The human immunodeficiency virus, *Med Clin North Am* 80:1247, 1996.

TABLE 1-2
HIV-1 Regulatory Proteins

Regulatory gene	Protein	Function
tat	p16/p14	Binds to RNA and increases primary viral transcription 1,000-fold
rev	p19	Necessary for expression of structural proteins and generation of new viral particles
vpu	p16	Promotes export (release) of viral particles
vif	p23	Enhances viral maturation
vpr	p10–15	Augments rate of virus production
nef	p25	Augments the infectivity of progeny virions; complete role undefined

Modified from Hardy WD: The human immunodeficiency virus, *Med Clin North Am* 80:1248, 1996.

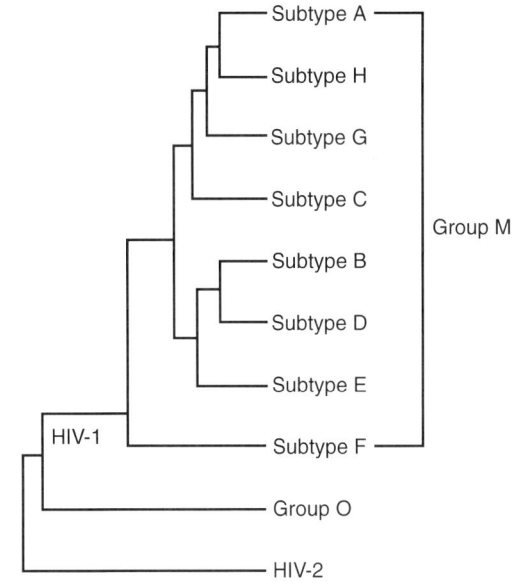

FIG. 1-2 A simplified phylogenetic tree of HIV-1. Group M represents the major group of HIV-1; group O consists of outliers. A ninth subtype I has been reported but is not included because it has not been characterized using the same sequence regions as other subtypes with group M. (Modified from Hardy WD: The human immunodeficiency virus, *Med Clin North Am* 80:1251, 1996.)

TABLE 1-3
Distribution of HIV-1 Subtypes Around the World

Region	A	B	C	D	E	F	G	H	I	O
Africa	+	+	+	+	+	+	+	+		+
Middle East									+	
Europe	+	+	+	+		+	+	+		+
Asia		+	+		+					
India	+	+	+							
Australia		+								
North America		+								
South America		+	+		+					

(GROUP M columns: A–H; then I; then O)

Modified from Hardy WD: The human immunodeficiency virus, *Med Clin North Am* 80:1251, 1996.

In general, people infected with HIV-1 virtually never have more than one subtype of virus. Although the sequences of the viral RNA genome isolated from an infected person vary continually, they are closely related, and the variation arises from mutation rather than from infection with different HIV-1 subtypes. There are characteristic HIV subtype geographic distribution patterns (see Table 1-3) that may relate to the predominant modes of HIV transmission in various regions. Subtype B predominates in North and South America and Europe, whereas subtype E is more prevalent in Southeast Asia, especially Thailand. In Thailand subtype E infects heterosexuals almost exclusively, but subtype B mainly infects injecting drug users (IDU). Subtype B is transmitted by blood among intravenous drug users (IVDU) and by homosexual sex in Europe and the United States. These differences may be at least partially due to the fact that some, but not all, reports have suggested that subtype E replicates more easily in Langerhans' cells, found in the reproductive tract, than does subtype B.

It is difficult to draw conclusions about relative transmissibility of different HIV-1 subtypes from available data, although large differences in transmissibility have been demonstrated between HIV-1 and HIV-2, with HIV-2 having much lower rates of sexual and mother-to-infant transmission. There is a lack of strong and consistent associations between transmission rates and particular HIV-1 subtypes. However, increasing evidence suggests that there are differences in HIV strains with regard to their cell tropism and host ranges. Some studies have shown enhanced disease progression with certain HIV-1 phenotypes, specifically with syncytium-inducing versus non–syncytium-inducing strains.

Epidemiology

AIDS was first identified in mid-1981, following reports of unusual clusters of *Pneumocystis carinii* pneumonia and Kaposi's sarcoma among homosexual men in New York City, Los Angeles, and San Francisco. Subsequent cases were noted among hemophiliacs, blood transfusion recipients, and heterosexual IDU, suggesting that a transmissible agent communicated by blood and sexual exposure was the etiologic agent. The transmissible retrovirus, HIV-1, was not isolated until 2 years after the initial AIDS cases were identified, and a reliable serologic test for HIV was not widely available until 1985. Currently, more than a decade after the original epidemiologic studies of AIDS were carried out, epidemiologic data throughout the world continue to strongly support three primary modes of transmission: sexual contact, exposure to blood, and perinatal transmission from mother to infant.

International Perspective

Since 1981, AIDS has reached almost every part of the inhabited world. The enormity of the worldwide HIV pandemic cannot be overstated. Although official reporting of HIV infections and AIDS cases varies widely, recent estimates suggest that there are 33.4 million HIV-infected people worldwide. Globally, about 12 million people have died of HIV-related diseases through 1997, including about 3 million children. The United Nations Joint Programme on HIV/AIDS and the World Health Organization (WHO) estimated that 5.8 million people, or 16,000 per day, were newly infected in 1997, including 580,000 children.

The greatest burden of disease is in developing countries. In many southern African countries, HIV/AIDS has reached emergent proportions, with 20% to 26% of people between the ages of 15 and 49 infected. It is estimated that in Botswana, Kenya, Malawi, Mozambique, Namibia, Rwanda, South Africa, Zambia, and Zimbabwe, HIV/AIDS will reduce life expectancy from 64 to 47 years by 2015.

Although HIV was introduced later into Asia, the rate of infection there is dramatically increasing. Asia, with its large populations, is expected to have the largest number of HIV-infected people in the world in the next decade. HIV prevalence and infection rates vary greatly among Asian nations.

WHO estimates that at least 6 million people are infected in the countries of southern and southeastern Asia, with the largest number of infections occurring in India and Thailand. Epidemiologic studies in Thailand illustrate the explosive nature that the epidemic can take on entering some new regional populations. In 1987, the seroprevalence of HIV in intravenous drug users in Thailand was reported as essentially zero. By 1988 the virus had entered the drug-using population of Bangkok, and by June of that year the seroprevalence in IVDU was almost 40%. The virus then spilled over into the population of brothel prostitutes, who had a seroprevalence of 45% in 1992. The next affected population was young men; HIV seropositivity among enlistees in the Thai army was 7.2% by 1993.

In Eastern Europe, the spread of HIV has differed in the states of the former Soviet Union versus central and southeastern countries. The cumulative number of HIV cases reported in Eastern Europe has increased fivefold between 1995 and 1997, from 9,111 to 46,573. The Ukraine, Russia, and Belarus accounted for about 90% of all new cases. Accompanying these trends are dramatic increases in the number of HIV-infected drug users in these countries, as well as in Moldova, the Baltic States, the Caucasus, and Kazakhstan. Countries of central Europe have had lower numbers of cases, and (other than Poland) most cases have been associated with homosexual transmission. In the Balkans, heterosexual transmission has been the most common route of spread. A significant increase in reported cases of syphilis has accompanied the rapid spread of HIV in the countries of the former Soviet Union.

In Latin America, an estimated 1.3 million people have HIV infection. Until recently, the major risk factors for transmission have been men having sex with men and injecting drug use. However, heterosexual transmission has been increasing, especially in Brazil. The ratio of AIDS cases in men versus women has declined from 16:1 in 1986 to 3:1 in 1996. Rates among pregnant women have increased to greater than 3%.

Epidemiology in the United States

Background. Monitoring the HIV/AIDS epidemic in the United States involves data that are available from several sources. Unique information is reported from (1) the national AIDS surveillance system, which monitors persons with severe HIV-related immunosuppression; (2) HIV reporting, a system that provides minimal estimates of HIV infections in the reporting area; (3) HIV serologic surveys that provide HIV prevalence and incidence data among targeted populations; (4) death registries that yield information about HIV-related mortality; and (5) specialized surveillance activities and epidemiologic studies that are available in defined populations. Data from these sources and through statistical modeling are used to estimate the magnitude of the HIV/AIDS epidemic, identify changes in patterns of HIV transmission, and quantify the impact of HIV/AIDS on mortality trends.

In the United States, AIDS cases are reported using a public health surveillance case definition developed by the Centers for Disease Control and Prevention (CDC). The initial case definition was designed in 1981 and was used to search medical records from earlier years to determine if AIDS was a new clinical entity or simply a newly recognized condition. This search clearly dated the start of the AIDS epidemic in the United States to the mid-to-late 1970s, with a few retrospectively identified cases occurring in the 1950s and 1960s. Early epidemiologic data identified sexual contact and blood exposures as risk factors for AIDS, suggesting that an infectious agent was involved. The etiologic agent, a previously unknown cytopathic retrovirus, was isolated from persons with lymphadenopathy and AIDS in 1983. In that same year persons with behavioral risk factors for AIDS were asked to refrain from donating blood, and AIDS became a notifiable condition. The serologic test to detect HIV antibody became available in 1985, allowing the recognition that many people were infected with HIV who had not yet developed AIDS and that there were many more conditions associated with HIV infection than had been originally understood. Consequently, the national AIDS surveillance case definition has been revised several times. Revisions in 1985, in 1987, and again in 1993 expanded the AIDS indicator conditions to include additional opportunistic infections (OIs) such as disseminated histoplasmosis, disseminated mycobacterial disease, and chronic isosporiasis, as well as conditions such as non-Hodgkin's lymphoma and HIV wasting syndrome. The 1993 revision (Box 1-1) aimed to include all persons with severe immunosuppression and HIV infection by including infected adults and adolescents with CD4+ T-lymphocyte counts of less than 200 cells/mm^3 or a total lymphocyte count of <14%. The criteria for pediatric AIDS case reporting were most recently revised in 1994 (Box 1-2).

All revisions to the AIDS surveillance definition have resulted in more patients being defined as having AIDS, but the 1993 additions had the greatest effect. Between 1992 and 1993, the number of AIDS cases in the United States increased by more than 100%, directly attributable to the change in definitions. Currently more than half of all AIDS cases are reported based on immunologic criteria alone. Changes in the AIDS case definition make direct observations of AIDS trends over time difficult, but AIDS surveillance continues to provide important information on the total number of AIDS cases and changes in the demographic characteristics and residences of persons with AIDS.

In the United States, there has been a marked decrease in deaths from AIDS and in new cases of AIDS opportunistic infections after 1995, reflecting the introduction of highly active antiretroviral therapy. This change has resulted in an increased number of persons living with AIDS and a decrease in AIDS incidence. AIDS incidence cannot provide unbiased information on HIV incidence, as it has in the past. Persons reported with newly diagnosed AIDS increasingly represent persons whose diagnosis was too late for them to benefit from therapy, persons who did not seek care or did not have access to care, or persons for whom treatment failed. In contrast, AIDS prevalence reflects the total number of persons living with AIDS, and thus is one surrogate measure of treatment resources needed. However, AIDS prevalence underestimates the actual number of HIV-infected persons requiring care. Because many persons will live for longer periods with HIV without developing AIDS, the ability to quantify the true scope of the HIV/AIDS epidemic is hampered. The CDC has become increasingly persistent in recommending that all states conduct surveillance

---

BOX 1-1
1993 Expanded Surveillance Case Definition for AIDS Among Adolescents and Adults*

AIDS INDICATOR CONDITIONS
- Candidiasis of bronchi, trachea, or lungs
- Candidiasis, esophageal
- Cervical cancer, invasive[†]
- Coccidioidomycosis, disseminated or extrapulmonary
- Cryptococcosis, extrapulmonary
- Cryptosporidiosis, chronic intestinal (>1 month's duration)
- Cytomegalovirus disease (other than liver, spleen, or nodes)
- Cytomegalovirus retinitis (with loss of vision)
- Encephalopathy, HIV-related
- Herpes simplex: chronic ulcer(s) (>1 month's duration), bronchitis, pneumonitis, or esophagitis
- Histoplasmosis, disseminated or extrapulmonary
- Isosporiasis, chronic intestinal (>1 month's duration)
- Kaposi's sarcoma
- Lymphoma, Burkitt's (or equivalent term)
- Lymphoma, immunoblastic (or equivalent term)
- Lymphoma, primary, of brain
- *Mycobacterium avium* complex or *M. kansasii,* disseminated or extrapulmonary
- *Mycobacterium tuberculosis,* any site (pulmonary[†] or extrapulmonary)
- *Mycobacterium,* other species or unidentified species, disseminated or extrapulmonary
- *Pneumocystis carinii* pneumonia
- Pneumonia, recurrent[†]
- Progressive multifocal leukoencephalopathy
- *Salmonella* septicemia, recurrent
- Toxoplasmosis of brain
- Wasting syndrome due to HIV

*HIV-infected persons with the AIDS indicator conditions in this box, as well as those with CD4+ T lymphocyte counts <200 cells/mm^3, are reportable as AIDS cases in the United States.
[†]Added in the 1993 expansion of the AIDS surveillance case definition.
Modified from Centers for Disease Control and Prevention: 1993 revised classification system for HIV infection and expanded surveillance case definition for AIDS among adolescents and adults, *MMWR* 41(No. RR-17):1–23, 1992.

---

for persons with a diagnosis of HIV, as well as collecting information on persons with AIDS.

Confidential name-based HIV infection reporting is conducted in 30 states; additionally, three states require HIV infection reporting only for pediatric HIV infection. These data are used to give a minimum estimate of the number of persons living with HIV infection. HIV infection reporting is particularly useful in evaluating HIV infection in adolescents and young adults, who will be underrepresented in AIDS surveillance. HIV infection reporting may also yield important information about persons with newly acquired HIV infection. However, HIV infection surveillance has limitations based on the timing of HIV testing at various stages of disease, the use of anonymous test sites and home test kits that are not included in surveillance data, and the limited number of areas where HIV reporting has been implemented. Seroprevalence studies provide similar data in specific subgroups. The CDC sponsors serosurveys in sexually transmitted disease (STD) clinics, drug treatment centers, women's reproductive health clinics, tuberculosis clinics, adolescent clinics, and sentinel

BOX 1-2
AIDS Indicator Conditions for Children (<13 Years of Age) Infected with HIV

- Serious bacterial infections, multiple or recurrent (i.e., any combination of at least two culture-confirmed infections within a 2-year period), of the following types: septicemia, pneumonia, meningitis, bone or joint infection, or abscess of an internal organ or body cavity) excluding otitis media, superficial skin or mucosal abscesses, and indwelling catheter-related infections)
- Candidiasis, esophageal or pulmonary (bronchi, trachea, lungs)
- Coccidioidomycosis, disseminated (at site other than or in addition to lungs or cervical or hilar lymph nodes)
- Cryptococcosis, extrapulmonary
- Cryptosporidiosis or isosporiasis with diarrhea persisting >1 month
- Cytomegalovirus disease with onset of symptoms at age >1 month (at a site other than liver, spleen, or lymph nodes)
- Encephalopathy (at least one of the following progressive findings present for at least 2 months in the absence of a concurrent illness other than HIV infection that could explain the findings): (1) failure to attain or loss of developmental milestones or loss of intellectual ability, verified by standard developmental scale or neuropsychological tests; (2) impaired brain growth or acquired microcephaly demonstrated by head circumference measurements or brain atrophy demonstrated by computerized tomography or magnetic resonance imaging (serial imaging is required for children <2 years of age); (3) acquired symmetric motor deficit manifested by two or more of the following: paresis, pathologic reflexes, ataxia, or gait disturbance
- Herpes simplex virus infection causing a mucocutaneous ulcer that persists for >1 month; or bronchitis, pneumonitis, or esophagitis for any duration affecting a child >1 month of age
- Histoplasmosis, disseminated (at a site other than or in addition to lungs or cervical or hilar lymph nodes)
- Kaposi's sarcoma
- Lymphoid interstitial pneumonitis (LIP)
- Lymphoma, primary, in brain
- Lymphoma, small, noncleaved cell (Burkitt's), or immunoblastic or large cell lymphoma of B-cell or unknown immunologic phenotype
- *Mycobacterium tuberculosis,* disseminated or extrapulmonary
- *Mycobacterium,* other species or unidentified species, disseminated (at a site other than or in addition to lungs, skin, or cervical or hilar lymph nodes)
- *Mycobacterium avium* complex or *M. kansasii,* disseminated (at site other than or in addition to lungs, skin, or cervical or hilar lymph nodes)
- *Pneumocystis carinii* pneumonia
- Progressive multifocal leukoencephalopathy
- Salmonella (nontyphoid) septicemia, recurrent
- Toxoplasmosis of the brain with onset at >1 month of age
- Wasting syndrome in the absence of a concurrent illness other than HIV infection that could explain the following findings: (1) persistent weight loss >10% of baseline, OR (2) downward crossing of at least two of the following percentile lines on the weight-for-age chart (e.g., 95th, 75th, 50th, 25th, 5th) in a child ≥1 year of age, OR (3) <5th percentile on weight-for-height chart on two consecutive measurements, ≥30 days apart PLUS (1) chronic diarrhea (i.e., at least two loose stools per day for ≥30 days) OR (2) documented fever (for ≥30 days, intermittent or constant)

Modified from Centers for Disease Control and Prevention. 1994 Revised classification system for human immunodeficiency virus infection in children less than 13 years of age, *MMWR* 43(No. RR-12):1–10, 1994.

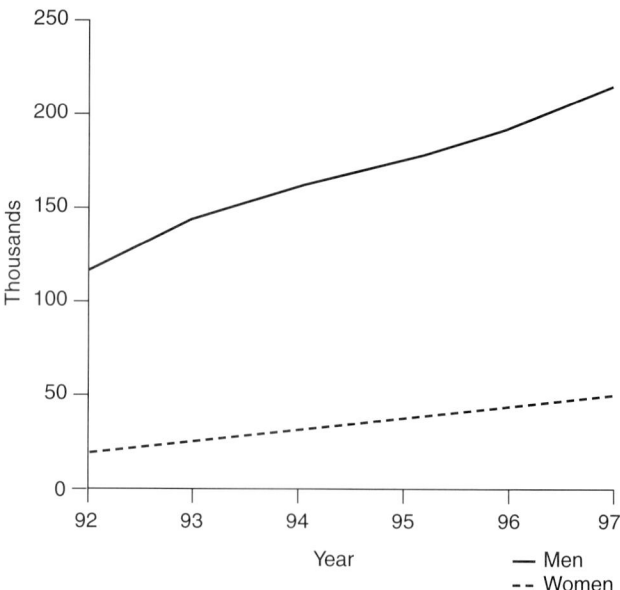

FIG. 1-3 Estimated number of persons living with AIDS by sex, 1992 through 1997, in the United States. (From Centers for Disease Control and Prevention: *HIV/AIDS Surveillance Report,* 10:1, 1998.)

hospitals. Seroconversion data from these groups can yield information on changing patterns of transmission and acquisition of HIV. It is important not to generalize the results of HIV serosurvey data to persons beyond the study groups.

Overview of AIDS Cases. Through December 31, 1998, the total number of men, women, and children with AIDS reported to the CDC was 688,200 cases. The total number of deaths for the same period was 410,800. During 1998, 48,269 persons were reported with AIDS, and 57% of these cases were from five states—New York, Florida, New Jersey, California, and Texas. In 1997, an estimated 270,841 persons were living with AIDS, a 12% increase from 1996. The increase in the number of persons living with AIDS was due to improved survival among patients receiving treatment and a substantial decrease in the number of deaths in 1997.

Of the 679,739 adult and adolescent AIDS cases reported through 1998, 84% were men. However, the proportion of AIDS cases reported each year among women is increasing. Among 47,884 AIDS cases reported in 1998, 23% were women compared with 20% in 1996 (Fig. 1-3).

HIV/AIDS is a major public health problem for racial and ethnic minorities. In 1998, 44% of reported AIDS cases were whites, 37% were blacks, and 18% were Hispanics. By late 1997, the number of blacks living with AIDS had increased from 32.7% of persons in 1992 to 39.2% in 1997, a number almost identical to whites living with AIDS (Fig. 1-4). From 1990 through 1995, the proportionate increases in AIDS incidence for black men (79%), Hispanic men (61%), American Indian and Alaskan Native men (77%), and Asian and Pacific Islander men (55%) were greater than the 14% increase for white men. A much larger proportion of black and Hispanic persons with AIDS have a history of injecting drug use and heterosexual transmission than have whites. Racial and ethnic minority

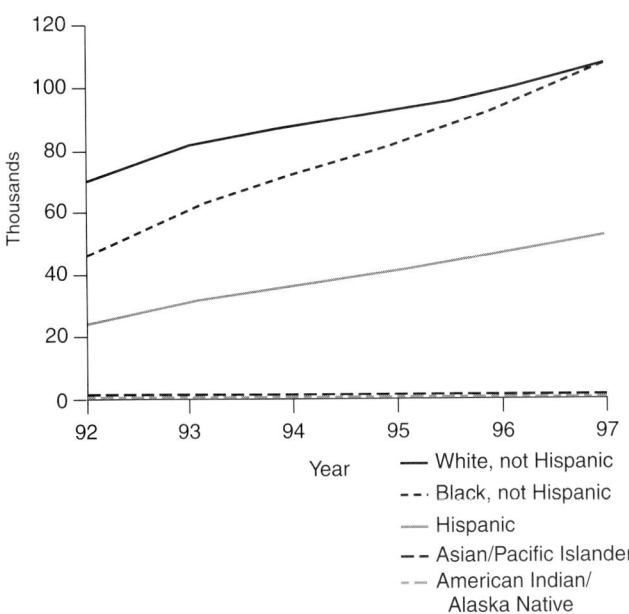

FIG. 1-4 Estimated number of persons living with AIDS by race/ethnicity, 1992 through 1997, in the United States. (From Centers for Disease Control and Prevention: *HIV/AIDS Surveillance Report,* 10:1, 1998.)

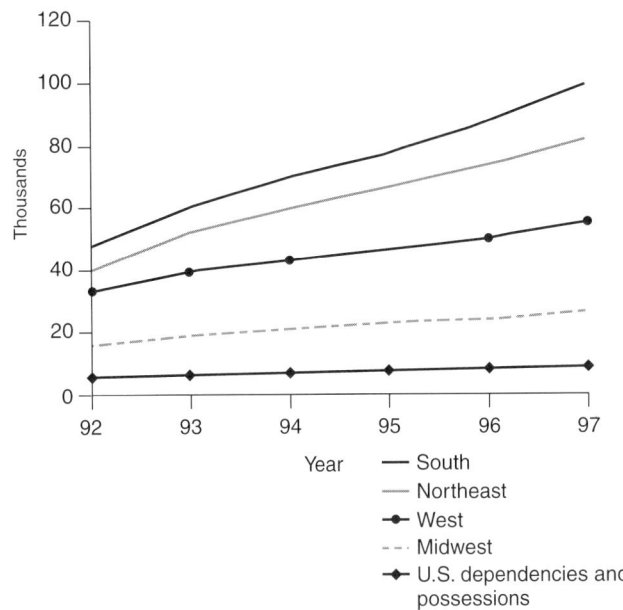

FIG. 1-5 Estimated number of persons living with AIDS by region, 1992 through 1997, in the United States. (From Centers for Disease Control and Prevention: *HIV/AIDS Surveillance Report,* 10:1, 1998.)

women have been disproportionately affected by AIDS. In 1998 the rates of AIDS reported for black women were 20 times higher than for white women, and the rates for Hispanic women were seven times higher than for white women.

Racial and ethnic minority communities differ in their risk profiles for acquiring HIV. The number of black men infected by injecting drug use is greater than the number infected by male sexual contact in the northeast and along the Atlantic Coast. However, in most other areas of the country, most black men are infected by male sexual contact. The incidence of AIDS and risks for HIV among Hispanics differ according to the country of origin. Among new AIDS cases reported in 1998, male sexual contact was the most commonly reported risk for Hispanics born in Mexico or Cuba; injecting drug use was the most common mode of transmission among Hispanics born in Puerto Rico.

Although all U.S. states and territories have reported AIDS cases, there are marked differences in AIDS case rates by state. In 1998, AIDS rates per 100,000 population were highest in the District of Columbia (189.1), New York (47.9), Puerto Rico (44.3), Florida (36.9), and Maryland (31.9). Five states (New York, California, Florida, Texas, and New Jersey) have reported more than half of the cumulative AIDS cases through 1998. In 1998, persons living in the southern and northeastern United States accounted for an increasing proportion of persons living with AIDS, while the proportion of persons living in the West declined (Fig. 1-5).

The highest AIDS case rates occur in the largest U.S. cities. In 1998 the AIDS case rate in cities with a population of 500,000 or more (23.0 per 100,000) was more than double the rate in cities with 50,000 to 500,000 population (10.3 per 100,000) and almost four times the rate in nonmetropolitan areas (6.3 per 100,000). Of cities with a population greater than 500,000, those with the largest AIDS case rates in 1998 were (per 100,000 population) New York, 86; Miami, 73; Jersey City, 59; San Francisco, 58; and Fort Lauderdale, 56.

During 1998, in the 33 states and territories that report HIV infection, 19,393 persons with HIV (but not AIDS) were reported. The total number of persons living with HIV in these states through December 1998 was 97,962. Since not all HIV-infected persons have been tested, this represents a minimum number of persons living with HIV infection in these states.

Men Who Have Sex with Men. HIV infection entered communities of homosexual and bisexual men in the United States in the mid-to-late 1970s—initially in the large coastal cities and then spreading rapidly to similar populations throughout the country. By the mid-1980s, the HIV seroprevalence among homosexual and bisexual men ranged from 36% in New York City and 42% in Los Angeles to 70% in San Francisco. In 1995 AIDS incidence among men who have sex with men (MSM) was unchanged from 1994. The national leveling of AIDS incidence among MSM was mainly a trend observed in the largest U.S. cities and among white MSM. From 1996 to 1997, AIDS incidence among MSM declined 18% and deaths declined 49%. As a reminder that MSM will continue to represent a significant proportion of the HIV-infected population, the highest HIV prevalence rates among populations at risk for HIV in 1997 were among MSM attending STD clinics. The median HIV prevalence among MSM in the 13 participating STD clinics around the country was 19.3% (Fig. 1-6). MSM represented the largest proportion (60%) of men diagnosed with AIDS in 1997.

Injecting Drug Users. The HIV epidemic among IDU exploded in the northeastern United States and along the Atlantic Coast early in the 1980s. Unlike the epidemic among

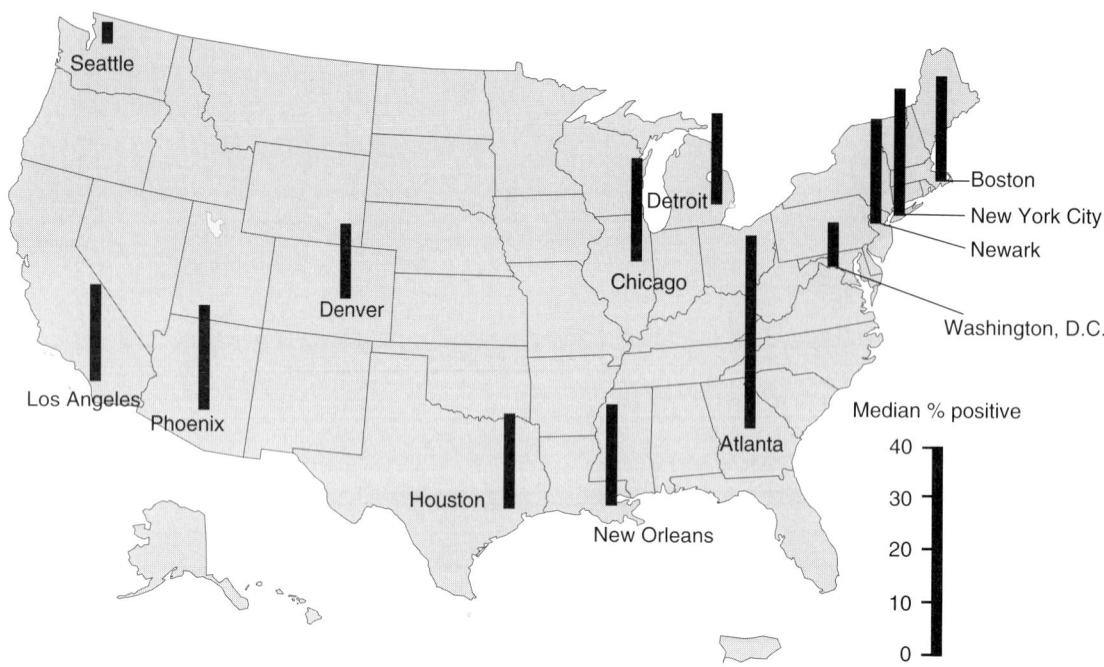

FIG. 1-6 HIV prevalence among men who have sex with men, sexually transmitted disease clinic surveys, 1997. The figure includes only areas with sufficient data for analysis. (From Centers for Disease Control and Prevention: *National HIV Prevalence Surveys, 1997 Summary,* Atlanta, 1998, Centers for Disease Control and Prevention.)

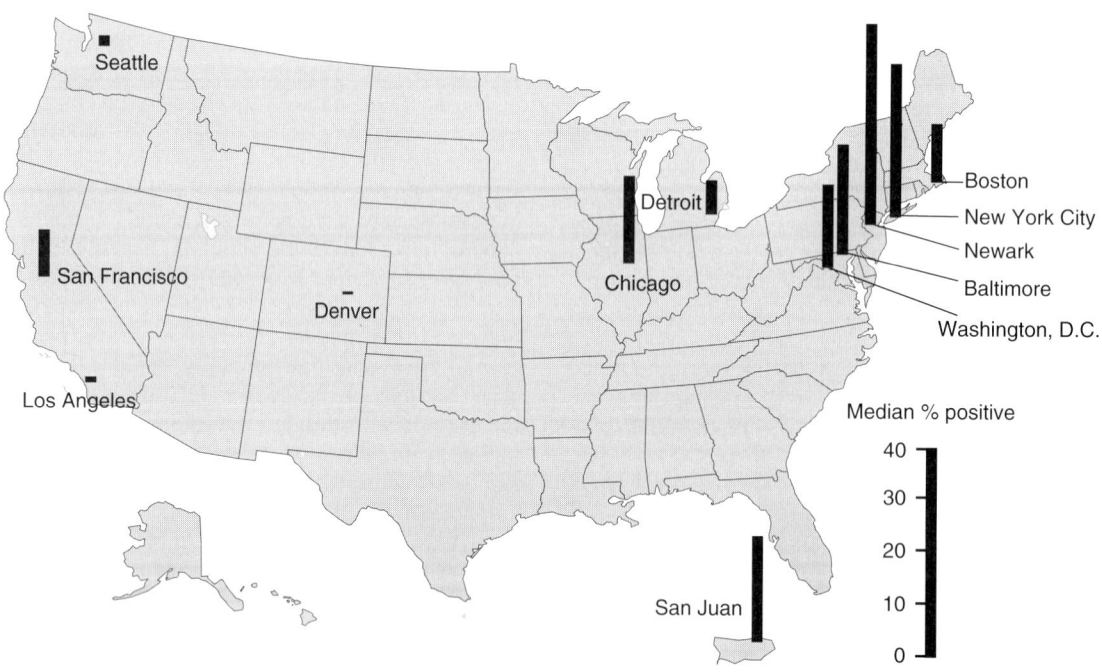

FIG. 1-7 HIV prevalence among injecting drug users, drug treatment center surveys, 1997. The figure includes only areas with sufficient data for analysis. (From Centers for Disease Control and Prevention: *National HIV Prevalence Surveys, 1997 Summary,* Atlanta, 1998, Centers for Disease Control and Prevention.)

homosexual and bisexual men, the epidemic among IDUs has remained largely in these geographic areas, although the south and Puerto Rico also have large numbers of infected IDUs (Fig. 1-7). HIV prevalence among black IDUs tends to be higher than among white IDUs. In the northeastern United States, where most Hispanics are of Puerto Rican origin, the HIV prevalence among Hispanics was about 30% in 1997; in the western United States, where most Hispanics are of Mexican origin, HIV seroprevalence among Hispanics was similar to whites (<5%) (Fig. 1-8). Among 21 drug treatment centers

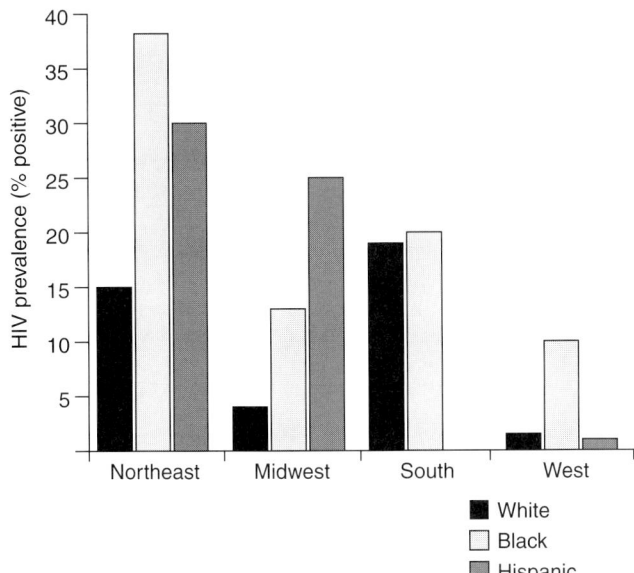

FIG. 1-8 HIV prevalence among injecting drug users, drug treatment center surveys, by race/ethnicity and region, 1997. (From Centers for Disease Control and Prevention: *National HIV Prevalence Surveys, 1997 Summary*, Atlanta, 1998, Centers for Disease Control and Prevention.)

evaluating HIV prevalence rates in 1997, the median prevalence rate was 14.8%. The highest median prevalence rates were in Newark (37.7%) and New York City (28.8%); IDU-associated prevalence rates were lowest in western cities (Denver, 0%; Los Angeles, 0.8%; Seattle, 1.8%; San Francisco, 8.8%). The reason why certain high prevalence areas have remained high (New York City) and others low (Los Angeles) has not been explained, particularly since high-risk behavior associated with IDU is practiced in both areas.

AIDS incidence and deaths among IDUs declined 15% and 45%, respectively, among men and 12% and 33% among women in 1997. IDUs diagnosed with AIDS represented 24% of AIDS cases in men and 47% of those in women in 1997.

Heterosexual Exposure. AIDS related to heterosexual contact with persons known to be infected with or at risk for HIV is increasingly represented among persons with AIDS. In 1997, 11% of AIDS cases among men were due to heterosexual transmission versus 59% of AIDS cases among women. An overall increase in the number of AIDS cases among women also reflects the increasing trend of heterosexual transmission. In 1998, 10,988 (23%) of 47,884 adult and adolescent AIDS cases were reported in women, an increase from 20% of cases in 1996 and 7% of cases in 1985. Heterosexual transmission accounts for most HIV infection among women. In 1997, among 6,824 women with AIDS attributable to heterosexual transmission, 30% reported sexual contact with an IDU(s). In 1997, 82% of women with heterosexually acquired AIDS were black or Hispanic. Serosurvey studies in STD clinics have shown a generally stable HIV prevalence over time. In 1997, the seroprevalence in STD clinics was 2.7% for men and 1.6% for women (excluding MSM and IDU); however, the prevalence varied by region and was >3% among women in Newark, Baltimore, Washington D.C., and Miami.

Studies of the heterosexual partners of HIV-infected persons have shown variable but appreciable rates of transmission. The risk for male-to-female transmission appears to be greater than the risk for female-to-male transmission. Other factors associated with enhanced heterosexual HIV transmission include increased numbers of high-risk sexual contacts, unprotected receptive anal intercourse, the stage of HIV infection in the contact (highest during acute infection and end-stage disease), and the presence of ulcerative or nonulcerative STDs in the infected contact or the partner.

Other Routes of Transmission. Other modes of transmission can account for HIV transmission. Of 688,200 persons reported with AIDS through 1998, 8,760 were recipients of blood, blood components, or tissue. To date, 5,145 persons with hemophilia or other clotting disorders requiring pooled plasma products have been diagnosed with AIDS. The incidence of AIDS related to blood products has been dramatically reduced in recent years due to prevention measures adopted in the mid-1980s. In 1983, persons at risk for HIV were asked to refrain from donating blood, and in 1985 HIV antibody testing of all blood and plasma donations and heat treatment of clotting-factor concentrates were begun. Rare cases of AIDS have been identified after these procedures were put in place. Through 1998, 37 adults/adolescents and two children had developed AIDS after receiving blood that screened negative for HIV antibody. The current risk of transmitting HIV through the transfusion of screened blood is as low as 1 in 450,000 to 600,000 donations. Organ and tissue donations are also screened using the same criteria as that established for the blood supply.

Health care workers and laboratory employees represent another small group of persons with HIV/AIDS. Occupationally acquired HIV/AIDS, reported through 1998, has been documented in 54 persons. The majority had percutaneous exposure to blood via a hollow bore needle, and most cases were among nurses and laboratory technicians.

Other rare exposures have resulted in HIV transmission, such as self-inoculation or human bites. The sexual abuse of children, particularly older children, has also resulted in HIV transmission.

Perinatal Transmission. Among 8,461 children (<13 years of age) reported with AIDS in the United States through December 1998, 91% acquired infection via transmission from mother to infant. Although the number of women with AIDS is increasing, the number of AIDS cases in children is decreasing. The declining trend in pediatric AIDS cases has been continuous since 1993 (Fig. 1-9) and is likely due to a reduction in perinatal transmission of HIV. Institution of guidelines for maternal use of zidovudine (AZT) before or at the time of birth and treatment of exposed infants in the postpartum period has likely been the major force behind the reduction of transmission to neonates. Continued efforts to encourage HIV counseling and testing of pregnant women are integral parts of the reduction in perinatal transmission as well.

Mortality. The cumulative number of deaths among persons reported with AIDS, through December 1998, was 410,800 or 60% of the cumulative number of reported AIDS cases. Among adults and adolescents, 405,816 deaths have occurred and 4,984 children under age 15 have died. However, mortality data from death certificates and AIDS surveillance reports show that HIV-related mortality has declined since 1996.

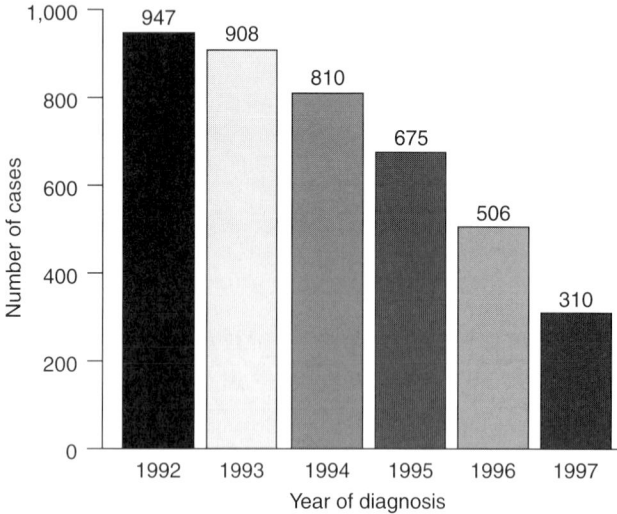

FIG. 1-9 Estimated pediatric AIDS incidence, by year of diagnosis, 1992 through 1997, in the United States. NOTE: These numbers do not represent actual cases of children diagnosed with AIDS. Rather, these numbers are point estimates based on cases diagnosed using the 1987 definition, adjusted for reporting delays. The 1993 AIDS surveillance case definition change affected only the adult/adolescent cases, not pediatric cases. *(From Centers for Disease Control and Prevention: HIV/AIDS Surveillance Report, 10:36, 1998.)*

Large annual increases in AIDS deaths occurred through 1994 when 49,311 deaths were reported. The number of deaths leveled in 1995 and declined by 25% in 1996 and 43% in 1997. Comparing data from 1997 with 1995, declines occurred in all demographic groups and in all major HIV transmission categories: 66% in MSM, 49% in IDU, and 41% in heterosexuals. This sudden decline in AIDS-associated mortality reflects a leveling of AIDS incidence and the introduction of highly active antiretroviral therapy.

Natural History of HIV Infection

The clinical spectrum of HIV infection ranges from acute infection to a prolonged period of clinical, but not viral, latency. The development of declining CD4+ counts and an increased susceptibility to opportunistic infections and certain neoplasms, such as lymphoma and Kaposi's sarcoma, follow. The median estimated time from seroconversion to development of AIDS varies widely but over a median of 8 to 10 years, 80% of HIV-1 infected persons will progress to AIDS. About 10% to 15% of HIV-1 infected persons are rapid progressors and will develop AIDS in 2 to 3 years. In contrast about 5% to 12% of infected persons are expected to remain free of AIDS for more than 20 years. One important study of the natural history of HIV infection was performed using a cohort of homosexual and bisexual men followed by the San Francisco Department of Public Health. This cohort consisted of men enrolled in a hepatitis B vaccine study in 1978 and followed forward with clinical and serologic evaluations. Among 489 men for whom seroconversion time could be reliably estimated, 13% developed AIDS (defined as presence of an opportunistic disease) within 5 years, 51% within 10 years, and 54% at 11 years. Among those who had been HIV positive for greater than 12 years, 19% had symptomatic HIV disease and 29% had CD4+ counts <200 cells/mm^3. Overall, after 11 years of follow-up, more than three quarters of HIV-infected homosexual men had progressed to advanced HIV disease or AIDS, or had died. After development of AIDS, clinical progression, without therapy, was initially found to ensue rapidly. Very early data from the first 505 AIDS cases in San Francisco found a median survival after AIDS diagnosis of 9 months.

The appearance of opportunistic infections, generally occurring at CD4+ counts below 200 cells/mm^3, has changed face with evolving prophylactic strategies. Large cohorts of HIV-infected persons studied early in the epidemic showed *P. carinii* pneumonia as the most common opportunistic infection, followed by cytomegalovirus disease and *Mycobacterium avium* complex disease. Kaposi's sarcoma was the most common neoplasm among this group of largely homosexual men. Among MSM in clinical care from 1990 through 1995, *P. carinii* pneumonia, *M. avium* complex disease, cryptococcosis, herpes simplex disease, toxoplasmosis, and encephalitis decreased while cytomegalovirus retinitis increased. The changes likely reflect the increased use of prophylactic regimens and perhaps longer survival at lower CD4+ counts.

Several studies have found that the introduction of highly active antiretroviral therapy and widespread use of prophylaxis against opportunistic infections, particularly *P. carinii*, have significantly altered the natural history of HIV infection. Use of these modalities has extended the clinical incubation period between HIV infection and progression to AIDS and has markedly improved survival. The incidence of all opportunistic infections has declined with the use of these agents as well.

Identifying methods to estimate prognosis for HIV-1–infected persons has been an area of particular interest since early in the epidemic. Clinical findings, such as the presence of oral candidiasis (thrush), have long been known to imply significant immunosuppression and even to predict an increased development of *P. carinii* pneumonia (independent of the CD4+ count). Laboratory markers that correlate with disease progression have been extensively studied. CD4+ lymphocyte counts have been found to correlate with the level of immunodeficiency. Baseline CD4+ counts of 200 cells/mm^3 or less have been associated with a 3-year progression rate to AIDS of 87%; with CD4+ counts of 200 to 400 cells/mm^3, 46% progressed; and for those with more than 400 cells/mm^3, a 15% progression rate was noted. Although CD4+ cell counts were a powerful tool, the ability to stage HIV disease, especially at higher CD4+ cell counts, was incomplete.

Attempts to use other virologic markers to stage infected patients, such as culture of HIV-1 from peripheral blood cells, isolation of HIV-1 from plasma, assay of HIV-1 p24 core antigen, and evaluation of anti-p24 antibody titers, were largely unsuccessful. Cultures of peripheral blood cells are positive for HIV-1 in almost 100% of infected persons. Isolation of HIV-1 from plasma is uncommon, except at the time of primary infection or late in disease when CD4+ lymphocytes have markedly declined. Assays for HIV-1 p24 core antigen were positive in only about two thirds of persons who went on to develop AIDS. Anti-p24 antibody titers were not more predictive than CD4+ counts in studies assessing multiple markers of infection.

However, with the development of technology that enabled quantification of HIV RNA in plasma in the mid-1990s, the dynamics of the viral replication cycle were defined. The methodology was also evaluated as a prognostic marker. Studies were performed in a number of different populations with differing routes of HIV-1 transmission, and high HIV RNA copy numbers were highly correlated with disease progression.

A retrospective analysis of data from the Multicenter AIDS Cohort Study (MACS) compared HIV RNA copy number with previously studied markers, including serum neopterin levels, serum β_2-microglobulin levels, and the number and percentage of CD4+ lymphocytes. The MACS was an investigation of the natural history of HIV-1 infection in MSM and enrolled 4,954 men in Baltimore, Pittsburgh, Chicago, and Los Angeles between April 1984 and March 1985. Participants returned to the clinic semiannually when a history and physical examination were obtained, as well as blood for immunologic and virologic studies. The substudy of HIV viral load included 1,604 participants. Plasma HIV RNA copy number was obtained by sensitive branched chain DNA assay; the lower limit of quantification was 500 copies/ml. Over the course of the study, through July 1, 1995, 62% of the participants developed AIDS and 53% died. HIV RNA copy number was clearly superior to other measured markers in predicting progression to AIDS and death. Baseline HIV RNA copy number correlated with the rate of decline of CD4+ lymphocytes; the higher the baseline viral load, the greater the rate of decline of CD4 at each year of the study. The effects were stratified as follows: 5.4% of persons with <500 copies of HIV RNA progressed to AIDS in the 6-year follow-up, 16.6% of those with viral loads of 501 to 3,000 copies/ml progressed, 31.7% of persons with baseline HIV-1 RNA of 3,001 to 10,000 copies/ml progressed, 55.2% with 10,001 to 30,000 copies/ml progressed, and 80% of persons with more 30,000 copies/ml progressed. In the five categories of viral load, highly significant differences in the percentage of participants who died of AIDS were noted (0.9%, 6.3%, 18.1%, 34.9%, and 69.5%, respectively).

Measures of viral burden (alternatively termed viral load, HIV-1 RNA copy number by RT polymerase chain reaction [RT-PCR], or branched chain DNA) define persons who progress at differing rates and also reflect differing rates of viral replication in the lymphatic tissue. Viral replication determines the rate of development of immunosuppression, clinical progression, and survival. Certain factors, such as viral genotype and phenotype, host characteristics, and concomitant infections, can interact with HIV to change the rate of virus production.

Viral genotypic changes occur during rapid viral replication and frequent viral mutations, resulting in swarms of viral variants, referred to as quasispecies. In persons with a vigorous immune response to infection, the number of viral variants is great and immunologic and clinical progression is slow. With a more "fit" virus and/or a less effective immune response, there is less variability of virus and more immunologic and clinical progression. Recent data have shown that host genotypic characteristics are also important contributors to viral replication. To infect a target cell, HIV-1 interacts with the CD4 surface protein and a coreceptor that is a chemokine. The most common phenotype for HIV-1 uses as its coreceptor a chemokine called CCR-5. About 1% of whites do not express CCR-5 on cell surfaces because they are homozygous for a mutation in the transmembrane receptor. Follow-up of such persons has revealed that, even in the presence of extensive sexual exposure to HIV-1, they remain largely uninfected. About 15% to 20% of whites are heterozygous for this mutation, and preliminary studies of these persons suggest that they have lower HIV-1 RNA copy numbers and are slower to progress. It has clearly been shown that concurrent infection in HIV-infected persons increases the rate of viral replication, likely due to antigenic stimulation and lymphocyte activation. The presence of opportunistic infections worsens the prognosis of HIV-infected persons with advanced disease.

Lastly, highly effective antiretroviral therapy that decreases viral replication results in decreased disease progression and improved survival. The durability of this suppression and its ability to alter the course of HIV-1 infection over time remain to be evaluated.

SUGGESTED READINGS

Centers for Disease Control and Prevention: HIV/AIDS Surveillance Report, 10:1-43, 1998. *http://www.cdc.gov/nchstp/hiv_aids/pubs*

Centers for Disease Control and Prevention: National HIV prevalence surveys, 1997 summary, 1-25, 1998. *http://wwwcdc.gov/nchstp/hiv_aids/pubs/hivsero.htm*

Dehne KL et al: The HIV/AIDS epidemic in Eastern Europe: recent patterns and trends and their implications for policy-making. *AIDS,* 13:741-749, 1999.

Hardy WD : The human immunodeficiency virus, *Med Clin North Am* 80:1239-1260, 1996.

Horowitz HW et al: Human immunodeficiency virus infection, Part I, *Dis Mon* 44:545-606, 1998.

Hu DJ et al: What role does HIV-1 subtype play in transmission and pathogenesis? An epidemiologic perspective, *AIDS* 13:873-881, 1999.

Mellors JW et al: Plasma viral load and CD4+ lymphocytes as prognostic markers of HIV-1 infection, *Ann Intern Med* 126:956-964, 1997.

Phair JP: Determinants of the natural history of human immunodeficiency virus type I infection, *J Infect Dis* 179(Suppl 2):S384-386, 1999.

Satcher D: The global HIV/AIDS epidemic, *JAMA* 281:1479, 1999.

Ward JW, Duchin JS: The epidemiology of HIV and AIDS in the United States, *AIDS Clin Rev* 1-45, 1997-1998.

2 Acute HIV-1 Infection

ELIZABETH M. COLSTON, R. MICHAEL BUCKLEY

Introduction

Acute or primary human immunodeficiency virus type I (HIV-1) infection is the stage of the disease when virus disseminates throughout a newly infected individual, resulting in seeding of lymphoid tissue and induction of an immune response. The high-level viremia and associated immune response during acute HIV-1 infection cause an abrupt-onset febrile illness in up to 80% of cases. Severe and prolonged symptoms are associated with a worse prognosis and more rapid progression to acquired immunodeficiency syndrome (AIDS). Unfortunately, the symptoms are relatively nonspecific; therefore the diagnosis of acute HIV-1 infection requires a high index of clinical suspicion. Identification of patients with acute infection is especially important given the benefit of early antiretroviral therapy.

Case Presentation

A 36-year-old heterosexual man was well until 3 weeks prior to admission when he developed fever, chills, sweats, nausea, vomiting, and diarrhea. He was seen in an emergency room where he was given intravenous fluids and sent home. He returned several days later with resolution of his gastrointestinal complaints but continued fever, chills, generalized malaise, and a new diffuse macular erythematous rash. He was admitted, treated with doxycycline, and discharged after 4 days. Over the next few days the rash resolved, but he developed low back pain, diffuse severe headache, photophobia, and neck stiffness, and sought medical attention at a second emergency room. His past medical history was unremarkable. He was on no medications and had no drug allergies. He was living with his girlfriend of 2 years and her 4-year-old son. He had a 30-packyear history of cigarette smoking, but had quit 1 month prior to admission. He did not use drugs or drink alcohol. He serviced outdoor pools for a living, reported numerous tick bites, and denied any recent travel. He had one sex partner for the past 2 years, denied sex with men or prostitutes, and denied blood transfusions. On physical examination his temperature was 99.4° F, blood pressure 118/68 mm Hg, pulse 79/min, and respiratory rate 16/min. In general he was an uncomfortable appearing young white man, lying in bed with the lights off, his eyes closed, and his head in his hands. The remainder of the physical examination was unremarkable. Specifically, there was no meningismus, lymphadenopathy, or rash. His white blood cell count was 6.1 THO/ml (normal 4.0 to 11.0 THO/ml), with 18% segmented neutrophils, 73% lymphocytes (normal 20% to 40%), 7% monocytes (normal 3% to 11%), hemoglobin 15.5 g/dl (normal 11.8 to 15.5 g/dl), and platelets 207 THO/ml (normal 150 to 400 THO/ml). A chemistry panel was normal except for slightly elevated transaminases, alanine aminotransferase (ALT) 164 U/L (normal 21 to 72 U/L), and aspartate aminotransferase (AST) 57 U/L (normal 17 to 59 U/L). Lumbar puncture had an opening pressure of 20 cmH$_2$O, 167 wbc/ml, 80% lymphocytes, 1 rbc/ml, glucose 57 mg/dl (normal 50 to 80 mg/dl), protein 98 mg/dl (normal 16 to 46 mg/dl), Gram's stain and culture negative, and cryptococcal antigen negative. Over the next 2 days the headache resolved, but the low back pain persisted. Additional work-up included Lyme titer (negative), Monospot (negative), blood cultures (negative), magnetic resonance imaging (MRI) of the brain (normal), repeat lumbar puncture (26 wbc/ml, 82% lymphocytes, 18% monocytes, 4 rbc/ml, glucose 62 mg/dl [normal 50 to 80 mg/dl], protein 67mg/dl [normal 16 to 46 mg/dl]), and CD4+ T cells 494 cells/mm^3 (normal 560 to 1,840 cells/mm^3). His HIV-1 enzyme-linked immunosorbent assay (ELISA) was negative, but his HIV-1 RNA polymerase was 1.2 million/ml, making the diagnosis of acute HIV-1 infection.

KEY POINTS

- Fever, chills, gastrointestinal symptoms
- Aseptic meningitis following above symptoms and signs
- Maculopapular rash
- "Viral" meningitis by lumbar puncture
- Negative HIV-1 ELISA antibody
- Positive HIV-1 viral load by RNA PCR

Human Immunodeficiency Virus–Type 1
Presentation and Progression

Virology of Acute HIV-1 Infection. The most common mode of HIV-1 infection is sexual transmission at the genital mucosa. A rhesus monkey model of intravaginal simian immunodeficiency virus (SIV) infection has elucidated the cellular events occurring at the earliest stage of infection. The virus first infects Langerhans' cells, tissue dendritic cells located in the lamina propria underlying the vaginal epithelium, which then fuse with CD4+ T cells and disseminate. Two days after infection virus can be detected in the draining iliac lymph nodes, and 5 days after infection virus can be detected in plasma. In humans the time from mucosal infection to initial viremia is 4 to 11 days. Disruption of the mucosal barrier caused by genital ulcers, urethritis, or cervicitis increases the risk of acquiring HIV-1 via sexual transmission. There are also reports of transmission across the oral mucosa as a result of genital-oral contact. In these cases, nasopharyngeal tonsillar and adenoid tissue, which are rich in dendritic cells, are the likely initial targets of infection.

The first step in viral infection is binding of the viral envelope protein gp 120 to the CD4+ molecule on cells, but this event alone is not sufficient to permit infection. Fusion and entry require the presence of coreceptor molecules CCR5 or CXCR4, cell surface chemokine receptors. Early experiments to characterize HIV-1 revealed that some strains were macrophage-tropic, and some were T cell–tropic, although the basis of this distinction was unclear. The identification of the coreceptors explained these differences. Macrophage-tropic strains utilize CCR5 and are now called R5 viruses. T cell–tropic strains utilize CXCR4 and are now called X4 viruses. Examination of the phenotypes of HIV-1 strains sampled during acute infection showed that the isolates were relatively homogenous and macrophage-tropic, now known to be R5 viruses. This observation suggested selective transmission of certain strains. Why are R5 viruses preferentially transmitted between individuals during acute infection, whereas X4 strains are rarely if ever transmitted and arise only later in the course of infection? One possible explanation is that the first cells that the virus encounters are macrophages that express CCR5 but not CXCR4, explaining the preferential transmission of R5 viruses. Another possibility is that both receptors are expressed on cells that virus initially infects, but only CCR5 can transduce signals required for viral replication. The importance of the observation of selective transmission of R5 viruses was supported by the discovery that a homozygous 32 base pair deletion in the CCR5 gene, present in approximately 1% of Caucasians, confers resistance to HIV-1 infection.

Although the acute retroviral syndrome was originally described in 1984, the significance of early virologic events to disease pathogenesis did not become clear until the development of methods to measure viral load in blood. The acute nature of the clinical syndrome and its resolution within 1 to 2 weeks suggest that the kinetics of HIV-1 replication in vivo change rapidly during acute HIV-1 infection. During primary HIV-1 infection there is a rapid rise in plasma viremia, often to levels in excess of 1 million RNA molecules per milliliter; widespread dissemination of the virus; seeding of lymphoid organs; and manifestation of an acute retroviral syndrome (Fig. 2-1). This stage of infection with high levels of replicating virus has important public health implications. According to widely accepted assumptions, as many as one half of HIV-1 transmissions occur during the acute infection interval. Therefore acute HIV-1 infection presents a window of opportunity in which prevention, counseling, and treatment efforts may exert a maximal effect on the spread of HIV-1.

After the initial rise in plasma viremia there is a tenfold to 1,000-fold decrease in viremia that correlates with emergence of a virus-specific host immune response and resolution of symptoms (see Fig. 2-1). After 6 to 12 months, the amount of circulating virus reaches a relatively stable baseline plasma

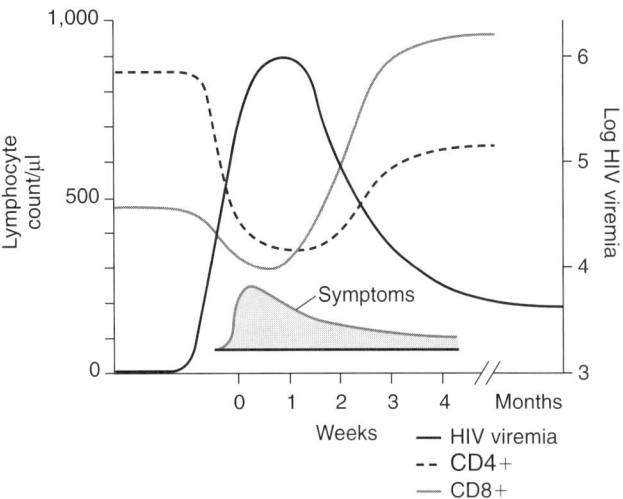

FIG. 2-1 Changes in lymphocyte subpopulations and HIV viremia during primary HIV infection. (Modified from Armstrong D, Cohen J, editors: *HIV and AIDS,* London, 1999, Mosby-Wolfe.)

HIV-1 RNA level, or set-point, where a steady-state level of viral replication is established. The viral set-point has clinical significance because it is a strong, CD4+ T cell–independent predictor of disease progression. Individuals with the highest plasma HIV-1 RNA levels have the most rapid rates of disease progression. For subjects with greater than 36,270 copies/ml, 62% progressed to AIDS and 49% died within 5 years; the median times to AIDS and death were 3.5 and 5.1 years, respectively. In contrast, among individuals with plasma HIV-1 RNA levels less than or equal to 4,530 copies/ml, only 8% progressed to AIDS and 5% died within 5 years; the median time to AIDS or death was greater than 10 years. The determinants of the set-point may be related to genetic differences in coreceptors, degree of sequestration of virus and infected CD4$^+$ T cells in the germinal centers of lymphoid tissue, effectiveness of the host's immune response, or differences in the virulence of viral strains.

KEY POINTS

- Infection is transmitted at the genital or oral mucosa
- Disruption of mucosal barrier increases risk
- Rapid rise, then fall of virus in blood
- After 6-12 months (if no treatment given) virus reaches a set-point
- The higher the set-point, the more rapid the disease progresses

The Immunology of Acute HIV-1 Infection. Vigorous HIV-1–specific humoral and cell-mediated immune responses are detected early during acute infection. The temporal association between the abrupt drop in viral titers, development of specific host immunity, and resolution of the acute retroviral syndrome suggests that early on the intact host immune system succeeds in limiting virus replication. However, the continued presence of HIV-1 RNA in plasma as measured in the set-point shows that host immunity is incomplete. A

BOX 2-1
Immunologic Responses to Acute HIV-1 Infection

HUMORAL
Immune complex formation
Neutralizing antibodies

CELLULAR
Reduction in CD4+ T cells
Increase in CD8+ T cells
Inversion of CD4+:CD8+ ratio
Soluble factors
Cytotoxic T lymphocytes

CYTOKINES AND CELL PRODUCTS
Increased neopterin
Increased β_2-microglobulin
Increased TNF-α
Increased IFN
Increased IL-10
Increased soluble IL-2 receptor

---

thorough understanding of the immune response in acute HIV-1 infection will provide information important to the development of an effective vaccine (Box 2-1).

During acute infection anti–HIV-1 antibodies are undetectable or barely detectable; however, during the period of seroconversion and down-regulation of viremia, high-titer anti–HIV-1 antibodies are detected (see Fig. 2-1). Antibodies produced during this period lack neutralizing activity, but may contribute to the down-regulation of viremia by mediating the formation of immune complexes that get trapped in the reticuloendothelial system, resulting in the removal of large numbers of virus particles from the circulation. Neutralizing antibodies are detected later in the course of infection, when the transition from acute to chronic infection has occurred. It has been suggested that these antibodies are directed against cryptic epitopes that are not exposed during primary infection.

HIV-1–specific cell-mediated immune responses are detected very early in acute infection. Cytokine responses are reflective of the general state of activation of the immune system. There are increased levels of neopterin, β_2-microglobulin, tumor necrosis factor (TNF)-α, interferon (IFN), interleukin (IL)-10, and soluble IL-2 receptor. The CD4+ T cell response is quantitatively and qualitatively impaired during acute HIV-1 infection. The number of CD4+ T cells decreases and there is a lack of HIV-1–specific proliferative responses. Along with the decrease in CD4+ T cells, there is an increase in CD8+ T cells, resulting in inversion of the CD4+:CD8+ ratio. CD8+ T cell responses occur by noncytotoxic and cytotoxic mechanisms. It has been shown that CD8+ T cells release soluble factors that suppress viral replication in vitro without direct cell killing. HIV-1–specific cytotoxic T lymphocyte (CTL) activity is found in the blood of infected individuals; however, the relationship between this response and the control of HIV-1 replication was not initially clear. There is indirect evidence in support of a role for the CTL response in controlling viremia. Studies have shown that HIV-1–specific CTL activity is induced during acute infection, prior to the decline in viremia, demonstrating a temporal relationship between these events. There are anecdotal reports of individuals who fail to develop a CTL response to HIV-1 experiencing a prolonged acute viral syndrome and persistent high levels of viremia. In addition, long-term nonprogressors, HIV-1–infected individuals with preserved CD4+ T cell counts and low viral loads in the absence of antiretroviral therapy, have been shown to have high levels of HIV-1–specific CTL activity compared with individuals with disease progression in whom CTL activity wanes or is lost. More direct evidence of the importance of the cellular immune response in controlling HIV-1 replication comes from CTL escape mutants. Several groups of investigators have demonstrated that the CTL response in infected individuals exerts a positive selective pressure, leading to the emergence of mutant viruses that are no longer recognized by autologous T cells. The accumulation of such mutations in the virus could provide a mechanism for immune evasion.

 KEY POINTS

- During acute HIV infection (first 1-3 weeks) antibodies to HIV are undetectable
- CD4+ lymphocytes decrease during acute infection
- Cytotoxic T lymphocyte (CTL) activity probably controls HIV-1 replication and results in recovery from acute infection
- Although the host immune system helps limit viral replication, it does not eliminate it entirely

Clinical Manifestations of Acute HIV-1 Infection. The clinical features of symptomatic acute HIV-1 infection were first described in 1984. A nurse caring for a patient with AIDS sustained a needle-stick injury and 13 days later developed a severe flu-like illness characterized by fever, malaise, headache, sore throat, myalgias, arthralgias, facial neuralgia, and generalized lymphadenopathy. Four days later a macular, nonpruritic rash developed on the trunk and spread to the face and neck. The symptoms resolved entirely by 3 weeks. Serum drawn 27 days after the needle-stick injury was negative for antibodies to HIV-III, but serum drawn on day 49 was positive. In 1985 a review of 12 cases of seroconversion among homosexual men described a sudden onset of mononucleosis-like illness associated with primary infection in 11 of the individuals. In 1986 the Centers for Disease Control and Prevention (CDC) defined acute infection as a mononucleosis-like syndrome with or without aseptic meningitis. Since then, there have been numerous descriptions of the protean clinical manifestations of acute HIV-1 infection.

Acute HIV-1 infection typically presents as an acute-onset, mononucleosis-like or flu-like illness within days to weeks after the initial exposure. The most common signs and symptoms include fever, lethargy, maculopapular rash, headache, lymphadenopathy, pharyngitis, myalgias, gastrointestinal distress, aseptic meningitis, retro-orbital pain, night sweats, and oral or genital ulcers (Box 2-2). An acute retroviral syndrome occurs in more than half of infected individuals. The acute illness usually resolves within 2 weeks, but may last from a few days to more than 10 weeks. Because of the relatively nonspecific signs and symptoms, acute HIV-1 infection is often confused with a

BOX 2-2
Clinical Manifestations of Acute HIV-1 Infection

GENERAL
Fever
Fatigue/malaise
Lymphadenopathy
Pharyngitis
Myalgia/arthralgia
Night sweats

NEUROLOGIC
Headache
Aseptic meningitis
Encephalitis/encephalopathy
Retro-orbital pain
Peripheral neuropathy
Radiculopathy
Brachial neuritis
Facial nerve palsy
Guillain-Barré syndrome

DERMATOLOGIC
Erythematous, maculopapular rash
Oral ulcers
Genital ulcers

GASTROINTESTINAL
Nausea/vomiting
Diarrhea
Anorexia/weight loss
Oropharyngeal candidiasis

BOX 2-3
Differential Diagnoses of Acute HIV-1 Infection

Infectious mononucleosis
Primary cytomegalovirus infection
Acute hepatitis A or B infection
Toxoplasmosis
Secondary syphilis
Measles
Rubella
Other viral illnesses

variety of other illnesses including infectious mononucleosis, primary cytomegalovirus (CMV) infection, acute hepatitis A or B, toxoplasmosis, secondary syphilis, measles, rubella, and other viral illnesses (Box 2-3). Acute HIV-1 infection should be considered in the differential diagnosis of any unexplained, severe febrile illness in a patient at risk.

Certain clinical manifestations are especially suggestive of acute HIV-1 infection in a person at risk and are valuable clues to the diagnosis. The finding of rash and/or mucocutaneous ulceration involving the oral, buccal, anal, or genital mucosa should prompt consideration of acute HIV-1 infection in a person at risk. The rash of acute HIV-1 infection classically appears as an erythematous, macular or maculopapular, nonpruritic, nonscaling eruption on the trunk and face (Fig. 2-2). Less often the rash is vesiculopapular. The skin lesions are nonspecific and resemble those seen in drug reactions and other infections, such as secondary syphilis and certain viral infections. Histopathology is also nonspecific, showing a normal epidermis and a lymphocytic infiltrate around superficial dermal vessels. Mucocutaneous ulceration is another useful clue to acute HIV-1 infection because it rarely occurs in most of the other infections in the differential diagnosis. In a series of 31 patients with acute HIV-1 infection, 68% of patients presented with rash and 43% presented with oral or genital ulceration (Fig. 2-3); 52% of patients with skin lesions had mucosal lesions, and 84% of patients with mucosal lesions had skin lesions. Therefore the finding of rash and mucocutaneous ulceration in a patient with a history of exposure should raise a strong suspicion of acute HIV-1 infection. In addition, an acute, self-limited aseptic meningitis, as described in the case presentation above, has been reported frequently as a symptom of acute HIV-1 infection. Other neurologic manifestations of acute HIV-1 infection include encephalitis, facial nerve palsy, brachial neuritis, acute myelopathy, seizure, and Guillain-Barré syndrome.

KEY POINTS

- Over 50% of patients with acute HIV infection have symptoms
- Acute-onset mononucleosis-like syndrome or flu-like illness days to weeks after exposure to HIV-1
- Fever, adenopathy, rash, with or without aseptic meningitis
- Rash and mucocutaneous ulcers in a patient at risk are particularly suggestive

Diagnosis of Acute HIV-1 Infection

An estimated 40,000 to 60,000 Americans contract HIV-1 each year. Assuming that over 50% of these infections are symptomatic, during any given week more than 500 people may present with symptoms consistent with acute HIV-1 infection. The diagnosis of acute HIV-1 infection requires a high index of suspicion and a basic understanding of the virologic and immunologic markers at this stage. It is important to diagnose acute HIV-1 infection because early diagnosis makes early treatment possible and leads to counseling to prevent further disease transmission.

The nonspecific presentation of acute HIV-1 infection makes diagnosis difficult and emphasizes the need for health care providers to obtain an accurate history of HIV-1 risk factors and maintain a high level of clinical suspicion. In a group of 23 patients who were at risk for HIV-1 infection and were enrolled in an HIV-1 surveillance program, 87% reported symptoms consistent with an acute retroviral syndrome, 95% sought medical attention for these symptoms, but only 26% were correctly diagnosed with acute HIV-1 infection when they first sought medical attention. This is an alarmingly low percentage, underscoring the need for a high index of clinical suspicion in a population with high-risk behavior and symptoms suggestive of acute infection.

Like the clinical manifestations, laboratory abnormalities during acute HIV-1 infection are nonspecific and can be seen

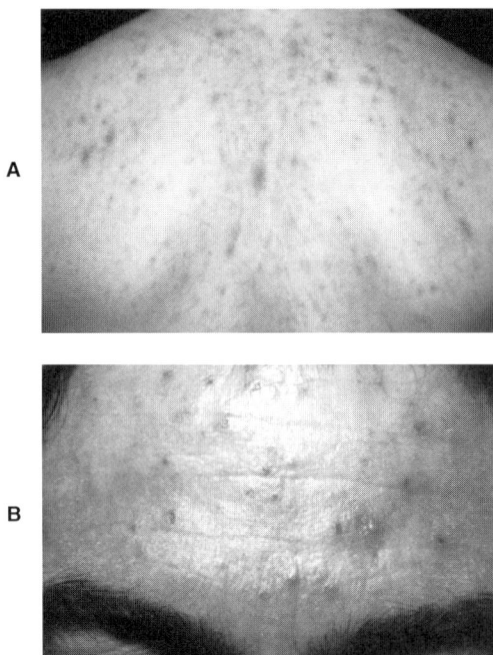

FIG. 2-2 Characteristic rash in acute HIV-1 infection. *A,* Trunk. *B,* Face. (From Armstrong D, Cohen J, editors: *HIV and AIDS,* London, 1999, Mosby-Wolfe.)

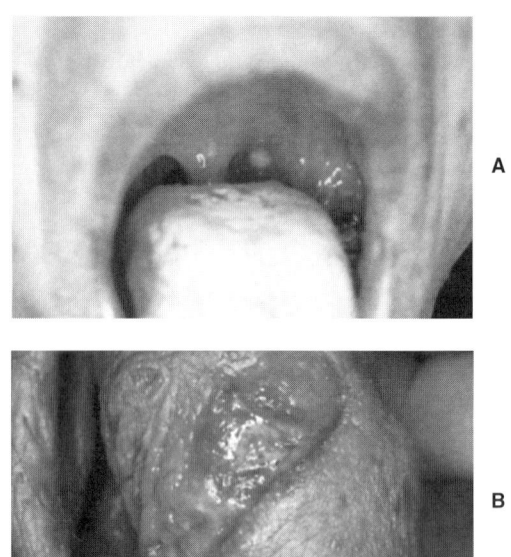

FIG. 2-3 Mucocutaneous ulceration in acute HIV-1 infection. *A,* Mucosal ulceration. *B,* Penile ulcer. (From Armstrong D, Cohen J, editors: *HIV and AIDS,* London, 1999, Mosby-Wolfe.)

in other acute viral illnesses. Laboratory tests performed during acute infection may show lymphopenia and thrombocytopenia, although atypical lymphocytes are uncommon. Some patients develop anemia and elevated transaminases. Cerebrospinal fluid (CSF) analysis often shows a lymphocytic pleocytosis with elevated protein. The CD4+ T cell count usually decreases during acute infection, but can remain in the normal range. Over the ensuing weeks the CD4+ T cell count decreases, the CD8+ T cell count increases, and the CD4+:CD8+ ratio inverts. Occasionally the CD4+ T cell count drops low enough during acute infection that opportunistic infections occur. Esophageal candidiasis, CMV pneumonitis, CMV colitis, *Pneumocystis carinii* pneumonia, tuberculous meningitis, and cerebral toxoplasmosis have been reported during acute HIV-1 infection.

Detecting viral DNA, high levels of viral RNA, or p24 antigen in a patient with a negative HIV-1 antibody test makes the diagnosis of acute HIV-1 infection. HIV-1–specific antibody assays are not positive until 4 to 6 weeks after infection and therefore are not used to diagnose acute HIV-1 infection. Standard serologic tests are used to determine if an individual has been exposed to HIV-1, to screen blood and plasma donations, and to conduct epidemiologic surveillance. Detection of p24 antigen has utility in the early diagnosis of HIV-1 infection. Levels of p24 antigen are high early in infection, and the test is positive in approximately 90% of acutely infected individuals who have not yet developed antibodies. Despite its high sensitivity, the p24 antigen test has been largely replaced by assays for integrated proviral DNA or viral RNA that are positive in virtually 100% of acutely infected individuals. Detecting proviral DNA in peripheral blood lymphocytes by a polymerase chain reaction (PCR) assay is extremely sensitive, detecting as few as 5 to 10 copies/ml. The viral DNA PCR test is a qualitative assay that provides a yes/no result. The quantitative viral RNA assay, or viral load assay, determines the number of copies of viral RNA per ml of plasma. Quantitative assays for HIV-1 RNA are extremely valuable for predicting disease progression, determining when to initiate antiretroviral therapy, monitoring response to treatment, and defining treatment failure. However, these assays are often used for diagnosis of acute HIV-1 infection, which can be problematic because of the false-positive rate. Reported cases of false-positives have had viral loads less than 5,000 copies/ml, whereas the viral load in an acutely infected individual is typically greater than 50,000 copies/ml and often greater than 1 million copies/ml.

KEY POINTS

⊃ High index of suspicion necessary
⊃ Negative antibody tests with positive tests for viral presence (HIV viral load) make diagnosis
⊃ Quantitative viral load usually very high (>50,000, often >1 million)

Natural History

It is unclear why some individuals have symptoms and some do not, but several studies indicate that severe and prolonged symptoms during acute HIV-1 infection are associated with a more rapidly progressive clinical course. Neurologic symptoms and fever for 7 or more days during acute infection are particularly ominous predictors of disease progression. Severe symptoms may be due to cytokine production or may be a marker of viral dissemination or an inadequate immune response. Other factors that may contribute to symptom severity include the quantity and virulence of the virus. For example, a study demonstrated that recipients of HIV-1–infected blood transfusions were more likely to develop an acute retroviral syndrome and progress rapidly to AIDS if the donor developed AIDS soon after donation.

Treatment of Acute HIV-1 Infection

An important reason to identify individuals with acute HIV-1 infection is to start antiretroviral therapy early. There are several arguments in favor of treatment during acute HIV-1 infection. Initial viral isolates are a relatively homogenous swarm of viruses that may be more susceptible to effective combination therapy, and early therapy may actually reduce the rate of viral mutation. Early treatment may limit the extent of viral dissemination and restore important HIV-1–specific cellular immune responses. Early treatment may further lower the viral set-point and thereby impact on disease progression. Finally, early treatment may reduce the risk of viral transmission.

Several small studies have evaluated the efficacy of treatment during acute HIV-1 infection. A retrospective, case-control study of patients with symptomatic acute HIV-1 infection investigated the effect of zidovudine monotherapy (1 g daily, a regimen considered inadequate by current standards). Over 12 months of follow-up there was a clear trend toward benefit in the zidovudine-treated group as measured by development of AIDS and CD4+ T cell count, although the results did not reach statistical significance. The only randomized, double-blind, placebo-controlled trial of antiretroviral therapy during acute HIV-1 infection examined the effect of 6 months of zidovudine (250 mg twice daily, a regimen considered inadequate by current standards) versus placebo. The zidovudine-treated group had a mean increase of 173 CD4+ T cells compared with a mean increase of six CD4+ T cells in the placebo group. The zidovudine-treated group also had a greater, although not statistically significant, reduction in plasma HIV-1 RNA levels. In neither of these studies was the duration of the acute antiretroviral syndrome affected. Several studies have investigated the effects of triple-drug regimens on patients with acute HIV-1 infection. Patients treated with three nucleoside reverse transcriptase inhibitors or two nucleoside reverse transcriptase inhibitors plus a protease inhibitor had rapid reductions in plasma HIV-1 RNA levels to less than 200 copies/ml and significant increases in the mean CD4+:CD8+ ratio. Compelling data in support of a beneficial effect of early therapy on the immune system come from a study of individuals treated with triple-drug therapy during acute HIV-1 infection. In six individuals treated with this regimen, HIV-1 RNA levels rapidly decreased to undetectable, and there was an associated vigorous HIV-1–specific CD4+ T cell lymphoproliferative response like that seen in long-term nonprogressors. An ongoing study is evaluating the efficacy of a potent four-drug regimen in patients with acute HIV-1 infection. Other potential treatments of acute HIV-1 infection include therapies directed at enhancing host responses to HIV-1, such as cytokines and adjuvant vaccines. As suggested by all currently available data, the goal of therapy for acute HIV infection should be suppressing HIV RNA levels to below detectable levels. There are insufficient data available to make firm recommendations, but to date most clinicians use the same drug combinations as those used to treat established infection (see Chapter 5).

Only combination regimens expected to maximally suppress viral replication should be used and compliance is essential. Since drug toxicity, cost, and a large number of pills, as well as the theoretic risk of drug resistance, are all potential drawbacks, the physician should carefully counsel the patient about the potential benefits and limitations of therapy. Based on available data to date it appears that the benefits outweigh the risks. If a decision to treat is made, then close follow-up is mandatory. HIV-1 RNA levels and CD4+ T cell counts should be checked on initiation of therapy, after 4 weeks of therapy, and every 3 to 4 months thereafter. The optimal duration of therapy is unknown, and ongoing clinical trials should answer this question. Until such data are available most experts continue to treat indefinitely.

KEY POINTS

Early treatment may
⊃ Limit the extent of viral dissemination
⊃ Restore and augment HIV-1–specific cellular immune response
⊃ Lower the eventual viral set-point
⊃ Decrease severity of acute disease
⊃ Reduce the risk of viral transmission

When to Refer

Primary care physicians need to have a high index of suspicion for acute HIV syndrome because by its very nature *they* will diagnose this syndrome, or not, a great majority of the time. Once the diagnosis is made, it is reasonable to seek consultation from an HIV treatment expert regarding therapy because these recommendations change rapidly.

Summary

Acute HIV-1 infection usually manifests as an acute, nonspecific febrile illness, and all physicians should consider this diagnosis in a sexually active or at-risk individual presenting with such symptoms. Early detection of acute HIV-1 infection is important because events during this period have an influence on disease progression. If acute HIV-1 infection is suspected, HIV-1 RNA and HIV-1 ELISA testing should be done. Once acute HIV-1 infection is diagnosed, aggressive antiretroviral therapy should be considered.

SUGGESTED READINGS

Daar ES: Virology and immunology of acute HIV type 1 infection, *AIDS Res Human Retro* 14(Suppl 3):S229-S234, 1998.
Kahn JO, Walker BD: Acute human immunodeficiency virus type 1 infection, *N Engl J Med* 339:33-39, 1998.
Russell ND, Sepkowitz KA: Primary HIV infection: clinical, immunologic, and virologic predictors of progression, *AIDS Reader* Nov/Dec:164-172, 1998.
Schacker T et al: Clinical and epidemiologic features of primary HIV infection, *Ann Intern Med* 125:257-264, 1996.
Schacker TW et al: Biological and virologic characteristics of primary HIV infection, *Ann Intern Med* 128:613-620, 1998.

3 Testing for the Virus

JAY R. KOSTMAN

Introduction

Laboratory diagnosis of human immunodeficiency virus (HIV) infection relies most commonly on the detection of antibodies to the virus in plasma. Currently available tests have a high degree of sensitivity and specificity in most clinical situations. This chapter will review currently available testing strategies, discuss the limitations of serology in detecting HIV-2 or unusual subtypes of HIV-1, and review new techniques that are useful in the diagnosis of acute HIV infection.

Antibody Response to HIV Infection

A complete understanding of the serologic tests available for HIV diagnosis requires a brief description of the antibody response to HIV infection. HIV viral proteins are divided into three groups: envelope proteins, which include the glycoproteins gp 120, gp 41, and gp 160; polymerase proteins, including the reverse transcriptase p66 and the integrase p31; and core proteins, including major structural proteins p24 and p18 and proteins p7 and p55. After transmission, the core HIV protein, p24 antigen, is the first marker to be detected in the serum, within 2 weeks of infection. Antibodies to p24 begin to appear in the serum within 1 to 2 months and their appearance correlates with a decline in p24 antigen. In addition, antibodies to the envelope glycoproteins (gp 160 and gp 120) and the transmembrane glycoprotein (gp 41) appear within 2 to 6 weeks of infection.

Screening for HIV Infection

Optimal use of available tests for HIV infection begins with a good understanding of who is at risk for infection. Recent estimates in the United States are that at most 60% of infected individuals are actually receiving care, implying that many infected individuals are not being tested and made aware of their HIV status. According to current recommendations, those who should be considered for HIV testing include: (1) persons with other sexually transmitted diseases; (2) persons in high-risk groups, such as injecting drug users, men who have sex with men, hemophiliacs, and individuals who are regular sexual partners of someone in a high-risk group; (3) pregnant women; (4) people at risk for occupational exposures, including source and recipient; (5) blood, organ, and semen donors; and (6) those with medical illnesses suggestive of HIV infection. Most states in the United States currently require that informed consent be obtained prior to HIV testing. Informed consent should be accompanied by appropriate pretest and posttest counseling. For individuals who continue to practice high-risk behavior, repeated serologic testing for HIV infection is indicated in order to detect seroconversion at as early a time point as possible. Data on annual seroconversion rates in different segments of the population include 0.02% in the general population, 0.5% to 2% in men who have sex with men, and 2% to 15% in injecting drug users.

The most common testing strategy used to confirm HIV infection is the combination of an enzyme immunoassay (EIA) with a confirmatory Western blot for specimens that are EIA-positive. This approach yields an overall sensitivity and specificity of greater than 99.5%. Positive serologies are reported if the EIA is repeatedly positive and the confirmatory Western blot is also positive. The EIA is performed by binding partially purified virus (from strains grown in infected cells) containing envelope and core proteins to a solid phase that is subsequently exposed to patient serum to allow for antigen-antibody binding. After washing away the unbound immunoglobulin, the solid phase with bound antigen-antibody is exposed to an enzyme-labeled anti-human globulin. The final complex is then exposed to an enzyme substrate, which leads to a colorimetric reaction that is proportional to the amount of bound anti-HIV antibody in the patient plasma. A positive EIA is confirmed by repeating the assay. Since the cutoff for a positive test is set low enough to make the test extremely sensitive, weak responses that fall close to the cutoff can present a problem (see the section on False-positive Serologic Tests).

The Western blot is performed by separating HIV proteins obtained from crude lysates of HIV grown in tissue culture by molecular weight onto a nitrocellulose strip. The strips are then exposed to patient serum and incubated with anti-human immunoglobulin that will produce a colored band at sites of antigen-antibody binding. Although there are several different rules for interpretation of Western blots, the Centers for Disease Control and Prevention and the Association of State and Territorial Public Health Laboratory Directors require that two of the following bands, p24, gp 41, and gp 120/160, be present for a blot to be positive. If one of the above bands is present or if there are other bands not corresponding to viral antigen, the blot is said to be indeterminate. If there are no bands present, the blot is negative.

False-negative Serologic Tests

False-negative serologic tests (EIA plus Western blot) are the result of several different circumstances including a delay in developing antibodies after acute infection, variation in HIV strain type, and loss of antibody late in infection. The "window" period refers to the time delay between acquisition of infection and the development of an antibody response. On average, this delay is of several weeks duration, although it may take up to 6 months to have detectable antibodies in rare cases. In a given population, the frequency of false-negative tests due to this window period depends on the seroprevalence in that population. If the prevalence is high, such as in certain groups of injecting drug users, the rate of false-negatives is 0.3% to 0.5%; in low-prevalence groups, such as those donating blood, the rate of false-negatives due to the window period is much lower. Modifications of traditional serologic tests have been suggested as one way to improve the diagnostic yield of serology in the window period (see the section on Diagnosis of Primary and Early HIV Infection).

HIV-1 is distributed worldwide and is characterized by groups and subgroups known as clades. The two major groups of virus are known as M and O. Group M is subdivided into subtypes, of which clade B is the dominant type in the United States and Western Europe. Many of the serologic tests have been designed to primarily detect clade B and will yield false-negative results in infections with non–clade B or group O strains of HIV-1. Other serologic tests are available to detect these less common strains, but they may need to be specifically requested.

HIV-2 has between 40% and 60% amino acid homology with HIV-1. HIV-2 has been found primarily in the West African countries of Cape Verde, Côte d'Ivoire, Gambia, Guinea-Bissau, Mali, Mauritania, Nigeria, and Sierra Leone. Most of the cases from the United States have occurred in individuals who were from West Africa. Since there is incomplete homology between HIV-1 and HIV-2, individuals infected with HIV-2 may have false-negative serologies unless an immunoblot assay with HIV-2 specificity is used. In individuals with a clinical syndrome compatible with HIV infection and a negative serology, testing for HIV-2 should be performed; in addition, HIV-2 infection should be suspected if a patient has had sexual partners with known HIV-2 infection or who were from a country where HIV-2 is prevalent, has received transfusions in a country where HIV-2 infection is prevalent, or is a child of a woman at risk for HIV-2 infection.

Occasionally, patients with late-stage HIV infection lose the ability to produce antibodies due to immune system collapse. If these individuals are tested for HIV infection, the serology may be falsely negative. The diagnosis of acquired immunodeficiency syndrome (AIDS) can be made on clinical grounds in these patients and confirmed by direct measurement of viral antigen or nucleic acid.

False-positive Serologic Tests

In the general population, the incidence of false-positive HIV serologic testing is very rare (0.0006%). False-positive reactions are most likely due either to recent vaccination or to co-morbid conditions that result in polyclonal hypergammaglobulinemia, such as systemic lupus erythematosus. In patients with one of these co-morbid conditions, a test for HIV antigen or nucleic acid should be used if the diagnosis is in question. For those who have a positive serology after recent vaccination (i.e., influenza vaccine), the HIV serology can be repeated at a later date to confirm that it is falsely positive related to vaccination. Alternatively, tests for HIV antigen or nucleic acid will be negative in these patients as well.

Indeterminate Western Blots

If a Western blot has evidence of some bands that do not meet the criteria for a positive reading, it is referred to as an indeterminate Western blot. In the general population, the incidence of indeterminate Western blots is approximately two in 10,000; however, in hospital laboratories, 10% to 15% of all specimens that are positive by EIA are subsequently indeterminate by Western blot. Most often, the indeterminate reading results from the presence of a single band due to p24 antigen. An indeterminate Western blot can result from testing during HIV seroconversion, cross-reacting antibodies produced in collagen vascular diseases or malignancies, or infection with non–clade B strains of HIV infection. In low-risk groups of individuals, an indeterminate Western blot is rarely associated with HIV infection. This can be confirmed by repeat testing at 3 and 6 months, which most likely will show persistence of the indeterminate pattern with no evolution of bands. By more specific testing for HIV antigen or nucleic acid, these individuals are almost always shown to not be HIV infected. If the indeterminate Western blot occurs in the setting of seroconversion, patients will usually have positive Western blots within 1 to 3 months of the original test. Current recommendations are to repeat the blot at 1, 3, and 6 months while using appropriate precautions to minimize viral transmission during this time period.

Alternative Methods for HIV Serologic Testing

In an effort to improve access to HIV testing, attempts have been made to develop alternative testing methodologies. These technologies include methods for home HIV testing as well as rapid HIV tests that could be employed easily in the field. Home HIV tests employ EIA technology with a confirmatory immunofluorescent assay. Blood is obtained by finger puncture and then fixed to a filter strip that is then mailed in with confidentiality assurances. Results are available in 3 days. Negative results can be obtained through an automated system; if a positive result is obtained, the result is communicated by an experienced counselor. In studies analyzing who uses home testing, results have shown that the majority of individuals tested have not been previously tested for HIV. The vast majority of tests are negative.

In addition to blood, other body fluids can be used for HIV antibody testing. The most widely used of these systems is the OraSure system, which uses saliva and a subsequent concentration step to collect antibodies for measurement by EIA and confirmatory Western blot, if necessary. OraSure is available for use by public health workers, medical practices, and HIV community service organizations for the purpose of HIV screening. After collection of saliva on a specialized pad, results are available generally within 3 days. Collection of antibodies in saliva may offer advantages in community-based settings where phlebotomy may be difficult or where individuals trained in phlebotomy may not be readily available. There is an extremely good correlation between the results of saliva-based testing and plasma testing for HIV antibodies, with comparable sensitivity and specificity. A urine-based antibody test for HIV antibodies has also been developed that offers similar advantages of ease of performance and reduced cost. All positive tests must be confirmed by a plasma antibody test, however, since the urinary test only measures antibodies by EIA.

All of the above-described methods for measuring HIV antibodies still require EIA and confirmatory Western blots, which require several days. Rapid tests for HIV antibodies offer the advantage of immediate turnover, especially important in cases of occupational exposures from a source patient of unknown HIV serology, in settings in which follow-up is likely to be difficult such as public health clinics, or in the assessment of pregnant women presenting in labor without prenatal care who may be candidates for antiviral therapy to prevent perinatal transmission. The rapid test that is currently Food and Drug Administration (FDA)-approved and available is the single use diagnostic system (SUDS) test, performed on serum. This test must be performed and interpreted by a trained technician; results can be obtained in 10 to 15 minutes. The sensitivity of the rapid test is comparable to standard serologic testing; thus negative tests can be reported definitively as negative without further confirmation. However, the specificity of the rapid test is slightly lower than standard plasma testing at 99.6%; thus positive rapid tests must be confirmed by standard testing. Since the major goal of the rapid test is to rule out HIV infection in settings in which empiric therapy could be avoided, such as occupational exposures or prevention of perinatal transmission, a slightly higher false-positive rate is acceptable. Currently, new rapid tests in development are expected to be able to be read directly by a provider and to be cheaper to perform.

Direct Detection of Virus

In certain situations, the diagnosis of HIV infection is established by direct detection of viral antigens, viral RNA or DNA, or by culture of the virus. The most common clinical scenarios in which direct detection is required include the window period after viral exposure (see above), disorders of globulin production, clarification of confusing serology results, primary HIV infection with an acute retroviral syndrome (see below), and neonatal infection. Although measurement of p24 antigen was commonly used for some of these situations, its lack of sensitivity (10% to 50%) and the increased availability of RNA and DNA assays have led to infrequent usage. The most sensitive of these tests is the DNA polymerase chain reaction (PCR) assay, which can detect between one and 10 copies of HIV proviral DNA. Quantitative measurement of HIV RNA is the preferred test for monitoring the effectiveness of antiretroviral therapy and for providing prognostic information on the rate of disease progression in therapy-naive individuals. When these measurements are used for HIV diagnosis, such as in the case with occupational exposures, the false-positive rate may be as high as 2% to 10%; these false-positive tests are usually low copy numbers of viral RNA (<100). Thus a low copy number in an untreated person should be suspect. Although viral isolation can be accomplished with high sensitivity and specificity by co-cultivation of patient peripheral blood mononuclear cells with donor cells, it is extremely expensive and labor intensive. Culture is rarely used in a clinical setting, the one exception being certain cases of potential neonatal infection.

Diagnosis of Primary and Early HIV Infection

As the virologic and immunologic events around primary HIV infection have become increasingly well understood, it has become apparent that timely diagnosis is imperative in order to initiate effective management. The acute infection period usually lasts from several weeks to several months, often with an accompanying clinical illness. In the classic presentation, this so-called acute retroviral syndrome is similar to a mononucleosis-like syndrome, with the most common signs and symptoms including fever, fatigue, myalgias, pharyngitis, lymphadenopathy, rash, and nonspecific gastrointestinal complaints, such as nausea, vomiting, and diarrhea. Less common findings include oral and/or genital ulcerations and neuritis. The differential diagnosis of such a syndrome is broad and includes other viral illnesses (such as infectious mononucleosis due to Epstein-Barr virus or cytomegalovirus; acute viral hepatitis due to hepatitis A, B, or C; acute parvovirus infection; or even influenza), bacterial illnesses (such as streptococcal pharyngitis or secondary syphilis), or rickettsial disease due to Rocky Mountain spotted fever or ehrlichiosis. The clinical diagnosis of acute HIV infection should always be suspected in such cases, and a thorough risk factor and potential exposure history is crucial to consideration for further laboratory testing. However, the lack of obvious risks does not rule out HIV infection, since the HIV epidemic is spreading most rapidly among heterosexuals in the United States, particularly in adolescents and young adults.

Laboratory Screening for Acute HIV Infection

Within weeks of infection with HIV, infected cells produce large amounts of virus, resulting in higher plasma viral loads than at any other time during the natural history of HIV infection. Since there is an average delay of 21 to 28 days between infection and seroconversion, the most common mistake made by health care providers evaluating patients with an acute retroviral syndrome is to miss the diagnosis of acute HIV infection due to a negative HIV EIA and Western blot. During this period, circulating levels of p24 antigen are very high (in excess of 100 pg/ml) and the average level of HIV RNA is 12 million copies/ml (as high as 95 million copies/ml in some patients). For this reason, a strategy of measuring either p24 antigen or HIV RNA has been recommended as a diagnostic test in suspected cases of acute HIV infection with a negative serologic evaluation. One recent study compared these two testing strategies and illustrates the potential advantages and disadvantages of the two tests. The sensitivity of plasma viral load testing was 100% compared with 88.7% for p24 antigen testing. On the other hand, the specificity of the p24 antigen test was 100% compared with 97.4% for the viral load test. The patients with acute HIV infection and negative serologic tests had plasma viral loads that exceeded 100,000 copies/ml; thus the false-positive tests demonstrated a low level of viremia (less than 10,000 copies/ml). There was also significant difference in cost: the p24 antigen assay resulted in a patient charge of $75 compared with $220 for the viral load assay. Thus, in employing one of these tests for large scale screening for acute HIV infection, the cost benefit ratio may favor the use of p24 antigen screening; although it will miss a small number of people with acute HIV infection, this test will not result in false-positive findings that would require extensive counseling and repeated testing, and produce an enormous emotional toll.

Diagnosis of Early HIV Infection

The ability to identify individuals who are in the early stages of HIV infection is important in order to estimate HIV incidence rates as well as to identify patients who may be appropriate candidates for early intervention and prevention efforts. Early infection is usually defined as the period immediately after seroconversion, and can be difficult to identify with a single blood test using traditional serologic testing. This period is different from the pre-seroconversion period outlined above in which measurement of p24 antigen or HIV RNA by PCR can be used for diagnosis.

One strategy that has been proposed for the detection of individuals with early infection has been the use of the "detuned" EIA, or a sensitive/less sensitive assay testing algorithm. In this algorithm, the less sensitive EIA is performed by modification of several elements of a standard EIA and of the cutoff used to determine a positive result. This concept utilizes the fact that seroconversion in the less sensitive assays will take a longer period of time after infection; thus the period of time between seroconversion in the two assays can be used to estimate the incidence of early infection in large cohorts of people at risk for HIV infection. This method has been validated in cohorts of blood donors as well as potential enrollees in a study of primary HIV infection. The detuned EIA may be useful in clinical trials and epidemiologic studies of early HIV infection, although its role in general clinical practice is still undefined.

SUGGESTED READINGS

Centers for Disease Control: Interpretation and use of the Western blot assay for serodiagnosis of human immunodeficiency virus type 1 infections, *MMWR* 38(supp l7):1-7, 1989.

Gurtler L: Difficulties and strategies of HIV diagnosis, *Lancet* 348:176-179, 1996.

Janssen RS et al: New testing strategy to detect early HIV-1 infection for use in incidence estimates and for clinical and prevention purposes, *JAMA* 280:42-48, 1998.

4 Initial Management of HIV Infection

STEPHEN J. GLUCKMAN

Introduction

Human immunodeficiency virus (HIV) infection is a chronic disease. As such its management should be an evolving partnership between the patient and the primary health care provider. The initial encounter is much more than a medical event; in fact, the pure clinical aspects are rather straightforward. It is a time to begin to establish a trusting therapeutic relationship. HIV infection is relatively unique in that its management combines the most cutting edge areas of the science of medicine with the most humanistic areas of the art of medicine—such things as easing emotional pain and fears, showing compassion and patience, and displaying the ability to educate and reassure patients and families. The initial encounter must initiate the inclusion of both the science and the art in the management of this disease. Two points of emphasis: it takes time to do it correctly and much of it has to be repeated. It is a lot of information to grasp at a time when a person's mind is preoccupied with the news of the recent HIV diagnosis.

Areas to cover during the initial encounter are summarized in Box 4-1. The encounter should not be rushed and may actually take several visits to complete.

Comprehensive History

HIV is a multisystem disease, so initially a complete history, review of systems, and physical examination are required. There are a number of particularly critical questions that should be asked regarding the patient's past history. The next sections give an overview of the questioning required.

HIV Testing

Among the questions the health care provider should ask in regard to HIV testing include: "When was the first positive test?" "Why was the testing done?" "Have there been prior negative tests?" and "Do you (the patient) have a copy of the test result?" It is a good idea to have proof of HIV positivity before initiating antiretroviral therapy. Therefore the health care provider should ask if there is information about the initial CD4+ cell count and viral load and about the most recent values.

Specific Diseases and Exposures

Certain diseases are particularly common and/or important in the history of HIV-positive persons and should be specifically inquired about including other sexually transmitted diseases, hepatitis, tuberculosis and tuberculosis exposure, chickenpox and zoster, international travel or travel to the southwestern United States, animal exposure, blood products receipt or donation, work, and hobbies.

General Past Medical/Surgical History

HIV-infected patients potentially have the same problems as any other patient. Knowledge of these non–HIV-related problems is often important in their overall management.

Current Medications and Treatments

The physician should inquire about any prescription, over-the-counter, and complementary medications and treatments the patient is using.

Medication Allergies and Side Effects

HIV-infected persons have an unusually high incidence of allergic reactions to medications.

Sexual History

The health care provider should inquire about sexual preferences, present partner(s), condom use, knowledge of the principles of safer sex, and prior sexually transmitted diseases.

Gynecologic History

The health care provider should ask if the patient is or has ever been pregnant and about any pregnancy outcome(s) and fertility status. The patient should also be asked about any history of abnormal Pap smears or cervical cancer and about when she had her last Pap smear.

Habits

Among the questions the health care provider should ask are: "Do you or have you ever used tobacco, alcohol, or illicit drugs?" and "Do you exercise regularly?"

Vaccination History

The health care provider should inquire about hepatitis B, pneumococcal, influenza, and tetanus/diphtheria immunizations.

Support Systems

The health care provider should find out who knows the HIV status of the patient, who he or she is planning to tell, and who is available to help the patient deal with HIV-related issues. The provider should also find out about the patient's insurance status and who pays for the medications, whether the patient is homeless, and whether the patient wants to (needs to) talk to a social worker.

BOX 4-1
Basics of the Initial Encounter

Comprehensive history and physical examination
Baseline laboratory testing
Indicated immunizations
Antiretroviral therapy and opportunistic infection prophylaxis
Possible referrals
Discussions of:
   Most recent information about the true prognosis
   Modes of transmission of HIV
   Who to tell
   Who not to tell
   Primer on CD4+ counts and viral loads for the patient
   Critical importance of adherence to a regimen
   Support systems
   Economic and social work issues
   Lifestyle issues such as exercise, diet, smoking, alcohol, and illicit drugs
   Complementary therapies
   Sex and HIV infection
   Syringe and needle cleaning and needle-exchange programs (when appropriate)
Monitoring the immune system
Frequency of follow-up visits

BOX 4-2
Comprehensive History

HIV TESTING
Date of the first positive test
Any prior negative tests? When?
Why was the testing done?
CD4+ cell counts?
Viral loads?

PAST MEDICAL HISTORY AND EXPOSURE HISTORY
Hepatitis
Tuberculosis or tuberculosis exposure
Chickenpox or zoster
International travel
Animal exposure
Blood products
Sexually transmitted diseases

CURRENT MEDICATIONS AND TREATMENTS
Prescribed medications
Over-the-counter medications
Complementary medications and treatments

MEDICATION ALLERGIES AND SIDE EFFECTS

SEXUAL HISTORY
Preferences
Condom use and knowledge of safer sexual practices

GYNECOLOGIC HISTORY
Pregnant?
Prior pregnancy outcomes
Last Pap smear? Results?
History of abnormal Pap smears?
Fertility status, method(s) of birth control

HABITS
Tobacco
Alcohol
Illicit drugs
Exercise

VACCINATION HISTORY
Tetanus/diphtheria
Hepatitis A, B
Pneumococcal
Influenza
Other

SUPPORT SYSTEMS AND ECONOMIC ISSUES
Who knows the diagnosis?
Who is the patient planning to tell?
With whom do they live?
Job information
Insurance issues
Who pays for the medications?
Does the patient want to talk to a social worker?

The comprehensive history is summarized in Box 4-2.

Since virtually any organ or organ system can be involved, the review of systems must be very comprehensive (Box 4-3).

Physical Examination

The physical examination needs to be equally comprehensive, with particular attention to the following.

General

There should be an overall assessment of nutritional status and appearance of well-being. The weight should be recorded along with the other vital signs.

Skin

Cutaneous problems are particularly common. Many common diseases such as seborrhea and psoriasis can be more highly expressed in patients with HIV infection. Pale conjunctiva and nail beds may reflect the common finding of anemia. Petechiae or ecchymoses may reflect thrombocytopenia. In addition, there are several skin findings that are relatively specific for HIV, such as Kaposi's sarcoma, bacillary angiomatosis, and cutaneous manifestations of disseminated cryptococcus.

Head, Ears, Eyes, Nose, and Throat

Intraoral findings are common including thrush, hairy leukoplakia, Kaposi's sarcoma, and herpes or aphthous ulcers. Periodontal disease can be very aggressive. An initial funduscopic examination should be routine and may reveal the nonspecific finding of cotton-wool spots or the characteristic findings of cytomegalovirus (CMV) retinitis.

Lymph Nodes

In addition to the generalized generally benign adenopathy that can be due to HIV itself, adenopathy can be due to a num-

BOX 4-3
Possible Signs and Symptoms Found in a Review of Systems

Anorexia
Cough
Depression symptoms
Diarrhea
Dyspnea
Fatigue
Fever
Headaches
Joint complaints
Menstrual problems
Mouth sores

Odynophagia or dysphagia
Paresthesias
Rashes
Sweats
Swollen lymph glands
Thinking problems
Vaginitis symptoms
Visual changes
Weakness
Weight loss

---

ber of associated diseases in HIV-infected persons, including mycobacterial infections, lymphoma, and Kaposi's sarcoma.

Cardiopulmonary

In addition to the possible findings associated with pulmonary infections, there may be evidence of myocarditis and/or pericarditis, both relatively common in HIV-infected persons. There may be evidence of endocarditis, particularly in injecting drug users.

Abdomen

Abdominal tenderness, particularly in the right upper quadrant, is a common concern, as are hepatomegaly and splenomegaly.

Genitourinary

A complete genital, pelvic, and rectal examination is essential due to the increased incidence of other sexually transmitted diseases and vaginitis. A Pap smear, if there has been none done in the past 6 months, and chlamydia test should be performed at this time. Perirectal herpes infection can be particularly aggressive and mistaken for a decubitus ulcer or a malignancy.

Neurologic

Specific evaluation is needed for evidence of peripheral neuropathy, weakness, and muscle wasting, and there should be a mini-mental status evaluation.

The physical examination summary is shown in Box 4-4.

Baseline Laboratory Testing

In addition to the testing suggested by the history, review of systems, and physical examination, there are several tests that are standard in all newly diagnosed patients (Box 4-5).

Liver function, renal function, complete blood count, syphilis serology, tuberculin skin test, lipid levels, and chest x-ray are all standard baseline tests. Routine anergy testing is no longer recommended because of the variability and poor predictive value, and because prophylaxis in anergic patients has been shown to prevent few cases of tuberculosis. If a patient's hepatitis B and C status are unknown, these should be checked. As mentioned above, all women should have a Pap smear and chlamydia test. Finally a CD4+ lymphocyte count and a quantitative HIV RNA (viral load) should be obtained. These tests are complementary and both need to be done. The former test reflects the degree of immune system impairment. It is used to determine the need for antiretroviral therapy, to establish the risk of specific HIV-associated complications, to guide the need for prophylaxis for opportunistic infections, and to some extent to evaluate the response to antiretroviral therapy. The latter test is used to assess prognosis, to determine the need for and the type of antiretroviral therapy, and to determine the response to therapy. Some experts recommend baseline serology for toxoplasma and CMV but this is controversial, since it is not clear that the information will be acted on. Although most patients do not lie about having a positive HIV test, there have been occasional patients who have. Therefore, if the specific laboratory results of the HIV test are unavailable and the viral load is undetectable, the HIV test result should be confirmed. A patient should not get antiretroviral therapy unless HIV infection has been formally documented.

Indicated Immunizations

Susceptible patients should be immunized for hepatitis B. All patients should receive the pneumococcal vaccine and an annual influenza immunization each fall. A tetanus/diphtheria booster should also be given if it has been 10 years since the last one. Some experts also recommend the *Haemophilus influenzae* B vaccine. The hepatitis A vaccine should be given to

---

BOX 4-4
Physical Examination

GENERAL
Nutritional status
Vital signs

SKIN
Kaposi's sarcoma
Bacillary angiomatosis
Seborrhea
Petechiae

OROPHARYNX
Thrush
Hairy leukoplakia
Kaposi's sarcoma
Periodontal and dental status
Ulcerations

EYES
Conjunctiva
Sclera
Fundus

LYMPH NODES

RESPIRATORY

CARDIOVASCULAR

BREAST

ABDOMEN
Liver and/or spleen enlargement

GENITAL
Ulcerations
Warts

NEUROLOGIC
Mental status
Neuropathy
Myopathy

BOX 4-5
Initial Laboratory Testing

Complete blood count with differential
Liver function testing
Serum creatinine and urinalysis
Hepatitis B and C testing
Serology for syphilis
Serum lipid levels
Pap smear and chlamydia probe of cervix
Intradermal tuberculin skin testing
CD4+ cell count
Viral load

---

carriers of hepatitis B and/or C. Most adults do not need the live virus vaccines (measles, mumps, rubella, yellow fever, oral polio, and varicella). Their administration is controversial in all immunosuppressed persons and should be individualized in HIV-positive persons, taking into consideration the exposure risk and the degree of immunosuppression.

Antiretroviral Therapy and Opportunistic Infection Prophylaxis

Antiretroviral therapy recommendations depend on the CD4 lymphocyte count, viral load, and specifics of the patient such as other medications and the ability to adhere to a complex regimen. In general, antiretroviral therapy should be initiated in all patients with signs or symptoms of opportunistic infections and in all patients with CD4+ T cell counts <350 cells/mm^3 with any plasma viral load, or counts >500 cells/mm^3 and a plasma viral load of greater than 20,000 copies HIV-1 RNA/ml (as determined by reverse transcriptase polymerase chain reaction [RT-PCR], or >10,000 copies/ml by branched DNA [bDNA]).

See Chapter 5 for a more complete a discussion about antiretroviral therapy. A general discussion should include a number of concepts. From the outset it is important to emphasize that there are now effective medications to treat HIV. It is the expectation that most patients will have their virus, and therefore their infection, controlled. All regimens utilize at least two and often three or more drugs and may not be easy to adhere to. However, it is very important that the patient do his or her utmost to take the medications as prescribed or these drugs might permanently lose their activity against the virus. Less than 95% adherence to the regimen has been associated with increased treatment failure rates. It should be made very clear to the patient that the physician and the pharmacist are willing to work closely with the patient to facilitate good adherence. Potential side effects for each prescribed medication, as well as plans for dealing with these side effects, should be reviewed.

Possible Referrals

Many patients do not need referrals to specialists at the time of the initial evaluation. Specific referrals depend on an individual patient's problems and CD4+ cell count. General considerations should be given to consultation with a social worker, mental health worker, nutritionist, dentist, and ophthalmologist, as well as an obstetrician if pregnant.

Educational Discussions

In addition to the medical aspects of the encounter, there is a great deal of HIV information that should be reviewed with a newly diagnosed patient. HIV infection has been around long enough that most persons have some concepts about this problem. Although often well meaning, that information has not always come from reliable sources. The physician should assume that it has not. Patients should be cautioned about future information. There is a lot of lay and professional material to which a patient has access. Newspapers, websites, friends, and family will often provide the patient with promises of a miracle treatment or other HIV-related revelations. The health care provider should pledge to be available to discuss such information in a nonjudgmental way.

Prognosis

Many people are unaware of the improvements in prognosis for HIV-infected persons. Although there is no cure, most people should expect to have their disease well controlled and should be able to function normally. It would be a mistake to not plan for the future. Patients should not make any major life decisions immediately after learning of their HIV infection because they are anticipating a "death sentence." This is also the time to start educating a patient about the meaning of CD4+ lymphocyte counts and viral loads, with particular attention to the normal fluctuations in these values. It is also important to emphasize that patients with HIV infection can and do get common medical problems. Every loose stool or cough does not reflect the start of an HIV-related illness. Patients should be assured that if their symptoms are too severe or last too long, they will be thoroughly evaluated, and that otherwise, they will be treated like any other (i.e., non–HIV-infected) patient. It should be emphasized to patients with CD4+ lymphocyte counts >500 cells/mm^3 that their immune systems are essentially normal and that they will not get any serious HIV-related problems as long as the counts remain in that range or higher. Most patients with counts between 200 and 500 cells/mm^3 also are asymptomatic, although there is an increased incidence of a number of problems, including herpes zoster, immune thrombocytopenia, HIV nephropathy, tuberculosis, lymphoma, recurrent bacterial pneumonias, sinusitis, and Kaposi's sarcoma. Most opportunistic infections do not occur unless the CD4+ lymphocyte count falls below 200 cells/mm^3, and it is rare to see CMV, disseminated *Mycobacterium avium,* cryptococcal meningitis, primary central nervous system (CNS) lymphoma, or cerebral toxoplasmosis with counts above 100 cells/mm^3.

Modes of HIV Transmission

The physician should review with patients how HIV can and cannot be transmitted. HIV may be transmitted via sex, sharing of needles, and contaminated blood products, and from an infected pregnant woman to her fetus. HIV is not transmitted by working or living with someone, by sharing food or utensils, or by nonsexual close contact. Therefore, other than the above cautions, persons infected with HIV should be allowed and encouraged to live and work normally.

Whom to Tell

Being infected with HIV is a heavy burden for most people to carry on their own. HIV-infected people should be advised to share this information with at least one person in whom they can confide. It is often helpful to offer to meet with the patient and important people in his or her life to answer all questions, so that everybody is up-to-date with the facts about HIV. Any persons who might have been infected by sexual contact or needle sharing with the patient should be notified. This can be an awkward situation for the patient. The health care provider should remind the patient that if one or more of the patient's contacts is unknowingly HIV positive, they are not getting the medical care that could save their life, and they may possibly transmit the virus to other persons. It should be explained to the patient that there is no real way to confirm if the HIV-infected patient is fully disclosing all contacts, but that he or she has a moral obligation to do so. If the patient is uncomfortable notifying contacts, the health care provider can do it anonymously.

Whom Not to Tell

Although things have improved remarkably in the past decade, there continues to be some uneasiness and frank discrimination toward HIV-infected persons. Since this infection is not transmitted by "casual" contact, there is no need to tell most people. In particular one should be careful about coworkers and employers. Although one cannot be fired for being HIV positive, there is the risk of having a very uncomfortable work environment.

Primer on CD4+ Cell Counts and Viral Load Measurements

Patients should have some understanding of the meaning of CD4+ cell counts and viral load measurements and how they are used to help determine the best treatment. The patient should be made aware of the range of variability of the test results so that he or she does not misunderstand the lack of significance of small changes (see the section on Monitoring the Immune System).

Critical Importance of Adherence to the Regimen

Many of the antiretroviral and prophylaxis regimens are complicated. Patients often are asked to take many pills and pay particular attention to meals. The medications have side effects. All of these things make adherence very difficult. Nonetheless, careful adherence is very important in the delay or prevention of the development of viral resistance. Patients need to understand that health care providers recognize how much they are asking of them; they also need to understand why the health care providers are asking it.

Support Systems

The health care provider should inquire about the possible support systems of the patient. Are there friends and/or family that are available and understanding? If there are physical needs such as housing, hospital beds, or transportation issues, then a social worker should be involved. Support groups are potentially helpful for some patients. They offer an opportunity to share concerns, fears, and triumphs with other persons dealing with HIV. Friends offer a less public form of support and some patients are more comfortable with this opportunity. These options should be discussed with the newly diagnosed patient.

Economic Concerns

Many patients are aware of how expensive antiretroviral medications are. A discussion of how the patient is to pay for medications is required. If there will be difficulties, a social worker should be consulted. For patients who do not have insurance coverage of medications, excellent treatment can often be arranged by enrolling them in a study. Specific work/income-related issues should also be reviewed with the patient.

Lifestyle Issues

In addition to taking medications, a patient can do a number of other things that might be beneficial for the immune system and for coping with infection. The patient should be encouraged to (1) stop smoking and be provided with the necessary support medications, (2) be very modest in alcohol intake, (3) stop the use of illicit drugs, and (4) get regular aerobic exercise. There are some data showing that exercise may benefit the immune system, and it improves the psychological state of many persons. Although there has been some concern in the past about pets, the only significant risk is with reptiles, which should be discouraged to prevent the acquisition of salmonella. Cats carry toxoplasmosis, but this does not seem to present a greatly increased risk for HIV-positive people; however, a person with HIV should not handle a litter box. Good nutrition and adequate sleep should be encouraged.

Complementary Therapies

Many patients partake of complementary medications and therapies. It is important to initiate the discussion about these options; otherwise the patient may believe that the physician is uncomfortable with this topic. The patient is likely to get advice to try such treatments and may wish to do so. The physician should discuss the following issues:

1. If these treatments were proven to work, they would be prescribed.
2. Whatever the patient chooses to do, the physician can and should give advice, but not be judgmental.
3. If the suggested treatments are expensive or potentially dangerous, the patient should be warned.
4. It is critical to know every medication that a patient is taking so that drug interactions can be avoided and potential side effects properly handled.

Sex

Although initially sex may not seem to be an important issue to a newly diagnosed patient, it is often useful to briefly mention to him or her that there will probably be a time when sex will again play an important role in the patient's life. An early mention of the topic by the health care provider may make the patient more comfortable with bringing it up in the future, and may add some reassurance that life will return to "normal." When a patient is ready, a very thorough discussion of sexual activity is crucial. It is not nearly enough to mention "safer sex" and "condoms." The specifics of safer sex need to be explicitly defined and the proper use of a condom needs to be described.

Needles

The topic of needles needs to be explicitly reviewed with the patient who is a needle user. Obviously, needle use should be discouraged, but it is also important to review methods for obtaining clean needles and for cleaning needles and syringes with bleach, and to discourage the sharing of needles or syringes.

Monitoring the Immune System

T lymphocytes can be separated into helper cells (CD4+) and suppressor or cytotoxic cells (CD8+). HIV infects and destroys the former. CD4+ cells decrease precipitously from a normal value of 800 to 1,000 cells/mm^3 during acute HIV infection, then generally rise over several weeks. The mean value at 1 year after infection is a little below 700 cells/mm^3. In most untreated patients these values progressively decrease at an average rate of about 50 cells/mm^3 per year. This represents a very high turnover rate, since about 10^9 CD4+ cells are destroyed and replaced daily. Patients and some physicians often develop a tendency to place too much emphasis on fluctuations in the CD4+ lymphocyte count. It is important to make sure that the patient is aware of these expected fluctuations so as not to be subjected to an unnecessary emotional roller coaster as the counts vary. The physician should emphasize that one looks for trends over many months to a year, not shorter-term fluctuations. A number of factors influence this variability. Of particular importance is the fact that the value is calculated as the product of three variables. The absolute CD4+ cell count is determined by multiplying the white blood cell count by the percentage of lymphocytes, and then by the percentage of CD4+ cells. As examples, in counts with a true value of 500 cells/mm^3, the 95% confidence range is between 300 and 850 cells/mm^3, while for counts that are truly 200 cells/mm^3, the 95% confidence range is 120 to 340 cells/mm^3! The CD4+ cell percentage is sometimes used instead of the absolute count since this is only a product of two variables and has a smaller standard deviation. Most laboratories report both values and they should be interpreted together. Corresponding values for the absolute count and the percent for the above examples are 500 cells/mm^3 (29%) and 200 cells/mm^3 (14%). HIV RNA quantitation (viral load) measurements should be routinely used in the management of infected persons. Viral load values are an independent predictor of time to progression to acquired immunodeficiency syndrome (AIDS) and death. They are used to help determine when to initiate antiretroviral therapy and to monitor the effect of the therapy. There are two widely available assays. The RT-PCR assay amplifies the substrate, while the bDNA assay amplifies the signal. Both assays measure HIV RNA in plasma. Ethylenediaminetetraacetic acid (EDTA) (purple top) collection tubes should be used to collect the blood specimen. Heparinized tubes and serum are unacceptable. Either test can be used, although it is generally a good idea to stick with one type of test in a patient, since the concentration of HIV RNA obtained with the RT-PCR is typically twofold higher than that measured by the bDNA. Both tests now have ultrasensitive assays that can detect down to about 50 copies/ml. Viral loads are the highest during acute infection, ranging to 10^6 copies/ml or more. Asymptomatic patients typically have levels between <50 and 10^5 copies/ml. Viral loads often transiently rise during intercurrent illnesses or after immunizations. Therefore HIV RNA values should not be determined within 1 month of such occurrences. As with the CD4+ counts, there is a great deal of variability in viral loads. A significant change is a change of at least 0.5 log.

Whereas CD4+ cell counts are primarily used to determine the status of a patient's immune system, viral load determinations are used to assess the adequacy of antiretroviral therapy. If the viral load does not decrease to <50 copies/ml by 4 to 6 months of therapy, consideration should be given to modifying the regimen. There may be a temptation to stop antiretroviral therapy in patients who have had undetectable viral loads for years. However, such patients have a reservoir of latently infected cells, and discontinuation of treatment will likely result in finding the viral RNA in the plasma in a matter of weeks. There are ongoing studies to determine if some form of intermittent treatment in such patients, termed "strategic treatment interruptions," might be of benefit, but this is not a standard approach at this time.

Frequency of Follow-Up Visits

Although the frequency of follow-up visits should be individualized, initially it is a good idea to see a new patient frequently. This gives the health care worker an opportunity to review much of the educational information, and the patient an opportunity to ask questions. It can also reinforce the need for compulsive adherence to the antiretroviral regimen. After the initial visit, the patient should be seen in 1 to 2 weeks. If all is going reasonably well, the next visit should be scheduled when the patient has been on antiretroviral therapy for about 1 month. At that time the viral load should be checked, with the expectation of at least a 0.5 to 0.7 log decrease. Failure to see such a decrease suggests that the patient is not taking the medication appropriately, there is a problem with absorption of the medication, or the patient's virus was resistant to one or more agents in the initial combination. Whatever the cause, it is a poor prognostic sign. Once a patient has settled into a stable regimen, visits can be gradually decreased to every 3 months.

The initial management of an HIV-positive patient is a time to assess the status of the immune system and get the viral replication under control with medications. It is also the first and often the best opportunity to establish a therapeutic lasting relationship with a patient and the family. A great deal of thoroughness and care at the beginning can mean the difference between successful control of HIV infection and a much more difficult clinical course.

SUGGESTED READINGS

Bartlett JG, Gallant J: *Medical management of HIV infection*, Baltimore, 2000, Johns Hopkins University.

Carpenter CCJ: Antiretroviral therapy in adults: updated recommendations of the International AIDS Society–USA panel, *JAMA* 283:381-390, 2000.

Ong KR, Iftikhar S, Glatt A: Medical management of the adult with HIV infection, *Infect Dis Clin North Am* 8:289-301, 1994.

5 Antiretroviral Therapy

IAN FRANK, AMY L. GRAZIANI

Introduction

Within the last 5 years, the development of new antiretroviral agents, a better understanding of their optimal use, and the use of plasma viral load monitoring have led to a dramatic decline in the number of individuals dying of human immunodeficiency virus (HIV) infection and experiencing opportunistic infections. Optimism that grew from these advancements and the description of the in vivo kinetics of HIV replication led to the hypothesis that HIV infection could potentially be cured if a patient were treated aggressively enough for a long enough period of time. Antiretroviral therapy was begun as early as possible following HIV diagnosis in order to "hit hard, hit early." However, a population of latently infected cells has been identified that can harbor HIV for years, if not decades, and it appears that currently available therapy cannot cure HIV infection. Studies of treatment-naive patients cared for in clinical practice have shown that only half of patients started on antiretroviral therapy are able to adhere to their medications at a level that is sufficient to maintain therapeutic success. Failure to maximally inhibit HIV replication leads to drug resistance, and because the available drugs are restricted to three therapeutic classes, cross-resistance among drugs within a class is common. Therefore, despite the proliferation of new anti-HIV drugs, the number of effective combinations that can be offered to a patient decreases each time a patient fails on a combination and develops resistant virus. Furthermore, a complicated array of drug toxicities is being recognized that may limit the ability of patients to continue on life-long therapy, if that is necessary to forestall damage to the immune system. For these reasons, treatment strategies for HIV-infected patients continue to evolve rapidly. This chapter will outline the current issues and therapeutic approaches.

When to Start Antiretroviral Therapy

The goals of antiretroviral therapy are to suppress HIV replication as much as possible; augment or preserve immunologic function; prevent the opportunistic infections, malignancies, and other morbidities associated with HIV infection; prolong survival; and improve the quality of life. In general, the decision to start therapy is based on the presence of symptoms, the risk for opportunistic infections and disease progression as predicted by CD4+ T cell counts and plasma viral load, and the patient's willingness to adhere to the complexities of pill taking required for success. However, special circumstances may influence the decision to start treatment. Two groups of expert panelists have established guidelines for the use of antiretroviral therapy that are listed in the reference section at the end of this chapter.

Acute HIV Infection

Approximately 70% of individuals recently infected with HIV will develop an acute illness characterized by a mononucleosis syndrome featuring fever, adenopathy, and pharyngitis; a skin rash; and neurologic signs or symptoms. The illness is nonspecific, and therefore many patients with acute HIV infection do not seek medical attention or are not suspected of having HIV infection. Recent studies of newly infected individuals have shown that patients treated within months of their clinical presentation with acute HIV infection are able to preserve their HIV-specific T helper immune responses. HIV-specific T helper responses are lost in patients once infection is established, and do not improve when patients with established infection are started on therapy. Studies of treatment interruption in patients treated shortly after their acute infection suggest that therapy may be stopped in some individuals, with persistence of viral loads at low levels not warranting therapy. Therefore it is recommended that patients with acute HIV infection be started on therapy as soon as possible following diagnosis.

Symptomatic HIV

Patients with HIV-associated opportunistic infections or signs or symptoms, including oral candidiasis, wasting, unexplained fever, or persistent diarrhea, should be urged to begin antiretroviral therapy, even if their CD4+ T cell counts are high. These individuals have already begun to experience some degree of morbidity associated with their disease. Antiretroviral therapy has been shown to provide clinical benefit to symptomatic individuals.

Asymptomatic Infection: Low CD4+ Cell Counts, High Plasma Viral Loads

For an asymptomatic patient, the exigency for starting antiretroviral therapy is based on the patient's current risk for an opportunistic infection, as suggested by his or her CD4+ T cell count, and the risk for progression to symptomatic disease, as suggested by the plasma viral load. Weighing against the potential immunologic benefits of therapy is the difficulty many patients have with adhering to pill taking, the tolerability of the medications, and potential long-term toxicities. In general, the lower the CD4+ T cell count and the higher the plasma viral load, the stronger the recommendation to start therapy.

Current guidelines suggest initiating antiretroviral therapy in asymptomatic patients based on epidemiologic data that predict the probability of an individual developing an acquired immunodeficiency syndrome (AIDS)-defining clinical condition within 3 years. Patients with CD4+ T cell counts <350 cells/mm^3 with any plasma viral load, or counts >500 cells/mm^3 and a plasma viral load of greater than 20,000 copies HIV-1 RNA/ml (as determined by reverse transcriptase polymerase chain reaction [RT-PCR], or >10,000 copies/ml by branched DNA [bDNA]) have about a 10% or greater risk of developing AIDS within 3 years, and therapy is recommended for these individuals. Patients with CD4+ T cell counts of 350 to 500 cells/mm^3 are recommended therapy by most experts, although some would defer therapy for patients whose plasma viral loads were <20,000 copies HIV-1 RNA/ml (as determined by RT-PCR, or >10,000 copies/ml by bDNA). Many expert HIV health care providers defer therapy for patients with CD4+ T cell counts >500 cells/mm^3 and plasma viral loads <20,000 copies HIV-1 RNA/ml (as determined by RT-PCR, or >10,000 copies/ml by bDNA), although some would treat these patients.

Pregnant Women

HIV-infected pregnant women in developed countries have an approximate 25% to 30% risk of transmitting their infection to their newborns if they go untreated during pregnancy. Studies of single drugs and combinations of drugs demonstrate dramatic decreases in the risk for vertical transmission to <2% when mothers receive antiretroviral therapy during pregnancy and delivery and their newborns receive therapy for a short period of time. The risk of transmission is directly related to the mother's plasma viral load at the time of delivery. Therefore all pregnant women should be offered therapy, irrespective of CD4+ T cell count, with the goal of decreasing the mother's viral load as much as possible prior to delivery.

Once the decision to initiate therapy has been made, patients need to be educated on the importance of adherence. Some studies have shown that the rates of achieving and maintaining a viral load below quantifiable levels decline rapidly if patients take less than 90% of the prescribed doses, and that optimal outcomes are most likely if patients take 95% or more of their doses. For that reason, patients who are reluctant to start therapy or those with active drug or alcohol use may benefit from a greater understanding of the importance of antiretroviral therapy or attention to psychosocial factors that may be impediments to adherence prior to the initiation of therapy.

Therapeutic Strategies for Antiretroviral-Naive Patients

Irrespective of when the decision was made to initiate therapy, the antiretroviral combination selected must be sufficiently potent to reduce the plasma viral load below quantifiable levels on the more sensitive assays that are commercially available (50 copies HIV-1 RNA/ml sensitivity). Failure to achieve a viral load below this threshold will usually result in a rebound in the viral load coincident with the selection of virus that is resistant to one, several, or all of the drugs used in the combination. The relatively poor success rate of second drug combinations in patients who have had a viral load rebound on their initial combination suggests that the initial regimen is the most likely to produce durable suppression of HIV replication. There is little data demonstrating the superiority of one potent antiretroviral combination over another, and virtually no data exist describing the most effective way to sequence drugs such that the maximum benefit is achieved from each combination used. Therefore the selection of a combination should be based on the potency of the combination in relationship to the patient's viral load, the ease of pill taking, the risk for adverse events, and alternative treatment options in the event that resistance develops to the initial combination. Each potential strategy and the use of specific agents have advantages and disadvantages. Tables 5-1, 5-2, and 5-3 list the individual drugs among the nucleoside reverse transcriptase inhibitors (NRTI), the non-nucleoside reverse transcriptase inhibitors (NNRTI), and the protease inhibitors (PI), as well as their dose, food effects on drug concentrations, and frequently associated adverse events.

The Food and Drug Administration (FDA)-approved NRTIs include zidovudine, didanosine, zalcitabine, stavudine, lamivudine, and abacavir. Most three- and four-drug antiretroviral combinations employ dual NRTIs. Preferred combinations of NRTIs (not listed in order of preference) include zidovudine plus didanosine, zalcitabine, or lamivudine; and stavudine plus didanosine or lamivudine. Abacavir, the most recently approved drug in this class, has been studied most widely in combinations of three NRTIs, typically used together with zidovudine and lamivudine. However, its potency and resistance profile suggest that in the future it will also be used as one of the two NRTIs in a three-drug combination that includes an NNRTI or PI. NRTI combinations that should be avoided included zidovudine plus stavudine because of their in vivo antagonism, zalcitabine plus didanosine or stavudine because of concerns for additive toxicities, and zalcitabine plus lamivudine due to the lack of clinical information with this combination.

Protease Inhibitor and Nucleoside Reverse Transcriptase Inhibitor Combinations

The FDA-approved PIs include saquinavir, ritonavir, indinavir, nelfinavir, amprenavir, and a lopinavir/ritonavir fixed-dose combination. Combinations of two NRTIs plus one PI have been shown to prevent the clinical progression of HIV infection, and the longest experience with sustained suppression of HIV replication has been with this strategic approach. In addition, the genetic barrier to resistance observed with some PIs results in the potential preservation of activity of the drugs in this class, even in the event of virologic failure on a PI-inclusive combination. The disadvantages of the PIs include a high rate of gastrointestinal adverse events, the need to coordinate pill taking and meals, the number of pills required, and the strong association with a group of metabolic and morphologic complications that will be described below.

Ritonavir has been shown to potentiate the activity of other PIs when used in PI-PI combinations because it inhibits the isoforms of cytochrome P450 responsible for metabolizing the PIs. Combinations of ritonavir with saquinavir, amprenavir, indinavir, and lopinavir (in a fixed-dose capsule) have

TABLE 5-1
Characteristics of Nucleoside Reverse Transcriptase Inhibitors

	Zidovudine (AZT, ZDV, Retrovir)	Didanosine (ddI, Videx, Videx EC)	Zalcitabine (ddC, HIVID)	Stavudine (d4T, Zerit)	Lamivudine (3TC, Epivir)	Abacavir (ABC, Ziagen)
Form	Capsules: 100 mg Tablets: 300 mg Solution: 10 mg/ml IV or po	Tablets: 25, 50, 100, 150, 200 mg Extended release capsules: 250, 400 mg Sachets: 167, 250 mg Oral pediatric suspension: 10 mg/ml	Tablets: 0.375, 0.75 mg Syrup: 0.1 mg/ml (investigational)	Capsules: 15, 20, 30, 40 mg Oral solution: 1 mg/ml	Tablets: 150 mg Oral solution: 10 mg/ml	Tablets: 300 mg Oral solution: 20 mg/ml
Pediatric dosing*	160 mg per m^2 q8h	90-150 mg per m^2 q12h	0.01 mg/kg q8h	1 mg/kg q12h, up to 30 kg	4 mg/kg bid	8 mg/kg bid, up to 300 mg bid
Adult dosing	300 mg bid, or 200 mg tid, or with 3TC as Combivir 1 bid, or with 3TC + ABC as Trizivir 1 bid	Extended release capsules: 400 mg qd if >60 kg 250 mg qd if <60 kg Tablets†: 200 mg, 2 qd, or 100 mg, 2 bid if >60 kg; 200 mg + 50 mg qd, or 100 mg + 25 mg bid if <60 kg	0.75 mg tid	40 mg bid if >60 kg 30 mg bid if <60 kg	150 mg bid, or with ZDV as Combivir 1 bid, or with ZDV + ABC as Trizivir 1 bid	300 mg bid, or with ZDV + 3TC as Trizivir 1 bid
Food effect	May be taken with or without food	Take 1 hr before meals or 2 hr after meals Separate from indinavir by 1 hr if using tablet form only	May be taken with or without food	May be taken with or without food	May be taken with or without food	May be taken with or without food Alcohol increases absorption by 41%
Adverse events	Anemia, neutropenia Headache, nausea, vomiting Lactic acidosis	Nausea, diarrhea Peripheral neuropathy Pancreatitis Increase amylase Lactic acidosis	Peripheral neuropathy Stomatitis Lactic acidosis	Peripheral neuropathy Increase LFTs Lactic acidosis	Well tolerated Lactic acidosis	Hypersensitivity reaction Nausea, vomiting Lactic acidosis

*These are the doses recommended for infants >90 days of age and children. For neonatal doses consult the Pediatric Guidelines listed in the Suggested Readings.
†If didanosine is administered in the tablet form, two tablets must be given at each dose administration to provide sufficient buffer to neutralize gastric pH.
LFT, Liver function tests.

TABLE 5-2
Characteristics of Non-Nucleoside Reverse Transcriptase Inhibitors

	Nevirapine (Viramune)	Delavirdine (Rescriptor)	Efavirenz (Sustiva)
Form	Tablets: 200 mg Oral suspension: 50 mg/5 ml	Tablets: 100, 200 mg	Capsules: 50, 100, 200 mg
Pediatric dosing*	120 mg per m² qd × 14 days, then 120 to 200 mg per m² q12h	Unknown	10 to <15 kg: 200 mg qd 15 to <20 kg: 250 mg qd 20 to <25 kg: 300 mg qd 25 to <32.5 kg: 350 mg qd 32.5 to <40 kg: 400 mg qd >40 kg: 600 mg qd
Adult dosing	200 mg qd × 14 days, then 200 mg bid	600 mg bid, or 400 mg tid May mix tablets in >3 oz water to produce slurry	600 mg qd Preferred administration at bedtime May divide dose 200 mg AM & 400 mg PM to improve tolerance
Food effect	May be taken with or without food	May be taken with or without food	May be taken with or without food, but avoid taking near high-fat meal, which increases absorption by 30%-50%
Adverse events	Rash Increased hepatic transaminases Hepatitis	Rash Increased hepatic transaminases Headache	Rash CNS symptoms: dizziness, confusion, trouble concentrating, depersonalization, abnormal dreaming, insomnia, somnolence Teratogenic in monkeys—avoid in pregnancy

*These are the doses recommended for infants >90 days of age and children. For neonatal doses consult the Pediatric Guidelines listed in the Suggested Readings.

proven to be potent, may allow for a reduction in the number of pills required and the number of daily doses, and eliminate the requirement to take indinavir on an empty stomach. PI-PI combinations have not been studied extensively in treatment-naive patients, but the pharmacokinetic and adherence advantages are certain.

Nelfinavir and amprenavir may have an advantage over the other PIs for treatment-naive patients because data suggest that virus resistant to nelfinavir and amprenavir is inhibited by other drugs in this class. Currently, indinavir is less often used as the sole PI in a combination because it must be given three times a day on an empty stomach. In combinations with ritonavir, it can be prescribed twice a day and can be taken with food. Saquinavir hard-gel should not be prescribed except in combinations with ritonavir because it has poor bioavailability. Saquinavir soft-gel and amprenavir are less often used as the initial PI because of pill burden.

Non-nucleoside Reverse Transcriptase Inhibitor and Nucleoside Reverse Transcriptase Inhibitor Combinations

There are three available NNRTIs: nevirapine, delavirdine, and efavirenz. Studies of efavirenz have shown similar, or superior, potency and equivalent increases in CD4+ T cell counts when used together with two NRTIs compared with indinavir plus two NRTIs. Based on these data, one of the published sets of HIV treatment guidelines includes efavirenz, but not the other NNRTIs, as a strongly recommended agent to be used in combinations as part of initial therapy. As a class, the NNRTIs have fewer dose-limiting adverse events compared with the PIs, have fewer limitations with respect to the need to take the drugs with or without food, and require fewer pills taken at a greater dosing interval. For these reasons, many practitioners favor starting therapy with NNRTIs in PI-sparing combinations. However, rapid resistance to NNRTIs is seen in patients experiencing virologic failure, and cross-resistance among all NNRTIs may lead to only a single opportunity to use any drug in this class. For this reason, some experts prefer to reserve the NNRTIs for use in patients who fail on an initial PI-inclusive combination.

Three–Nucleoside Reverse Transcriptase Inhibitor Combinations

Initial therapy employing a three-NRTI combination has been studied in a limited number of trials, most often with a focus on the combination of zidovudine, lamivudine, and abacavir. This combination has been shown to be convenient and well tolerated. However, the durability of the virologic response is not as well proved as other strategic approaches, and it is not as potent as other combinations in patients with pretreatment viral loads greater than 100,000 copies HIV-1 RNA/ml. The conse-

TABLE 5-3
Characteristics of Protease Inhibitors

	Saquinavir (Invirase, Fortovase)	Ritonavir (Norvir)	Indinavir (Crixivan)	Nelfinavir (Viracept)	Amprenavir (Agenerase)	Lopinavir/Ritonavir (Kaletra)
Form	Capsules: 200 mg in each variety	Capsules: 100 mg Oral solution: 600 mg/7.5 ml	Capsules: 200, 333, 400 mg	Tablets: 250 mg Oral powder: 50 mg/g	Capsules: 50, 150 mg Oral solution: 15 mg/ml	Capsules: 133/33 mg Oral solution: 400/100 mg/5 ml
Pediatric dosing*	Unknown	350 to 400 mg per m² q12h	500 mg per m² q8h	30 mg/kg tid	22.5 mg/kg bid oral solution, or 20 mg/kg bid capsules	7 to <15 kg: 12 mg/kg bid 15 to 40 kg: 10 mg/kg bid >40 kg: adult dose
Adult dosing	Fortovase 1,200 mg tid, or Fortovase 1,600 mg bid (lower trough concentrations and AUC than 1,200 bid, though clinical significance is not known), or Fortovase or Invirase 400 mg bid + ritonavir 400 mg bid	600 mg bid	800 mg q8h, or 400 mg bid + ritonavir 200 mg or 100 mg bid 1,000 mg q8h if given with efavirenz or nevirapine	1,250 mg bid	1,200 mg bid, or 600 mg bid + ritonavir 200 mg or 100 mg bid	400/100 mg bid 533/133 mg bid if given with efavirenz or nevirapine
Food effect	Take following meals No food effects if taken with ritonavir	Take with food	Take 1 hr before or 2 hr after meal Can be taken with food if administered with ritonavir	Take with food	Take with or without food, but avoid high-fat meal	Take with food
Adverse events	Nausea, vomiting, diarrhea Headache Increased transaminases Hyperlipidemia	Nausea, vomiting, diarrhea, taste perversion Oral paresthesia Increased transaminases Hyperlipidemia Increased CK Increased uric acid	Nausea, vomiting Nephrolithiasis Increased indirect bilirubin Hyperlipidemia	Diarrhea Nausea, vomiting Hyperlipidemia	Nausea, vomiting, diarrhea Oral paresthesia Increased transaminases Hyperlipidemia Rash	Nausea, vomiting, diarrhea Increased transaminases Hyperlipidemia

*These are the doses recommended for infants >90 days of age and children. For neonatal doses consult the Pediatric Guidelines listed in the Suggested Readings.
AUC, Area under the curve.

quences of resistance to a three-NRTI combination with respect to the subsequent activity of the remaining NRTIs are unknown.

Selecting the Initial Combination

Other circumstances may influence the selection of the initial combination. Therapeutic success rates are lower in patients starting therapy with CD4+ T cell counts less than 50 cells/mm^3 or plasma viral loads greater than 100,000 copies HIV-1 RNA/ml. PI-PI combinations or other four-drug treatment strategies should be considered in these circumstances. Patients with HIV-related peripheral neuropathy may experience a worsening of symptoms on stavudine, didanosine, or zalcitabine. Bone marrow suppression due to zidovudine may exacerbate preexisting anemia. Patients with chronic hepatitis B or C infections are more likely to experience hepatotoxicity if prescribed a PI, and nevirapine should be used with caution in patients with underlying liver disease. Patients on methadone may experience withdrawal symptoms when started on a PI or NNRTI because of drug-drug interactions (see the section on Drug-Drug Interactions). Patients requiring a rifamycin for treatment of tuberculosis should not, in general, receive rifampin together with a PI. Most of the PIs can increase rifabutin concentrations to toxic levels, and rifabutin, conversely, can lower serum concentrations of PIs to ineffective levels. Rifabutin used at reduced doses is a therapeutic alternative for patients with active tuberculosis requiring a PI.

After an antiretroviral combination has been selected for a patient, written instructions should be provided listing medications, how many pills should be taken at what dosing intervals or suggested times for pill taking, whether the medication should be taken with food or on an empty stomach, and common side effects that may be encountered. All medications should be started at the same time, rather than beginning drugs sequentially, because resistance to some agents can emerge within days or weeks when given as monotherapy or in subinhibitory combinations. For an analogous reason, patients should also be instructed to not stop one medication and continue on others, even in the event of an adverse experience, without notifying their provider. Therefore, if a patient must stop a medication because of an adverse experience, it is better to stop all drugs, rather than the single offending agent.

Monitoring Patients on Antiretroviral Therapy
Assess Adherence

Following the initiation of therapy, patients should be seen in follow-up within 2 to 4 weeks. This provides an opportunity to learn about any impediments to adherence, including early side effects, difficulty in remembering to take medication, trouble coordinating pill taking with meal times, and other obstacles. A repeat plasma viral load should also be obtained at this visit. For asymptomatic patients, seeing improvements in laboratory tests such as declines in viral loads or increases in CD4+ T cell counts may be the only or principal positive reinforcement of treatment.

Measure Plasma Viral Load Frequently

An early follow-up viral load also provides the clinician with an assessment of the initial response to therapy. Failure to observe a 0.5 to 0.7 log$_{10}$ copies HIV-1 RNA/ml decline in viral load after 4 weeks of treatment is indicative of a poor virologic response and suggests that the patient is not taking the medication appropriately, there is a problem with absorption of the medication, or the patient's virus was resistant to one or more agents in the initial combination.

Some experts suggest that patients have viral load monitoring at monthly intervals until the viral load falls below quantifiable levels in order to observe a leveling off of the viral load decline or an early increase in viral load, suggesting early treatment failure. Patients with higher pretreatment viral loads take longer to achieve a viral load below quantifiable levels, and it may take 24 weeks or longer for some patients' viral loads to become undetectable. Once a patient's viral load becomes undetectable, patients should have viral load and CD4+ T cell counts monitored at 3-month intervals.

Inquire About Adverse Events

Many side effects of medication (see the section on Adverse Events Associated with Antiretroviral Therapy) occur early after the initiation of medication. Patients should be informed of possible side effects prior to starting medication and have strategies in place to deal with them. A number of these early side effects resolve within several days to weeks while patients continue on medication, and patients should be encouraged to try to tolerate early side effects without an interruption in treatment.

Follow Laboratory Tests for Safety

Many HIV medications cause laboratory abnormalities including anemia, liver function abnormalities, increases in serum lipid concentrations, hyperamylasemia, and lactic acidosis. Some of these may occur early following the initiation of treatment, whereas others are seen more commonly after prolonged therapy. At a minimum, patients should have a complete blood count with differential, platelet count, and serum chemistries evaluated at the first follow-up visit to detect any idiosyncratic reactions, and similar monitoring at 3- to 6-month intervals thereafter.

Adverse Events Associated with Antiretroviral Therapy

Tables 5-1, 5-2, and 5-3 list the adverse events associated with the available antiretroviral drugs. Some adverse events are encountered with all drugs within a class of agents, whereas others are unique to specific drugs.

Gastrointestinal Side Effects

Gastrointestinal side effects, especially nausea and vomiting, may interfere with adherence. All of the PIs are associated with gastrointestinal side effects. Saquinavir, indinavir, amprenavir, and lopinavir/ritonavir cause nausea, vomiting, and dyspepsia. Ritonavir is rarely given as the only PI in a combination because few patients can tolerate it at its full dose due to nausea, vomiting, dyspepsia, and abdominal pain. Nelfinavir causes loose stools or diarrhea in the majority of patients, although this is usually easily controlled with over-the-counter antimotility agents. Diarrhea is associated with the other PIs to a lesser extent. Among the NRTIs, zidovudine and abacavir can cause nausea and vomiting early in the course of therapy that typically resolves with continued use. Didanosine in tablet form causes nausea, vomiting, dyspepsia, and diarrhea, although these adverse effects may be less frequent with a new enteric-coated capsule formulation.

Rash/Hypersensitivity Reactions

Rash is a common side effect with all of the NNRTIs. Patients begin on nevirapine at one-half the daily dose, and then increase to bid after 2 weeks of treatment to lessen the incidence of rash. Rash is less common with delavirdine and efavirenz than with nevirapine, and severe rash including Stevens-Johnson reaction is more common with nevirapine than the other two NNRTIs. Frequently NNRTI-induced rashes will resolve with continued therapy, so patients with rashes of mild or moderate severity should continue on medication under close observation. Patients who develop a rash on nevirapine that requires cessation of the drug may not develop a rash on rechallenge with efavirenz or delavirdine. Antihistamines and acetaminophen may improve some of the discomfort associated with drug rashes but will not prevent them. In addition, studies have shown that prophylactic therapy with corticosteroids is not effective in preventing rash, nor is it effective as interventional therapy when rash has occurred. Among the PIs, amprenavir and indinavir are most likely to cause rash.

Abacavir may cause a systemic hypersensitivity reaction in approximately 3% to 5% of recipients that most commonly occurs 1 to 3 weeks after starting the medication. Clinical features of this reaction include fever in approximately 80% of cases; rash in 70%; nausea or vomiting in 35%; malaise in 25%; and headache, fatigue, myalgias, pruritus, oral ulcers, and pulmonary symptoms in 5% to 20%. Symptoms continue to worsen if patients continue the medication, and fatalities have occurred if patients continue the medication or discontinue and restart. Patients receive a warning about the hypersensitivity reaction when filling a prescription for abacavir, and should be forewarned. Patients who experience the hypersensitivity reaction should be instructed to bring the unused portion of the medication to their provider for disposal, because some fatalities have occurred when patients have mistakenly taken another dose of the drug despite being told to throw away the remainder of the prescription.

Neurologic Adverse Effects

Peripheral sensory neuropathy is associated with the use of the dideoxynucleoside reverse transcriptase inhibitors didanosine, zalcitabine, and stavudine, and is manifest as a symmetrical numbness, tingling, or pain that begins in the feet and/or hands and progresses proximally. Signs consistent with peripheral neuropathy include decreased bone vibratory sensation and decreased or absent ankle jerk reflexes. Patients with more advanced disease are more likely to experience peripheral neuropathy than patients treated at early stages. If the offending agent(s) is stopped early, symptoms will improve or may resolve completely. Amitriptyline, nortriptyline, gabapentin, and lamotrigine have been used to control symptoms with varying success, and narcotic analgesia may be required in severe cases. Perioral paresthesia is associated with amprenavir and ritonavir use. Patients starting efavirenz should be informed that up to half of patients experience one or more central nervous system adverse events, including dizziness, confusion, concentration difficulty, drowsiness, insomnia, abnormal dreaming, or depersonalization. These symptoms usually occur after the first dose of the drug, but resolve over the following few days or weeks, and patients infrequently discontinue the drug due to these symptoms. Patients should take the drug near bedtime to minimize the effects, and should avoid eating a fatty meal in proximity to taking the drug, which increases efavirenz concentrations. Zidovudine, delavirdine, and efavirenz can cause headache.

Fat Redistribution and Metabolic Complications

A group of metabolic and morphologic abnormalities are being experienced by patients on antiretroviral drugs that may limit the ability of patients to continue on life-long therapy. Morphologic changes include a redistribution of body fat, with fat atrophy observed in the nasolabial folds and malar regions of the face, the extremities, and the buttocks. Prominent veins in the arms and legs are common. In addition to fat wasting, visceral fat accumulation occurs in the abdomen; women may experience breast enlargement; gynecomastia may occur in men; and fat deposits in the dorsocervical region (buffalo humps, similar to those seen with Cushing's disease), supraclavicular fossae, and lipomas can be observed. These cosmetically disfiguring changes can adversely affect patients' quality of life. However, these abnormalities are not restricted to purely physical effects. The majority of patients also experience hyperlipidemia with elevated triglycerides, total cholesterol, and low-density lipoprotein (LDL) cholesterol, and decreased high-density lipoprotein (HDL) cholesterol. Reports of coronary artery disease in patients have raised concerns that accelerated atherosclerosis may accompany these derangements and that increasing numbers of individuals with heart disease will be encountered in the future.

Lipodystrophy. Redistribution of body fat and hyperlipidemias are often lumped into a single syndrome termed "lipodystrophy," although many investigators favor a broader classification of these abnormalities. There is no definition of this syndrome, so prevalence of these abnormalities in cross-sectional studies varies widely. However, many experts believe that the majority of patients on potent antiviral combinations who maintain viral loads below quantifiable levels have some manifestation of these disorders.

The etiology or etiologies of this syndrome are unknown. It is not known whether these complications are a direct effect of specific drugs or are caused by a modification of metabolic consequences of HIV infection or its immunologic dysfunction. Fat redistribution and hyperlipidemias were originally observed in patients on combinations that included PIs. Elevated triglycerides and cholesterol levels have been observed with some PIs as single agents in phase I studies that included HIV-uninfected individuals. However, hyperlipidemia is also observed in patients on PI-sparing therapy, so no single drug or class of agents can be implicated as the cause of these changes. Patients on NNRTIs tend to have slight increases in HDL cholesterol on NNRTI-inclusive and PI-sparing combinations, whereas HDL cholesterol levels do not change or decrease in patients on PI-inclusive and NNRTI-sparing combinations, suggesting that there are biochemical differences between these two classes of agents. More recent data have suggested that the NRTIs may contribute to fat redistribution, with some studies suggesting that patients on stavudine may be more likely to experience fat wasting than patients on other NRTIs. This observation has yet to be confirmed in prospective trials. Risk factors for this syndrome that have been identified include increased age, duration of HIV infection, duration of time on therapy, and CD4+ T cell count nadir at the time therapy was begun.

Trials comparing different strategies to treat fat redistribution and hyperlipidemia are underway. Early results suggest that modification of the antiviral regimen does not greatly alter fat redistribution or lipid levels, although HDL cholesterol concentrations generally increase a small amount if patients are switched from a PI to an NNRTI or NRTI. Diet and exercise are not effective in modifying hyperlipidemia in these patients. Lipid-lowering agents including fibrates and HMG-coA reductase inhibitors are being studied to treat hyperlipidemia. Early results suggest that patients do not respond as completely to these agents as HIV-uninfected individuals. Atorvastatin is the preferred HMG-coA reductase inhibitor because it is least likely to have significant drug-drug interactions with the PIs.

Glucose Intolerance, Lactic Acidosis, and Osteopenia. Metabolic complications of therapy include insulin resistance in up to 30% of patients, with a small fraction manifesting type II diabetes mellitus; lactic acidosis, which has been fatal in some cases; and osteopenia. Data on insulin resistance should be viewed with caution because a high prevalence of impaired glucose tolerance was observed in a longitudinal study prior to starting therapy. Insulin resistance has been primarily associated with the use of PIs, although cases of insulin resistance and new-onset diabetes have been reported in patients on PI-sparing combinations. Thioglitazone derivatives and metformin are being studied as treatment for insulin resistance.

Lactic acidosis has been linked to all of the NRTIs, although it may be more common with stavudine than other drugs in the class, and is thought to be due to mitochondrial toxicity caused by the inhibition of mitochondrial gamma DNA polymerase. Patients may present with asymptomatic elevated blood lactate levels or with fatigue with or without nonspecific gastrointestinal symptoms including nausea, vomiting, and abdominal pain. Symptomatic patients with high serum lactate levels should have their antiretroviral therapy held, since deaths due to lactic acidosis have been reported. Most experts are not monitoring lactate levels in asymptomatic patients.

Osteopenia has recently been described in patients on PIs. The etiology of osteopenia is not known, and its consequences are also yet to be determined.

Laboratory Abnormalities

Antiretroviral agents can also cause laboratory abnormalities other than those described above. Zidovudine may cause anemia or neutropenia. Didanosine may cause hyperamylasemia. Abnormalities in hepatic transaminases can be seen in patients on stavudine, nevirapine, saquinavir, ritonavir, and amprenavir. Patients with underlying liver disease, especially hepatitis C infection, are more likely to experience worsening of liver function tests on these drugs. Indinavir causes an indirect hyperbilirubinemia that has no clinical consequence. Ritonavir and zidovudine can cause an increase in creatine kinase levels.

Other Adverse Events

Other common side effects not mentioned above include pancreatitis caused by didanosine. Patients on didanosine should be alerted to stop their medication if they develop severe abdominal pain or nausea, and patients with a history of pancreatitis or heavy alcohol consumption should be monitored carefully if prescribed didanosine. Indinavir can cause nephrolithiasis. For that reason, patients on indinavir should be advised to increase their fluid consumption, especially during hot weather or when exercising. Zidovudine may cause myopathy. Pregnant monkeys given efavirenz delivered offspring with defects of brain and spinal cord development. For that reason, efavirenz should not be given during pregnancy.

If a patient develops intolerance to a specific drug, an alternative agent, preferably within the same class of inhibitors, should be substituted. If a patient develops a side effect that requires interruption of therapy, all drugs should be temporarily held rather than just the drug thought to be causing the problem. Following resolution of the side effect, the combination can be resumed, with an appropriate modification made.

Defining Failure of Therapy
Virologic Failure

As described above, viral load monitoring is essential following the initiation of antiretroviral therapy in order to evaluate response. The probability that a patient will achieve a viral load that is below quantifiable levels is directly related to the rapidity of the viral load decline over the first several months of therapy. If a patient's viral load declines by less than 1.0 $\log_{10}$ copies/ml after 2 months of treatment, that patient is unlikely to achieve a viral load below quantifiable levels. Virologic failure can also be defined as failing to achieve a viral load below quantifiable levels after 4 to 6 months of therapy.

Patients who achieve a viral load below quantifiable levels and then have confirmed quantifiable viral loads are experiencing virologic failure. The exception to that rule is the low level (<1,000 copies HIV-1 RNA/ml) "blips" in viral load that some patients periodically experience. These viral load blips are transient and are not a sign of virologic failure. If the viral load reaches a nadir, and is repeatedly 0.5 $\log_{10}$ copies/ml (threefold) above the nadir, that patient likely has virologic failure. Patients should not be considered to have virologic failure if they have signs or symptoms of an intercurrent illness or have had a recent vaccination, factors that can be associated with a transient increase in viral load.

Immunologic Failure

Patients occasionally experience persistent declines in CD4+ T cell counts despite having undetectable viral loads, a phenomenon some term "immunologic failure." Immunologic failure may be caused by cytotoxic effects of medications that lower absolute lymphocyte counts, such as zidovudine or hydroxyurea. Occasionally, patients who start on therapy with low CD4+ T cell counts fail to experience a significant increase in counts. These individuals may have a diminished capacity for immune reconstitution.

Clinical Failure

Clinical failure refers to the situation in which a patient develops new signs or symptoms of an opportunistic infection or a recurrence of a previous one despite having a viral load that is below quantifiable levels. This is most commonly seen in individuals who start on therapy with low CD4+ T cell counts. Studies of patients with low CD4+ T cell counts have shown that a significant risk for opportunistic infections persists in the first 3 months of therapy. In addition, the incidence of lymphomas has not changed during the era of potent antiviral therapy. Therefore opportunistic infections diagnosed soon after medication is started or a diagnosis of lymphoma should not be considered to be failure of therapy.

In general, patients should be evaluated for a change in their antiretroviral therapy when experiencing virologic failure, rather than immunologic or clinical failure. Practitioners may wish to observe patients with virologic failure with viral loads that are persisting at a low level (<5,000 copies HIV RNA/ml) rather than switch therapy. Patients experiencing virologic failure may continue to maintain CD4+ T cell counts above pretreatment levels despite an increase in the viral load. However, the disadvantages of delaying a change in therapy include the risk of the additional selection of drug resistance. Studies have shown that patients experiencing virologic failure are more likely to achieve a viral load below quantifiable levels if their viral load is low at the time their treatment was modified. The decision to switch therapy also must be based on the number of new treatment options that exist for the patient. At times, it may be better to continue a patient on a failing combination than to switch to a regimen that is not likely to be successful. In particular, NNRTIs should not be used unless there is a good chance that the patient's viral load can be reduced below quantifiable levels because resistance to NNRTIs develops quickly in the face of suboptimal therapy. In addition, studies have shown that patients who have failed multiple combinations and have virus that is broadly resistant to many drugs in each therapeutic class will experience an increase in viral load and decline in CD4+ counts if they stop therapy. Therefore there is value in continuing therapy that is being tolerated in patients without better treatment options.

Patients with immunologic failure who have viral loads below quantifiable levels should continue on therapy if their CD4+ T cell counts are above the levels that require prophylaxis for the prevention of opportunistic infections. Patients with immunologic failure who have other treatment options could be tried on alternative medications, especially if they are on an agent known to depress lymphocyte counts. Patients should continue on prophylactic therapies until their CD4+ T cell counts rise above the thresholds used to decide when to begin prophylaxis. When CD4+ T cell counts rise above these levels, prophylaxis can be safely discontinued, assuming the viral load is undetectable. This therapeutic strategy decreases the probability that clinical failure will occur.

Strategies for Patients Requiring Treatment Modification

Treatment Intensification

When a patient has experienced virologic failure and the decision has been made to alter the patient's combination, two strategies are typically followed. In one strategy, termed "treatment intensification," a single drug is added to the existing regimen. The advantage of treatment intensification is that drugs that remain active are continued. The disadvantage is that if the intensification strategy does not work, the patient's virus may become resistant to a greater number of agents. The other strategy is to change all of the drugs in the combination. The disadvantage of this approach is the abandonment of drugs that are still active and the introduction of new drugs that may cause side effects.

Treatment intensification is employed in two situations. The first is when a patient has begun an antiretroviral combination, his or her viral load has declined, but the slope of the viral load decline has flattened and it appears that it will not decline below quantifiable levels. Because the viral load has not increased, it is presumed that resistant virus has not emerged. However, it is possible that the incomplete response to therapy is due to the presence of virus resistant to one or more drugs selected in the combination at baseline. Rather than switch to a new combination and give up on drugs that are working, one hopes the addition of another drug will provide enough added activity to reduce the viral load below quantifiable levels. If not present in the initial combination, abacavir is often chosen as the drug for intensification because of its favorable toxicity profile, the ease of administration, its potency, and the fact that it maintains activity against virus that is resistant to lamivudine. Another intensification option to consider if the patient is on a PI-containing combination is the addition of a low dose (100 mg or 200 mg bid) of ritonavir to boost the serum concentrations of the accompanying PI. As explained above, ritonavir inhibits the metabolism of other PIs, so when used in PI-PI combinations, ritonavir slows the clearance of the accompanying PI, increasing concentrations through most of the dosing interval and hopefully enhancing potency.

The second clinical scenario when an intensification strategy may be employed is shortly after observing a viral load rebound in a patient receiving a PI-containing regimen. In this case, it is assumed that the virus is resistant to one or more components of therapy, including the PI, but that this "low-level" resistance can be overcome by adding an additional agent. Again, the strategy most often used is the addition of ritonavir for the same reasons described above.

Changing the Entire Regimen

Accompanying an increase in plasma viral load is the selection of resistant virus. Resistance occurs because HIV has a rapid replication rate (approximately 1 to 10 billion viral particles are produced every day in the average infected individual), and as the virus replicates, it mutates. Roughly one mutation is introduced into proviral DNA each time the HIV genome is reverse transcribed. Because HIV reverse transcriptase has no proofreading function, all mutations are carried in the progeny virions that emerge from that infected cell. When specific substitutions occur at certain codons in the part of the HIV genome that encodes the reverse transcriptase and protease enzymes that are the targets of current therapy, these mutations can alter the binding of the drug to the enzyme or produce other biochemical changes that result in some degree of resistance to the therapy. Mutations occur whether or not a patient is taking medication, and probably exist prior to the initiation of treatment. Because mutations in these viral enzymes impede the efficiency of HIV replication, the resistant virus is present at concentrations that are too low to measure in the absence of treatment. However, once the patient starts on therapy, if incomplete suppression of HIV replication occurs, the virus with the resistance mutations that provide a survival advantage is selected for, and it rapidly becomes the dominant population of virus. When a patient has an increasing viral load on therapy, the strategy that is most commonly employed is to change at least two of the drugs used in the combination or to select an entirely new combination.

Resistance Monitoring Assays

HIV develops resistance in an ordered fashion. Early on when the viral load is increasing, the virus is likely to be resistant to only a single drug in the combination. The probability that virus will develop resistance to any particular drug is influenced by the activity of the combination, the number of mutations needed for the virus to become resistant (it often requires several in combination), and the impact of the mutations on the "fitness" of the virus. Fitness refers to the efficiency of viral replication. Mutations that adversely influence the virus' fitness will develop more slowly than others that have less impact.

There are two ways to characterize resistance in clinical practice, genotypic and phenotypic. Genotypic resistance refers to the mutations that are selected for by drugs when a patient has virologic failure. Phenotypic resistance refers to the concentration of drug required to inhibit a given amount of virus replication in vitro. Phenotypic resistance data typically cite an IC_{50} or IC_{90}, the concentration of drug that is required to inhibit 50% or 90% of virus replication. There are advantages and disadvantages of analyzing resistance from either perspective. Genotypic resistance only gives data on mutations that are associated with loss of activity of a drug. Occasionally, certain mutations that are associated with resistance when drugs are used individually can interact to restore sensitivity when present together. Unfortunately, this positive effect of interacting mutations cannot be determined a priori in the absence of phenotypic data. In addition, new mutations associated with resistance are frequently being recognized, especially as we study the effects of more drugs in new combinations. As a result of these factors, expert interpretation of genotypes is required to guide clinicians in their therapeutic decision making. There are also several disadvantages to analyzing resistance by phenotyping. Phenotyping assays have a variability of 250% or 400% (2.5-fold to fourfold), depending on the methodology used. Therefore, unless the change in IC_{50} or IC_{90} exceeds those thresholds, virus is reported as wild type or sensitive. Some drugs require several mutations in order for a phenotypic change in sensitivity to be observed. This suggests that these assays may not be sensitive enough to detect small changes in phenotype that may be early markers of resistance. In addition, we do not know the level of phenotypic resistance that correlates with the loss of a specific drug's activity in vivo. Some drugs may no longer be effective if there has been a twofold or fourfold phenotypic change, while other drugs with good pharmacokinetic profiles may maintain activity even if there is tenfold change in phenotype.

Unfortunately, HIV cross-resistance among drugs within a class of inhibitors is common. Cross-resistance means that the virus has developed resistance to a drug that the patient has not taken. Understanding the patterns by which virus acquires sequential resistance and patterns of cross resistance is important when considering how to optimally sequence combinations of drugs and when selecting a combination for a patient with virologic failure requiring a complete change in therapy. Resistance to lamivudine requires only a single mutation, at codon 184, and this mutation can be selected for within a matter of weeks if lamivudine is used as monotherapy. When lamivudine is used in the initial combination with a PI and zidovudine or stavudine, the initial mutation encountered is most often the 184V mutation associated with lamivudine resistance. The virus typically has no mutations associated with resistance to the PI or the other NRTI. If the patient continues on the same combination with a quantifiable viral load, over time the virus will develop resistance to the other agents in the combination. Resistance to the other NRTIs emerges more slowly.

Resistance to didanosine also requires only a single mutation, at either codon 74 or 184. Despite the fact that both didanosine and lamivudine may both select for virus with the same mutation, mutant virus emerges more slowly against didanosine than lamivudine. In one study that sequenced virus from patients with virologic failure on combinations of zidovudine or stavudine plus lamivudine and indinavir versus stavudine plus didanosine and indinavir, the mutations encountered were associated with lamivudine resistance when that drug was used in the combination. Patients receiving stavudine, didanosine, and indinavir developed virus with mutations associated with PI resistance, rather than NRTI resistance. Patients failing on abacavir most commonly have virus that also has the 184V mutation, but paradoxically abacavir maintains complete phenotypic sensitivity versus virus with only the codon 184 mutation. Recent data suggest that the mutational path to resistance to zidovudine and stavudine may be similar. It typically takes months before virus develops resistance to these drugs.

Resistance to the NNRTIs also develops rapidly. Patients on NNRTI monotherapy may develop resistant virus within 1 week of beginning therapy. Patients with virologic failure on NNRTIs will usually have virus that is NNRTI resistant. The pattern of mutations associated with NNRTI resistance is slightly different among the three drugs in this class. However, a mutation at codon 103 that is almost always seen in patients failing on efavirenz and seen in half of patients failing nevirapine or delavirdine gives rise to virus that is resistant to all of the drugs in this class. Patients with a mutation at codon 181 that can be seen in patients failing nevirapine or delavirdine may be inhibited to some extent by efavirenz, but the limited data that exist from patients treated with efavirenz who have a codon 181 mutation are not encouraging. Many experts consider there to be total cross-resistance among

NNRTIs, so a patient may have only a single opportunity to use one of these agents.

Resistance to the PIs is complicated. The initial mutation associated with PI resistance influences the binding of the drug to the enzyme. These mutations slow the activity of the enzyme. Subsequent mutations called secondary or compensatory mutations are the virus' attempt to restore the efficiency of the enzyme. In general, the more PI-associated mutations that the virus has acquired, the less likely that any drug in this class will be effective. That said, there are considerable data suggesting that there is the opportunity to effectively sequence drugs in this class. There are unique primary mutations associated with nelfinavir resistance at codon 30 and amprenavir resistance at codon 50. Patients with nelfinavir-resistant virus associated with a codon 30 mutation will respond to combinations of ritonavir plus saquinavir and lopinavir/ritonavir. Patients with amprenavir-resistant virus will respond to indinavir or lopinavir/ritonavir. Complete cross-resistance between indinavir and ritonavir occurs. However, ritonavir should still be considered in its role as a pharmacokinetic potentiator together with another PI in a patient with indinavir or ritonavir resistance. Preliminary results with the newest protease inhibitor, Kaletra, a fixed-dose lopinavir/ritonavir combination, suggest that this drug is effective against virus that is resistant to any PI individually, and maintains some activity against virus with as many as 10 PI-associated mutations. Combinations of amprenavir plus ritonavir or indinavir plus ritonavir are also being studied in patients with multiple PI-resistant virus.

Assays that assess genotypic and phenotypic resistance are now commercially available. Genotypic assays were the first available, and as a consequence, more clinical experience exists evaluating treatment strategies that follow genotypic paradigms. Neither the genotypic nor phenotypic assay is good at detecting mutant virus that is present in low concentrations. In addition, the tests are only helpful at detecting virus with resistance relative to the combination that the patient is currently taking. Mutations or phenotypic resistance to a drug can be undetectable when a patient switches to another combination, only to rapidly emerge if the patient is rechallenged with the drug later on. Early concerns with commercial phenotyping assays regarding reproducibility and turn-around time have improved, and these tests are being more widely used in clinical practice. Phenotyping assays are approximately twice the cost of genotyping assays, an obstacle to their more generalized acceptance.

Several studies in patients with virologic failure have compared the outcomes of combinations that were selected based on genotyping or phenotyping virus versus combinations that were selected by patients' treatment history alone. Each trial has shown that having the resistance data available influences the antiretroviral combination that is selected. In three of four large trials that have been published, patients who had a combination selected on the basis of resistance testing had a greater reduction in viral load, and were more likely to have an undetectable viral load, compared with patients whose combination was based solely on knowledge of the treatment history. These benefits have been seen even in patients failing on their initial combination, a group that many expert practitioners would have predicted would not require a resistance test to guide the selection of an effective combination. Studies comparing treatment decisions based on genotyping versus phenotyping are underway, and more data are needed to examine the utility of these assays in patients who have failed multiple combinations.

Guidelines have been established that suggest when resistance testing should be obtained. Resistance testing is recommended for patients who have virologic failure in order to select the next combination in a more informed way. Individuals with acute HIV infection have been found to be infected with resistant virus in a minority, but substantial proportion, of cases. Because resistant virus can be transmitted, resistance testing should be considered for patients diagnosed with acute HIV infection. Resistant virus is not recommended for patients coming into care with established infection or those who have been off medication for a month or more. Following the discontinuation of therapy, the proportion of mutant virus in a patient declines; is overtaken by the wild type, sensitive virus; and is no longer detectable with the presently available resistance testing. The longer a patient is off medication, the less likely resistant virus, although still present, will be detected.

Patients with virologic failure have better responses the more active drugs used in second or third combinations. Therefore a patient with a virologic rebound should ideally receive a new combination of three or more drugs to which the virus is sensitive. Patients failing on an initial PI-sparing combination that includes an NNRTI should receive two new NRTIs plus one PI or a PI-PI combination. Patients failing on a PI-inclusive NNRTI-sparing combination should receive two new NRTIs plus an NNRTI and possibly another PI in addition. Patients started on NNRTI- and PI-sparing combinations should receive an NNRTI plus a PI or a PI-PI combination together with two new NRTIs. Resistance testing should guide these decisions. Occasionally patients with a viral load rebound have a genotype or phenotype that reveals no mutations and wild type virus. Most likely, these patients are not taking their medication or there is a problem with their absorption of the medication.

Any time patients experience a rebound in their viral load, a clinician should determine to what extent drug nonadherence has influenced the treatment failure. If a patient describes side effects on a combination, every effort should be made to select a new combination with agents that are unlikely to cause that same side effect, even if the patient swears that the side effect did not influence his or her adherence. When prescribing a new combination for a patient with treatment failure, it should be emphasized to the patient that with each failure the chance of therapeutic success diminishes, so the patient must make pill taking a priority.

Drug-Drug Interactions, Contraindicated Medications, Dose Adjusting

There is considerable potential for drug-drug interactions between many classes of compounds and the PIs and NNRTIs because both the PIs and NNRTIs are metabolized by the hepatic cytochrome p450 enzyme system. Classes of compounds that require judicious use after referral to a dosing guide include calcium channel blockers, lipid-lowering agents, oral contraceptives, anticonvulsants, ergot alkaloids, antidysrhythmics, antimycobacterial agents, selective serotonin receptor inhibitors, sildenafil, cisapride, benzodiazepines, warfarin, and some herbal medicines. In addition to the drug interactions that affect metabolism, the potential exists for drug-drug interactions that result from interference with gastric absorption or renal excretion. Although some interactions are minor and rarely result in clinically significant adverse effects, many can cause serious adverse reactions or death. In addition, drug-drug interactions can lower the effective concentrations of the antiretrovirals, leading to treatment failure and drug resistance.

For these reasons, great care should be taken to ensure that patients are on the appropriate doses of medication and are not taking drugs that should be avoided. Providers that do not care for many HIV-infected patients should review all of the medicines a patient is prescribed at each visit. Patients should be interviewed and asked specifically about current prescription medications, medications prescribed by other health care professionals, nonprescription medications, investigational drugs, injectable medications, and nutritional supplements and herbal remedies. Because patients often think the medication review is only for oral medications prescribed for illnesses, they may not volunteer that they are taking oral contraceptives, transdermal ("patch") preparations, or injectable medications unless specifically asked.

Careful scrutiny of the medication profile is also necessary when patients discontinue certain medications. Supratherapeutic or subtherapeutic drug concentrations can occur at the time of discontinuation of a drug that has induced or inhibited the metabolism of another agent. For example, ritonavir can induce the metabolism of morphine. If the dose of the narcotic has been increased during ritonavir therapy to compensate for the increased clearance, supratherapeutic levels may develop, leading to narcotic-related adverse effects if ritonavir is discontinued.

Table 5-4 lists drugs that are contraindicated for use with PIs and NNRTIs. Many of the drugs listed are contraindicated when used with all of the antiretrovirals within a class or with either the PIs or NNRTIs. Rather than remembering contraindicated drugs, it may be simpler to remember what agents within a class of drugs are safe to use. Alternatives to simvastatin and lovastatin include atorvastatin, pravastatin, and fluvastatin. Alternatives to rifabutin for *Mycobacterium avium* complex treatment include azithromycin, clarithromycin (azithromycin, rather than clarithromycin, should be used if patients are taking efavirenz), or ethambutol. Loratadine, fexofenadine, and cetirizine can be used in place of astemizole or terfenadine. Temazepam and lorazepam are safe benzodiazepines.

The acid buffer containing dihydroaluminum sodium carbonate and magnesium hydroxide in didanosine can affect the absorption of many medications that require an acidic pH for absorption or those that can be chelated by divalent cations. Such drugs include dapsone, delavirdine, indinavir, itraconazole, ketoconazole, ritonavir, quinolone antibiotics, and tetracyclines. Dramatic reductions in the bioavailability of these agents can occur and can lead to treatment failure. Separating administration times by several hours can help minimize the effects. Indinavir and delavirdine should be separated from didanosine by at least 1 hour. Quinolones should be taken at least 2 hours before or 6 hours after didanosine. Itraconazole and ketoconazole should be taken at least 2 hours before didanosine. The newly available enteric-coated formulation of didanosine that lacks a buffer should alleviate the need for these precautions.

Several medications commonly used by HIV-infected patients may be affected by their antiretroviral drugs. Methadone can interact with many antiretrovirals in different ways. Methadone decreases the plasma concentrations of didanosine by 41% and that of stavudine by 27%, although methadone levels appear unchanged. No guidelines exist for dose modification. Many of the NNRTIs or PIs may decrease methadone levels substantially, and contact with methadone maintenance programs should be made to support the need to increase a patient's methadone dose if the patient experiences symptoms of withdrawal. Birth control pills may not be effective when taken with certain NNRTIs and PIs. Dilantin and phenobarbital, drugs that induce cytochrome P450 enzymes, may reduce the effective concentrations of the NNRTIs and PIs, and alternative antiseizure medications should be sought for patients requiring antiretroviral therapy.

Patients often do not think to mention the herbal medications they are taking, but the potential exists for significant drug-drug interactions. St. John's wort *(Hypericum perforatum)* can reduce indinavir serum concentrations by 57%, a result of induction of the CYP 3A isoenzyme and/or the induction of intestinal p-glycoprotein drug transporters. Because the effects of St. John's wort have not been studied with other PIs or NNRTIs, it should be avoided by patients receiving PIs or NNRTIs until more data are available.

It is virtually impossible to memorize all of the possible drug interactions and to keep up with the new information that is constantly becoming available. Although retail pharmacies may identify some of the interactions, their systems do not catch all interactions, particularly recently recognized interactions. Furthermore, if patients use more than one retail pharmacy or receive sample medications, the drug interaction check systems in the retail pharmacies may be circumvented. Therefore clinicians caring for patients with HIV should have access to an updated, preferably on-line drug interaction reference.

When to Refer

Studies show that the more experienced the provider, the more likely an HIV-infected patient receives appropriate antiretroviral therapy and timely prophylactic therapy to prevent opportunistic infections or death. HIV-infected individuals do not all need to be cared for by infectious disease specialists, but a practitioner who elects to make antiretroviral therapy decisions needs to make the commitment to keep up with this rapidly changing field. The recognized complications of antiretroviral therapies are increasing in number, and HIV-infected patients are living longer and developing other medical problems unrelated to their HIV infection. In the future, HIV-infected patients will need to be cared for by a team of practitioners. Currently, all patients prescribed antiretroviral therapy should receive the benefit of an evaluation by a provider who is expert in the management of HIV infection.

TABLE 5-4
Contraindicated Drugs

	Saquinavir	Ritonavir	Indinavir	Nelfinavir	Amprenavir	Lopinavir/Ritonavir	Nevirapine	Delavirdine	Efavirenz
DRUG CATEGORY									
Calcium channel blocker	None	Bepridil	None	None	Bepridil	None	None	None	None
Cardiac	None	Amiodarone Flecainide Propafenone Quinidine	None	None	None	Flecainide Propafenone	None	None	None
Lipid-lowering agents	Simvastatin Lovastatin	Simvastatin Lovastatin	Simvastatin Lovastatin	Simvastatin Lovastatin	Simvastatin Lovastatin	Simvastatin Lovastatin	None	Simvastatin Lovastatin	None
Antimycobacterial	Rifampin Rifabutin	None	Rifampin	Rifampin	Rifampin	Rifampin	None	Rifabutin Rifampin	None
Neuroleptic	None	Clozapine	None	None	None	Pimozide	None	None	None
Psychotropic	Midazolam Triazolam	Midazolam Triazolam	Midazolam Triazolam	Midazolam Triazolam	Midazolam Triazolam	Midazolam Triazolam	Midazolam Triazolam	Midazolam Triazolam	Midazolam Triazolam
Ergot alkaloids	Dihydro-ergotamine Ergotamine (various forms)	Dihydro-ergotamine Ergotamine (various forms)	Dihydro-ergotamine Ergotamine (various forms)	Dihydro-ergotamine Ergotamine (various forms)	Dihydro-ergotamine Ergotamine (various forms)	Dihydro-ergotamine Ergotamine (various forms)	None	Dihydro-ergotamine Ergotamine (various forms)	Dihydro-ergotamine Ergotamine (various forms)
Gastrointestinal	Cisapride	Cisapride	Cisapride	Cisapride	Cisapride	Cisapride	Cisapride	Cisapride H-2 blockers Proton pump inhibitors	Cisapride

SUGGESTED READINGS

Bartlett JG, Gallant J: *Medical management of HIV infection,* Baltimore, 2000, Johns Hopkins University.

Carpenter CCJ et al: Antiretroviral therapy in adults: updated recommendations of the International AIDS Society–USA Panel, *JAMA* 283:381-390, 2000.

Department of Health and Human Services (DHHS) and the Henry J. Kaiser Family Foundation: Guidelines for the use of antiretroviral agents in HIV-infected adults and adolescents, January 28, 2000. http://www.hivatis.org.

Hirsch MS et al: Antiretroviral drug resistance testing in adult HIV-1 infection: recommendations of an International AIDS Society–USA Panel, *JAMA* 283:2417-2426, 2000.

Mullin SM, Jamjian CM, Spruance AL: Antiretroviral adverse effects and interactions: clinical recognition and management. In Sande MA, Volberding PA, editors: *The medical management of AIDS,* ed 6, Philadelphia, 1999, WB Saunders.

Working Group on Antiretroviral Therapy and Medical Management of HIV-Infected Children: Guidelines for the use of antiretroviral agents in pediatric HIV infection, *HIV Clin Trials* 1:59-99, 2000.

6 Prevention of Opportunistic Infections

KARA JUDSON, NEIL O. FISHMAN

Introduction

Patients infected with the human immunodeficiency virus (HIV) may become immunosuppressed as a result of the disease and subsequently may be at risk for infections by opportunistic pathogens. This chapter will review the current recommendations for prophylaxis to prevent opportunistic infections in persons infected with HIV. The majority of information will be based on the 1999 U.S. Public Health Service (USPHS) and the Infectious Diseases Society of America (IDSA) Guidelines for the Prevention of Opportunistic Infections in Persons Infected with Human Immunodeficiency Virus.

Patients who receive a combination of adequate chemoprophylaxis, timely vaccinations, and appropriate therapy for both acute and chronic infections, and who adhere to certain hygiene recommendations and appropriate antiretroviral drug regimens, may substantially reduce the occurrence of many life-threatening opportunistic infections. Chemoprophylaxis is implemented in two ways; primary prophylaxis prevents the initial episode of an opportunistic infection, and secondary prophylaxis prevents these infections from recurring once the patient has recovered from the initial episode.

The development of highly active antiretroviral therapy (HAART), which includes protease inhibitors and non-nucleoside reverse transcriptase inhibitors, has enabled HIV-infected patients to maintain or reconstitute adequate immune systems, and subsequently the incidence of opportunistic infections has decreased and the quality of life has improved. Most of the information in this chapter will apply to adults and adolescents, including pregnant women. Recommendations for children will not be covered.

Primary Care Office Visits
Initial Visit

History. During the initial interview with an HIV-infected individual, the provider must obtain a detailed history of previous infections and malignancies. Screening for opportunistic infections is important to help the provider stage the HIV infection and determine the level of immunocompetence. History should be obtained about abnormal Pap smears, sexually transmitted diseases, tuberculosis, pneumonia, meningitis, gastrointestinal problems, and hepatitis A, B, and C. The patient should be asked directly about a history of oral thrush or ulcers. It is also important to gather information about exposure risk to opportunistic infections at home and at the workplace. A travel history can be helpful to assess the risk for fungal infections that are endemic to certain geographic areas.

Patient Education. While gathering a detailed history, it is also important to assess the level of understanding a patient has about HIV and how the disease can be transmitted. Many patients will need education about primary prevention.

HAART was developed in the mid-1990s. This treatment had a huge impact on the frequency of opportunistic infections in the HIV-infected population. Some patients may be started on HAART therapy soon after diagnosis. Their HIV RNA levels may have decreased while their CD4+ T lymphocyte counts may have increased in a matter of weeks. The risk of new opportunistic infections may be reduced after HAART therapy, but patients should still receive an extensive education about signs and symptoms for the common opportunistic infections because this could be the first sign that the disease is progressing and their HAART regimen is no longer adequate. In addition, certain patients may be unable to tolerate or will adhere poorly to HAART regimens and will require closer monitoring for risk of disease progression and the need for prophylaxis.

Initial Work-up for Newly Diagnosed HIV-Infected Patients

Blood Tests. There are numerous blood tests that will assist the provider in determining the level of immunocompetence and in making decisions about prophylactic therapy. The patient's absolute CD4+ T lymphocyte count, which is a strong predictor of the likelihood of developing opportunistic infections, needs to be documented and trends need to be closely followed. The patient's medical record should have a chart demonstrating these trends. Both the CD4+ count and the percentage of total lymphocytes that are CD4+ cells should be followed. The percentage of CD4+ T lymphocytes can be measured with greater reliability than the absolute number, but the majority of medical research has used the absolute number; so this is the number typically followed. Plasma viral levels are not currently recommended for use as a determinant for the starting or stopping of prophylactic therapy. Most opportunistic infections occur when the CD4+ count falls below 200 cells/mm^3. However, some opportunistic infections require greater levels of immunosuppression and typically occur at lower CD4+ counts. For example, disseminated *Mycobacterium avium* complex (MAC) infections and cytomegalovirus (CMV) retinitis usually occur when the CD4+ count falls below 100 or 50 cells/mm^3.

A question arises about what to do when an HIV-infected person's CD4+ count rises in response to HAART therapy. Is the recent CD4+ number an adequate marker for making management decisions for primary prophylaxis and do these cells represent effective immune reconstitution? More simply, will this great number of cells work to fight infection? Recent studies have demonstrated that the CD4+ count continues to be the best predictor for the development of opportunistic infections. Therefore it appears as though primary prophylaxis may be discontinued once the CD4+ count remains above 200 cells/mm³ for approximately 6 months. Studies are ongoing to determine whether similar guidelines may be applied to secondary prophylaxis, but preliminary results are promising.

Serologies for particular antibodies to opportunistic pathogens can be useful in determining the level of risk a patient has for the development of infection and for other interventions. After the initial diagnosis of HIV infection, a patient should be tested for immunoglobulin G (IgG) antibody to detect the presence of a latent infection with *Toxoplasma gondii*. Patients whose CD4+ T lymphocyte cell count drops below 100 cells/mm³ should be retested for *T. gondii* antibody. HIV-infected patients who belong to risk groups with low rates of seropositivity for CMV should be tested for the CMV antibody (anti-CMV IgG). Patients who are seronegative will benefit from CMV-negative and leukocyte-reduced blood products if a transfusion becomes necessary. Low-risk groups for seropositivity include patients who have not had male homosexual contact and are not injecting drug users. Patients who have a questionable history of chickenpox can be tested for the varicella-zoster antibody.

HIV-infected patients should be screened for viral hepatitis serologies. For hepatitis B, antihepatitis B core antigen (anti-Hbc) and the hepatitis B surface antibody (HbsAb) are sufficient. Hepatitis C can be screened for by testing for the antibody to hepatitis C virus (HCV) (anti-HCV). Positive anti-HCV results should be verified with additional testing such as recombinant immunoblot agency (RIBA) or reverse transcriptase polymerase chain reaction (RT-PCR) for HCV RNA. Advanced HIV-infected patients may not be able to make sufficient antibodies. For those with chronic liver disease and with undetectable antibody, a test for the presence of HCV RNA may be used.

Other Tests. A patient with newly diagnosed HIV infection should receive a tuberculin skin test by administration of intermediate-strength (5-TU) purified protein derivative (PPD) unless a positive test result is already known. Testing should be repeated annually. Induration greater than 5 mm is defined as positive in this population. Any individual with a positive tuberculin skin test should have a chest radiograph performed.

Immunizations. An HIV-infected patient needs to receive a number of important vaccinations. It is critical to give these vaccinations early, since as the disease progresses, immunosuppression worsens and the response to these vaccinations will diminish. HIV-infected patients should receive vaccines with live viruses or bacteria with caution, particularly if they have low CD4+ cell counts. Patients should receive the 23-valent pneumococcal vaccine (Pneumovax) against *Streptococcus pneumoniae* once every 5 years. Hepatitis B vaccine should be administered to all seronegative individuals. It is given as a series of three muscular injections at 0, 1, and then 6 months. Hepatitis A vaccine also should be given to all seronegative patients, but particularly to those also infected with hepatitis C. Hepatitis A occurring in the setting of chronic hepatitis C disease can result in fulminant and potentially deadly disease. The influenza vaccine should be given annually between the months of October and December. The vaccine generally causes a slight reversible increase in HIV viral load, but influenza infection is potentially fatal. Therefore we support the administration of the influenza vaccine in our practice. Lastly, a tetanus booster needs to be given once every 10 years.

Disease-Specific Recommendations

The opportunistic infections discussed below are described in greater detail elsewhere in this text. The purpose of the following discussion is to present guidelines and recommendations for the primary care physician when caring for persons infected with HIV. Patient education, initiation of prophylaxis, and appropriate medications, including the most commonly prescribed drugs for chemoprophylaxis, will be described. For more complete information, including alternative regimens, see Table 6-1 at the end of the chapter.

Protozoan infections

Pneumocystis carinii *Pneumonia*. *Pneumocystis carinii* is an opportunistic pathogen that is transmitted by inhalation. The organism is found worldwide, and many individuals have asymptomatic infections. Symptomatic pneumonia occurs in the setting of immunosuppression.

Prevention of Exposure. There is no recommendation with sufficient supportive data to decrease the risk of *P. carinii* pneumonia (PCP) exposure, although some authorities suggest that a person at risk should not share a hospital room with a patient who has PCP because of the high risk for reinfection with a new strain. There are no recommendations for avoiding PCP exposure in the ambulatory setting.

When? Prophylaxis against PCP should begin when the CD4+ T lymphocyte count falls below 200 cells/mm³ or after the patient has an initial episode of oropharyngeal candidiasis. If a person has a CD4+ T lymphocyte percentage of less than 14% or has a history of an acquired immunodeficiency syndrome (AIDS)-defining illness other than oropharyngeal candidiasis, prophylaxis should be strongly considered. Patients with a history of PCP should receive chronic maintenance therapy. If a patient's CD4+ T lymphocyte count cannot be monitored every 3 months, the patient should be considered high risk and prophylaxis should be initiated when the count falls below 250 cells/mm³. Pregnant women should receive prophylaxis following these same guidelines.

What? Trimethoprim-sulfamethoxazole (TMP-SMX), one double-strength tablet per day, is the recommended prophylactic agent. If this dose is poorly tolerated, one single-strength tablet per day or one double-strength tablet three times a week is also effective. Although side effects, especially rash and gastrointestinal symptoms, are common, most patients can continue the medication, and over the course of several days to weeks things generally resolve. If the side effects are so severe that TMP-SMX must be stopped, patients who suffer a non–life-threatening adverse reaction should restart therapy once the reaction has resolved. There are published dose-escalation guidelines that improve the likelihood of the patient tolerating the medication on rechallenge. TMP-SMX also provides protection against toxoplasmosis and some bacterial respiratory infections. Pregnant women may use TMP-SMX as recommended or may consider aerosolized pentamidine since there is little systemic absorption.

How long? Patients on HAART with a sustained increase in their CD4+ T lymphocyte count greater than 200 cells/mm^3 for 3 to 6 months, especially in those patients with no history of PCP infection, may discontinue primary prophylaxis. In patients with a history of PCP infection, it is recommended that secondary prophylaxis be continued for life since there are insufficient data to support discontinuing therapy at this time. As noted above, studies are ongoing.

Toxoplasma gondii

Prevention of Exposure. *T. gondii* infection is often acquired by ingestion of the cysts in undercooked meat or of the oocysts found in cat feces. After the initial infection, cysts remain dormant in their host, often in the central nervous system. With the onset of immunodeficiency, these dormant infections may be reactivated, resulting in encephalitis or other clinical manifestations. Providers can counsel patients with a few simple dietary and household guidelines to avoid initial exposure to *T. gondii* reservoirs. All patients, especially those with a negative IgG antibody test result, should be advised to avoid consuming raw or undercooked meat, including pork, lamb, and venison. Meat should be cooked until it is no longer pink inside and thus has reached an internal temperature of 150° F (65.5° C). Patients should be advised to pay close attention to hand washing after contact with raw meat and with soil from activities such as gardening. In addition, raw fruits and vegetables need to be thoroughly cleaned before consumption.

HIV-infected patients who are cat owners should be advised that the litter box needs daily changing, preferably by a member of the household who is not immunocompromised. If this is not an option, patients should wash their hands thoroughly after contact with the litter box. Cats preferably should be kept inside and fed canned, dried, or well-cooked table food. Patient contact with stray cats should be avoided. Cats, however, do not need to be tested for toxoplasmosis.

When? Prophylaxis against *T. gondii* should be considered for individuals who are known to be seropositive with the *Toxoplasma* IgG antibody and who have a CD4+ T lymphocyte count of less than 100 cells/mm^3. Patients who are seronegative should be retested for the *Toxoplasma* IgG antibody when their CD4+ T lymphocyte count drops below 100 cells/mm^3. If the patient has seroconverted, they should be started on chemoprophylaxis.

What? TMP-SMX, one double-strength tablet daily, is the recommended regimen against toxoplasmic encephalitis. This same regimen is active for PCP prophylaxis.

Patients who have had toxoplasmic encephalitis require chronic maintenance therapy because the relapse rate is extremely high. The combination of pyrimethamine and sulfadiazine (with or without leucovorin) is recommended and is also active against PCP.

Pregnant women can receive TMP-SMX, which is effective against both PCP and toxoplasmic encephalitis. Pyrimethamine should not be used during pregnancy for primary prophylaxis because of the low risk for teratogenicity; however, if it is being used as chronic maintenance therapy, the benefits of lifelong therapy for the mother outweigh the risk of teratogenic effects to the fetus.

How Long? There is limited evidence to suggest that patients who discontinue prophylaxis when their CD4+ T lymphocyte counts increase to greater than 100 cells/mm^3 in response to HAART have a low risk for toxoplasmic encephalitis, but the sample of patients is small. At this time, it is recommended to continue prophylaxis once a patient has met the initial criteria. Patients who survive an episode of toxoplasmic encephalitis should receive chemoprophylaxis for life, although this is also an area that is evolving. Some experts believe that as with *Pneumocystis*, a sustained elevation in CD4+ cell count to greater than 200 cells/mm^3 allows for stopping prophylaxis.

Cryptosporidiosis.

Cryptosporidium is a cyst-forming protozoan parasite of the gastrointestinal tract. Infection is acquired by fecal-oral transmission from humans or animals.

Prevention of Exposure. HIV-infected patients should avoid contact with others infected with *Cryptosporidium*. They should take particular care to avoid children in diapers and any direct contact with human or animal feces. If they have contact, they should wash their hands thoroughly. In addition, patients should avoid sexual practices that may result in oral exposure to feces.

Patients should not consume water or food that may be contaminated with *Cryptosporidium*. This also refers to ice and fountain beverages made from tap water that may come from a contaminated source; precautions should be taken in restaurants, bars, and other places. Nationally distributed brands of bottled or canned soft drinks are typically safe. Juice that does not require refrigeration until after it has been opened is safe as is concentrated frozen juice if prepared with safe water. Pasteurized juices, beer, and other beverages are safe, but unpasteurized drinks are not. There is no information available about cyst survival in wine. In addition, patients should not eat raw oysters. Patients infected with *Cryptosporidium* should not work as food handlers, especially with food that will not be cooked before being consumed.

Patients should not come into contact with contaminated water through recreational activities such as swimming. Many lakes, rivers, swimming pools, salt-water beaches, recreational water parks, and ornamental water fountains may be contaminated with human or animal waste and may be infected with *Cryptosporidium*. There have been outbreaks reported that have been traced to municipal water supplies. If an outbreak occurs in the community and a "boil-water" advisory is issued, water should be boiled for 1 minute prior to consumption. There are personal water filters that may be used but they should meet all of these following requirements: remove particles 1 μm in diameter, work by reverse osmosis, be labeled as absolute 1 μm filters, and meet National Sanitation Foundation standard no. 53 for cyst removal. An optional recommendation for bottled water may reduce the risk of cyst transmittal, but the patient should be aware that some bottled water may still contain cryptosporidial cysts. In general, water from wells and springs is less likely to be contaminated than water from rivers and lakes. If water is treated by distillation or by reverse osmosis, the cysts will likely be removed.

Newborn and young pets have a small risk of transmitting *Cryptosporidium*. If a patient wants to purchase a pet, it is recommended that an animal with diarrhea not be brought into the home. Additionally, dogs and cats should be greater than 6 months of age, and strays should be avoided. If a patient wants to assume the risk of acquiring a pet less than 6 months of age, a veterinarian may check the animal's stool for *Cryptosporidium* before the patient has contact with the animal. In addition, patients should avoid exposure to calves and lambs and to locations where these animals are raised.

In a hospital, hand washing and gloves are sufficient to prevent transmission from an infected patient to other patients.

Although there is little evidence, it is recommended that HIV-infected patients should not share a hospital room with an infected patient because of the potential for fomite transmission.

What? There are no agents available for chemoprophylaxis for primary or chronic maintenance therapy against *Cryptosporidium* infection. Patients should carefully follow recommendations to prevent exposure.

Microsporidiosis

Prevention of Exposure. Microsporidia are also cyst-forming protozoa that may be a cause of diarrhea in immunosuppressed patients. Some species can also produce disease in other organs. Patients should practice good hygiene practices such as hand washing to reduce exposure.

What? There are no agents for chemoprophylaxis for primary or chronic maintenance therapy against microsporidiosis.

Tuberculosis. *M. tuberculosis* are acid-fast bacilli that are transmitted by respiratory aerosol. Primary infection typically occurs in the lungs. Prior infection can be detected with a tuberculin skin test using PPD, as discussed above.

Prevention of Exposure. Patients with HIV may increase their chance of exposure to tuberculosis if they work in health care facilities, correctional institutions, homeless shelters, or other high-risk facilities. The patient and the provider should determine the risk of exposure, the precautions that need to be taken, and the prevalence of tuberculosis in the community to determine if the patient's activities need to be limited. Depending on these factors, the frequency of screening can be determined.

The tuberculin skin test should be administered with the initial diagnosis of HIV, and annual testing should be considered in patients who test negative, especially in high-risk groups. Patients whose immune system has improved with HAART therapy to a CD4+ T lymphocyte count greater than 200 cells/mm^3 should be considered for retesting. An HIV-infected patient should never receive the bacille Calmette-Guérin (BCG) vaccine because of the potential for disseminated disease.

What? If a patient tests positive with a tuberculin skin test result greater than 5 mm of induration, a chest radiograph and clinical evaluation to rule out active tuberculosis should be performed immediately. If the patient has a positive test, no evidence of active tuberculosis, and no history of treatment for tuberculosis, he or she should begin chemoprophylaxis. In addition, if a patient has close contact with a person with infectious tuberculosis, the patient should receive preventive therapy once active disease has been ruled out.

There are a number of options for treatment including isoniazid daily or biweekly for 9 months, or rifampin and pyrazinamide daily for 2 months. The latter regimen has been associated with an increased incidence of hepatotoxicity, however. Patients receiving isoniazid should also receive pyridoxine, since they are at risk for peripheral neuropathy. There are potential drug interactions between rifampin or rifabutin and the protease inhibitors and non-nucleoside reverse transcriptase inhibitors (Box 6-1).

Pregnant women should receive prophylaxis for tuberculosis if they have a positive skin test or have been exposed to a person with active tuberculosis. Once active disease has been excluded, the drug regimen of choice is isoniazid with pyridoxine daily or twice weekly. Rifampin and pyrazinamide should be avoided. Therapy may be postponed until after the first trimester.

If the patient has been exposed to isoniazid- and/or rifampin-resistant tuberculosis, other agents should be considered in conjunction with public health authorities. Directly observed therapy should be used if possible, especially with regimens that are not administered daily.

How long? After completion of therapy for a positive tuberculin test, there is no indication for chronic maintenance therapy to prevent tuberculosis.

Disseminated Infection with Mycobacterium avium Complex

Prevention of Exposure. MAC is composed of multiple species of *Mycobacterium* that typically cause a febrile and wasting syndrome and rarely pulmonary disease in immunocompromised hosts. These organisms are common in the environment, and there are no recommendations to avoid exposure at this time.

When? Patients should begin chemoprophylaxis when their CD4+ T lymphocyte count is below 50 cells/mm^3. Before beginning chemoprophylaxis, disseminated MAC disease may need to be excluded with blood cultures.

What? Clarithromycin and azithromycin are the therapies of choice to prevent disseminated MAC disease. These agents also protect against bacterial respiratory infections. If clarithromycin or azithromycin cannot be tolerated, rifabutin is an alternative. See Box 6-1 for considerations on rifabutin dosing. Active tuberculosis needs to be ruled out because rifabutin monotherapy can cause resistance to rifampin. Pregnant women should also receive chemoprophylaxis, with azithromycin being the preferred drug. Clarithromycin should be used with caution during pregnancy. Azithromycin plus ethambutol is the preferred regimen for secondary prophylaxis.

How long? Although sufficient data are lacking, a patient who responds to HAART therapy with a rise in CD4+ T lymphocyte count to greater than 100 cells/mm^3 for 3 to 6 months and a sustained suppression of HIV plasma RNA may discontinue prophylaxis. Patients who have been treated for and survived disseminated MAC disease should receive treatment for life regardless of their response to HAART therapy.

Bacterial Infections
Bacterial Respiratory Infections

Prevention of Exposure. *S. pneumoniae* is the leading cause of bacterial respiratory disease in patients with HIV infection. Because *S. pneumoniae* and *Haemophilus influenzae* are common in the environment there is no effective way to reduce exposure.

BOX 6-1
Potential Interactions

- Rifampin should not be used with protease inhibitors and non-nucleoside reverse transcriptase inhibitors because both drugs are cleared by cytochrome P450
- Rifabutin may be used with caution with soft gel saquinavir but not with hard gel saquinavir
- Rifabutin can be administered at half the usual daily dose with indinavir, nelfinavir, or amprenavir, and at one fourth the daily dose with ritonavir
- Rifabutin should not be used with delavirdine
- Rifabutin at an increased dose can be used with efavirenz
- There is no information about rifabutin's interactions with nevirapine
- Nucleoside reverse transcriptase inhibitors are okay: zidovudine, didanosine, zalcitabine, stavudine, lamivudine, and abacavir

When? After HIV diagnosis, patients with CD4+ T lymphocyte counts greater than 200 cells/mm^3 should receive a single dose of 23-valent polysaccharide pneumococcal vaccine if they have not received this within the last 5 years. For patients with CD4+ T lymphocyte counts less than 200 cells/mm^3, vaccination may be offered, although the efficacy is likely diminished. Revaccination may be considered every 5 years and may also be useful for patients who have responded to HAART therapy with a rise in the CD4+ T lymphocyte count to greater than 200 cells/mm^3.

The incidence of *H. influenzae* type B infection in adults is low, so vaccination is not recommended.

Pregnant women may receive the pneumococcal vaccine, although providers may want to wait until after the initiation of antiviral therapy because of the transient viremia that has been shown to be associated with the administration of the vaccine.

What? TMP-SMX when used for PCP prophylaxis also reduces the frequency of bacterial respiratory infections, but this drug should not be given for the sole reason of preventing primary infection with bacterial respiratory pathogens because of the concern for the development of resistant organisms. Similarly, clarithromycin or azithromycin for MAC prevention may also lower the frequency of bacterial respiratory infections. Providers should be cautious with chemoprophylaxis for individuals who have frequent recurrences of bacterial respiratory infections because of the potential for the development of drug-resistant organisms.

Bacterial Enteric Infections

Prevention of Exposure. Patients can lower their chances of acquiring a bacterial enteric infection by avoiding certain foods. This includes raw or undercooked eggs, poultry, meat, or seafood, and unpasteurized dairy products. Meat should be cooked to an internal temperature of 165° F (65.5° C), which has occurred once the meat is no longer pink inside. Produce should be washed thoroughly. Patients should prevent the cross-contamination of food by cleaning all utensils and cutting boards carefully when cooking. Patients who are severely immunocompromised should be aware that soft cheeses and ready-to-eat foods such as hot dogs have been linked to listeriosis. Patients should limit their contact with reptiles because of the risk of salmonellosis.

Patients who travel to developing countries should avoid raw fruits and vegetables that cannot be peeled, raw or undercooked seafood or meat, tap water, ice, unpasteurized milk and dairy products, and food items sold by street vendors. Food that is safe includes steaming hot food, fruits peeled by the patient, hot coffee or tea, beer, wine, and water boiled for 1 minute. If water cannot be boiled, an alternative treatment is iodine or chlorine, but this method is not as effective in reducing the risk of infections with gastrointestinal protozoa.

HIV-infected patients who have salmonellosis or shigellosis may consider having household contacts evaluated for asymptomatic carriage. If they are found to be carriers, they require appropriate antimicrobial therapy.

What? Prophylactic antimicrobials are not usually recommended for travelers to prevent the development of bacterial enteric infections. However, some patients may benefit based on their level of immunosuppression and duration of travel. Options include a fluoroquinolone such as ciprofloxacin or TMP-SMX, if already being given for PCP prophylaxis. Patients may be given ciprofloxacin 500 mg bid for 3 to 7 days to be taken empirically if traveler's diarrhea develops. If their diarrhea is severe or contains blood, if they have fever or shaking chills, or if they are suffering from dehydration, they should seek the care of a physician. Antiperistaltic agents should only be used if the diarrhea lasts less than 48 hours. These agents should be avoided in patients with fever and blood in the stool.

Pregnant women should not take ciprofloxacin. They should be treated for *Salmonella* gastroenteritis with ampicillin, cefotaxime, ceftriaxone, or TMP-SMX, since infection of the placenta or amniotic fluid may result in fetal loss.

How long? Only patients who have had *Salmonella* septicemia require chronic maintenance therapy, typically with ciprofloxacin.

Bartonella

Prevention of Exposure. *Bartonella* are bacteria that are part of the oral flora of cats and may be transmitted from pets or strays. Immunocompromised patients are at higher risk for developing severe disease from *Bartonella*. If patients are considering purchasing a cat, they should choose an animal that is in good health and greater than 1 year of age. Patients should avoid any rough play with cats. Cats should not be able to lick open wounds of immunocompromised patients. It is also recommended that cats receive proper flea control.

What? There is no current recommendation for prophylaxis to prevent either primary or recurrent *Bartonella* infection.

Fungi
Candidiasis

Prevention of Exposure. *Candida* organisms are opportunistic fungi that are part of the normal flora found on mucosal surfaces and skin, and therefore there are no recommendations to prevent exposure.

What? It is not recommended to provide primary prophylaxis against candidiasis because current treatments for acute infection are effective and mortality from mucosal candidiasis is low. In addition, there is a concern for the development of drug-resistant strains, and prophylaxis can be quite costly. Secondary prevention for oropharyngeal or vulvovaginal candidiasis also is unnecessary for similar reasons. If patients suffer from frequent or severe infections, fluconazole or itraconazole solution may be considered. Patients with multiple frequent episodes of documented esophageal candidiasis may benefit from chronic suppressive therapy with fluconazole 100 to 200 mg daily. Azole therapy has the potential to be teratogenic; thus pregnant women should not receive chemoprophylaxis for candidal infections.

Cryptococcosis

Prevention of Exposure. *Cryptococcus neoformans* is a budding yeast that is found throughout nature, especially in soil that contains bird droppings. Because of its large presence in the environment, there is no recommendation to avoid exposure to *C. neoformans*.

What? It is generally not recommended to provide routine antifungal prophylaxis to prevent cryptococcosis because of the relative infrequency of the disease, lack of survival benefits associated with prophylaxis, potential for drug resistance, and high cost. If used, fluconazole at doses of 100 to 200 mg daily is reasonable for patients with CD4+ T lymphocyte counts less than 50 cells/mm^3.

Patients who have completed treatment for cryptococcosis should receive lifelong suppressive therapy; fluconazole is superior to itraconazole. Patients who respond to HAART might continue to receive suppressive therapy due to lack of evidence suggesting that they will be protected from systemic mycosis with a rise in T lymphocyte count; however, many clinicians now discontinue secondary prophylaxis when the CD4+ count is sustained over 100 cells/mm^3. Studies are ongoing to help definitively answer this question.

Pregnant women should not receive prophylaxis with fluconazole or itraconazole due to the teratogenic effects of these drugs. Women on lifelong suppressive therapy who become pregnant should be switched to amphotericin B during the first trimester.

Histoplasmosis

Prevention of Exposure. *Histoplasma capsulatum* is a fungus that is found in soil rich in bird droppings and is endemic to the central and eastern United States, especially the Ohio and Mississippi River valleys. HIV-positive patients with CD4+ T lymphocyte counts less than 200 cells/mm^3 who live in histoplasmosis-endemic areas should avoid activities known to be associated with higher risk of exposure such as creating dust when working with surface soil; cleaning chicken coops; cleaning, remodeling, or demolishing old buildings; or exploring caves.

When? In general, it is not recommended to provide primary prophylaxis to prevent histoplasmosis. Providers may consider giving itraconazole to those patients who have CD4+ T lymphocyte counts less than 100 cells/mm^3 and who are at an especially high risk of disease because of occupational exposure or who live in a community with a hyperendemic rate of histoplasmosis (approximately 10 or more cases per 100 patient-years).

What? Patients who have had histoplasmosis should receive lifelong suppressive therapy with itraconazole 200 mg twice a day. This should be continued despite a good response to HAART therapy. Pregnant women should not receive itraconazole secondary to teratogenic potential. Amphotericin B is an alternative therapy.

Coccidioidomycosis

Prevention of Exposure. *Coccidioides immitis* is a fungus that is endemic to arid regions of the southwestern United States. There are few recommendations for HIV-infected patients to avoid exposure to *C. immitis* in endemic areas; however, they should avoid high-risk activities such as excavation sites or dust storms.

What? Primary prophylaxis for HIV-infected patients to avoid coccidioidomycosis is not recommended. Lifetime suppressive therapy for patients who have been treated for coccidioidomycosis should be fluconazole 400 mg daily or itraconazole 200 mg twice a day. Patients who have had meningeal disease require consultation with an expert. Patients who have responded to HAART therapy should continue lifetime suppressive therapy despite increases in CD4+ T lymphocyte counts. Pregnant women on lifetime suppressive therapy should not receive azoles as discussed for other fungal infections.

Viruses

Cytomegalovirus Disease

Prevention of Exposure. CMV is a member of the herpesvirus family with a life cycle similar to that of the herpes simplex virus (HSV). CMV is a common virus, and it is difficult to avoid exposure to it. In particular, patients need to be aware that CMV is shed in semen, cervical secretions, and saliva. Physicians should teach patients to engage in safe sex practices by using latex condoms to lower the risk of exposure to pathogens. Patients who are child-care providers or parents of children at child-care facilities are at an increased risk for acquiring CMV infection. This risk may be diminished by the practice of good hygiene such as frequent hand washing. In nonemergent situations, HIV-infected patients who are known to be CMV-negative should receive CMV antibody-negative or leukocyte-reduced cellular blood products.

When? The most important method for preventing severe CMV disease is early detection. The most common manifestation of severe CMV disease is retinitis. Patients should be taught to check their visual acuity regularly by reading newsprint, and they need to call their health care provider if they notice increased floaters.

What? Providers may opt to have regular funduscopic examinations for patients with CD4+ T lymphocyte counts less than 50 cells/mm^3. Providers may consider offering oral ganciclovir for those patients who are CMV-positive and have a CD4+ T lymphocyte count of less than 50 cells/mm^3. Things to consider with this decision include the risk of ganciclovir-induced neutropenia, anemia, conflicting reports of efficacy, lack of proven survival benefit, and the risk of developing ganciclovir-resistant CMV. Valganciclovir was recently approved as a more bioavailable agent against CMV, but this drug has not been studied for primary prophylaxis. Acyclovir and valacyclovir are not active against CMV and therefore should not be offered. Pregnant women should not receive ganciclovir for primary prophylaxis. For patients on chronic maintenance therapy who become pregnant, ganciclovir should be continued and an expert needs to be consulted.

CMV disease is not curable with current medications. Lifetime therapy is recommended once induction therapy has been completed. An expert should be consulted for therapy options, which may include parenteral or oral ganciclovir, parenteral foscarnet, combined parenteral ganciclovir and foscarnet, or parenteral cidofovir. For retinitis only, intraocular implant of ganciclovir plus oral ganciclovir is an option. The intraocular implant only provides protection to the affected eye. For retinitis, an ophthalmologist should be consulted. Oral valganciclovir is an effective option for treatment and secondary prophylaxis.

Maintenance therapy may be discontinued in patients with CMV retinitis whose CD4+ T lymphocyte count has increased to greater than 100 to 150 cells/mm^3 for a 3- to 6-month period and whose HIV plasma RNA levels have been suppressed in response to HAART therapy. Maintenance therapy should likely be restarted when the CD4+ T lymphocyte count has decreased to less than 50 cells/mm^3.

Herpes Simplex Virus

Prevention of Exposure. HSV may come in two types that are distinguished by antigenicity and likely location of infection. The virus becomes latent after initial exposure, and there may be recurrences characterized by the development of a vesicular rash. HIV-positive patients should be advised to avoid sexual contact when herpetic lesions are present, since the risk of transmission of both HSV and HIV with lesions present may be higher.

What? There is no primary prophylaxis to prevent initial episodes of HSV disease. After an acute episode of HSV has resolved, chronic therapy with acyclovir is unnecessary. Patients who have frequent or severe recurrences may benefit from daily suppressive therapy with acyclovir, valacyclovir, or famciclovir. If patients have an acyclovir-resistant strain of HSV, intravenous foscarnet or cidofovir is the agent of choice. Pregnant women should receive acyclovir suppressive therapy if they have frequent or severe episodes of HSV. This therapy does not reduce the risk of neonatal transmission and should not be given for that reason only.

Varicella-Zoster Virus Infection

Prevention of Exposure. Varicella-zoster virus (VZV) is a member of the herpesvirus family with a similar life cycle and is typically transmitted by respiratory droplets or by direct contact with a lesion. Therefore HIV-infected patients who have no history of chickenpox or shingles or are seronegative for VZV should avoid exposure to any person with chickenpox or shingles. Household contacts, especially children, who have no history of chickenpox and are HIV-negative should receive the VZV vaccine.

What? Giving the VZV vaccine to an HIV-positive person who is seronegative for VZV is complicated because it is a live virus vaccine. It may be considered for persons with normal CD4+ cell counts, but should be avoided if there is evidence of immunosuppression. There are very little data about the safety and efficacy in this particular population. If a susceptible HIV-infected patient, including a pregnant woman, is exposed to a person with chickenpox or shingles, the patient should receive varicella-zoster immunoglobulin within 96 hours to prevent the development of chickenpox. There are no established measures to prevent shingles.

Human Herpesvirus 8 Infection

Prevention of Exposure. The mechanism of transmitting human herpesvirus 8 (HHV-8), the herpesvirus associated with Kaposi's sarcoma, is unknown. There is some epidemiologic evidence suggesting that sexual transmission occurs more commonly among men who have sex with men and can occur among heterosexuals as well. In addition, the virus has been detected in saliva more frequently than semen in HHV-8 seropositive HIV-infected patients.

What? Lower rates of Kaposi's sarcoma have been observed among AIDS patients treated with ganciclovir or foscarnet for CMV retinitis. In addition, HHV-8 replication in vitro is inhibited by these drugs. The efficacy and clinical use of these drugs in preventing Kaposi's sarcoma have not been established; thus it is not recommended to use these drugs to prevent the disease. Antiretroviral medication that suppresses HIV replication reduces the frequency, progression, and development of new lesions of Kaposi's sarcoma.

Human Papillomavirus Infection

Prevention of Exposure. Some types of human papillomavirus (HPV) have been linked to the development of cervical cancer. There is little supporting evidence that condom use prevents the transmission of HPV, but safe sexual practices are recommended to lower the risk of transmission of all sexually transmitted diseases.

What? HIV-infected women should ideally be followed by a gynecologist with HIV interest and experience, since the management can be a bit complicated. Briefly, HIV-infected women should have a Pap smear test biannually after initial diagnosis. If the results are normal, the frequency of the Pap smear test may be reduced to annually. If the Pap smear is interpreted as atypical squamous cells of undetermined significance (ASCUS), there are a few management options. If the study is believed to represent a reactive process, follow-up Pap tests should be performed every 4 to 6 months for 2 years until there are three consecutive smears that are negative. If during this 2-year period there is a second report of ASCUS, then a colposcopic examination should be done. If women are diagnosed with unqualified ASCUS associated with severe inflammation, they should be evaluated for an infectious process. After treatment, the Pap test should be repeated after 2 to 3 months.

If women are diagnosed with ASCUS and are suspected of having a neoplastic process, they should be treated as if they have a low-grade squamous intraepithelial lesion (LSIL). If this patient is at high risk because of a previous history of positive Pap tests or poor adherence to follow-up, colposcopy should be considered. Patients who have LSIL should have Pap tests every 4 to 6 months if they are reliable for follow-up. If repeat Pap smears demonstrate persistent abnormalities, then colposcopy and directed biopsies should be obtained. Women with evidence of high-grade squamous intraepithelial lesions (HSILs) or squamous cell carcinoma should undergo colposcopy and directed biopsy. The risks for recurrence of these lesions are higher in HIV-infected women, and thus frequent follow-up Pap smears and colposcopic examinations when necessary are important.

There is evidence that HPV-positive men who have sex with men are at an increased risk for the development of anal HSILs and might be at an increased risk for anal cancer. Based on this evidence, further studies of screening and treatment programs for this lesion in men are currently underway. At this time routine anal cytology screening is not yet recommended.

Hepatitis C Infection

Prevention of Exposure. HCV is a member of the *Flavivirus* family and typically invades hepatocytes when a person becomes infected. It may be transmitted by injecting drug use. Patients should be advised to stop injecting drug use and to complete a substance abuse program. Patients who continue injecting drug use should be advised to never reuse or share syringes, needles, water, or drug preparation equipment. If they reuse equipment, they should first clean it with bleach and water. They should only use sterile syringes obtained from a reliable source, and use boiled water to prepare drugs or clean water from a reliable source. They should use a new or disinfected container and a new filter to prepare drugs, and clean the injection site with alcohol before each injection. Individuals should also be instructed on the safe disposal of needles after use. Intranasal drug use also has been associated with HCV transmission; therefore patients should not share straws.

Body piercing and tattooing are methods of HCV transmission. Sterile equipment and proper infection control procedures should be used at all times. Patients should not share dental appliances, razors, or other personal care articles.

Persons with HIV and HCV infection should avoid drinking excessive amounts of alcohol. Even moderate alcohol use has been associated with an increase in the incidence of cirrhosis. Patients with chronic hepatitis C should be vaccinated with hepatitis A to decrease the risk of fulminant hepatitis. If the patient is greater than 40 years of age, prevaccination screening for hepatitis A antibody is considered cost-effective. Patients with both infections have a higher incidence of chronic liver disease and should be screened accordingly.

Guidelines for Thinking about Prophylaxis Reliability

Physicians should be able to lower the incidence of opportunistic infections in HIV-infected persons by providing recommendations to avoid exposure to certain pathogens, and by initiating primary and secondary prophylaxis when appropriate, based on the trends of the CD4+ T lymphocyte counts. The individual patient's ability to follow complicated drug regimens and avoidance of exposure should also be taken into account. A physician-patient partnership should be developed to provide adequate patient education and counseling in order to maximize the patient's health and adherence to complex drug regimens.

Summary

HIV is a complicated infectious disease to manage because of the wide array of opportunistic pathogens that may cause disease as an individual's immune system becomes depressed. Careful monitoring of CD4+ counts and frequent office visits with patient education as a major focus can improve the management of these patients. Review of the guidelines for prophylaxis can ensure that treatment is consistent with the latest recommendations as well.

TABLE 6-1
Recommendations for Chemoprophylaxis

Pathogen	PRIMARY PROPHYLAXIS First-choice regimen	PRIMARY PROPHYLAXIS Alternative regimen	SECONDARY PROPHYLAXIS First-choice regimen	SECONDARY PROPHYLAXIS Alternative regimen
Pneumocystis carinii	1. TMP-SMX 1 ds tab po qd 2. TMP-SMX 1 ss tab po qd	1. Dapsone 50 mg po bid 2. Dapsone 100 mg po qd 3. Dapsone 50 mg po qd + pyrimethamine 50 mg po qw + leucovorin 25 mg po qw 4. Dapsone 200 mg po qw + pyrimethamine 75 mg po qw + leucovorin 25 mg po qw 5. Aerosolized pentamidine 300 mg qm via Respirigard II nebulizer 6. Atovaquone 1,500 mg po qd 7. TMP-SMX 1 ds po tiw	1. TMP-SMX 1 ds po qd 2. TMP-SMX 1 ss po qd	1. Dapsone 50 mg po bid 2. Dapsone 100 mg po qd 3. Dapsone 50 mg po qd + pyrimethamine 50 mg po qw + leucovorin 25 mg po qw 4. Dapsone 200 mg po qw + pyrimethamine 75 mg po qw + leucovorin 25 mg po qw 5. Aerosolized pentamidine 300 mg qm via Respirigard II nebulizer 6. Atovaquone 1,500 mg po qd 7. TMP-SMX 1 ds po tiw
Toxoplasma gondii	1. TMP-SMX 1 ds po qd	1. TMP-SMX 1 ss po qd 2. Dapsone 50 mg po qd + pyrimethamine 50 mg po qw + leucovorin 25 mg po qw 3. Atovaquone 1,500 mg po qd +/− pyrimethamine 25 mg po qd + leucovorin 10 mg po qd	1. Sulfadiazine 500-1,000 mg po qid + pyrimethamine 25-75 mg po qd + leucovorin 10-25 mg po qd	1. Clindamycin 300-450 mg po q6-8h + pyrimethamine 25-75 mg po qd + leucovorin 10-25 mg po qd 2. Atovaquone 750 mg po q6-12h +/− pyrimethamine 25 mg po qd + leucovorin 10 mg po qd

Note: those entries marked with C denote an optional recommendation. See below.
Categories reflecting the strength of each recommendation for or against the use of a product or measure for the prevention of opportunistic infection

Category	Definition
A	Both strong evidence and substantial clinical benefit support a recommendation for use.
B	Moderate evidence—or strong evidence for only limited benefit—supports a recommendation for use.
C	Poor evidence supports a recommendation for or against use.
D	Moderate evidence supports a recommendation against use.
E	Good evidence supports a recommendation against use.

Categories reflecting the quality of evidence forming the basis for recommendations regarding the use of a product or measure for the prevention of opportunistic infection

Category	Definition
I	Evidence from at least one properly randomized, controlled trial.
II	Evidence from at least one well-designed clinical trial without randomization, from cohort or case-controlled analytic studies (preferably from more than one center), or from multiple time-series studies or dramatic results from uncontrolled experiments.
III	Evidence from opinions of respected authorities based on clinical experience, descriptive studies, or reports of expert committees.

Continued

TABLE 6-1—cont'd
Recommendations for Chemoprophylaxis

	PRIMARY PROPHYLAXIS		SECONDARY PROPHYLAXIS	
Pathogen	First-choice regimen	Alternative regimen	First-choice regimen	Alternative regimen
Cryptococcus neoformans	1. Fluconazole 100-200 mg po qd (CI)	1. Itraconazole 200 mg po qd	1. Fluconazole 200 mg po qd	1. Amphotericin B 0.6-1.0 mg/kg iv qw-tiw 2. Itraconazole 200 mg po qd
Mycobacterium avium complex	1. Azithromycin 1,200 mg po qw 2. Clarithromycin 500 mg po bid	1. Rifabutin 300 mg po qd 2. Azithromycin 1,200 mg po qw + rifabutin 300 mg po qd (CI)	1. Clarithromycin 500 mg po bid + ethambutol 15 mg/kg po qd +/- rifabutin 300 mg po qd (CI)	1. Azithromycin 500 mg po qd + ethambutol 15 mg/kg po qd +/- rifabutin 300 mg po qd (CI)
Histoplasma capsulatum	1. Itraconazole capsule 200 mg po qd (CI)		1. Itraconazole capsule 200 mg po bid	1. Amphotericin B 1.0 mg/kg iv qw
Cytomegalovirus	1. Oral ganciclovir 1 g po tid (CI)		1. Ganciclovir 5-6 mg/kg iv 5-7 days/wk 2. Ganciclovir 1,000 mg po tid 3. Foscarnet 90-120 mg/kg iv qd For retinitis: 1. Ganciclovir sustained release implant q 6-9 mo + ganciclovir 1.0-1.5 g po tid	1. Cidofovir 5 mg/kg iv qow + probenecid 2 g po 3 hrs before dose + probenecid 1 g po 2 hrs post dose + probenecid 1 g po 8 hrs post dose (total 4 g probenecid) 2. Fomivirsen 1 vial injected into the vitreous, then repeat q 2-4 wks
Varicella-zoster virus	1. Varicella-zoster immunoglobulin (VZIG) 5 vials (1.25 ml each) im, given within 96 hours of exposure			
Hepatitis B virus	1. Hepatitis B vaccine: 3 doses; 0, 1, and 6 months			
Influenza virus	1. Whole or split virus 0.5 ml im/yr	1. Rimantadine 100 mg po bid (CIII) 2. Amantadine 100 mg po bid (CIII)		

Note: those entries marked with C denote an optional recommendation. See below.
Categories reflecting the strength of each recommendation for or against the use of a product or measure for the prevention of opportunistic infection

Category	Definition
A	Both strong evidence and substantial clinical benefit support a recommendation for use.
B	Moderate evidence—or strong evidence for only limited benefit—supports a recommendation for use.
C	Poor evidence supports a recommendation for or against use.
D	Moderate evidence supports a recommendation against use.
E	Good evidence supports a recommendation against use.

Categories reflecting the quality of evidence forming the basis for recommendations regarding the use of a product or measure for the prevention of opportunistic infection

Category	Definition
I	Evidence from at least one properly randomized, controlled trial.
II	Evidence from at least one well-designed clinical trial without randomization, from cohort or case-controlled analytic studies (preferably from more than one center), or from multiple time-series studies or dramatic results from uncontrolled experiments.
III	Evidence from opinions of respected authorities based on clinical experience, descriptive studies, or reports of expert committees.

TABLE 6-1—cont'd
Recommendations for Chemoprophylaxis

Pathogen	PRIMARY PROPHYLAXIS First-choice regimen	PRIMARY PROPHYLAXIS Alternative regimen	SECONDARY PROPHYLAXIS First-choice regimen	SECONDARY PROPHYLAXIS Alternative regimen
Hepatitis A	1. Hepatitis A vaccine: 2 doses			
Mycobacterium tuberculosis				
Isoniazid-sensitive	1. Isoniazid 300 mg po qd + pyridoxine 50 mg po qd for 9 mths 2. Isoniazid 900 mg po + pyridoxine 100 mg po biw for 9 mths 3. Rifampin 600 mg po + pyrazinamide 20 mg/kg po qd for 2 mths	1. Rifabutin 300 mg po qd + pyrazinamide 20 mg/kg po qd for 2 mths 2. Rifampin 600 mg po qd for 4 mths		
Isoniazid-resistant	1. Rifampin 600 mg + pyrazinamide 20 mg/kg po qd for 2 mths	1. Rifabutin 300 mg + pyrazinamide 20 mg/kg po qd for 2 mths 2. Rifampin 600 mg po qd for 4 mths 3. Rifabutin 300 mg po qd for 4 mths (CIII)		
Isoniazid- and rifampin-resistant	1. Consult public health authorities			
Streptococcus pneumoniae	1. Pneumococcal vaccine 0.5 ml im			
Salmonella species			1. Ciprofloxacin 500 mg po bid for several mths	1. Antibiotic prophylaxis with another active agent (CIII)
Candida Oropharyngeal or vaginal			1. Fluconazole 100-200 mg po qd	1. Itraconazole solution 200 mg po qd (CI) 2. Ketoconazole 200 mg po qd (CIII)
Esophageal			1. Fluconazole 100-200 mg po qd	1. Itraconazole solution 200 mg po qd 2. Ketoconazole 200 mg po qd (CIII)
Coccidioides immitis			1. Fluconazole 400 mg po qd	1. Amphotericin B 1.0 mg/kg iv qw 2. Itraconazole 200 mg po bid
Herpes simplex virus			1. Acyclovir 200 mg po tid 2. Acyclovir 400 mg po bid 3. Famciclovir 500 mg po bid	1. Valacyclovir 500 mg po bid (CIII)

SUGGESTED READINGS

Centers for Disease Control and Prevention: USPHS/ IDSA Guidelines for the prevention of opportunistic infections in persons infected with human immunodeficiency virus, *MMWR* 48(No. RR-10):1-66, 1999. Available online at http://www.cdc.gov/mmwr/PDF/RR/RR4810.pdf. A draft version of the 2001 updated guidelines may be found at http://www.hivatis.org

Kovacs JA, Masur H: Prophylaxis against opportunistic infections in patients with human immunodeficiency virus infection, *N Engl J Med* 342(19):1416-1429, 2000.

Part II

SYMPTOMATIC PROGRESSIVE INFECTION

Section 1 **Opportunistic Infections**

7 *Pneumocystis Carinii* Pneumonia

JAMES TANG, JOHN J. STERN

Presentation and Progression
Cause

Pneumocystis carinii pneumonia (PCP) is a variant of pneumonia that typically infects immunosuppressed patients such as those undergoing chemotherapy or suffering from the acquired immunodeficiency syndrome (AIDS). Since its discovery in 1981, AIDS has been closely linked with PCP. It was the unexplained occurrence of PCP that year in five previously healthy homosexual men in Los Angeles that helped in the first recognition of AIDS, and in the following years before the introduction of highly active antiretroviral therapy (HAART), PCP was widely known to be the most common presenting manifestation of AIDS and was responsible for the vast majority of AIDS-related deaths. Today, PCP is the initial AIDS-defining illness in close to 20% of human immunodeficiency virus (HIV)-infected patients, and it is estimated that 50% of all HIV-infected patients experience at least one episode of PCP in the course of their disease. In addition, because of the AIDS epidemic, PCP now must also be considered in evaluating patients with community-acquired pneumonia. With the development of HAART and effective prophylactic regimens in the past decade, however, we have seen the progressive decline in the frequency of PCP infection and its contribution to morbidity and mortality in the HIV-infected population. Medical research has made tremendous strides in both the diagnosis and treatment of PCP, and collectively it has made the disease less common in AIDS and has greatly improved the outcome of infected patients.

PCP remains a significant problem in the realm of AIDS-related opportunistic infections, particularly in those who have limited access to medical care, are diagnosed with HIV late in the course of their disease, choose not to treat their HIV disease consistently, or do not respond to HIV therapy. Therefore it can be seen that although the incidence and mortality associated with PCP have steadily decreased in the past years, its importance as an opportunistic infection in AIDS has not. Its patient population has shifted, and without proper treatment or prophylaxis, PCP can become just as devastating a disease as before.

P. carinii has a worldwide distribution and has been found in a number of animals in addition to humans, including rodents, horses, and nonhuman primates. Although the organisms found in different species are morphologically identical, there is evidence that different strains of *P. carinii* do exist and that each infects a distinct animal species. Transmission from animals to humans does not appear to occur. The organism is extremely difficult to propagate by laboratory culture methods, and little is known of its basic biologic structure and life cycle. Current research suggests that the life cycle of *P. carinii* consists of asexual replication of a tachyzoite form and sexual reproduction of a cystic form, which then ends in the release of a sporozoite form. No intracellular stage has been discovered yet. Adding to the difficulty of the study of *P. carinii* is that the exact taxonomy of the organism has been controversial; although its morphology and response to certain antiparasitic drugs once led to its classification as a protozoan, recent studies of its messenger RNA (mRNA) sequences, enzyme structure, and cell wall favor its placement with the fungi. Treatment with antifungal regimens for PCP is ineffective, however.

Although PCP occurs in many hosts including premature and malnourished infants, children with primary immunodeficiency diseases, and patients receiving immunosuppressive therapy, most of the patients stricken with PCP are those infected with HIV. Although B cell dysfunction plays a small role, the major common predisposition to infection with *P. carinii* is impaired cellular immunity. Clear associations between the risk of pneumocystosis in HIV-infected patients with markedly reduced CD4+ cell counts (<200 cells/mm^3) have supported this belief. With impaired immunity and subsequent *P. carinii* infection, organisms in the lung attach preferentially to alveolar type I pneumocytes. From there the organisms migrate into the alveoli and cause an increase in alveolar-capillary permeability, defects in surfactant phospholipid and protein levels, and damage to type I cells. Through this mechanism PCP causes pulmonary dysfunction, manifested by cough and shortness of breath. Although a number of other clinical manifestations such as otitis, thyroiditis, and ascites have been reported, these represent extremely rare occurrences.

In the past, it was thought that infection with PCP was primarily due to reactivation of latent infection, since serologic studies demonstrated that most healthy children are exposed to the organism by the ages of 3 or 4. Recently, though, it has been speculated that some episodes of the disease are due to new infection. Animal models have demonstrated airborne transmission of *P. carinii,* with an incubation period of 4 to 8 weeks. Person-to-person spread has been suggested by hospital pneumocystosis outbreaks among immunosuppressed patients, but this is rare.

In HIV-infected patients, as the CD4+ count declines, the risk of acquiring PCP increases; most cases of PCP are seen in those who either have had a previous episode of the disease or have a CD4+ count of less than 200 cells/mm^3.

Current data show that the risk of PCP in nonprophylactically treated patients with prior PCP is 60% to 70% per year, and risk in nonprophylactically treated PCP-naive patients with CD4+ counts <100 cells/mm^3 is 40% to 50% per year. In a recent study that followed 1,182 HIV-infected subjects over a 52-month period, 79% of PCP cases occurred in patients with CD4+ counts of less than 100 cells/mm^3, and 95% occurred with CD4+ counts of less than 200 cells/mm^3. Overall, the average CD4+ count is ~100 cells/mm^3 for first-episode PCP in patients not on prophylaxis, and is ~20 cells/mm^3 in patients receiving prophylaxis. PCP can occur over a wide range of CD4+ counts, however, and a significant number of cases have been reported with CD4+ counts of 300 to 500 cells/mm^3. Estimates have suggested that in total, only 5% of PCP cases occur in patients with a CD4+ cell count >200 cells/mm^3.

Besides prior disease and falling CD4+ counts, other risk factors have also been proposed. One of the most important is the absence of prophylactic therapy use. In the same study of 1,182 HIV-infected patients, it was found that subjects whose CD4+ counts had fallen below 200 cells/mm^3 and who were not receiving prophylactic therapy were nine times more likely to develop PCP within 6 months compared with those on such therapy. Also, relationships were also found between increased PCP risk and race (black subjects were found to have one third the risk of PCP than white subjects), a falling diffusing capacity of carbon monoxide (DLCO), and the presence of constitutional signs and symptoms in patients with CD4+ counts <200 cells/mm^3.

Presentation

Clinical. In early disease, PCP often presents with subtle symptoms that can easily be missed by both clinicians and patients. Patients often complain of a mild, unproductive cough, exertional dyspnea, and retrosternal chest pain often described as a burning sensation. Arterial blood gases may be normal at rest, the patient may be afebrile, and up to 10% of chest radiographs show no signs of disease. Thin-section computed tomography (CT) scans can demonstrate pulmonary infiltrates. Likewise, a bronchoalveolar lavage (BAL) or induced sputum sample may show numerous organisms at this stage of the disease. Often, a desaturation with mild exercise is the only objective laboratory finding. Because of the seemingly benign nature of the disease and lack of findings on physical examination and preliminary laboratory values, the disease may go unrecognized in its early stages. Further confounding diagnosis is that early manifestations of PCP can often mimic other diseases as well, most notably bacterial pneumonia and tuberculosis. Current studies have speculated on independent predictors of these three diseases. For PCP, they include exertional dyspnea plus interstitial infiltrate on chest radiograph and presence of oral thrush; predictors for bacterial pneumonia include lobar infiltrate plus fever >7 days and a clinically "toxic" appearance, and those for tuberculosis are cough for >7 days plus night sweats, weight loss, and cavitary lesions (CD4+ counts must be >300 cells/mm^3 for the development of cavitary lesions, however). Although diagnosing PCP is challenging at best, many studies have shown that the best prognosis, with avoidance of hospitalization, complications, and death, is associated with recognition and treatment of PCP as early in the course of the disease as possible. For this reason, clinicians must always be suspicious of PCP when presented with any HIV-infected patient with pulmonary signs or symptoms and an appropriate CD4+ count.

More often than not, however, PCP presents later in the course of the disease. Patients complain of several weeks of the above-mentioned symptoms, which have progressed to fever, shortness of breath, and a cough that either remains nonproductive or becomes productive of small amounts of white sputum. Physical findings may include tachypnea, tachycardia, and cyanosis, but lung auscultation often reveals few abnormalities besides possible diminished breath sounds. Late findings include weight loss, unexplained fevers for weeks, and fatigue.

In approximately 2% of cases, PCP is complicated by pneumothorax. This complication is usually more common in patients with prior bouts of PCP or those who have received aerosolized pentamidine for prophylaxis, which has been attributed to the predilection of these patients to present with apical cavitary disease. PCP may also present with multiple small pneumatoceles, which predispose to pneumothorax. Aggressive therapy is required for these patients, since the estimated mortality of this complication is 10%.

Radiographic. Although PCP has often been characterized classically by diffuse interstitial pulmonary infiltrates beginning in the perihilar regions, this finding is associated more commonly with non–HIV-associated PCP. Thus this x-ray presentation may not be expected in HIV-infected patients. The most common findings with HIV-associated PCP are either a normal chest film or faint bilateral interstitial infiltrates, although numerous other conceivable patterns—including nodular lesions, cavitary lesions, and asymmetrical patterns—have been reported as well. As described above, of particular interest are patients either with prior history of PCP or on aerosolized pentamidine prophylaxis, since an increased frequency of upper-lobe infiltrates similar to tuberculosis and pneumothoraces has been reported in these patients.

Laboratory. Laboratory values often show a characteristic increase of the alveolar-arterial O$_2$ gradient with exercise, and arterial blood gases also will usually demonstrate hypoxemia and a respiratory alkalosis. Measurements of arterial blood gases also assist in assessing the severity of infection and directing treatment. Although a mild leukocytosis is common, a white blood cell count is of minimal value, since it is somewhat variable in PCP and usually is affected by the patient's underlying HIV disease. Diffuse increased uptake in both lung fields has been noted in nuclear gallium scans, but this study has generally been replaced by bronchoscopy. In addition, elevations in serum concentrations of lactate dehydrogenase (LDH) have been reported and are quite useful in making an early presumptive diagnosis of PCP prior to bronchoscopy.

Atypical Presentations. In extremely rare cases *P. carinii* can cause extrapulmonary disease as well. In many of these cases, it has been found that patients have been using aerosolized pentamidine as prophylaxis for PCP. This finding can be explained by the relative ineffectiveness of pentamidine in preventing disease outside the lung; subsequently this form of prophylaxis has largely been replaced by oral systemic prophylaxis with trimethoprim-sulfamethoxazole (TMP-SMX), dapsone, or atovaquone.

Spread of *P. carinii* to extrapulmonary organs is thought to be through hematogenous spread from the lungs. Ear involvement, however, differs in that it is most often a primary infection without concurrent pulmonary involvement. Otic disease often presents as a unilateral polypoid mass that involves the external auditory canal but can also extend into the middle ear and even into the mastoid. Ear pain and decreased hearing are the most common complaints, and in over half of cases, tympanic membrane perforation has been reported. Other forms of extrapulmonary disease are associated with patients with a history of PCP. The most common of these are ophthalmic lesions of the choroid, which present as multiple, bilateral, asymptomatic lesions that appear as slightly elevated yellow-white plaques on physical examination. Reports of a Buerger's disease–like necrotizing vasculitis, intestinal obstruction, and retinitis have also been attributed to *P. carinii* infections. Additional possible manifestations of extrapulmonary infection include visceral cystic calcifications, lymphadenopathy, bone marrow abnormalities, ascites, and thyroiditis; additional organ involvement can include the spleen, liver, kidney, pancreas, pericardium, heart, bone marrow, and adrenals. The most common sites of extrapulmonary involvement are the lymph nodes (40% to 50%), followed by the spleen, liver, and bone marrow (30% to 40%). As stated before, however, these manifestations are all very uncommon.

Diagnosis

Because the clinical features of PCP can easily be confused with other disease entities—most importantly bacterial or viral pneumonias and tuberculosis—definite diagnosis is based solely on visualization of organisms in pulmonary samples or tissue, which is usually done through histopathologic staining. The most widely used stain is methenamine silver, but other common stains include toluidine blue and cresylecht violet; all three selectively stain *P. carinii* cyst walls. In contrast, Wright-Giemsa, Diff-Quick, and direct immunofluorescent stains can identify all developmental stages. Serum antibody detection through Western blot techniques or other serologic approaches has not been shown to be effective in diagnosing acute disease or monitoring therapy response.

The most important step in the diagnosis of PCP is the collection of proper pulmonary samples. Sensitivities can range widely based on which technique is used. Organism yields can also vary greatly from patient to patient, since HIV-infected patients with PCP will typically have much higher organism burdens than non–HIV-infected patients. Currently, sample collection techniques include fiberoptic bronchoscopy with BAL and biopsy, percutaneous needle aspiration, and induced sputum collection.

Bronchoalveolar Lavage

At most medical institutions, PCP is diagnosed using BAL, which, although invasive, has become the standard of PCP diagnosis due to its consistently high sensitivity and relative safety. When performed properly, BAL should be close to 95% to 99% sensitive. In contrast, bronchial washings or brushings, which do not sample as many alveoli as BAL, can diagnose PCP in only 30% to 70% of cases. This disparity is thought to be related to the fact that PCP is an almost exclusively alveolar disease and that BAL samples a much larger alveolar volume than other diagnostic tests. Some reports suggest that the lack of routine upper lobe lavage in BAL is a possible weakness of the procedure, especially when evaluating patients receiving aerosolized pentamidine, who often present with upper lobe disease. Overall, BAL is a highly sensitive, safe, and relatively well-tolerated procedure with a few rare complications, even in AIDS patients with significant thrombocytopenia. Immediately following BAL, a chest radiograph may demonstrate a new infiltration at the site of lavage. This finding should disappear within 24 hours. Also, in the first 2 to 12 hours following BAL, it is not uncommon for patients to experience marked yet transient temperature elevations, chills, or rigors. More significant complications such as hemorrhage or pneumothorax occur infrequently.

Sputum Induction

Recent research has increased the popularity of sputum induction as a simple, noninvasive technique that has had sensitivities as high as 75% to 95% in some reports. This procedure is extremely institution-variable, however, and requires well-trained technicians and scrupulous laboratory processing in order to be an effective diagnostic technique. In most institutions, it is used mainly as a second option for sample collection behind BAL. Expectorated sputum, which has an extremely low yield, should not be used in PCP diagnosis.

Lung Biopsy

If a patient is thought to be hematologically stable, with adequate pulmonary function, a transbronchial lung biopsy is occasionally performed during diagnostic BAL. This procedure serves many functions. While providing a tissue sample to aid in diagnosis, more importantly transbronchial biopsy will often determine if additional pathologic processes (i.e., *Mycobacterium avium* complex, cytomegalovirus) are present. Also, although BAL is usually positive in AIDS patients with PCP due to their higher organism burdens, in non-AIDS patients BAL is often negative; for these patients biopsy is therefore crucial in determining a diagnosis. Finally, by performing the transbronchial biopsy during the initial bronchoscopy, the patient is spared from another bronchoscopy if the BAL proves to be nondiagnostic. Although extremely unusual, if both BAL and transbronchial biopsy are nondiagnostic, it may be necessary to perform an open lung biopsy in order to obtain a diagnosis. As would be expected, if a substantial piece of affected lung is obtained, the yield for this procedure is superior to all other diagnostic procedures. One of the few populations in which an open lung biopsy may be useful is patients with extensive pulmonary Kaposi's sarcoma, although CT scanning and endobronchial examinations may be sufficient in these cases as well. In most cases, however, when both BAL and transbronchial biopsy are negative for PCP, a disease process other than PCP is the cause of the patient's symptoms. For this reason, and because of its invasive nature, open lung biopsy should be performed as a last resort for diagnosis, only after other etiologies have been explored.

Needle Aspiration

If focal lesions are present and BAL proves to be nondiagnostic, occasionally percutaneous needle aspiration is performed in order to obtain tissue for diagnosis. Most often, however, focal pulmonary lesions are a result of some other process besides PCP, so investigation into alternative etiologies should be initiated as well.

Polymerase Chain Reaction

Recent research has created interest in the use of polymerase chain reaction (PCR) in PCP diagnosis. Using PCR, it has been speculated that *Pneumocystis* could be detected in urine, blood, BAL, oral washings, or sputum samples with an extremely high sensitivity. However, the data on PCR diagnosis, although promising, are currently inconclusive. Reported sensitivities and specificities of PCR testing of urine samples have been extremely low. Testing of BAL, sputum, and oral washings has shown some favorable results; PCR can detect *Pneumocystis* in all three samples. Also, for BAL and sputum samples, it appears that PCR provides more sensitivity than histopathologic staining. However, the important question of whether or not the detection of *P. carinii* in respiratory secretions correlates to clinically significant disease has yet to be investigated, particularly given the fact that most of us are colonized with *P. carinii*. In both *P. carinii*-naive patients and those who have been successfully treated for previous bouts of PCP, it is often possible to detect *Pneumocystis* in respiratory secretions using highly sensitive techniques. Thus it is entirely possible to detect subclinical levels of *Pneumocystis* in asymptomatic patients. Unless these data could then be used to predict patients' risk of acquiring active, symptomatic disease (i.e., the ability to quantitate patients' *P. carinii* burden and make direct associations with symptomatic disease), they are clinically of little use to physicians at this time.

Natural History

The natural course of untreated PCP is a progressive decline in pulmonary function that ultimately leads to death. If treatment can be initiated before there is alveolar damage, prognosis is greatly improved. It is widely accepted that the best prognostic indicator at the time of diagnosis is the alveolar-arterial O_2 gradient; this value has implications in the staging of *P. carinii* infection and treatment regimens. Second and subsequent episodes of PCP have been reported to have worse prognosis than initial episodes. However, in a 5-year prospective study by Dohn et al that investigated 222 PCP occurrences, it was concluded that survival rates of first, second, and third episodes were close to equal (86%, 84%, and 88%, respectively), whereas the survival rate of a fourth episode was markedly decreased at 67%. In this study, a greater majority of mild PCP occurred during the second and third episodes. Other indicators currently thought to affect patient survival are the arterial O_2 pressure, organism burden, neutrophil % in lavage fluid, chest radiographic findings, serum LDH and albumin levels, and the individual physician's and hospital's experience with AIDS patient care.

PCP is an entirely treatable disease, but one of the most important determinants of treatment success rate is the speed at which a diagnosis is made and treatment initiated. If the disease goes unnoticed or is treated late in its course and the patient survives, this may lead to a weakening of the pulmonary function of the patient and a consequent greater susceptibility to future bouts of the disease, especially in HIV-positive patients.

Treatment

The importance of early diagnosis and aggressive therapy in the treatment of PCP cannot be stressed enough. In most instances, it is advisable to begin empiric therapy before a definitive diagnosis is made. In all instances, however, unless a patient has a history of life-threatening intolerance, TMP-SMX (Bactrim) is the mainstay of treatment for both pulmonary *Pneumocystis* and extrapulmonary disease, regardless of the severity of the disease. Other forms of treatment—trimethoprim plus dapsone, aerosolized or intravenous pentamidine, atovaquone, trimetrexate, eflornithine, and clindamycin plus primaquine—exist as well, but in every study performed to date TMP-SMX has been either as effective or superior than alternative drugs. Also of great importance is the concurrent use of steroids in PCP treatment, which will be discussed later in this section.

Empiric therapy for PCP can be appropriate when an individual presents with cough, fever, and a chest X-ray consistent with PCP, and is known or presumed to be HIV-positive. These patients should be clinically stable, with a room air O_2 pressure >70 mm Hg. In these situations, it is reasonable to begin therapy at usual therapeutic dosages until a definitive diagnosis is established. In most cases, the addition of another broad-spectrum antibiotic is not needed, since TMP-SMX, the first line agent for PCP, is also effective against most community-acquired pneumonias except those caused by *Mycoplasma*.

Trimethoprim-Sulfamethoxazole

TMP-SMX is always the preferred medication for PCP treatment and is effective in approximately 90% of patients. The drug is absorbed well orally, is generally safe, and is inexpensive. Available in IV and PO forms, each 5 ml of IV infusion and each single-strength (SS) tablet of TMP-SMX contains 80 mg of trimethoprim and 400 mg of sulfamethoxazole; double-strength (DS) tablets contain twice as much of each drug. Therapeutic dosing of TMP-SMX for patients with PCP is calculated by administering 15 mg/kg of trimethoprim daily in 3 to 4 divided doses. Because of the fixed TMP-SMX ratio in all forms of the drug, this dosing method will provide accurate sulfamethoxazole doses as well. A 21-day course of therapy is standard, although no evidence exists proving that it is more effective than a 14-day regimen. Unless a patient develops drug-induced cytopenias, concurrent use of leucovorin is not needed. Compliant patients with mild disease (defined as a room air O_2 pressure >80 mm Hg), slowly progressing disease, and no major gastrointestinal dysfunction or intolerance to the drug can be managed on an outpatient basis with regular follow-up.

The only major disadvantage of TMP-SMX therapy is the high incidence of side effects in the HIV-infected population. Although there is a 10% incidence of adverse effects in non–HIV-infected patients with PCP, the incidence is 50% to 65% in the HIV-infected population. Relatively benign adverse reactions to TMP-SMX usage include nausea, rash, fever, pruritus, and crystalluria, and these have been reported to occur in 95% of HIV-infected patients in a study by Medina et al. More serious side effects, found to occur in 57% of HIV-infected patients in the same study, include pancytopenia, hyperkalemia (due to the amiloride effect of high-dose TMP-SMX), hepatitis, pancreatitis, interstitial nephritis, renal failure (due to sulfa-induced crystalluria), and aseptic meningitis. Life-threatening hypersensitivity reactions such as Stevens-Johnson syndrome or a sepsis-like reaction have been occasionally reported as well. In addition, it often may be necessary to discontinue other myelosuppressive drugs such as zidovudine during TMP-SMX therapy. These adverse reactions tend to be dose-related, so minimizing side effects can sometimes be accomplished by slightly reducing dosage. Although many of these toxicities cause a large number of patients to discontinue their therapeutic regimen, less serious side effects should not be indications for switching to less effective therapeutic regimens. Because of these potentially serious toxicities, a complete blood count, electrolytes, liver function tests, and creatinine should be monitored two to three times a week. Similarly, clinical symptoms and signs should be reevaluated two to three times a week as well. Unless a patient is deteriorating on therapy or is clinically unstable, repeat chest radiographs or arterial blood gases are not needed. A pulse oximetry evaluation at rest and with exercise is often all that is required to assess the patient's progress. In order to provide a baseline for future use, a chest radiograph at the end of therapy is recommended but often demonstrates persistent infiltrates and/or minimal fibrosis.

Pentamidine Isethionate

Second-line therapy for PCP treatment is pentamidine isethionate, an antiprotozoal drug that must be administered parenterally. Currently, pentamidine is given intravenously. Aerosolized pentamidine is not recommended for acute PCP due to a high failure rate; as mentioned previously, it is ineffective against extrapulmonary forms of *Pneumocystis* and is recommended only for prophylaxis for those patients unable to tolerate systemic prophylaxis. Intramuscular delivery of pentamidine is also not recommended due to the possibility of sterile abscess development following injections. Of all alternative treatment regimens, only intravenous pentamidine appears to have an efficacy equal to TMP-SMX. Dosages of 3 or 4 mg/kg (4 mg has been used more frequently) have been promising, but a number of possibly serious side effects have made this drug less desirable than TMP-SMX in PCP treatment. In practice, many experts quickly reduce the dose of pentamidine from 4 mg/kg to 3 mg/kg once the patient has shown signs of improvement from PCP. Side effects such as nephrotoxicity, pancreatitis, dysglycemia (14% of patients), thrombocytopenia, and cardiac abnormalities (torsades de pointes) have been reported. In order to prevent cardiovascular effects, pentamidine must be administered slowly. Also, there is some evidence that patients who have received either didanosine (ddI, Videx), stavudine (d4T, Zerit), or zalcitabine (ddC, HIVID) are at increased risk for pancreatitis. The ensuing pancreatic injury may be severe and is thought to be the etiology of the variable hyperglycemic or hypoglycemic events, which have the potential to lead to the development of insulin-requiring diabetes. These glucose metabolism disorders also have a propensity to affect patients with renal damage and to develop in patients taking total doses higher than 4 grams or those with previous pentamidine exposure. Instances of hypoglycemia often occur late in the course of therapy and have been reported as late as 2 weeks following discontinuation. Patients must therefore be warned about the possibility of hypoglycemia once they have been discharged from the hospital off therapy, and it is our recommendation that IV pentamidine *not* be administered at home.

Trimethoprim-Dapsone

For those with severe reactions to TMP-SMX and who are intolerant to or unable to take pentamidine, trimethoprim plus dapsone is an alternative regimen that is often better tolerated than TMP-SMX. Although it is known that this regimen has an efficacy close to TMP-SMX, it is unknown how many patients truly intolerant to TMP-SMX can tolerate this regimen. Problems with trimethoprim-dapsone arise from its inconvenience and potential for compliance issues: whereas dapsone must be taken once per day, trimethoprim must be taken three times per day. Used alone, dapsone is not effective for acute PCP. Also of note is the infrequent incidence of methemoglobinemia in some patients, or the incidence of hemolysis in patients with underlying glucose-6-phosphate dehydrogenase (G6PD) deficiency taking dapsone. Although these adverse reactions are serious, screening for G6PD deficiency is not necessary unless there is clear reason for suspicion of the condition, such as Mediterranean ancestry. This treatment can only be given orally, and recommended dosages are trimethoprim 320 mg q8 hours with dapsone 100 mg qD.

Atovaquone

Another well-tolerated drug for use in PCP is atovaquone (Mepron). A hydroxynapthoquinone that interferes with mitochondrial oxidative phosphorylation and disrupts pyrimidine synthesis in protozoa, it is highly efficacious, although not as potent a drug as TMP-SMX or intravenous pentamidine. It can only be administered orally. Side effects are less common with use of atovaquone than with TMP-SMX, but response rates are lower and relapses more frequent. Also, at the recommended dosage several days are needed in order to achieve therapeutic levels. Absorption from the gastrointestinal tract is variable (although it is increased with ingestion of a high-fat meal), and many patients report that the drug is unpleasant to taste. The use of atovaquone suspension has significantly improved the bioavailability of the drug. In practice, it is recommended that atovaquone be used in instances of mild, stable disease in patients without gastrointestinal dysfunction who are intolerant to TMP-SMX.

Trimetrexate

Trimetrexate is a well-tolerated drug that is 1,500 times more potent than trimethoprim as a dihydrofolate reductase inhibitor. It is similar to methotrexate, and its toxic effects (e.g., bone marrow suppression, mucous membrane ulceration, renal impairment) are less severe and managed well with concomitant use of folinic acid (leucovorin). Available parenterally, trimetrexate is associated with a response rate of approximately 69% in patients who have failed both TMP-SMX and pentamidine. When it was compared with TMP-SMX for moderate to severe episodes of PCP, trimetrexate plus leucovorin was found to be effective but far inferior to TMP-SMX for PCP treatment. Regarding their respective side effects, however, trimetrexate plus leucovorin was better tolerated. Although not to be used as an initial PCP therapy, it does have a role in patients unable to tolerate or who are failing other forms of treatment.

Clindamycin-Primaquine

In one large study, clindamycin plus primaquine was shown to be comparable to TMP-SMX and trimethoprim-dapsone in efficacy. Like the trimethoprim-dapsone, however, it is an inconvenient regimen in that two drugs are needed to be taken instead of the single tablet of TMP-SMX. Clindamycin is also associated with a number of adverse reactions such as rash, diarrhea, and hepatic dysfunction; primaquine, like trimethoprim-dapsone, has been associated with G6PD deficiency–related hemolysis. Like most alternative regimens, clindamycin plus primaquine is currently recommended for patients with mild PCP who do not have gastrointestinal dysfunction and are intolerant to both TMP-SMX and atovaquone.

Eflornithine

Eflornithine is yet another alternative drug for use in PCP that is currently not available in the United States. It is an irreversible inhibitor of decarboxylase that interferes with protozoal synthesis of polyamines, and its main side effect is thrombocytopenia. Like trimetrexate, it is less effective than TMP-SMX and has been recommended for use in patients in whom other drug regimens are failing or have failed.

Role of Glucocorticoids

The use of glucocorticoids along with antimicrobial therapy has become standard for moderate to severe PCP. Whereas most patients usually either stabilize or improve within 24 to 48 hours of initiation of antimicrobial therapy, AIDS patients with PCP tend to worsen for the first 3 days of treatment, especially in moderate to severe cases. Improvement is often not noted until the end of the first week. This phenomenon is thought to be attributed to the body's inflammatory response to the high number of killed organisms in the lungs. For patients with more serious cases of PCP, this potentially dangerous response has resulted in increased morbidity rates during early stages of treatment. The addition of glucocorticoids to treatment regimens has been found to markedly reduce this inflammation and its adverse clinical consequences. Current indications for steroid use are for any HIV-infected patient with moderate to severe PCP, defined by a room air O_2 pressure less than 70 mm Hg or an alveolar-arterial O_2 gradient greater than 35 mm Hg. When used in this setting, PCP clinically improves faster with glucocorticoids than without. Many clinical trials have affirmed the benefits of glucocorticoid use, with an estimated 50% decrease in mortality of hospitalized patients (from 40% to 20%) and a 50% decrease in mortality of patients requiring ventilatory support. Common side effects include irritability and oral thrush. Studies have shown that when used correctly for relatively short periods (1 to 3 weeks), long-term adjunctive use of steroids has not been found to increase either the mortality or risk of most common HIV-associated complications.

Glucocorticoid therapy, similar to any anti-PCP regimen, should be started as soon as possible once an empiric diagnosis is made, preferably no later than 36 to 72 hours. This time period is important, since glucocorticoid therapy added later in the course of PCP has not been found to confer any benefits to infected patients and has actually been associated with an increased risk of additional opportunistic infections. Also, if at any time during the course of the illness a room air O_2 pressure measures below 70 mm Hg or an alveolar-arterial O_2 gradient measures above 35 mm Hg, it is recommended to initiate glucocorticoid therapy regardless of the time elapsed since diagnosis. It is not known whether there is any benefit of glucocorticoid use in patients whose room air O_2 pressure is greater than 70 mm Hg, since the mortality rates of this population are so low already. The standard recommendation for duration of glucocorticoid therapy is 21 days, although many clinicians rapidly taper steroids over 7 to 10 days in patients demonstrating an adequate response to treatment (Table 7-1).

Role of Respiratory Isolation

For hospitalized patients with PCP, the necessity of respiratory isolation is an issue that often arises. Although rodent studies have proven that *Pneumocystis* is an airborne pathogen that can be transmitted to other animals of the same species, human *Pneumocystis* is immunologically distinct from the rodent species; it is unknown whether the organisms can be transmitted through the airborne route. This mode of infection has been suggested, however. Studies have demonstrated human *Pneumocystis* present in random air samples, and higher numbers of organisms have been found in samples drawn near patients with active PCP. Current evidence has also proposed that patients who have suffered multiple episodes of PCP are infected with different strains of *Pneumocystis*, which would suggest that the disease could be due to exposure to new strains and not to reactivation of latent infection. However, while it appears that patient-to-patient transmission is a possibility, the general approach in most U.S. hospitals and the current guidelines of the Centers for Disease Control and Prevention are not to place PCP patients in respiratory isolation.

Salvage Therapy

In general terms, once a diagnosis of PCP is either suspected or established, appropriate systemic therapy with one of the above regimens should be initiated as soon as possible. Most clinicians will begin PCP therapy empirically prior to tissue diagnosis. TMP-SMX should always be the first choice in therapy unless there is a history of life-threatening reaction. For patients with moderate to severe disease, a glucocorticoid such as methylprednisolone (Solu-Medrol) at 40 mg IV q6 to 12 hours should also be included in the regimen within 36 to 72 hours. Physicians should expect clinical or physiologic improvement within 4 to 8 days using the recommended treatment regimens described above. Because of this delay, any switch of therapy before day 6 would be considered premature and is not recommended.

Although no organized studies have been performed investigating the optimal time to switch therapy or the best regimens to use, it is advisable to treat suspected PCP aggressively while always searching for other possible etiologies. If a patient deteriorates on adequate therapy, one should carefully investigate other pulmonary processes that are occurring concurrently or are the primary etiology of the disease. This assessment can be quickly accomplished through a repeat chest radiograph and a careful history and physical examina-

TABLE 7-1
Therapy for Acute PCP Infection

Drug	Dosage	Toxicities	Comments
Trimethoprim-sulfamethoxazole (TMP-SMX, Bactrim)	Trimethoprim 15 mg/kg IV or PO qD in 3-4 divided doses (TMP/SMX ratio fixed with all forms)	Nausea, rash, fever, pruritus, GI intolerance, anaphylaxis, pancytopenia, hyperkalemia, hepatitis, pancreatitis, renal failure, tremor, ataxia, aseptic meningitis	First-line therapy Effective in 90% of patients Side effects dose-related May be necessary to hold myelosuppressive drugs (i.e., zidovudine)
Pentamidine (Pentam)	3 or 4 mg/kg IV qD	Fever, rash, urticaria, anaphylaxis, nephrotoxicity, pancreatitis, dysglycemia, thrombocytopenia, cardiac abnormalities, hypotension	Administer slowly to reduce cardiac effects and hypotension Increased pancreatitis risk with ddI, d4T, ddC Hypoglycemia can occur up to 2 weeks after discontinuation Do not administer at home
Trimethoprim + dapsone	Trimethoprim 15 mg/kg IV or PO qD Dapsone 100 mg PO qD	Rash, pruritus, GI intolerance, headache, hepatitis, agranulocytosis, methemoglobinemia, hemolysis (G6PD deficiency–related), peripheral neuropathy	Less convenient than TMP-SMX
Atovaquone (Mepron)	750 mg PO BID	Rash, GI intolerance, fever, insomnia	For mild-moderate PCP (A-a O_2 gradient <45 mm Hg, Pao_2 >70 mm Hg) No life-threatening side effects
Trimetrexate (Neutrexin)	45 mg/m^2 IV qD over 60-90 min Leucovorin 20 mg/m^2 IV or PO q6 hours	Bone marrow suppression, oral and GI ulceration, renal impairment, hypotension, pancreatitis, dysglycemia, hepatic toxicity	Decreased bone marrow, oral, GI, renal, and hepatic effects with use of leucovorin (folinic acid)
Clindamycin + primaquine	Clindamycin 600-900 mg IV or 300-450 mg PO, q6-8 hrs Primaquine 15 mg PO qD	Diarrhea, nausea, vomiting, rash, anorexia, hepatic dysfunction, hemolysis (G6PD deficiency–related)	Less convenient regimen Recommended for mild PCP infection
Glucocorticoids	Methylprednisolone (Solu-Medrol) 40 mg IV q6-12 hrs or prednisone 40 mg PO qD Taper according to patient response	Thrush, irritability	For moderate-severe PCP (A-a O_2 gradient >35 mm Hg, Pao_2 <70 mm Hg) Should be started as soon as possible (within 36-72 hrs) No increase in mortality or opportunistic infection risk

tion to search for other possible processes. Repeat bronchoscopy is recommended only if 10 to 14 days of adequate therapy are shown to be failing. Suspected community-acquired pneumonias can be treated empirically with a fluoroquinolone, and empiric therapies for other possible bacterial infections can be considered as well. Noninfectious processes, such as heart failure, bronchospasm, adult respiratory distress syndrome (ARDS), or pulmonary emboli, must also be considered and investigated if suspected. Finally, even if a patient's oxygenation status does not dictate its use, the addition of glucocorticoids would not be unreasonable when treatment appears to be failing.

If no improvement is noted after 7 to 10 days of therapy, it would then be reasonable to consider a change in therapy. If the patient is on TMP-SMX, it is recommended to first switch to intravenous pentamidine due to the high efficacy of the regimen. Side effects can potentially be more serious with this drug, and it has been reported that patients exposed to didanosine, zalcitabine, or stavudine are at a higher risk for pentamidine-induced pancreatitis. Therefore care must be taken with administration of this regimen. Trimetrexate is the drug of choice following failure of both TMP-SMX and intravenous pentamidine. As above, bone marrow suppression with its use can be controlled with concurrent use of leucovorin. If a patient on an initial regimen other than TMP-SMX is failing after 7 to 10 days of therapy, it is strongly recommended that TMP-SMX be started in the patient, even if desensitization in the intensive care unit is required. For both scenarios, clindamycin plus primaquine has been reported to help in some cases of salvage therapy, but the limitation of the exclusive oral administration of primaquine and the ineffectiveness of clindamycin used alone have made regimens such as trimetrexate a more popular third-drug alternative behind TMP-SMX and intravenous pentamidine.

Mechanical Ventilation

In severe cases of PCP, mechanical ventilation is often required to prevent respiratory failure. Although not appropriate for many end-stage AIDS patients, it may be a viable option for some if the disease is believed to be reversible. Patients who should be considered for mechanical ventilation include those who have had a good quality of life prior to the onset of PCP, who have received less than 7 to 10 days of therapy, who have not received glucocorticoids, and who have reversible processes such as heart failure, concomitant bacterial pneumonia, or pneumothorax complicating their disease. For those patients on mechanical ventilation, the long-term goals of this intervention and a realistic prognosis must be reevaluated daily. Of utmost importance, however, is that physicians discuss the option of mechanical ventilation, along with other options, with their patients before its use is mandated.

Prophylaxis

Over the past decade, HIV-infected patient care has moved out of hospitals and into physicians' offices. Opportunistic infections that were once primarily treated in the hospital are now prevented with effective prophylactic regimens and HAART. Of all prophylactic regimens, PCP prophylaxis has been one of the most successful and has become one of the cornerstones of HIV management. In compliant patients the incidence of the disease and associated mortality have dropped dramatically. There has been a substantial amount of evidence that PCP is a preventable disease. In addition, numerous studies have shown that the risk of acquiring PCP is inversely related to a patient's CD4+ count and viral load, that PCP occurring in patients on prophylactic therapy is usually less severe and is associated with reduced mortality rates, and that PCP prophylaxis is highly cost-effective. In addition, daily use of TMP-SMX prophylaxis substantially reduces the risk of toxoplasma encephalopathy as well. A recent Johns Hopkins retrospective study reported that all PCP cases that were lethal or required admission to the intensive care unit occurred in patients who had not received prophylaxis. Further analysis of these data speculated that PCP prophylaxis would save an average of 60 lives per year and $5 million in health care costs annually.

For patients with CD4+ counts below 200 cells/mm^3, chemoprophylaxis for PCP has long been considered standard management. Other indications for prophylaxis are patients with a CD4+ percentage of 15 or lower, a past history of PCP, HIV-associated oropharyngeal thrush, or unexplained fevers >100° F (37.8° C) for more than 2 weeks. Although helpful, these criteria only provide a guideline and are by no means absolute, as evidenced by the substantial number of patients who still acquire PCP today. These patients are usually atypical in presentation in that they usually do not manifest with oral thrush or fevers, and their CD4+ counts are usually above 200 cells/mm^3. Because of these instances, other predictors for those at risk for PCP or criteria for prophylaxis initiation would undoubtedly be helpful for clinicians. In practice, viral load levels serve as a marker for disease activity and antiretroviral efficacy in individual patients. Although there are no established guidelines by which to use viral load levels in prophylaxis initiation, it would not be unreasonable to use this parameter as a rough marker for PCP risk in an HIV-infected patient. For example, a patient with a high viral load of >50,000 copies/ml and a current CD4+ count between 200 and 300 cells/mm^3 would be a good candidate for PCP prophylaxis. Likewise, it would also be reasonable to consider rapidly falling CD4+ levels in the face of high viral loads as an indicator for possible PCP risk. Additional possible predictors of PCP risk are clinical markers such as the occurrence of a past AIDS-defining event or AIDS-related wasting. Although there currently are insufficient data on the use of these parameters as predictors of PCP risk, they can certainly be of some help to physicians presented with possible high-risk patients who do not fit any major criteria for prophylaxis initiation.

The absolute use of a CD4+ count below 200 cells/mm^3 as an indication for PCP prophylaxis has caused a considerable amount of confusion and has raised many as of yet unresolved questions. First, a definitive interpretation of CD4+ levels as a marker of risk for opportunistic infections has yet to be established, especially for those patients on HAART with or without a protease inhibitor. It is not known whether or not antiretroviral therapy conveys any additional protection against PCP, and it is not known whether the risk of developing an opportunistic infection at a certain CD4+ cell count is equivalent between patients receiving antiretroviral therapy and those who are not. Another common issue of debate presents itself when physicians are confronted with patients who at one time had a CD4+ count less than 200 cells/mm^3, and due to a change in their antiretroviral regimen rebounded their CD4+ count to a level greater than 200 cells/mm^3. Should PCP prophylaxis be continued in these patients? In a recent retrospective study in the *New England Journal of Medicine*, Furrier et al demonstrated that prophylaxis could cautiously be discontinued in these patients provided that their viral load was stable or decreasing. In their study, 262 patients whose CD4+ counts had risen above 200 cells/mm^3 or to at least 14% of their total peripheral lymphocytes for at least 12 weeks while on combination antiretroviral therapy were studied. These patients discontinued

TABLE 7-2
Chemoprophylactic Regimens for PCP

Drug	Dosage	Comments
Trimethoprim-sulfamethoxazole (TMP-SMX, Bactrim)	1 double-strength (DS) tablet qD Alternatively: 1 single-strength tablet qD 1 DS tablet TIW	First-line prophylaxis Higher patient tolerance with gradual dosage increases over 6-14 days Can rechallenge after 2 weeks if reaction not life-threatening
Dapsone (+ pyrimethamine, leucovorin)	Dapsone 100 mg PO qD *or* 50 mg PO BID Pyrimethamine 50-75 mg PO q week *or* 50 mg PO BIW Leucovorin 25 mg PO q week	Second-line prophylaxis Pyrimethamine adds *Toxoplasma* prophylaxis Leucovorin decreases side effects
Aerosolized pentamidine	300 mg q month	Third-line prophylaxis No protection from other pathogens Albuterol pretreatment decreases bronchospasm
Atovaquone (Mepron)	750 mg PO qD	Third-line prophylaxis Can use up to 1,500 mg qD No antibacterial activity, sufficient *Toxoplasma* prophylaxis, costly

their *P. carinii* prophylaxis and were followed a median of 11.3 months. During this time, while prophylaxis was resumed in nine patients and two patients died, no cases of PCP were reported. Incidence of PCP in these patients was calculated to be 1.9 cases per 100 patient-years (Table 7-2).

Trimethoprim-Sulfamethoxazole

As in acute PCP treatment, TMP-SMX is the drug of choice for PCP prophylaxis. When compared with other regimens, it is more effective, relatively better tolerated, and less expensive. Every study to date has demonstrated that TMP-SMX is either superior to or as effective as all other drugs used for PCP prophylaxis. In a controlled trial comparing TMP-SMX with aerosolized pentamidine for prophylaxis, recurrence rates at 18 months were 11.4% (14/154) with TMP-SMX, and 27.6% (36/156) with aerosolized pentamidine, with one extrapulmonary recurrence. Other more recent studies have reported failure rates due to PCP breakthrough ranging from 0% to 18% using standard prophylactic dosages in large populations of PCP naive patients with CD4+ <200 cells/mm^3. Another advantage of trimethoprim-sulfamethoxazole is that clinical research has shown that it offers protection from bacterial respiratory infections and toxoplasmosis in HIV-infected patients as well. Susceptible pathogens include *Isospora, Salmonella, Listeria, Nocardia, Legionella, Haemophilus influenzae, Streptococcus pneumoniae, Staphylococcus aureus*, and many gram-negative bacilli. In contrast, as stated above the use of aerosolized pentamidine has been associated with increased incidence of pneumothorax and disseminated pneumocystosis, while a study of dapsone was prematurely stopped when it was observed that a greater number of patients on dapsone died of bacterial infection when compared with those on TMP-SMX.

True PCP infection in compliant individuals who are on TMP-SMX prophylaxis is very uncommon, with most disease occurring in hosts with CD4+ counts below 50 cells/mm^3. In these cases of breakthrough, a poor host response is speculated to be the culprit rather than organism resistance to TMP-SMX. Although the difficulty in growing *P. carinii* in vitro has made it close to impossible to detect resistance, current genetic research has shown that mutations can occur that could create drug resistance. These data are preliminary at this point, however, and as of yet *P. carinii* resistance has not been proven.

Again, as in PCP treatment with TMP-SMX, side effects for TMP-SMX prophylaxis are quite common, with 25% to 50% of patients requiring complete discontinuation of the drug, usually due to rash, fevers, and nausea. Less common side effects include pruritus, hepatitis, pancreatitis, anemia, neutropenia, thrombocytopenia, aseptic meningitis, interstitial nephritis, crystalluria, and gastrointestinal toxicity. These adverse reactions appear to be dose-related, and whether they are allergic or IgE-mediated is not clear.

The most common dosing regimen for PCP prophylaxis is a single DS tablet once daily, although preliminary studies have shown no change in efficacy in patients using the better-tolerated SS tablets instead. In TMP-SMX–sensitive patients, it would therefore be reasonable to begin therapy with one SS tablet qD. Currently, two other alternatives are available to TMP-SMX–sensitive patients. First, studies have reported higher patient tolerance to gradual dosing "desensitization" regimens that slowly increase dosages of TMP-SMX over 6 to 14 days rather than beginning with full doses. Secondly, when used for PCP prophylaxis, one DS tablet three times a week has been reported to be as effective in both primary (PCP-naive) and secondary (previous PCP) prophylactic regimens as one DS tablet daily. This regimen is not without risk, however, since significant increases in toxoplasmosis and bacterial infections such as sinusitis and pneumonia were also reported in patients receiving one DS tablet three times a week. Because of these complications of the latter regimen, gradual dosing of TMP-SMX is most commonly used in practice in patients with Bactrim intolerance. Rechallenging of patients previously intolerant to TMP-SMX has a role in PCP prevention as well. Current recommendations of the U.S. Public Health Service Task Force on PCP Prophylaxis call for discontinuation of TMP-SMX for 2 weeks, with resumption of the same dose or lower dose if the reaction was not life-threatening. During rechallenging, a gradual dose-escalating regimen can also be used to reduce the possibility of adverse reaction formation. If a patient has a history of life-threatening reaction to TMP-SMX, however, rechallenging is not recommended. The AIDS Clinical Trial Group 021 study showed that rates of reaction to TMP-SMX during rechallenge were essentially the same between patients with a previous history of reaction and those without such history (31% vs. 26%, respectively). Other rechallenge studies show that close to half of patients with mild to moderate reactions will be able to tolerate TMP-SMX after a 2-week drug holiday.

Dapsone

For those who cannot tolerate any dosing regimen of TMP-SMX, dapsone prophylaxis is considered the best alternative. A sulfone, as opposed to TMP-SMX, which is a sulfonamide, dapsone is tolerated in close to 80% of patients intolerant to TMP-SMX. Dapsone prophylaxis is still associated with relatively severe side effects, however, and in 25% to 40% of cases they lead to its discontinuation. These side effects are the same as those seen with PCP therapy with dapsone and include rash, fever, methemoglobinemia, and particularly in patients with G6PD deficiency, hemolysis. Also as in PCP therapy with dapsone, routine testing of G6PD deficiency or monitoring of methemoglobinemia is generally not practiced in dapsone-treated patients despite these side effects. Usual dapsone dosing for PCP prophylaxis is 50 mg orally bid or 100 mg orally qD. Unlike TMP-SMX, reductions in dapsone dosage are not associated with improved tolerability and are not recommended because of the loss of effectiveness with less than full doses. Also, as stated above, another limitation of dapsone prophylaxis is that alone it does not have any antibacterial activity. Antitoxoplasma activity is gained when dapsone is administered with pyrimethamine, which has been given in doses of 50 to 75 mg orally once per week or 50 mg orally twice per week. Leucovorin is effective in reducing adverse reactions associated with dapsone when used in doses of 25 mg orally once per week. Many experts use this combination of dapsone, pyrimethamine, and leucovorin as an effective alternative for patients intolerant to TMP-SMX.

Aerosolized Pentamidine

Aerosolized pentamidine is another alternative for PCP prophylaxis that is especially effective for patients with CD4+ counts above 100 cells/mm^3. The drug is usually delivered with a Respirgard II nebulizer (Marquest, Englewood, CO) in doses of 300 mg monthly, although some uncontrolled studies have shown greater efficacy with a monthly dose of 600 mg or biweekly doses of 300 mg. Aerosolized pentamidine is better tolerated than TMP-SMX, with only 2% to 4% of patients with adverse reactions severe enough to discontinue its use. Its efficacy as a prophylactic regimen is below that of TMP-SMX, however, with reported failure rates ranging from 5.1% to 23.1%. A modest number of patients experience bronchospasm, which can be minimized with albuterol pretreatment. Rarely, aerosolized pentamidine has been reported to produce pancreatitis, although a causal relationship between aerosolized pentamidine and pancreatitis has yet to be established. Its use is known to cause an increased risk of pneumothorax, however. A major disadvantage of aerosolized pentamidine is that it provides no protection against other pathogens, including extrapulmonary *Pneumocystis*. Also, the bronchospasm created by its use has the potential to be a possible source of respiratory pathogen transmission to other patients in an unprotected environment. In some reports, tuberculosis outbreaks have been associated with aerosolized pentamidine facilities. In order to protect against the possibility of such an event, the drug must be delivered in a negative pressure room in the hospital or at the patient's home.

Atovaquone

Little data are available on the use of atovaquone as PCP prophylaxis. In two recent trials, atovaquone in a daily dose of 1,500 mg of liquid suspension had an efficacy comparable to aerosolized pentamidine or oral dapsone. Currently, however, 750 mg/day of atovaquone suspension is an acceptable regimen. Although atovaquone has no antibacterial activity, its effectiveness in preventing toxoplasmosis is good. Two disadvantages of atovaquone prophylaxis are its poor taste and high cost. Atovaquone averages $7,000 to $9,000/year compared with TMP-SMX or dapsone, which costs <$100/year.

The above-described PCP prophylaxis agents are currently the only regimens with established efficacy. However, some studies have reported relative amounts of success with other alternative regimens such as pyrimethamine plus sulfadiazine, azithromycin plus standard PCP prophylaxis, intravenous pentamidine, clindamycin plus primaquine, and clindamycin plus pyrimethamine. Although usually given as therapy for toxoplasmic encephalitis, pyrimethamine plus sulfadiazine has been shown to be effective PCP prophylaxis as well. Intravenous pentamidine has shown some efficacy as a prophylactic regimen in some studies but not in others; substantial toxicity has been suggested in all studies, however. Finally, clindamycin plus either primaquine or pyrimethamine is often complicated by diarrhea and has not been shown to be effective.

When to Refer

Because of the efficacy of the available treatment regimens for PCP, in most cases clinicians can diagnose and treat patients with the disease in the outpatient setting. If, however, patients present late in the course of the disease or are suffering from repeated episodes of PCP and exhibit severe respiratory compromise, it would be advisable to refer them to an infectious disease specialist. Although PCP will most likely remain one of the most common diseases associated with AIDS, due to today's diagnostic and treatment modalities there should be no reason for PCP to cause significant mortality in the HIV-positive population.

Summary

Despite the recent decline in the number of cases of PCP that are seen by most clinicians, the disease remains a relatively common manifestation of HIV. Some characteristics of PCP have changed, however, with the improved diagnostic methods and treatment options available. Once a disease usually seen in its late stages in the hospital, PCP is now almost primarily seen and treated in outpatient settings. If recognized quickly and treated aggressively, it is easily treated and can be avoided with the strict use of prophylactic regimens. TMP-SMX remains the drug of choice for both treatment and prophylaxis of PCP, but many other options exist for those patients who are unable to tolerate it. Concurrent use of steroids in therapy has also been found to greatly improve outcome in those patients with moderate to severe PCP and should be used when necessary. Overall, PCP is an easily treatable disease, and as long as clinicians are vigilant and are able to recognize PCP in symptomatic patients there is no reason for patients with PCP to have the poor outcomes seen in the past.

KEY POINTS

- PCP is still extremely common in the HIV-positive patient population
- *Prompt* diagnosis and treatment dramatically improve prognosis
- First-line therapy: trimethoprim-sulfamethoxazole
- Glucocorticoid use improves prognosis in moderate to severe cases
- First-line prophylaxis: trimethoprim-sulfamethoxazole

SUGGESTED READINGS

Castro M: Treatment and prophylaxis of *Pneumocystis carinii* pneumonia, *Semin Respir Infect* 13(4):296-303, 1998.

Donlin R, Masur H, Saag MS: *AIDS therapy,* Philadelphia, 1999, Churchill Livingstone, pp 291-307.

Furrer H et al: Discontinuation of primary prophylaxis against *Pneumocystis carinii* pneumonia in HIV-1-infected adults treated with combination antiretroviral therapy: Swiss HIV Cohort Study, *N Engl J Med* 340(17):1301-1306, 1999.

Limper AH: Diagnosis of *Pneumocystis carinii* pneumonia: does use of only bronchoalveolar lavage suffice? *Mayo Clin Proc* 71(11): 1121-1123, 1996.

Schneider MME et al: Efficacy and toxicity of two doses of trimethoprim-sulfamethoxazole as primary prophylaxis against *Pneumocystis carinii* pneumonia in patients with human immunodeficiency virus, *J Infect Dis* 171:1632, 1995.

8 Mycobacterial Infections

ROB ROY MacGREGOR

Introduction

It should come as no surprise that tuberculosis (TB) and the nontuberculous mycobacteria represent a major threat to HIV-infected individuals, given the ubiquitous distribution of these microbes, the specialized defenses that our species has evolved against them, and the relentless progressive attack on that arm of defense represented by multiplying human immunodeficiency virus (HIV). TB has become the most common cause of death among HIV-positive individuals living in areas of the world where TB is endemic, underscoring the normally effective defense exerted by an intact cell-mediated immune (CMI) system. In areas such as the United States where endemic TB infection is low, a high incidence of disseminated infection with *Mycobacterium avium* complex (MAC) occurs only in the subgroup of HIV-infected patients who have reached the stage of profoundest immunosuppression, indicating how little CMI function is ordinarily necessary to protect against this minimally invasive organism.

The genus *Mycobacterium* is made up of at least 53 different species of slow-growing bacilli. These bacilli are characterized by a cell wall with a high lipid content that includes characteristic high-molecular-weight mycolic acids, which makes them hydrophobic and difficult to stain with standard aniline dyes. However, once stained with the aid of heating or detergents, they resist decoloration with acid-alcohol mixtures, leading to the name acid-fast bacilli (AFB). This unique cell wall structure is also thought to be responsible for the slow growth rate of the genus, with doubling times of 2 to 24 hours compared with 20 to 30 minutes for most bacteria. The best-known pathogens are *M. tuberculosis* and *M. leprae;* most of the other species are free-living environmental saprophytes, occurring in humans mainly as opportunistic pathogens, and are commonly referred to as nontuberculous mycobacteria (NTM), mycobacteria other than tuberculosis (MOTT), or historically as atypical mycobacteria. The NTM have been further divided into four groups by Runyon, based on pigment production and speed of growth. Closely related species have been grouped into complexes; hence the *M. tuberculosis* complex contains *M. tuberculosis, M. bovis, M. microti,* bacille Calmette-Guérin (BCG), and others, and the MAC includes *M. avium* and *M. intracellulare.*

In this chapter, we will first review the interaction between *M. tuberculosis* and HIV in the human host, stressing aspects of pathogenesis, diagnosis, treatment, and prevention, and then discuss nontuberculous mycobacterial infections, primarily those caused by MAC.

Tuberculosis
Pathogenesis

Lesions consistent with TB can be found in Stone Age human skeletons, and mummified remains have been shown to carry genetic sequences of *M. tuberculosis.* Thus the organism can be viewed as one of the selective pressures on the evolving human immune system, which helps to explain why cell-mediated immune mechanisms are normally quite effective in controlling primary tuberculous infection in most healthy adults. During initial infection, the organisms are ingested by macrophages and carried to regional nodes, where the process of antigen presentation leads to development of an expanding population of T-lymphocytes with specific ability to recognize the organism's lipid-rich cell wall antigens. Production of Th-1 cytokines, such as interleukin-2 (IL-2), interferon-γ, and tumor necrosis factor (TNF), by CD4+ cells that recognize *M. tuberculosis* antigens appears critical to effective lymphocyte/macrophage control of infection, although details of these interactions remain ambiguous. Normally, this robust cell-mediated immune response induces a granulomatous inflammatory reaction at sites of infection, with caseous necrosis, control of bacterial proliferation, and killing of most but not all organisms. With healing of the primary infection, patients are left with latent tuberculous infection. This state of latent infection can be detected by the intradermal injection of purified protein extract (PPD) from cultured *M. tuberculosis,* which induces accumulation of sensitized lymphocytes at the injection site. This is detected as palpable induration—a "positive" tuberculin test. Infected patients are thought to remain at life-long risk for reactivation of their infection, related to local tissue factors and reduced cell-mediated immune activity; when this occurs, one then has active tuberculous disease.

HIV infection modifies the normal cell-mediated immune responses to *M. tuberculosis* in several ways. CD4+ cells are progressively reduced, and those remaining have decreased capacity to secrete interferon-γ; moreover, macrophages from HIV-infected patients have a reduced ability to kill intracellular mycobacteria. Active TB infection also promotes HIV replication: lymphocytes and macrophages taken from HIV-infected individuals and exposed to *M. tuberculosis* in vitro have increased viral production, probably secondary to augmented TNF-α production by macrophages. The impact of HIV-induced depression of CD4+ lymphocyte counts is demonstrated in multivariate analyses that show a reduced CD4+ count to be the strongest predictor for the development of reactivation TB in dually infected subjects; in addition, TB mortality correlates directly with the degree of immunosuppression. Also, development of active TB in HIV-positive patients accelerates the course of HIV disease progression, doubling the risk of death compared with CD4+-matched patients without TB.

The outcome of dual infection with HIV and *M. tuberculosis* in an individual patient depends on which pathogen arrived first. If latent TB infection is established before the acquisition of HIV (the common situation in areas of the world where TB is endemic and primary infection is usually acquired in childhood), the subsequent acquisition of HIV infection begins the process of progressive immunosuppression, which gradually increases the likelihood of reactivation disease. Risk of reactivation begins to increase with early HIV infection but increases as the CD4+ count falls. The yearly risk of developing active TB in such patients is estimated at 5% to 10%, with a cumulative risk of >50% by time of death from AIDS. In contrast, HIV-negative subjects have an estimated yearly risk of reactivation of 0.1% to 0.2%, or 5% over their lifetime. In the AIDS Clinical Trials Group/Community Programs for Clinical Research on AIDS (ACTG/CPCRA) combined treatment trial for active TB in HIV-positive subjects, although some cases had CD4+ cell counts above 700 cells/mm^3 at the time of TB diagnosis, the median CD4+ cell count was only 70 cells/mm^3. This very high risk of reactivation over the time course of HIV infection has made TB the most common opportunistic infection among HIV-positive patients in areas of the world where TB is endemic, and the most common cause of death.

In contrast, if HIV infection occurs before primary TB is acquired, the course of TB infection is dependent on the degree of immunosuppression at the time that TB infection is acquired. When the CD4+ cell count is near normal, TB tends to behave in a manner similar to that in HIV-negative subjects, but with advanced immunosuppression, primary TB infection cannot be controlled, and subjects acquiring new infection have progressed from diagnosis of their active TB infection to death in 1 to 3 months in the absence of effective therapy. Explosive epidemics of primary disease have been documented among acquired immunodeficiency syndrome (AIDS) patients in hospital clinics, prisons, and shelters. In addition, the likelihood of extrapulmonary disease, often with positive blood cultures, rather than pulmonary disease increases as the CD4+ cell count falls, indicating more profound immunosuppression. This vulnerability to TB dictates a high index of suspicion for the disease in patients with advanced HIV disease, including use of pressure-negative hospital isolation rooms and empirical treatment (see below).

Epidemiology

It is estimated that one third of the world's population is infected with *M. tuberculosis,* with tuberculin reactor rates of up to 80% in parts of Africa and the Far East. The World Health Organization (WHO) estimates that >95% of all HIV-infected people live in the Third World and that more than half have also been infected with *M. tuberculosis.* The coexistence of malnutrition and other chronic diseases among these people increases the risk of active TB even further, making it the "epidemic within the epidemic" and responsible for about 30% of deaths among AIDS patients in the developing world. In the United States, a yearly 5% to 6% reduction in the number of newly reported TB cases that began in the 1950s leveled off in 1985 and began to climb, reaching a peak of 26,673 cases in 1992 (10.5 cases/100,000 population). This reversal of the downward trend was largely attributable to AIDS-related cases. The situation was complicated by a deteriorating public health infrastructure that allowed up to 90% of patients with active TB who were admitted to some inner city hospitals to be lost to follow-up, leading to a surge of multidrug-resistant (MDR) cases. Particularly in New York City and in prison settings, these MDR cases occurred in the same social strata as HIV, creating epidemics of rapidly progressive, often poorly responsive TB. This public health threat galvanized the public and their elected officials to recommit needed funds to TB control measures. Fortunately, these efforts, particularly the use of directly observed therapy (DOT), have been successful in stemming the tide of new cases (drug-susceptible and MDR) and reestablishing the downward trend of the last 50 years: in 1998, the annual incidence in the United States fell to 18,361 cases, or 6.8/100,000 population, the lowest in history.

TB in the United States is a disease that disproportionately affects people living in poverty and social disorganization. Tuberculin reactor rates have been found as high as 30% in inner city methadone clinic populations compared with less than 2% among suburban school children. Similarly, HIV is also increasingly affecting our country's disadvantaged inner city and rural poor subpopulations: minority group members account for two thirds of newly reported adult AIDS cases and >80% of pediatric cases. The Centers for Disease Control and Prevention (CDC) has recommended that all newly diagnosed cases of TB be HIV tested. A Miami study found that 31% of new cases were seropositive for HIV, even though only 28% had any symptoms suggestive of HIV infection. A CDC study found rates of 46% in New York City and 13% to 33% elsewhere on the East Coast, and San Francisco reported that 28% of new TB cases were HIV-positive. The positive subjects were more likely to be male, to be between 18 and 45 years old, to be a minority group member, and to have a history of injecting drug use or male-male sexual activity. Noteworthy is the fact that most had no signs or symptoms of their HIV infection. Unfortunately, many TB programs have a poor record of obtaining HIV tests in their new TB cases; this should be an important priority because of the high yield when performed and the implications of dual infection for the patient.

Data on the percent of AIDS patients for whom TB was the initial opportunistic infection are available from the CDC's "Spectrum of HIV Disease" project. Between 1992 and 1997, of 10,658 men reported on, 4.8% had pulmonary TB and another 2.0% had extrapulmonary disease. For women, the percentages were 6.6% and 3.0%, respectively. Thus discovery of latent TB infection in HIV-positive individuals by tuberculin testing, and intervening with preemptive prophylactic treatment, is another priority in good HIV-infected patient management (see below).

MDR TB—defined as resistance to at least isoniazid and rifampin—broke on the national consciousness between 1990 and 1992, when the CDC and local investigators reported six outbreaks of MDR TB involving more than 200 patients. Most patients had HIV infection, with advanced immunosuppression, and had rapid progression of their disease, often dying 4 to 12 weeks after diagnosis, before it was clear that their organisms were resistant to standard treatment. Clear person-to-person transmission of MDR strains was documented in hospital wards, outpatient settings, and prisons, with rapid spread among patients lacking normal immune defenses. The fact that the outbreaks occurred among such defenseless patients and caused such rapidly fatal disease actually allowed for the earlier discovery of the epidemic than would have been possible had the secondary cases mounted a normal immune response. Fortunately, the initiation of appropriate measures to isolate infectious patients and to individualize effective multidrug treatments has resulted in containment of these outbreaks. Moreover, their explosive destructive nature sobered the nation so that excellent diagnostic and multidrug treatment programs have been established, and the widespread use of directly observed therapy has greatly reduced the potential for development of new MDR strains. Data from 1998 indicate that MDR strains accounted for 1.1% of isolates tested (down from 2.8% in 1993).

Clinical Presentation

Because *M. tuberculosis* disseminates during primary infection, sites of clinical disease can be anywhere in the body, and manifestations can be protean. Therefore TB should at least be *considered* in any progressive wasting, especially when associated with fever and complaints related to virtually any organ system. This general caution is magnified the lower the CD4+ cell count is in an HIV-positive patient.

TB that develops early in HIV infection usually has a typical presentation and course: a majority of cases are pulmonary and should not present a diagnostic challenge. As immunosuppression progresses, the clinical presentations are often less typical, and the incidence of extrapulmonary disease, although often associated with concomitant pulmonary TB, can be >50%. A study from the Los Angeles County Medical Center of 97 HIV-positive patients admitted with positive cultures for *M. tuberculosis* found that 46% had only pulmonary disease, 44% had pulmonary and extrapulmonary infection, and 10% had only extrapulmonary sites of active infection. The frequency of extrapulmonary disease was quite dependent on the patient's level of immunosuppression, varying from 70% (30/43) in those with CD4+ cell counts below 100 cells/mm^3 to only 28% (5/18) in those with CD4+ counts above 300 (Table 8-1). Blood was the most common extrapulmonary site for positive cultures, and was very CD4+-dependent: 49% in those with CD4+ counts <100 cells/mm^3, 20% in those in the 100 to 200 cell range, 7% in those in the 200 to 300 cell range, and 0 in those >300 cells/mm^3—demonstrating how important CD4+ cell function is in preventing bacteremia/dissemination. After blood, lymph nodes are the next most common extrapulmonary site of infection, with the central nervous system (CNS), pleura, pericardium, genitourinary tract, and even skin reported as significant sites of infection. CNS disease can present as ring-enhancing or hypodense mass lesions without pulmonary disease or as tuberculous meningitis; often both are present together. Positive cerebrospinal fluid (CSF) cultures and/or AFB smears can occur without CSF leukocytosis.

Tuberculin skin tests demonstrated >10 mm induration in 39% of patients with AIDS and TB in a San Francisco General study, compared with 91% in pre-AIDS TB cases. The Los Angeles County study reported PPD reactions >5 mm in 0/13 TB patients with CD4+ counts <100 cells/mm^3, 8/13

TABLE 8-1
Los Angeles County Medical Center Study of Pulmonary and Extrapulmonary (EP) TB

CD4+ range	With EP infection	Blood +	Blood only EP site
<100 cells/mm^3	70%	49%	43%
100-200 cells/mm^3	50%	20%	10%
200-300 cells/mm^3	44%	7%	0%
>300 cells/mm^3	28%	0%	0%

(61%) in the 100 to 200 CD4+ stratum, 5/12 (42%) at 200 to 300, and 10/11 (91%) at >300. In a similar fashion, biopsies from infected tissues have granulomata in only about 50% of cases, again related to the patient's CD4+ cell count.

Chest radiographs can show changes typical for reactivation apical cavitary disease, a progressive primary infection picture, or any phase in between, depending on the stage of HIV disease. Patients with advanced disease often have a picture of progressive primary TB, with hilar and/or mediastinal adenopathy, pleural effusions, and infiltrates either in the lower lung fields or in a diffuse miliary pattern. A diffuse infiltrate in a patient with a very low CD4+ cell count often suggests *Pneumocystis carinii* pneumonia (PCP), but PCP rarely causes hilar adenopathy or pleural effusions. Although the presence of adenopathy is typical of primary infection in an immunocompetent person, molecular strain typing of isolates from patients with HIV infection indicates that adenopathy also occurs with reactivation disease when patients have poor cell-mediated immunity. In fact, a study of 135 cases in HIV-infected patients showed that the CD4+ cell count was a sensitive predictor of adenopathy: adenopathy was present in 30% of patients with CD4+ cell counts below 200 cells/mm^3, compared with 7% of those with higher counts (odds ratio of 5.9). The typical x-ray appearance of reactivation TB, apical cavitary infiltrates, without adenopathy occurs in <10% of patients with advanced HIV infection. Several series report that 5% to 10% of patients with bacteriologically proven active pulmonary TB had normal chest radiographs, although some of these show disease on computed tomography (CT).

Diagnosis

Diagnostic methods for identifying mycobacteria have advanced considerably in the past 10 years, so that it now is possible to isolate and identify specific organisms from sputum and other body sites in days to weeks rather than months. Generally, it is not more difficult to culture *M. tuberculosis* from HIV-infected patients than from those without HIV. Smears of sputum, now generally examined with fluorescent stains (which are faster and more sensitive than Kinyoun staining), are positive in approximately half of pulmonary cases, including some with negative chest x-rays. Some studies have reported a smaller percentage positive, perhaps owing to the low frequency of cavitary disease. When smears are positive, the use of rapid TB nucleic acid amplification tests directly on sputum can provide specific identification of *M. tuberculosis* in 24 to 48 hours, with a specificity and sensitivity of >95%. It has recently been approved for use with negative smears, but the positive and negative predictive values are considerably worse than with positive smears. Because of their expense, use of the molecular probes should be limited to situations in which the diagnosis is strongly in doubt and empirical therapy is problematic. Critical in patient evaluation is understanding that *a negative smear does not eliminate the diagnosis of active TB.* Traditionally, cultures have been performed on solid medium and normally take 3 or more weeks to produce testable growth. Liquid growth systems have now become generally available that can detect growth in 1 to 2 weeks. Isolates from either system can now be submitted to nucleic acid probe tests, which can give rapid identification of *M. tuberculosis, M. kansasii, M. avium* complex, and *M. gordonae,* without waiting for slower biochemical testing. Thus current technology will permit specific diagnosis of *M. tuberculosis* from positive sputum smears within 24 to 48 hours, and from culture growth in 1 to 2 weeks. Molecular probing of tissue specimens is still under development. Because of the threat of MDR TB, all isolates should undergo drug susceptibility testing. Conventional testing takes 3 weeks after the primary isolate is obtained, whereas rapid liquid systems can yield results in 5 to 7 days. When smears are positive, direct testing can be attempted by inoculation of the primary specimen onto conventional solid medium, potentially shortening the testing process by 3 weeks. At present, the rapid liquid method is not effective with primary specimens. As noted above, blood cultures are often positive, particularly in patients with low CD4+ cell counts, and should be performed in cases in which the diagnosis of TB is unclear. The method is called lysis-centrifugation, in which blood is drawn into special Isolator tubes in which the cells are lysed and the centrifuged lysate plated onto solid medium; growth is usually demonstrable in 3 to 4 weeks. Clinicians should be aware of another new technique, called restriction fragment length polymorphism (RFLP), which enzymatically cleaves an isolate's DNA into smaller segments, producing a "DNA fingerprint" pattern unique to each organism, making it possible to trace which isolates come from a common source. Although not useful in the individual patient, it is an extremely powerful tool for determining whether or not a common source outbreak is occurring, so that resources can be focused on containing it. This technique has identified common source outbreaks in hospitals, communal housing, and a dialysis unit; studies indicate that up to 50% of cases in large urban areas represent recent primary infections from several small common foci rather than reactivation of infections acquired years before.

Tuberculin testing is worthwhile in suspected cases: if reactions are >5 mm, this is consistent with prior or current infection; if nonreactive, particularly in patients with CD4+ cell counts >350 cells/mm^3, TB is less likely. (Frequency of tuberculin reactions >5 mm in patients with culture-proven active disease has been reported as 91% for patients with CD4+ counts >300 cells/mm^3, 52% for those between 100 and 300 cells/mm^3, and 0% for those below 100.)

Treatment

The response of HIV-infected patients to standard four-drug antituberculous therapy is excellent, even in those with far-advanced immunosuppression. Clinical improvement and conversion of cultures to negative appear to occur at similar rates as for HIV-negative patients. Concerns and complications in the HIV-infected population relate to duration of therapy, rates of relapse, adverse experiences from treatment drugs, and drug-drug interactions between antituberculous and antiretroviral drugs.

CDC guidelines for treating TB, independent of HIV status, call for use of four drugs for the first 2 months or until the organism is shown to be sensitive to standard drugs, followed by 4 months of isoniazid (INH) and rifampin. Use of DOT is strongly recommended, and intermittent (two or three times weekly) treatment is often used from the beginning or after an initial course of daily therapy (Table 8-2). Response to treatment of extrapulmonary TB is as good as for pulmonary disease, and the recommended duration of treatment is the same. Although 6 months of treatment has proven sufficient in most reviews of HIV-positive patients with TB, potential problems with compliance and concern that relapse rates may be higher have caused some experts to recommend a 9-month course. The guidelines from the CDC Conference on HIV-Related Tuberculosis, September 1997, recommend a minimum duration of 6 months, with 4 months of treatment after cultures convert to negative. The 9-month course is also favored for patients with advanced immunosuppression or whose clinical response to treatment is slow. Adverse reactions to antituberculous drugs have been reported to be more common among HIV-infected patients, varying from rates near normal in those with early HIV infection to three times higher in those with advanced HIV disease. Diagnosis of adverse reactions is often difficult in patients who are taking multiple other drugs and who may have coincident problems with HIV-related gastrointestinal (GI), liver, hematologic, and CNS disease. When possible, continuation of the antituberculous drugs should be attempted while potential medication-related symptoms are being evaluated.

Drug-drug interactions, particularly between rifamycins and the protease inhibitors (PIs) and non-nucleoside reverse transcriptase inhibitors (NNRTIs), are the biggest challenge in treating dually infected patients. The problem stems from the fact that rifampin and, to some extent, rifabutin are inducers of the cytochrome P450 system that metabolizes PIs and NNRTIs (Table 8-3). Rifampin causes such rapid metabolism of PIs and some NNRTIs that the CDC recommendations state that its use is *contraindicated* with these drugs because of concern that their resultant low levels will be ineffective and lead to resistance mutations in the viral population. Rifabutin is a much less active inducer of the CYP450 system, and is the recommended rifamycin for treating TB in patients receiving PI therapy. Because its coadministration lowers indinavir and nelfinavir levels by a mean of one third, their doses should be adjusted up accordingly. Rifabutin seems to have the least effect on the newer PI, amprenavir, lowering its mean levels by approximately 15%. Several clinical trials have shown rifabutin to be of comparable effectiveness to rifampin in treatment of TB.

Acute uveitis is another serious complication of rifabutin treatment in patients receiving antiretroviral therapy. The inhibition of CYP450 by PIs leads to markedly increased levels of rifabutin, normally metabolized by this system. This caused a significant incidence of uveitis in patients receiving PIs and rifabutin before the mechanism was recognized. The Depart-

TABLE 8-2
Dosage Recommendation for the Initial Treatment of Tuberculosis in Children* and Adults

	DAILY DOSE		TWICE-WEEKLY DOSE		THRICE-WEEKLY DOSE	
	Children	Adults	Children	Adults	Children	Adults
Isoniazid	10-20 mg/kg (max 300 mg)	5 mg/kg (max 300 mg)	20-40 mg/kg (max 900 mg)	15 mg/kg (max 900 mg)	20-40 mg/kg (max 900 mg)	15 mg/kg (max 900 mg)
Rifampin	10-20 mg/kg (max 600 mg)	10 mg/kg (max 600 mg)	10-20 mg/kg (max 600 mg)	10 mg/kg (max 600 mg)	10-20 mg/kg (max 600 mg)	10 mg/kg (max 600 mg)
Pyrazinamide	15-30 mg/kg (max 2 g)	15-30 mg/kg (max 2 g)	50-70 mg/kg (max 4 g)	50-70 mg/kg (max 4 g)	50-70 mg/kg (max 3 g)	50-70 mg/kg (max 3 g)
Ethambutol[†]	15-25 mg/kg	15-25 mg/kg	50 mg/kg	50 mg/kg	25-30 mg/kg	25-30 mg/kg
Streptomycin	20-40 mg/kg (max 1.0 g)	15 mg/kg (max 1.0 g)	25-30 mg/kg (max 1.5 g)	25-30 mg/kg (max 1.5 g)	25-30 mg/kg (max 1.5 g)	25-30 mg/kg (max 1.5 g)

*Children < 12 yr of age.
[†]Ethambutol is generally not recommended for children whose visual acuity cannot be monitored (< 8 yr of age). However, ethambutol should be considered for all children with organisms resistant to other drugs when susceptibility to ethambutol has been demonstrated or susceptibility is likely.

ment of Health and Human Services (DHHS) Guidelines for Antiretroviral Therapy, January 2000, recommend reduction of the rifabutin dose to 150 mg qd (or 300 mg twice or thrice weekly with DOT) when it is used with the PIs indinavir, nelfinavir, or amprenavir, or reduction to 150 mg qod or thrice weekly when used with ritonavir. Use of rifamycin with saquinavir is contraindicated. Fluconazole also inhibits the hepatic cytochrome P450 system. Thus, when fluconazole and rifabutin are coadministered, the rifabutin area under the curve (AUC) increases by 80%, and the rifabutin active metabolite increases over twofold, while fluconazole levels are unaffected. This interaction is thought to be responsible for the increased incidence of rifabutin-related uveitis in patients receiving both rifabutin and fluconazole. Clarithromycin can similarly raise rifabutin levels; azithromycin has much less effect. Patients receiving rifabutin along with PIs, clarithromycin, and/or fluconazole should be warned about the signs and symptoms of uveitis: red, painful eye or blurred vision, photophobia, or floaters.

Use of the NNRTI nevirapine with rifabutin causes modest reductions in the circulating levels of both drugs. Efavirenz reduces rifabutin levels by about 40%, and so it is recommended to increase the daily dose of rifabutin to 450 mg when efavirenz is used without a PI. Efavirenz doses do not need to be adjusted. Fortunately, the nucleoside RTIs (zidovudine [AZT], didanosine [ddI], lamivudine [3TC], stavudine [d4T], and abacavir) do not require dose adjustment when used with rifamycins, nor do doses of INH, ethambutol, pyrazinamide, or streptomycin need to be changed when they are used with PIs and NNRTIs. Owing to the complicated nature of these drug-drug interactions and fears that their coadministration may compromise their effectiveness, many experts counsel that, when both infections are discovered simultaneously, it may be prudent to treat the TB first and withhold antiviral treatment for the first few months, thereby easing the pill burden on the newly diagnosed patient and simplifying the interpretation of possible drug reactions. When TB develops in an individual already taking PIs, to reduce drug-drug interactions it may be possible to change to efavirenz and to increase the dose of rifabutin to 450 mg, but antiviral treatment should *not* be interrupted. Whenever rifabutin is used with PIs or the NNRTI delavirdine, patients should be warned of the possibility of acute uveitis symptoms—pain, decreased vision, photophobia, and conjunctivitis. Because of the infrequency of insidious onset chronic uveitis, regular ophthalmologic screening is not recommended. Ritonavir should be avoided, because it is the most potent inducer of CYP450 among the PIs. Clearly, this is a complicated therapeutic area. Physicians not experienced with the use of these drugs in combination should consult with specialists who are.

To summarize drug choices for the dually infected: rifabutin should be used instead of rifampin in the antituberculous regimen, and HIV can be treated using two NRTIs (e.g., AZT/3TC) plus efavirenz, nevirapine, or nelfinavir 1,250 bid without too much risk of untoward drug-drug interactions. When efavirenz is the third drug of combination therapy, the dose of rifabutin should be increased to 450 mg daily; when nelfinavir is the third drug, rifabutin doses are reduced to 150 mg daily.

Clinical Course

Critical to any treatment strategy is placing a suspected case in isolation until sputum smears have been examined for presence of AFB. If the clinical presentation is compelling or if the smear is positive, empirical treatment is warranted awaiting culture results. Because of the danger of transmission, especially in a hospital setting, a low threshold is used for isolation on suspicion: HIV-positive patients with fever, productive

TABLE 8-3
Effects of Coadministering Rifamycins and Antiretroviral (AV) Drugs on the Systemic Exposure of Each Drug

	RIFAMPIN (RIF)		RIFABUTIN (RFB)	
Drugs	Rif effect of AV	AV effect on Rif	Rfb effect of AV	AV effect on Rfb
Saquinavir	80% decrease	Not reported	45% decrease	Not reported
Ritonavir	35% decrease	Unchanged	Not reported	293% increase
Indinavir	92% decrease	Not reported	34% decrease	173% increase
Nelfinavir	82% decrease	Not reported	32% decrease	200% increase
Amprenavir	81% decrease	Unchanged	14% decrease	200% increase
Nevirapine	37% decrease	Unchanged*	16% decrease	Decrease*
Delavirdine	96% decrease	Unchanged*	80% decrease	342% increase*
Efavirenz	13% decrease	Unchanged*	Decrease*	Decrease*

*Predicted effect based on knowledge of metabolic pathways for the two drugs.

cough, and/or pulmonary infiltrate. As a result, high numbers of patients are put into respiratory isolation for every patient who turns out to have pulmonary TB (>100:1 in our institution), and there is a pressing need for a new approach that can move patients through the isolation process faster than the current 4 to 7 days spent waiting for three sputum smears to be obtained and examined.

Isolation is continued in smear-positive cases until both clinical and microbiologic responses have been seen. This usually requires a drop in fever, improved appetite and sense of well-being, and a decrease in the number of AFB organisms seen on sputum smears. Because response rates to treatment are as good in HIV-positive patients as in the normal population, a failure to see prompt improvement should raise the concern of infection with an MDR strain. In such cases, consideration should be taken for early intervention with second-line drugs, in consultation with a TB specialist.

Once patients are released from the hospital, it is critical that they be monitored closely for medication use and clinical course; unless there are pressing reasons to the contrary, this should be done in a public health facility that administers treatment under DOT and has the legal empowerment to pursue patients who do not come for treatment. Ultimately, to avoid development of MDR strains, the public health system must have the option to use court-ordered care.

Paradoxical ("Reversal") Reactions

Approximately one third of patients who start effective antiretroviral regimens simultaneously to or soon after initiation of treatment for TB will develop a paradoxical worsening of their TB, with new adenopathy, increasing infiltrates, and fevers. This correlates with return of tuberculin skin test reactivity and is thought to result from improved immune response to the organisms in the tissue because of control of HIV production. Although these reactions usually resolve in 2 to 6 weeks, they can be severe and interfere with a patient's rate of recovery. In such cases, after confirming that the new symptoms are not due to a second HIV-related process, clinicians can utilize a short course of prednisone therapy to lessen the inflammatory symptoms without adversely affecting the patient's response to antituberculous therapy.

Screening for Inactive Infection and Preventive Treatment

Because the risk of reactivation of dormant TB infection is >50% over the course of HIV infection, all HIV-infected patients should have a Mantoux skin test to look for delayed hypersensitivity to tuberculoprotein, indicating prior mycobacterial infection. Because responsiveness wanes with advancing HIV immunosuppression (raising the risk of reactivation and lowering the likelihood of a positive skin test response), all patients should be tested as early in their HIV infection as possible. Mantoux testing uses the intradermal injection of 0.1 ml (5 tuberculin units) of intermediate strength PPD reagent; induration of ≥5 mm after 48 to 72 hours is considered a specific positive reaction to tuberculoprotein, and evidence for prior TB infection (up to 5 mm can occur nonspecifically due to injection trauma). Although nontuberculous mycobacterial infections can also cause small positive reactions, the possibility of blunted reactions related to HIV immunosuppression and the dire implications of failure to use preventive treatment in this population have resulted in the CDC's recommendation that 5 mm of induration should be the threshold for recommending prophylactic treatment in HIV-infected patients. Such patients should have a chest x-ray to look for evidence of active pulmonary disease and should be questioned for symptoms consistent with extrapulmonary sites of active TB. Anergy testing in subjects with ≥5 mm of induration is not recommended because of poor reproducibility of reactions to repeat testing and uncertainty regarding interpreting results. Patients who are PPD-negative on initial testing are recommended for retesting periodically if they are members of groups with significant ongoing risk of exposure (e.g., prisoners, homeless or living in shelters, addicts). In addition, patients whose negative tuberculin tests were obtained at a time when their CD4+ lymphocyte counts were profoundly depressed and who subsequently have recovered to above 200 cells/mm^3 on highly active antiretroviral therapy (HAART) may warrant repeat tuberculin testing.

Numerous clinical trials have shown the effectiveness of prophylaxis in PPD-positive/HIV-positive subjects. INH given daily or twice weekly for 6 to 12 months has reduced clinical TB in subsequent years by 60% to 83% versus placebo treatment, and improved 5-year survival rates. In addition, combination prophylaxis with short-course rifampin plus pyrazinamide has proven as effective as longer treatment with INH alone, at lower calculated cost per case prevented. The largest trial was the Community Programs for Clinical Research on AIDS/AIDS Clinical Trials Group (CPCRA/ACTG) protocol 004/177, which compared 12 months of daily INH (300 mg/day) with the regimen of daily rifampin (600 mg) plus pyrazinamide (20 mg/kg) for 2 months in patients with ≥5 mm tuberculin reactions. Rates of tuberculosis were equal in the two treatment groups: 0.9 cases/100 patient years in the rifampin plus pyrazinamide group compared with 1.1/100 patient years for the INH group. A similar study performed in Haiti demonstrated equal efficacy with the regimens in a twice-weekly DOT mode: rifampin plus pyrazinamide (450 to 600 mg/1,500 to 2,500 mg) for 2 months or INH (600 to 800 mg) plus pyridoxine (25 mg) for 6 months. In both studies, compliance was better with the 2-month regimens. Drawbacks to the rifampin plus pyrazinamide combination include drug-drug interactions with rifampin, including opiate withdrawal reactions in patients on methadone maintenance programs, and contraindication to use of PIs. Rifabutin has been proposed as an alternative to rifampin, although its effectiveness in the short-course prophylaxis regimen has not been studied. Also, it should *not* be used with ritonavir or delavirdine. Many experts recommend the 9-month INH regimen for people on PIs, to avoid drug-drug interactions. The 1999 Guidelines from the U.S. Public Health Service and the Infectious Diseases Society of America recommend that HIV-positive subjects with tuberculin tests of ≥5 mm receive 9 months of 300 mg INH daily or 900 mg twice weekly (directly observed), or 2 months of rifampin (600 mg) or rifabutin (300 mg) plus pyrazinamide (2 g). For patients receiving PI therapy, the rifabutin dose should be reduced to 150 mg daily. Recommendations for monthly monitoring include attention to possible rifamycin interactions with PIs and NNRTIs, questioning for symptoms of hepatitis and uveitis, and reminder to the patient that symptoms should cause immediate consultation with the care team for advice. Monitoring of liver function tests is not recommended unless the patient has underlying liver disease, has baseline values ≥ three times normal, is over 35 years of age, or is pregnant.

INH prophylaxis has not been shown to reduce TB attack rates significantly when given to anergic HIV-positive subjects and is not recommended. The choice of prophylaxis in MDR-exposed patients is problematical; the CDC's Expert Conference recommends the use of at least two drugs to which the MDR strain is susceptible (if that many can be found), with emphasis on levofloxacin, pyrazinamide, and ethambutol.

Nontuberculous Mycobacterial Infections
Mycobacterium avium Complex

Microbiology. MAC is made up of *M. avium,* a pathogen in birds, and *M. intracellulare,* initially reported to be a significant cause of a pulmonary TB–like illness in humans at the Battey State TB sanitarium in Georgia—hence the name Battey bacillus. It also causes self-limited cervical adenitis in children. The complex was known as *M. avium-intracellulare* (MAI) until the recent MAC designation. These organisms were in Runyon Group 3, so-called nonphotochromogens, due to their failure to produce pigment in light or dark, although it is now recognized that many of the strains that cause disease in AIDS patients may produce a yellow pigment. The frequency of clinical illness with MAC increased dramatically with the advent of the AIDS epidemic. More than 90% of isolates from AIDS patients are *M. avium.*

Epidemiology. The organisms are ubiquitous in the environment worldwide, being resident in soil; fresh, sea, and municipal water; and plumbing fixtures such as faucet aerators and showerheads. They can also be isolated from domestic livestock and wild animals, although direct transmission from animals or person-to-person has not been documented. Genetic examination of isolates from patients in the same city indicate that most are unique and distinct strains, and not suggestive of common-source origins.

Race, gender, and lifestyle do not appear to affect the risk for clinical MAC infection in HIV-infected patients. Horsburgh and colleagues examined numerous environmental factors for potential risk for MAC infection and found that only consumption of hard cheese and exposure to sawdust were associated with MAC disease; no risk was found with other foods, drinking water, bathing or showering, soil or animal exposure, or prior hospitalization. The most important risk factor for development of disseminated MAC (DMAC) disease is the CD4+ lymphocyte count. Nightingale and colleagues in Dallas monitored patients with monthly lysis-centrifugation blood cultures from the point when they had developed an AIDS-defining illness; 21% developed MAC bacteremia by 12 months' observation, and 41% by 24 months. The median CD4+ cell count at diagnosis of DMAC was 13 (mean 36 ± 4) and 93% had <100 cells/mm^3. Table 8-4 shows the 6- and 12-month incidence of MAC bacteremia related to entry CD4+ cell count. For patients who entered the study with counts below 10 cells/mm^3, the risk at 1 year was 39%. Data from the 1980s estimated that up to 15% to 30% of AIDS patients developed DMAC prior to death, and postmortem studies suggested that the actual infection rate was as high as 50%. Clinical DMAC frequently appeared at a point where other opportunistic infections (particularly cytomegalovirus [CMV] disease) and wasting had already occurred, with the patient's CD4+ cell count below 30 cells/mm^3, and its advent shortened subsequent life span to a mean of 5.6 months compared with 10.8 months in CD4+-matched AIDS patients without DMAC. Fortunately, as with other opportunistic infections, since the general use of HAART regimens and spe-

TABLE 8-4
Incidence of MAC Bacteremia by CD4+ Cell Count in Patients Not on MAC Prophylaxis

	INCIDENCE OF MAC BACTEREMIA	
CD4+ Range at entry	After 6 months	After 12 months
0-9	28 ± 5	39 ± 6
10-19	13 ± 3	30 ± 5
20-39	7 ± 2	20 ± 4
40-59	5 ± 2	15 ± 4
60-99	2 ± 1	8 ± 3

TABLE 8-5
Frequency of Symptoms, Physical Findings, and Laboratory Abnormalities Among Patients with DMAC Infection

Finding	Number of patients	Percent positive
Fever	120	87
Night sweats	85	78
Diarrhea	92	47
Abdominal pain	54	35
Nausea/vomiting	31	26
Weight loss	37	38
Lymphadenopathy		
Intraabdominal	54	37
Mediastinal	49	10
Hepatosplenomegaly	38	24
<8.5 g hemoglobin/dl	39	85
Elevated alkaline phosphatase	38	53

From Benson CA, Ellner JJ: *Mycobacterium avium* complex infection and AIDS: advances in theory and practice, *Clin Infect Dis* 17:7-20, 1993.

cific MAC prophylaxis (see below), the incidence of DMAC as a first opportunistic infection has fallen dramatically: from 101.4 cases per 1,000 person years in 1992 to 15.6 in 1997.
Pathogenesis. Unlike TB, in which many cases represent reactivation of foci of prior infection, it is thought that most DMAC cases are primary infections. The GI and respiratory tracts are the likely portals of entry: in patients with CD4+ cell counts below 50 cells/mm³, respiratory tract colonization confers a > twofold increased risk of DMAC infection, and GI tract colonization raises the risk by sixfold compared with noncolonized patients. In one study, more than half of subjects found to be colonized with MAC developed DMAC within the following 6 to 8 months. However, only 30% to 40% of patients who develop DMAC can be shown to be colonized, suggesting either poor sensitivity of the culture, possibility of intermittent colonization, or other routes of entry. Colonization does not necessarily lead to disseminated disease, but a likely scenario is that repeated environmental exposures lead to transient or protracted colonization, with the immune system's containment efficiency deteriorating as the individual's CD4+ cell count drops below 50 cells/mm³ of blood. Transient bacteremias may ensue, with potential for infecting components of the reticuloendothelial system such as marrow, lymph nodes, spleen, and liver, whose fixed macrophages phagocytize the circulating bacteria. Such extravascular infection then slowly worsens until symptoms occur and a sustained blood stream infection is established. Supporting this thesis, transient MAC bacteremias have been demonstrated, as well as instances of marrow infection with concurrent blood cultures failing to grow the organism.

Mimicking the pathology of lepromatous leprosy, the organisms excite very little inflammatory response in the infected tissues. Macrophages become distended with organisms that they are unable to kill, with resultant disruption of normal organ architecture, but with little cellular infiltration. Granuloma formation is rare. The primary immune defect appears to be a failure of the host's ability to mount a normal inflammatory response and to effect intracellular killing of the organisms. Failure to produce macrophage-activating cytokines, such as IL-2, interferon-γ, and IL-12, and the action of immunosuppressant cytokines, such as transforming growth factor (TGF)-β, have been proposed as pathogenic mechanisms.

Presentation and Progression. Patients with DMAC have characteristic though not specific symptoms, signs, and laboratory abnormalities that include fevers, night sweats, weight loss, GI distress, hepatosplenomegaly, adenopathy, anemia, and elevated serum alkaline phosphatase (Table 8-5). Symptoms usually are of vague onset, but unless diagnosed and treated, they progress over weeks to months to profound wasting, inanition, and punishing fevers. The differential diagnosis includes non-Hodgkin's lymphoma, other disseminated carcinomas, and fungal infections. Fevers can be >39° C daily.

Adenopathy can be predominantly mediastinal or retroperitoneal, requiring CT or magnetic resonance imaging for detection. The anemia can be isolated and profound, requiring repeated transfusion. Similarly, elevated alkaline phosphatase can be the main chemical abnormality to suggest presence of DMAC. Despite chronic symptoms and high concentrations of MAC persisting in multiple organs, patients can tolerate this continually bacteremic state for months with only a gradual decline in health, much like a patient with metastatic cancer. Experience with the syndrome before development of adequate treatment showed that, although not abruptly lethal, DMAC reduced survival time by at least half versus matched patients without DMAC.

In addition to the disseminated picture of infection, some patients have a predominantly intestinal illness characterized by chronic crampy abdominal pain, nausea and vomiting, diarrhea, malabsorption, and weight loss progressing over several months. Biopsy of the mucosa demonstrates intense infiltration of the small and/or large bowel with MAC. Although uncommon, MAC can also produce diffuse pulmonary infiltrates, localized pneumonitis, nodules, and cavitary disease. MAC tuberculomas of CNS and elsewhere, local adenopathy, and skin lesions have also been reported.

Diagnosis. Clinical suspicion should be aroused in any AIDS patient with a CD4+ cell count below 75 to 100 cells/mm³ who also has unexplained fever, anorexia and weight loss, or abdominal pains (with or without diarrhea) for more than 2 weeks; who develops progressive anemia or thrombocytopenia; or who has progressive elevation of serum alkaline phosphatase. Although blood is the most commonly cultured body compartment, growth of MAC from any normally sterile body site (liver, lymph node, marrow, bowel biopsy) confirms the diagnosis of DMAC infection. Blood can be inoculated either into broth or onto solid medium. Several effective semiautomated broth culture systems employing various growth sensors can detect organism growth within 7 to 14 days following direct inoculation of blood, and a single culture is recommended because of a sensitivity reported to be >90%. When an acid-fast stain of the broth is positive, DNA-RNA hybridization can confirm the presence of MAC, *M. tuberculosis,* or other mycobacteria within 48 hours. The solid medium systems generally take a week longer to demonstrate visible colonies and employ lysis of whole blood specimens (releasing phagocytized organisms) and culture of centrifuged sediment. For tissues other than blood, direct AFB staining can provide useful rapid information, although with certain drawbacks: first, high organism concentrations are required (10^4 to 10^5/ml), and a positive result does not permit differentiation among the various mycobacteria. Specific direct molecular probing for rapid diagnosis of organisms in tissue is still experimental.

Culturing of respiratory secretions or stool is not recommended for diagnosis of DMAC because studies show that less than one third of patients with positive cultures of blood or marrow grow the organism from sputum or stool prior to diagnosis of bacteremia. On the other hand, patients with a CD4+ cell count below 50 cells/mm³ who have the organism isolated from stool or sputum have a 60% likelihood of developing DMAC within the next 12 months, most within the next 4 months.

Treatment. In the first decade of the AIDS epidemic, response to therapy was generally poor and, owing to major drug toxicities and the frail nature of most patients with DMAC, many experienced AIDS clinicians elected not to treat the infection. Then, in the early 1990s several careful studies demonstrated that patients given four to five anti-MAC agents (and able to take them) were able to reduce their bacteremic colony counts by >1 log, or to sterilize their blood transiently in over half of cases. Initially, the use of intravenous amikacin was believed key to the success of these regimens, but subsequent studies showed that similar success rates could be achieved with all-oral regimens including rifampin, ethambutol, ciprofloxacin, and clofazimine. Soon thereafter, clarithromycin and azithromycin, two new macrolide antibiotics, were found to have excellent activity against most strains of MAC. When studied as monotherapy, both showed a dose-dependent rate of bloodstream clearing over 12 weeks of study. However, the more rapid microbiologic success with high doses was achieved at the expense of unacceptable toxicity (GI upset, and even higher mortality). Moreover, as one might suspect, relapse with resistant organisms was encountered in up to 50% of cases when the drugs were used as monotherapy. Therefore, current practice is to use 500 mg of clarithromycin twice daily or 600 mg of azithromycin once daily, in association with at least one other effective agent (Box 8-1).

> **BOX 8-1**
> **Current Recommended Treatment and Prophylaxis vs DMAC in HIV-Infected Persons**
>
> **TREATMENT**
> Clarithromycin 500 mg po q12h
> or
> Azithromycin 600 mg po qd
> plus
> Ethambutol 15 mg/kg qd
> and/or
> Rifabutin 300 mg po qd
>
> **PROPHYLAXIS**
> Clarithromycin 500 mg po q12h
> or
> Azithromycin 1,200 mg po once weekly
> or
> Rifabutin 300 mg po qd

Both ethambutol and rifabutin have been demonstrated to be effective with either of the macrolides, but clofazimine, although active in vitro, should not be used to treat DMAC because it has been shown to increase mortality in recipients. The largest and most comprehensive trial of treatment of DMAC has been ACTG 223 in which all 160 eligible patients received clarithromycin 500 mg po bid; equal numbers were randomized to additionally receive ethambutol 15 mg/kg po qd, rifabutin 450 mg po qd, or both rifabutin *and* ethambutol in these doses. Clearing of MAC bacteremia occurred by 12 weeks' treatment in 40% of clarithromycin plus ethambutol patients, 42% of clarithromycin plus rifabutin patients, and 51% of clarithromycin plus ethambutol plus rifabutin patients (p = 0.44). Clinical improvement was also similar. There was a trend for the triple therapy group to have a better response rate, lower rate of adverse drug effects, and lower relapse rate, with the clarithromycin plus rifabutin group doing the worst. Finally, the median survival time was significantly greater for the three-drug arm compared with either of the two-drug arms. Therefore the study authors recommend that the three-drug regimen be utilized whenever possible for DMAC. Because feasibility in these brittle patients often means balancing tolerability, drug-drug interactions, and pill fatigue, some experts often limit their initial treatment to clarithromycin plus ethambutol. Susceptibility testing is not generally recommended to guide the choice of initial treatment (most isolates appear to be susceptible initially). When microbiologic relapses occur (12% in the ACTG 223 trial), susceptibility testing can be used as a guide, although no general laboratory standards exist. If testing indicates that the organism now has a high minimum inhibitory concentration for macrolides, most experts advocate the addition of two new drugs (e.g., ciprofloxacin, amikacin) and extended therapy.

The usual response to treatment is one of slow clinical and microbiologic improvement. It usually takes several weeks for fevers to resolve, and may take up to 8 weeks; bacteremia colony counts fall slowly to undetectable by week 12 to 16. Even though most patients with DMAC have far-advanced AIDS, often with wasting and other opportunistic infections, studies have shown that effective anti-MAC treatment extends life expectancy. Until the current era of truly effective antiretroviral therapy, recommendation was for life-long continuation of anti-MAC treatment at the same dose used initially. Currently, although the data are still sparse, it appears that it may be safe to discontinue treatment in patients whose response to potent antiretroviral therapy has raised their CD4+ counts to >100 cells/mm^3 for ≥6 months. A confirmatory trial is underway.

Prevention. Because the occurrence of DMAC is limited to those with far-advanced immunosuppression from HIV, and because it results in significant morbidity and mortality, prophylaxis is a reasonable goal. Fortunately, clarithromycin, azithromycin, and rifabutin have each been shown to be effective in this role. The two macrolides are of equal effectiveness, whereas rifabutin should be restricted to patients who cannot tolerate either macrolide. Rifabutin was the first agent shown to be effective, 300 mg/day reducing the incidence of MAC bacteremia by 50% and prolonging life in one study. Thereafter both clarithromycin and azithromycin were studied either alone or in combination with rifabutin: both macrolides were approximately twice as effective in reducing DMAC incidence as the rifabutin arms. In the clarithromycin study, combining clarithromycin plus rifabutin did not significantly reduce DMAC compared with clarithromycin alone; in the azithromycin study, combined azithromycin plus rifabutin *did* provide additional protection over azithromycin alone (DMAC incidence of 2.8% versus 7.6%), but owing to greater toxicity, cost, and drug-drug interactions, the combination is not recommended. Both clarithromycin and azithromycin prophylaxis also reduce the incidence of bacterial infections significantly. It appears that DMAC developing in the face of clarithromycin prophylaxis may be slightly more likely to demonstrate macrolide resistance than similar cases developing on azithromycin, but the overall incidence of developing macrolide-resistant DMAC is <3%. The 1999 USPHS/IDSA guidelines for the prevention of opportunistic infections in HIV-positive persons recommend that all patients with CD4+ cell counts ≤50 cells/mm^3 receive either clarithromycin 500 mg bid or azithromycin 1,200 mg q week (see Box 8-1). It is prudent to obtain a blood culture to confirm absence of MAC bacteremia prior to initiating prophylaxis in patients with any signs or symptoms that suggest DMAC.

Based on a growing number of reports as well as case experience, it appears to be safe to withdraw prophylaxis in patients whose CD4+ cell count has risen to above 100 cells/mm^3 of blood for at least 6 months on effective HAART. For example, the Swiss HIV Cohort Study recently reported on 253 patients whose median nadir CD4+ had been 10 cells/mm^3 and whose median time with counts ≤50 was 12 months. MAC prophylaxis was discontinued after their CD4+ count on HAART had risen to ≥100 for at least 3 months and they were followed for an aggregate of 364 patient years. No cases of DMAC have occurred.

Mycobacterium kansasii

Infection with *M. kansasii* is the third most commonly reported mycobacterial infection among AIDS patients. A 1989 CDC report calculated a prevalence of 138 cases/100,000 AIDS cases, and a 1998 review from Northern California found an incidence of 115 cases/100,000 HIV-infected population and 638 cases/100,000 AIDS patients. It has been associated with poverty and homelessness, although documented cases of person-to-person transmission are rare, and it is not commonly isolated from environmental sources. Approximately 90% of isolates are from sputum, with blood being the most common documented site of dissemination, being positive in about 20% of pulmonary patients who have blood cultured. Several large retrospective studies have shown that isolation of the organism from sputum is usually associated with convincing clinical and radiologic evidence of active pulmonary infection. The chest x-ray can show focal upper lobe infiltrates, diffuse interstitial infiltrates, nonspecific chronic pneumonitis, and thin-walled cavitary lesions.

Most clinical *M. kansasii* infections occur in patients with advanced immunosuppression: median CD4+ cell counts have been reported as ≤25 cells/mm^3 and >90% of patients have already had an AIDS diagnosis made. Sputum smears are positive for AFB in half of cases, and multiple positive cultures are the norm. However, it is unwise to disregard even a single sputum culture positive for *M. kansasii* in a clinical setting compatible with pulmonary infection. An interesting phenomenon reported in several series has been concomitant isolation of other pathogens, particularly MAC (blood and/or sputum), *P. carinii, Cryptococcus neoformans,* and CMV. We have had two patients who were admitted with typical PCP who resolved their clinical pneumonia with co-trimoxazole therapy, but whose sputa also grew *M. kansasii* and who developed nodular pneumonitis 4 to 8 weeks after initiating HAART; on evaluation, they were smear and culture-positive for *M. kansasii* and responded to treatment with INH, rifabutin, and ethambutol. Some series report poor response to treatment, although others have had excellent success with standard drugs. It is prudent to perform susceptibility testing on all isolates as a guide, particularly in the event that response to initial treatment appears to be poor. Initial therapy is usually with INH plus rifabutin plus ethambutol or INH plus rifabutin plus pyrazinamide and an 18-month treatment duration is recommended.

Mycobacterium xenopi

M. xenopi has been reported in increasing frequency isolated from sputum and extrapulmonary sites in AIDS patients. A Runyon Group II organism, it grows best at 42° to 45° C, and has been grown from hospital hot water systems. Clusters of pulmonary colonization and disease have been linked epidemiologically to hospital exposures, and colonized hot water tanks and faucets have been thought to be reservoirs. In HIV-negative subjects, most isolates are from sputum specimens and are considered to be nonpathogenic, although pulmonary disease has been documented in patients with underlying chronic lung disease. In HIV-positive patients, pulmonary isolates also predominate, but blood, bone marrow, lymph node, bone, and subcutaneous abscess have all been reported as sources of *M. xenopi*. Instances of true tissue infection appear to be limited to lung or are found in lung plus extrapulmonary sites (usually blood) in approximately equal proportions. In general, isolated pulmonary disease occurs at higher CD4+ cell counts, whereas the disseminated cases usually have counts below 50 cells/mm^3. Although the large majority of pulmonary isolates represent colonization, clinical syndromes of chronic cough, fever, dyspnea, and weight loss, with chest radiographs showing abnormalities including multinodular densities, bilateral interstitial infiltrates, upper lobe infiltrates with or without cavitation, fibrosis, and hilar adenopathy, have been reported. The organism is easy to grow and identify in the laboratory, and, although in vitro susceptibility tests should be considered only a guide, susceptibility to clarithromycin, azithromycin, and ciprofloxacin is common, with INH, rifampin, ethambutol, and pyrazinamide showing variable susceptibility. Clinical responses to multidrug therapy can be expected.

Other Nontuberculous Mycobacteria

A number of other organisms have been reported to cause disease in HIV-positive patients, including *M. haemophilum*, *M. gordonae*, *M. marinum*, *M. scrofulaceum*, *M. fortuitum*, *M. chelonei*, *M. genavense*, *M. malmoense*, and *M. celatum*. Both pulmonary and disseminated diseases occur, with the latter associated with advanced immunosuppression and symptoms similar to DMAC. *M. genavense* and *M. haemophilum* are difficult to grow and should be suspected in cases showing organisms in biopsies but with negative cultures. Most isolates have been from blood and other sterile sites. Susceptibility of these unusual organisms to antibiotics is variable and often hard to determine, and multidrug regimens including a macrolide, a rifamycin, and a quinolone are rational initial choices.

SUGGESTED READINGS

Benson CA, Ellner JJ: *Mycobacterium avium* complex infection and AIDS: advances in theory and practice, *Clin Infect Dis* 17: 7-20, 1993.

Benson C et al: ACTG 223: an open prospective, randomized study comparing efficacy and safety of clarithromycin plus ethambutol, rifabutin, or both for treatment of MAC disease in patients with AIDS [Abstract 249], 6th Conference on Retroviruses and Opportunistic Infections, Chicago, Ill, 1999.

Bloch KC et al: Incidence and clinical implications of isolation of *Mycobacterium kansasii*: results of a 5-year population-based study, *Ann Intern Med* 698-704, 1998.

Dooley SW et al: Multidrug-resistant tuberculosis, *Ann Intern Med* 117:257-258, 1992.

Furrer H et al: Discontinuing or withholding primary prophylaxis against *M. avium* in patients on successful antiretroviral combination therapy: the Swiss HIV Cohort experience. [Abstract 246], 7th Conference on Retroviruses and Opportunistic Infections, San Francisco, January 30-February 2, 2000.

Horsburgh CR et al: Environmental risk factors for acquisition of *Mycobacterium avium* complex in persons with HIV infection, *J Infect Dis* 170:362-367, 1994.

Johnson JL et al: Instability of tuberculin and candida skin test reactivity in HIV-infected Ugandans, *Am J Respir Crit Care Med* 158:1790-1796, 1998.

Nightingale SD et al: Incidence of *Mycobacterium avium-intracellulare* complex bacteremia in human immunodeficiency virus–positive patients, *J Infect Dis* 165:1082-1085, 1992.

Perlman DC et al: Variation of chest radiographic patterns in pulmonary tuberculosis by degree of HIV-related immunosuppression, *Clin Infect Dis* 25:242-246, 1997.

Prevention and treatment of tuberculosis among patients infected with human immunodeficiency virus: principles of therapy and revised recommendations, *MMWR* 47(RR-20):1-58, 1998.

Rose DN: Short-course prophylaxis against tuberculosis in HIV-infected persons: a decision and cost-effectiveness analysis, *Ann Intern Med* 129:779-786, 1998.

Whalen C et al: Accelerated course of HIV infection after tuberculosis, *Am J Respir Crit Care Med* 151:129-135, 1995.

1999 USPHS/IDSA Guidelines for the Prevention of Opportunistic Infections in Persons Infected with Human Immunodeficiency Virus. US Public Health Service and Infectious Diseases Society of America. Supplement to *MMWR* 48(RR-10):1-66, 1999.

9 Fungal Infections

DANIEL K. MEYER, MINDY SCHUSTER

Introduction

From the earliest days of the acquired immunodeficiency syndrome (AIDS) epidemic, fungal infections resulting from profound immunosuppression due to the human immunodeficiency virus (HIV) have been recognized. As knowledge of immune compromise and opportunistic infection has increased, so has the understanding of how normal hosts are able to prevent infection by fungi. It is now recognized that fungal illnesses in HIV infection cover a spectrum from superficial dermatomycoses to localized mucosal infection to disseminated invasive infection, with increased incidence of invasion occurring at lower CD4+ counts.

In general, the fungi are human colonizers and have a limited ability to cause disease in normal hosts. Humans have evolved multiple strategies to prevent fungal invasion and thus disease. The presence of fungal infection implies a defect in the normal host defense. The defect may be localized or systemic, and disseminated disease represents dysfunction on several levels of immunity.

Host Defense

Normal host defenses include natural barriers to invasion by bacterial and fungal pathogens, including intact skin. Normal bacterial flora present in the human gastrointestinal and genitourinary tract inhibits fungal growth by competition for nutrients and perhaps also by elaborating antifungal substances. Fungal overgrowth has been noted to occur when bacterial colonization is reduced by administration of broad-spectrum antibiotics.

Invasive fungal disease is prevented by a complex interaction of several immune system strategies. Fungi are resistant to lysis by the terminal components of the complement system. However, antibody and complement contribute to the host defense by opsonization of fungi. The phagocytic defenses of neutrophils and mononuclear phagocytes are important defenses against invasive fungal infections. The hyphae of *Candida albicans* and *Aspergillus fumigatus* stimulate neutrophils to undergo a respiratory burst and degranulate, releasing oxidants including hydrogen peroxide and hypochlorous acid, which have been demonstrated to damage and kill hyphae in vitro. Cell-mediated immunity plays a significant role in the normal host defense against fungi. The antigen presenting cells process and present fungal antigens to T lymphocytes, which then proliferate and elaborate the cytokines required for the inflammatory response and fungal killing.

The development of a significant fungal infection requires dysfunction of these defenses. Additionally, with impaired cell-mediated immunity there is limited ability to mount an inflammatory response, and symptoms of invasive fungal disease may be either mild or absent.

Risk Factors

The primary risk factor for developing invasive fungal disease is the profound cell-mediated immune dysfunction that develops during the natural history of HIV infection. The incidence of fungal diseases increases as the CD4+ levels fall. Patients with CD4+ levels less than 50 cells/mm^3 are at the greatest risk. Additional risk factors include neutropenia, malnutrition, and concomitant infections.

Fungal pathogens include normal human commensal organisms, such as *Candida* species, and the environmental molds associated with invasive fungal diseases, such as *Aspergillus* species and the endemic mycoses. When pursuing a diagnosis, obtaining pertinent residence and travel histories is important to assist in formulating the differential diagnosis.

Superficial Fungal Infections
Seborrheic Dermatitis

Presentation and Progression. Seborrheic dermatitis is probably the most common dermatitis in AIDS, and has been postulated to represent superficial fungal infection. The incidence is estimated at 50% in patients with HIV compared with 10% in the normal population. The evidence for a fungal pathogen is not conclusive, yet the response to topical antifungal therapy is well documented, and *Malassezia furfur* has been isolated from patients with seborrheic dermatitis, although its role in the pathogenesis is not clear. Seborrheic dermatitis presents as mildly erythematous patches with a yellowish greasy scale. These patches are commonly located on the face, scalp, and chest areas. They may also be found in the groin and axillae, and may be confused with superficial candidiasis in those locations. Occurrences typically are worse at lower CD4+ levels, and may be quite pruritic when on the trunk.

Treatment. Treatment is usually with topical ketoconazole, with the addition of topical steroids when there is severe inflammation associated with it. Oral itraconazole is useful when patches are extensive or refractory to topical therapy.

Other Dermatologic Mycoses

Other dermatologic mycoses also have increased incidence in AIDS. These include tinea versicolor, tinea capitis, tinea pedis, tinea cruris, and tinea corporis. These are caused by the dermatophytes *Trichophyton, Microsporum,* and *Epidermophyton,* and treatments include topical antifungal agents or oral itraconazole or terbinafine.

Candidiasis

The *Candida* species are commensal yeast organisms that colonize the gastrointestinal and genitourinary tracts of healthy humans. Localized mucosal infections that can occur in otherwise healthy persons are associated with the use of antibiotics, corticosteroids, immunosuppressive therapy, or extremes of age.

In HIV disease, infection with *Candida* species covers a spectrum from localized oropharyngeal or vaginal candidiasis to more invasive esophageal and, rarely, disseminated systemic candidiasis.

Mucocutaneous Candidiasis

Mucocutaneous candidiasis is a prominent opportunistic infection in HIV disease, and commonly occurs as CD4+ levels decline to less than 200 cells/mm^3. The earliest manifestation is usually oropharyngeal candidiasis, which may be an early marker for HIV disease and has been reported to occur at CD4+ counts greater than 500 cells/mm^3.

Oropharyngeal Candidiasis. Oropharyngeal candidiasis may be seen with the acute immunosuppression associated with acute HIV seroconversion. The incidence of oropharyngeal candidiasis increases as CD4+ levels fall below 200 cells/mm^3, and approaches 90% for patients with CD4+ counts less than 200 cells/mm^3.

Frequently asymptomatic in mild cases, candidiasis of the oral mucosa may have a variable appearance, from white patches on the tongue or uvula—termed pseudomembranous— that are easily scraped off to white-yellow hyperplastic plaques that cannot be scraped off. Erythematous candidiasis, which manifests as bright red erosions on the oral mucosa, may be missed because of the lack of the characteristic plaque or may be confused with other oral ulcer–producing processes. Diagnosis of oropharyngeal candidiasis is primarily by physical examination, supported by a wet mount showing budding yeast or hyphae. Cultures may be performed if the diagnosis is in question, particularly if refractory to therapy. Recommended initial treatment is with topical agents such as nystatin or clotrimazole, reserving the use of oral fluconazole for cases in which the plaques are extensive or not responding to topical therapy. Fluconazole treatment is initiated with 200 mg orally on day one, followed by 100 mg daily thereafter, for a 14-day course. Improvement in symptoms is usually within 1 week. In patients who do not improve in this period, higher doses of fluconazole may be tried—400 to 800 mg daily. Although fluconazole has been used for suppression of candidiasis, extended courses of fluconazole have resulted in the development of resistance to fluconazole, and in this setting, sending isolates for susceptibility testing is important. In cases of fluconazole-resistant candidal infections, alternative treatments include the use of itraconazole oral solution at 100 to 200 mg twice daily or the use of intravenous amphotericin B at 0.5 mg/kg/day for a 14-day course.

Vulvovaginal Candidiasis. Vulvovaginal candidiasis is also a common manifestation of early HIV disease, and frequently occurs in conjunction with oropharyngeal candidiasis in women with HIV disease. The severity and frequency of vulvovaginal candidiasis are increased in HIV-infected women compared with normal hosts. Clinical presentation includes pruritus and vaginal discharge, and diagnosis is made by physical examination showing typical white plaques and discharge with erythematous vaginal mucosa, supported by a wet mount demonstrating yeast forms or pseudohyphae. Treatment options include topical preparations such as clotrimazole or miconazole, with oral fluconazole reserved for severe or refractory cases, dosed at 100 to 200 mg daily for a 7- to 10-day course. Candidal resistance to fluconazole has also been reported in vulvovaginal candidiasis, and in patients who are refractory to therapy, obtaining specimens for susceptibility testing is appropriate. Refractory cases may be treated with either itraconazole oral solution 100 to 200 mg twice daily or intravenous amphotericin B at 0.5 mg/kg/day.

Esophageal Candidiasis. As CD4+ levels fall below 100 cells/mm^3, significant mucosal invasion by *Candida* species increases, with the development of esophageal candidiasis. This has been an AIDS-defining illness from the earliest descriptions of the epidemic, with median CD4+ counts at presentation of less than 50 cells/mm^3. Symptoms may be absent or mild to severe, with dysphagia, odynophagia, and retrosternal chest pain common presenting complaints. A history of these complaints in conjunction with seeing oropharyngeal candidiasis may be enough to make a presumptive diagnosis. Initial empiric therapy with fluconazole is reasonable in this setting, beginning with 100 to 200 mg daily. Improvement should occur within the first week of treatment; in patients who are continuing to have symptoms, or in the absence of oral lesions, esophagogastroduodenoscopy (EGD) may be required to confirm the diagnosis and obtain specimens for susceptibility testing. Characteristic appearance in the esophagus is large yellow-white plaques, which may be solitary or multiple to diffuse. Differential diagnosis for esophageal ulcers includes not only *Candida*, but also herpes simplex virus (HSV), cytomegalovirus (CMV), and aphthous ulcers, which may be difficult to differentiate by upper gastrointestinal radiography alone. Biopsy is often required to confirm the diagnosis, and will show the characteristic mucosal invasion by the pseudohyphae of *Candida*.

Treatment for esophageal candidiasis with oral fluconazole 100 to 200 mg daily is often begun empirically if symptoms are consistent with the diagnosis. However, esophageal candidiasis may be seen in conjunction with other opportunistic pathogens, including CMV, HSV, and histoplasmosis, and these need to be ruled out if symptoms do not resolve with initial therapy for *Candida*. There is an increasing incidence of resistance to fluconazole, especially in patients who have received prolonged courses of fluconazole previously. In these cases, confirming the diagnosis by EGD is preferable, and treatment with intravenous amphotericin B 0.5 mg daily is used for refractory cases of esophageal candidiasis.

Bloodstream infections with *Candida* species do occur in HIV disease and are associated with the use of central venous catheters, prolonged antibiotics, and neutropenia. Treatment is with removal of catheters and the use of either amphotericin B or intravenous fluconazole if the isolate is susceptible.

> **KEY POINTS**

- Seen most commonly with CD4+ count below 200 cells/mm^3
- Mucocutaneous disease includes oropharyngeal and vulvovaginal
- As CD4+ counts fall below 100 cells/mm^3 and particularly below 50 cells/mm^3, esophageal disease becomes more common
- Treatment with oral fluconazole is indicated, but increasing resistance to fluconazole is being observed

Cryptococcosis

Cryptococcosis is caused by the encapsulated yeast *Cryptococcus neoformans*, which has been associated with exposure to birds, particularly pigeons, and soil contaminated by them. In most cases of cryptococcal infections, however, no exposure history can be elicited. The incidence of cryptococcosis is approximately 6% to 10% in patients with AIDS in the United States, and approaches 30% in AIDS patients in Africa. Although the portal of entry for *Cryptococcus* is through the lung, pulmonary symptoms are rare, and the primary manifestation of this disease is often meningitis, which occurs in 85% to 90% of those infected with *Cryptococcus*. Other sites affected can include bloodstream, liver, skin, lymph nodes, and adrenal glands. The majority of cases of cryptococcal meningitis occur in those patients with CD4+ counts less than 50 cells/mm^3, although it may occur at any level, and in rare cases may occur in the normal host as well.

Presentation and Progression

Patients occasionally may present primarily with pulmonary symptoms—fever and cough—and an abnormal chest radiograph. More commonly the presentation is a subacute illness with headache and fever, which may or may not include a change in mental functioning. There are usually no signs of meningismus, and the level of suspicion must be high to pursue the diagnosis in subacute cases. There may be associated skin findings, including subcutaneous nodules, herpetiform, Kaposi's sarcoma–like lesions, or molluscum-like lesions.

Diagnosis

Diagnosis is usually made by examination and culture of spinal fluid. The opening pressure is generally elevated, and may exceed 200 mm H$_2$O. Typical cerebrospinal fluid (CSF) findings include a low-grade lymphocyte-predominant pleocytosis, with an elevated protein and mildly lowered glucose. India ink preparation showing the encapsulated yeast forms is positive in approximately 75% of cases. A more sensitive and specific test is the cryptococcal antigen test on the CSF, which approaches 100% sensitivity and specificity. Fungal culture of the CSF will confirm the diagnosis, usually within a few days.

Treatment

Mortality in the acute treatment phase of cryptococcal meningitis is significant, in the range of 10% to 25%. Indicators of poor outcome include impaired mental status at presentation, with confusion, lethargy, and obtundation, which indicate increased intracranial pressure. An elevated cryptococcal antigen titer in the CSF of greater than 1:1,1024 and low cell count in CSF are also associated with poor outcome. Current treatment strategy includes an initial treatment phase with intravenous amphotericin B 0.7 mg/kg/day with or without 5-flucytosine for a 2-week course to sterilize the CSF, followed by oral fluconazole 400 mg daily for an additional 8 to 10 weeks. Lifelong maintenance therapy is then required with fluconazole 200 mg daily to prevent relapse of disease. The role of flucytosine in the initial treatment phase, standard for normal hosts, is less clear in AIDS patients, with some studies demonstrating no clear benefit.

An important part of the management of cryptococcal meningitis involves recognition of the management of the increased intracranial pressure, which often occurs in this disease. These patients either may present with a change in mental status and obtundation or may develop these signs and symptoms after therapy is initiated. Imaging of the brain by computed tomography (CT) scan is important in establishing this diagnosis. CSF pressures may exceed 500 mm H$_2$O. Treatment requires the use of repeated lumbar punctures to maintain pressure less than 300 mm H$_2$O, with neurosurgical consultation for placement of ventricular shunts in refractory cases.

Occasionally there are patients who demonstrate ongoing infection or relapse with *Cryptococcus* while on therapy. The prostate has been reported to serve as a reservoir of infection, and *Cryptococcus* has been cultured from prostatic secretions, even while on appropriate therapy.

> **KEY POINTS**

- Most cases occur in those with CD4+ counts below 50 cells/mm^3
- Meningitis is the primary manifestation in 85%-90% of those infected
- The most common presentation is fever and headache without meningismus
- Cryptococcal antigen testing of the CSF is the diagnostic test of choice
- Most experts treat with amphotericin B initially followed by oral fluconazole, and then maintenance therapy is required lifelong

Endemic Mycoses and AIDS

The endemic mycoses are fungal diseases associated with specific geographic regions. All are found as molds in soil in these areas that has been contaminated by animal or bird droppings. An increasingly mobile global population has necessitated broadening the differential diagnosis of fungal illnesses, and detailed residence and travel histories are required to establish an individual patient's risk for these diseases. The pathophysiology for the endemic mycoses is similar, and all have the ability to cause disease in the normal host. The portal of entry for the organisms is the lung, and in the normal host usually results in a self-limited pulmonary infection. Cell-mediated immunity is important in controlling the infection, since the fungal elements are not susceptible to neutrophil-mediated killing in the lung. Because of impaired cell-mediated immunity, the tendency to cause disseminated disease is greatly increased in AIDS, and the disseminated endemic mycoses were recognized as AIDS-defining illnesses early in the epidemic. The endemic mycoses include histoplasmosis, coccidioidomycosis, blastomycosis, and penicilliosis. Paracoccidioidomycosis and sporotrichosis are also reported to cause disseminated disease in AIDS patients.

Histoplasmosis

Presentation and Progression. Histoplasmosis is caused by the dimorphic fungus *Histoplasma capsulatum,* which is found as a mold in the environment and converts to an intracellular yeast form in human infection. The organism is endemic in the Ohio and Mississippi River valleys, including the states of Missouri, Kentucky, Tennessee, Illinois, and Ohio, although it has been reported elsewhere. The mold grows in soil that has been contaminated by bird or bat droppings, and can commonly be found in caves and old buildings.

Histoplasmosis is a common opportunistic infection complicating the course of AIDS in approximately 5% of patients from endemic areas. Disseminated histoplasmosis may present with either primary infection or reactivation of quiescent disease. About 95% of AIDS patients with histoplasmosis present with disseminated disease, with fever, weight loss, and skin and oral lesions. Skin findings are typically erythematous maculopapular lesions, although cutaneous ulcers and purpura are also reported. Pneumonia and pulmonary symptoms are present in 50% at presentation, and if present, often will have pulmonary pathology demonstrated by chest radiography. The chest x-ray typically will demonstrate diffuse patchy interstitial infiltrates with nodular appearance. The central nervous system may also be involved, with change of mental status present in 10% to 20% of AIDS patients. Histoplasmosis may cause lymphocytic meningitis, as well as focal brain lesions or a diffuse encephalitis. About 10% to 20% of patients present with septic shock, multisystem organ failure, and disseminated intravascular coagulation (DIC).

Diagnosis. Diagnosis may be made from routine blood culture, although incubation for 19 to 24 days is required. Isolator blood cultures will be positive in 8 to 13 days. The organism has been isolated from all sites in postmortem examinations. Diagnosis is frequently made by fungal stains of pathology specimens—examination of bone marrow biopsy, lymph node biopsy, or liver biopsy. Fungal forms in circulating phagocytic cells may be seen on peripheral smears. Recently the *H. capsulatum* polysaccharide antigen test of urine has been helpful in early diagnosis, with 90% positive in patients with disseminated histoplasmosis. The antigen test will be positive less frequently—25% to 50%—in patients with less severe disease.

Treatment. Although often no treatment is recommended for normal hosts with minimal disease, the increased likelihood of dissemination in AIDS patients warrants treatment when the diagnosis is likely. In mild disease, treatment may be initiated with oral itraconazole 300 mg twice daily for 3 days then 200 mg twice daily for 12 weeks, followed by maintenance therapy with 200 mg daily. In severe illness, the treatment is high-dose therapy with intravenous amphotericin B at 0.8 to 1.0 mg/kg/day for 7 days, then every other day to a total dose of approximately 1 g, followed by maintenance therapy with itraconazole. Oral fluconazole 400 mg per day has also been used for maintenance therapy, but may have a higher relapse rate.

▶ KEY POINTS

⊃ Most common in Ohio and Mississippi River valleys
⊃ 95% of AIDS patients with histoplasmosis present with disseminated disease; 10%-20% present with septic shock picture
⊃ Diagnosis is confirmed by histoplasmosis antigen testing on urine or by seeing histoplasmosis in biopsy material
⊃ Mild disease is treated with itraconazole; all others are treated initially with amphotericin B then put on itraconazole for life

Coccidioidomycosis

Presentation and Progression. Coccidioidomycosis is caused by the dimorphic fungus *Coccidioides immitis,* endemic in the southwestern United States (California, Arizona, New Mexico, and Texas) and northern Mexico. In rare instances the fungus may be encountered outside the endemic area by carriage of the organism by fomites or wind-borne soil. Infection develops after inhaling the arthroconidia found in soil, which convert to form endosporulating spherules in the human host. In the normal host coccidioidomycosis may be asymptomatic or may cause mild respiratory symptoms as a subacute pneumonia, associated with migratory arthralgias and skin rashes, particularly erythema nodosum and erythema multiforme. As with the other endemic mycoses, the fungi are not susceptible to neutrophil-mediated killing, and an intact T cell–mediated immunity is required to clear the infection. In HIV-infected patients with CD4+ counts less than 200 cells/mm^3, coccidioidomycosis presents as a more severe and life-threatening illness, associated with a high mortality approaching 70% within 1 month of diagnosis. Eighty percent of AIDS patients will present with pulmonary disease, usually with reticulonodular pulmonary infiltrates and pneumonia. When disseminated, coccidioidomycosis can cause a meningoencephalitis, which is universally fatal if untreated. Skin manifestations are less common in HIV patients, occurring in only 5%. Other infections include arthritis and osteomyelitis.

Diagnosis. Diagnosis is made by fungal stains of biopsy specimens. It is imperative to alert microbiology laboratory personnel when *Coccidioides* is a potential pathogen, since it is considered a significant laboratory hazard. *Coccidioides* may be isolated in fungal culture of sputum, bronchoalveolar lavage, or biopsy specimens. Isolation of *Coccidioides* from blood is less reliable. Diagnosis may also be made by serologic testing, which is positive in greater than 80% of AIDS patients with the disease. Complement fixation of antibody is the diagnostic test of choice and correlates with disseminated disease. Titers are followed throughout the treatment course, with a rising titer indicative of treatment failure or relapse.

Treatment. Treatment of coccidioidomycosis is associated with a significant failure rate of approximately 50% and a significant relapse rate, which are roughly equal for the antifungals available. Intravenous amphotericin B and fluconazole have been tried, as well as oral fluconazole and itraconazole. Current recommended strategies include high dose intravenous amphotericin B at 1.0 to 1.25 mg/kg/day or fluconazole 400 to 800 mg/day for severe pulmonary disease, and either fluconazole or itraconazole 200 mg twice a day for less severe disease. There is some evidence that fluconazole may be superior to amphotericin B, and most clinicians will initiate therapy with fluconazole. Maintenance therapy with fluconazole or itraconazole is recommended.

KEY POINTS

- Endemic in southwest United States
- 80% of AIDS patients present with pulmonary disease
- Disseminated disease can also cause meningoencephalitis
- Diagnosis is made by serologic testing or by fungal stains of biopsy specimens
- Treatment is not highly successful, and either amphotericin B or fluconazole is used

Blastomycosis

Presentation and Progression. Blastomycosis is caused by the dimorphic fungus *Blastomyces dermatitidis*, which grows as a mold in the moist, acidic soil of the Ohio River valley, the geographic region generally overlapping that of *H. capsulatum*. After inhalation, the mold converts to a yeast form in the lung and has the ability to cause disseminated disease in those with impaired cell-mediated immunity. In the normal host, blastomycosis can cause a pulmonary syndrome with pulmonary infiltrates and nodules similar to tuberculosis. Disseminated disease occurs in HIV-infected individuals with CD4+ counts less than 200 cells/mm^3. Clinical presentation is primarily of pulmonary symptoms, with fever, cough, dyspnea, and chest pain, often associated with weight loss and failure to thrive. The chest radiographic appearance can be variable, showing focal or diffuse infiltrates, bilateral nodules, cavitary lesions, or pleural effusions. In disseminated disease multiple organ involvement is common, involving the liver, spleen, lymph nodes, and kidney. Forty percent of patients with disseminated disease will have a lymphocyte-predominant meningitis. Ulcerated cutaneous lesions are seen less commonly in patients with AIDS than in normal hosts.

Diagnosis. Diagnosis is suggested by history and chest radiographs, and confirmed by fungal culture of pertinent body fluids: bronchoalveolar lavage specimens, blood, CSF, or biopsy specimens.

Treatment. Treatment of severe blastomycosis is with intravenous amphotericin B, dosed at 0.5 mg/kg/day continued for a total dose of 1.5 g or more, with itraconazole 200 to 400 mg daily for 6 months an effective alternate for less severe disease. Maintenance therapy is required, and oral itraconazole is the treatment of choice.

KEY POINTS

- More common in Ohio River Valley
- Disseminated disease is most common presentation in HIV-infected patients with CD4+ counts = 200 cells/mm^3, and 40% of these will have meningitis
- Diagnosis is generally by culture of body fluids or stains of biopsies
- Treatment is generally with amphotericin B followed by maintenance fluconazole

Penicilliosis

Presentation and Progression. Penicilliosis is the most common mycosis infection in patients with AIDS from the southeast Asian countries of Burma, southeast China, northern Thailand, Vietnam, and Indonesia, and is the third most common opportunistic infection after tuberculosis and cryptococcal meningitis in these areas. In northern Thailand, one third of AIDS patients with CD4+ counts less than 100 cells/mm^3 present with disseminated penicilliosis. It is caused by the dimorphic fungus, *Penicillium marneffei*, which is found as a mold in the environment. Infection is established by inhalation of the mold, which converts to the yeast form in the host.

Clinical presentation is usually that of a severe systemic illness, with fever, weight loss, cough, and dyspnea prominent. Lymphadenopathy, hepatosplenomegaly, pericarditis, or peritonitis may be present. Typical skin lesions of papules, acneiform pustules, nodules, or ulcers may be present.

Diagnosis and Treatment. Diagnosis is made primarily by blood culture. *Penicillium* is less susceptible to amphotericin B and fluconazole, although intravenous amphotericin B is the recommended agent for the seriously ill. Oral itraconazole 200 to 400 mg daily is used for less severe disease, and for maintenance therapy.

Other fungal pathogens have been reported to cause disseminated disease in AIDS patients. These include *Sporothrix schenckii* and *Paracoccidioides brasiliensis*. Although seen rarely, they are important to remember as potential causes of disseminated fungal disease in AIDS patients.

Other Invasive Fungal Infections

Aspergillus species, which are associated with invasive disease in neutropenic patients, are occasionally seen in late-stage AIDS. They may take the form of an aspergilloma in those with extensive destructive pulmonary disease, as well as invasive sinus or pulmonary disease in those with very low CD4+ counts. Similarly invasive disease with the Zygomycetes has also been reported to occur in end-stage AIDS. Treatment with amphotericin B or itraconazole along with surgical debridement is recommended.

Antifungal Therapy

In response to the recognition of the increasing importance of fungi as pathogens, improved antifungal therapies are being developed. Current agents include amphotericin B and the azoles (Table 9-1).

Amphotericin B

Amphotericin B has been the mainstay of treatment for disseminated fungal disease, but has been associated with significant toxicity, including infusion-related sensitivities, nephrotoxicity, and electrolyte disturbances. Newer lipid-containing delivery systems, including amphotericin B lipid complex (ABLC) and liposomal amphotericin B (AmBisome), have been developed to alleviate some of this toxicity. Although patients have been demonstrated to tolerate the agents better than the standard amphotericin B preparation, no improvement in efficacy has been established.

TABLE 9-1
Systemic Antifungal Agents

	Route	Usual dosage	Uses
AZOLES			
Ketoconazole	Oral	200-800 mg daily	Nonmeningeal mycoses; poor absorption when used with H_2 blockers
Fluconazole	Oral, IV	100-800 mg daily	*Candida, Cryptococcus,* coccidioidomycosis
Itraconazole	Oral, IV	100-400 mg daily	*Aspergillus,* coccidioidomycosis, histoplasmosis, blastomycosis, penicilliosis, fluconazole-resistant *Candida*
AMPHOTERICIN B PREPARATIONS			
Amphotericin B	IV	0.5-1.0 mg/kg/day	*Cryptococcus* meningitis, histoplasmosis, blastomycosis, coccidioidomycosis, penicilliosis
Amphotericin B lipid complex	IV	5 mg/kg/day	
Amphotericin B cholesteryl complex	IV	3-4 mg/kg/day	
Liposomal amphotericin B	IV	3-5 mg/kg/day	
Amphotericin B suspension	Oral	100 mg 4 times daily	Fluconazole-resistant thrush
OTHERS			
Flucytosine	Oral	150 mg/kg/day, divided q6h	Used in combination with amphotericin B for cryptococcal meningitis

The development of the antifungal azoles has reduced the reliance on amphotericin B and offered oral options for treatment and maintenance therapy. These agents are generally well tolerated, but carry important precautions for drug-drug interactions that need to be remembered. Significant interactions occur with nonsedating antihistamines such as astemizole and terfenadine, which can lead to cardiac dysrhythmias. Additional interactions occur with cyclosporine, warfarin, phenytoin, and oral hypoglycemics, among others. Consultation with a pharmacist is advised when using these agents.

Fluconazole

Fluconazole is the only azole preparation currently available in both oral and intravenous form, and has an important role in the treatment of *Candida* and *Coccidioides* infections and cryptococcal meningitis.

Itraconazole

Itraconazole is an oral azole with activity against *Aspergillus* and is useful in cases of fluconazole-resistant fungal infections.

SUGGESTED READINGS

Diamond RD: The growing problem of mycoses in patients infected with the human immunodeficiency virus, *Rev Infect Dis* 13:480-486, 1991.

Hood S, Denning DW: Treatment of fungal infection in AIDS, *J Antimicrob Chemother* 37(suppl B):71-85, 1996.

Macher AM et al: AIDS and the mycoses, *Infect Dis Clin North Am* 2:827-839, 1988.

Powderly WG: Recent advances in the management of cryptococcal meningitis in patients with AIDS, *Clin Infect Dis* 22 (suppl 2):S199-223, 1996.

Wheat J: Endemic mycoses in AIDS: a clinical review, *Clin Microbiol Rev* 8(1):146-159, 1995.

10 Cytomegalovirus and Other Herpes Family Viral Infections

KATHLEEN BRADY

Cytomegalovirus
Presentation and Progression

Cause. Cytomegalovirus (CMV) is a common cause of opportunistic infections and increased morbidity, and is a predictor of death in patients with the human immunodeficiency virus (HIV). CMV is a large, double-stranded DNA virus in the herpesvirus family. Humans are the only reservoir for infection with CMV. Transmission occurs through direct contact with any body secretion including saliva, urine, feces, genital secretions, breast milk, and blood. Primary infection in the immunocompetent host results in a minor mononucleosis-like syndrome or asymptomatic disease. Approximately 90% or more of HIV-infected individuals have antibodies to CMV, indicating prior infection. Prior infection is more common among men who have sex with men, where seroprevalence approaches 100%, than among heterosexuals, where seroprevalence may be only 70% or 75%. Therefore disease in the HIV-infected host results not from primary infection but from reactivation of latent infection. End organ disease develops after hematogenous dissemination. CMV disease among patients with acquired immunodeficiency syndrome (AIDS) increased after the institution of prophylaxis against *Pneumocystis carinii* pneumonia due to improved survival. Prior to the widespread use of highly active antiretroviral therapy (HAART), CMV infection was commonly recognized in up to 40% of patients with advanced AIDS. HAART has drastically changed the face of HIV infection by increasing survival time and improving CD4+ counts by controlling HIV replication. In recent years, numerous studies have found a declining incidence of CMV infections due to HAART. CMV retinitis accounts for approximately 85% of cases of CMV infections in HIV-infected patients. An additional 10% of cases involve the gastrointestinal tract and the remainder of cases involve the lung or the nervous system.

Presentation

Retinitis. The first cases of CMV retinitis were reported in 1982. It occurs late in the course of HIV infection typically when peripheral blood CD4+ T lymphocyte counts (CD4+) drop below 50 cells/mm^3.

Symptoms from CMV retinitis are wide ranging and depend on the location of involvement on the retina. Visual symptoms of peripheral lesions include floaters and loss of peripheral vision. Lesions closer to the macula and/or optic nerve often result in paracentral scotomas. In one study, however, less than 50% of AIDS patients with CMV retinitis had visual symptoms. As many as 13% to 19% of patients with less than 50 CD4+ cells/mm^3 have asymptomatic CMV retinitis, stressing the importance of routine ophthalmologic examinations. At the time of presentation, CMV retinitis is unilateral in approximately 50% of cases. Without treatment, 60% of the initially unilateral cases will become bilateral. Systemic symptoms such as fever, myalgia, and weight loss may also be present. Symptoms such as eye pain, scleral injection, photophobia, and discharge are not associated with CMV retinitis.

Visual loss in CMV retinitis occurs for several reasons. First, retinal necrosis from direct infection of the retinal cells by CMV may occur. This type of loss is irreversible and does not respond to antiviral therapy. Second, macular edema secondary to the retinitis near the macula may also result in reduction of visual acuity. This type of loss is potentially reversible with immediate treatment with antiviral therapy. Third, retinal detachment occurs frequently in patients with CMV retinitis due to thinning of the retina. Patients may present with the sudden onset of floaters, flashing lights, visual field loss, and diminished visual acuity. The incidence of retinal detachment may be as high as 50% at 1 year after diagnosis. The risk of retinal detachment is greater in the presence of large peripheral lesions and continued active retinitis.

Direct invasion of the retinal cells by CMV results in full-thickness retinal necrosis, which appears as multiple granular or fluffy white lesions with varying amounts of hemorrhage. If untreated, the lesions enlarge and coalesce over time. Advancement of the retinitis usually leaves behind a zone of chorioretinal atrophy in which the choroidal vasculature is more easily visualized. The retinitis progresses in a characteristic "brushfire" pattern, with the zone of atrophy located centrally in the lesion and the active necrosis peripherally. On examination, minimal vitreal inflammation is characteristic, which helps to distinguish it from other pathogens, specifically toxoplasmosis.

In addition to toxoplasmosis the differential diagnosis of retinitis in a patient with AIDS includes several other diagnoses. Cotton-wool spots are microinfarctions of the retinal nerve fiber layer that occur commonly in persons with HIV infection and may resemble early CMV. These lesions do not affect visual acuity and commonly regress spontaneously over time. Acute retinal necrosis is caused by recurrence of varicella zoster (see the section on Herpes Zoster). Patients typically present with rapidly progressive visual loss and peripheral retinal vascular occlusion overlying a white, necrotic retina. Intraocular lymphomas are also in the differential of retinitis in patients with AIDS. Patients may present with small chorioretinal infiltrates. Other less common entities in the differential diagnosis include *P. carinii* chorioretinitis, syphilis, *Mycobacterium tuberculosis, Cryptococcus,* and *Candida.*

Gastrointestinal Cytomegalovirus. Gastrointestinal disease from CMV in patients with AIDS usually occurs as esophagitis or colitis but any part of the gastrointestinal tract can be involved. Dysphagia and odynophagia are the typical presenting symptoms of esophagitis. The differential diagnosis of esophagitis in AIDS patients includes *Candida,* herpes simplex, gastrointestinal reflux disease, lymphoma, and Kaposi's sarcoma. Less commonly it can be caused by infections with *M. tuberculosis* or *M. avium,* histoplasmosis, and cryptosporidia.

Symptoms of CMV colitis include systemic symptoms of fever, malaise, and weight loss, and can also include anorexia, abdominal pain, and severe diarrhea. Life-threatening complications such as gastrointestinal bleeding and perforation can occur. The symptoms of CMV colitis are not unique, and the differential diagnosis is broad and includes other infectious causes of diarrhea such as *Cryptosporidium, Microsporidium, Cyclospora, Giardia, Entamoeba histolytica, Salmonella, Shigella, Campylobacter, M. avium,* lymphoma, or Kaposi's sarcoma.

Pneumonitis. CMV is frequently isolated from bronchoalveolar lavage fluid in patients with AIDS and pulmonary symptoms or pneumonia. Despite this finding, CMV pneumonia is a rare cause of pneumonia in patients with AIDS. In most of the cases in which either CMV is isolated or CMV inclusion bodies are identified from a pulmonary specimen, another pathogen is isolated. These patients usually make a complete and rapid recovery without specific therapy directed at CMV. CMV has been identified as the pathogen in only 4% of AIDS patients with active pneumonitis.

Patients with AIDS and CMV pneumonia usually have CD4+ counts less than 75 cells/mm^3. Symptoms usually develop subacutely (over 1 to 4 weeks) but more acute onset (<1 week) has been reported. Systemic symptoms are common and include fever, dyspnea, and cough. Chest pain is uncommon. Chest x-ray usually reveals bilateral interstitial infiltrates that can have a ground-glass, nodular, or reticular pattern. Hypoxemia with a Pao$_2$ less than 75 mm Hg is found in 50% to 75% of cases. Extrapulmonary CMV is frequently documented (50% to 60% of cases) prior to or at the same time as the presentation with CMV pneumonia.

Central Nervous System Disease. CMV has been associated with ventriculoencephalitis and ascending polyradiculopathy in patients with AIDS. Symptoms of ventriculoencephalitis include memory deficits, apathy, difficulty with balance, headache and fever. On examination, impaired memory, psychomotor retardation, ataxia, cranial nerve abnormalities, or dementia may be apparent. Magnetic resonance imaging (MRI) examination of the brain frequently reveals periventricular enhancement. Cerebrospinal fluid (CSF) analysis may be unremarkable with the exception of an elevated protein.

Patients with CMV polyradiculopathy present with bilateral leg weakness and areflexia. CSF analysis in these patients may show a pleocytosis with a neutrophilic predominance. Without treatment, symptoms are progressive and can result in urinary retention and flaccid paraplegia.

Patients with CMV ventriculoencephalitis usually present with confusion, lethargy, fever, cranial nerve abnormalities, and ataxia. CSF analysis shows an elevated protein in 60% of cases and a high cell count in 25% to 30% of patients. In the remainder of cases the CSF analysis is normal. MRI typically shows periventricular enhancement.

Diagnosis

The diagnosis of CMV retinitis is based solely on clinical findings. Due to the high seroprevalence of past CMV infection in this population, CMV-specific antibodies are not helpful in making the diagnosis of CMV retinitis. Other diagnostic studies, including CMV cultures from other body sites, CMV antigenemia, and CMV DNA polymerase chain reaction (PCR), are also insufficient to establish a diagnosis of CMV retinitis. In order to make the diagnosis, clinicians must be alert to the symptoms and signs of CMV retinitis.

The diagnosis of CMV esophagitis is typically made by biopsy. Due to the high incidence of *Candida* esophagitis, endoscopy with biopsy is usually reserved for patients who have continued symptoms after empiric treatment for *Candida* esophagitis. Although both CMV and *Candida* occur when CD4+ counts are less than 50 cells/mm^3, only *Candida* esophagitis typically can occur when the CD4+ count is greater than 50 cells/mm^3. On endoscopy large, shallow ulcers are observed at the distal esophagus. On biopsy, the diagnosis is confirmed by characteristic large intranuclear inclusion bodies, which are seen in the endothelial cells at the edge of the ulcer.

Due to the nonspecific nature of symptoms in CMV colitis, colonic or rectal biopsy by colonoscopy or flexible sigmoidoscopy is required to make the diagnosis. Characteristic intranuclear and intracytoplasmic inclusions on pathologic specimens confirm the diagnosis.

The diagnosis of CMV pneumonia in AIDS patients is made by either transbronchial biopsy or open biopsy or needle aspiration. The diagnosis should be made only in the setting of clinically compatible symptoms and signs, by the identification of multiple CMV inclusion bodies on lung tissue, and when all other potential pathogens have been excluded.

CMV neurologic disease should be considered in any AIDS patient with a CD4+ count less than 50 cells/mm^3 who presents with diffuse or focal signs in the absence of focal parenchymal lesions on imaging. Any evidence of other end organ disease due to CMV is supportive of the diagnosis. Quantification of CMV by PCR is a reliable means of diagnosis of CMV central nervous system (CNS) disease. CMV PCR is positive in 75% to 100% of cases of CMV CNS disease. Lower sensitivity has been reported in series in which postmortem samples were used.

CMV culture including the more rapid shell-vial method correlates poorly with clinical disease and is therefore not useful in the diagnosis of CMV disease. Other newer methods of CMV detection may be of use in predicting the development of CMV disease. The CMV antigenemia test is a rapid method to assess CMV viremia by detecting the pp65 antigen of CMV in circulating neutrophils using monoclonal antibodies. The antigenemia test and the CMV PCR have both been evaluated in predicting the development of CMV disease in patients with AIDS and a CD4+ count less than 50 cells/mm^3. The CMV antigenemia test can predict the onset of CMV disease a median of 34 days prior to the development of CMV disease with 92% sensitivity and 88% specificity. The CMV PCR can predict the onset of disease somewhat earlier, with a median of 46 days before disease onset with a sensitivity of 95% and a specificity of 85%. Whether these tests can be used to identify a higher risk subgroup for whom preemptive preventive therapy would be cost-effective has not been determined.

Natural History

Without treatment, CMV retinitis is progressive and ultimately ends in irreversible blindness. There are very few data on the natural history of the other presentations of CMV disease.

Treatment

Methods. The drugs that are currently available for treatment of CMV infections include ganciclovir, valganciclovir, foscarnet, and cidofovir.

Ganciclovir or dihydroxypropoxymethyl guanine is a nucleoside analogue of guanosine. The drug requires triphosphorylation for activation. The first of these phosphorylations is carried out by a CMV kinase (encoded by the UL97 gene), with the subsequent two completed by cellular enzymes. It competitively inhibits CMV DNA polymerase and viral proliferation. It is poorly absorbed orally; therefore it is often given intravenously. A permanent intravenous catheter is required for administration. It is virustatic in nature against CMV, so long-term maintenance therapy is required following induction to prevent recurrence. Side effects include neutropenia, thrombocytopenia, anemia, elevation of transaminases, and line infections due to the need for a permanent intravenous catheter.

Ganciclovir can also be administered in the form of intravitreal injections and by an implantable tablet. The ganciclovir implant allows for slow, continuous release of ganciclovir into the vitreous cavity. The higher intraocular levels of ganciclovir result in a longer period to progression than can be achieved with systemic therapy. The main disadvantages to the implant are the requirement for surgery and the potential surgical complications. Endophthalmitis, retinal detachment, vitreous hemorrhage, malposition of the implant, temporary decreased vision, hypotony, and cataract have all been reported in association with the use of the ganciclovir implant. An additional disadvantage of any of the local therapies is the failure to protect against systemic disease, including the development of CMV retinitis in the contralateral eye.

Valganciclovir, a hydrochloride salt of the L-valyl ester of ganciclovir, has recently been Food and Drug Administration (FDA)-approved for the treatment of CMV retinitis in patients with AIDS. The orally administered drug is converted to ganciclovir by intestinal and hepatic esterases. The drug is well absorbed from the gastrointestinal tract, resulting in a higher area under the curve (AUC) compared with oral ganciclovir. In clinical trials, valganciclovir was equivalent to intravenous ganciclovir in delaying progression of CMV retinitis in HIV-infected patients with newly diagnosed CMV retinitis. The side effect and drug interaction profile is similar to that of ganciclovir.

Foscarnet or trisodium phosphonoformate hexahydrate is a pyrophosphate analogue that inhibits CMV DNA polymerase. Side effects include nephrotoxicity, anemia, hypocalcemia or hypercalcemia, hyperphosphatemia or hypophosphatemia, hypokalemia, hypomagnesemia, and line infections due to the need for a permanent intravenous catheter.

Cidofovir or hydroxyphosphonomethoxypropyl cytosine is a nucleotide analogue that is a competitive inhibitor of CMV DNA polymerase. Cidofovir requires diphosphorylation by cellular enzymes for activation. It has a long half-life, which makes intermittent dosing possible. Side effects include nephrotoxicity, uveitis, and hypotony.

Treatment recommendations for CMV disease differ based on the organ that is infected. The recommendations described here are based on guidelines published by the International AIDS Society (IAS). These guidelines have not been updated to include oral valganciclovir. Valganciclovir would be a reasonable substitution for systemic induction and maintenance therapy in addition to the ones described below.

Since visual loss due to retinal necrosis is irreversible in CMV retinitis, the goal of treatment is to prevent further loss of vision. A number of factors need to be considered when making treatment decisions for CMV retinitis including the location of the retinal lesions, the visual acuity of the patient, the risk of toxicity, and quality of life issues. Daily intravenous infusions of ganciclovir or foscarnet, or weekly then biweekly intravenous infusions of cidofovir, are appropriate choices for induction and then maintenance therapy for CMV retinitis. The ganciclovir intraocular implant is also an appropriate choice for initial therapy for CMV retinitis. It should be strongly considered in patients with sight-threatening disease. It should be cautioned that in addition to any local therapy, systemic treatment is recommended. Oral ganciclovir should not be used for induction in any patient and should not be used for maintenance therapy in patients with sight-threatening disease. Oral ganciclovir may be an option for patients whose retinitis is not immediately sight-threatening.

Prior to HAART, relapse of CMV retinitis occurred in virtually all patients. Most relapses occur due to the poor intraocular penetration of the systemic antivirals that are currently available. Further decline in the patient's immunologic status and antiviral resistance also needs to be considered. In cases of relapse, reinduction with any of the available antivirals is recommended, even if the same drug was being used for maintenance.

Relapse must be distinguished from refractory CMV disease. Refractory disease is defined as disease that remains active despite appropriate therapy for 6 to 8 weeks or where frequent relapses occur, suggesting inadequate control. For refractory disease, reinduction with combination therapies including a different induction drug or with local therapy is recommended.

The IAS treatment guidelines also include recommendations for the follow-up of patients with CMV retinitis. Ophthalmologic examinations are recommended immediately prior to treatment initiation, after induction has been completed, and then monthly. Examination schedules should be individualized to the patient and should take into consideration severity of disease and treatment response. Patients should be counseled that they should return for immediate follow-up if they experience any change in their visual acuity or if they develop new symptoms. Retinal photographs in conjunction with clinical examinations are considered the optimal method for patient monitoring.

For CMV gastrointestinal disease and pulmonary disease, a 3- to 6-week course of intravenous therapy with ganciclovir or foscarnet is recommended. The benefit of maintenance therapy has not been established for either of these conditions. However, maintenance therapy after reinduction for a relapse should be considered.. The efficacy of oral ganciclovir in this situation has not been established but it should be considered as a reasonable option. Patients with either gastrointestinal or pulmonary disease should undergo frequent ophthalmologic examinations to evaluate for CMV retinitis.

Treatment of CMV neurologic disease should include intravenous ganciclovir or foscarnet or a combination of both drugs. Combination therapy should be considered in patients who have received prior CMV therapy. There are no data regarding the use of cidofovir in this setting. It should be noted that there is no evidence that treatment for CMV neurologic disease extends survival. As with gastrointestinal and pulmonary disease, patients with CMV neurologic disease should undergo frequent ophthalmologic examinations to evaluate for CMV retinitis.

The initiation of HAART alone does not prevent the development of CMV retinitis. Patients with AIDS and no evidence of CMV end organ disease who have measurable CMV viremia at the initiation of HAART have been found to have reductions in CMV viral loads without any anti-CMV specific therapy. Despite this, case reports of the development of CMV retinitis after the initiation of HAART have been reported. All of the cases have been diagnosed within 7 weeks of starting HAART. Response rates to treatment in these cases were better than in the pre-HAART era.

Expected Response. The expected response to treatment for CMV is dependent on the antiretroviral treatment that a patient is receiving. With patients not on HAART, 90% of patients with CMV infection will initially respond to CMV treatment. Relapse rates are high, however. On cessation of CMV therapy, the average time to progression of retinitis is 2 weeks. With patients not on HAART, the disease will reactivate and progress in nearly all patients with current CMV treatment regimens. The median time to progression is 2 months in patients treated with intravenous ganciclovir or foscarnet, 2 to 4 months in patients treated with intravenous cidofovir, and up to 7 months in patients treated with intravitreal ganciclovir implants.

With a patient with AIDS and CMV-related retinal detachment, the determination of benefit of surgery is not clearly defined, and the decision to operate requires special consideration of such factors as the overall clinical status and life expectancy of the patient, the status of the other eye, and the wishes of the patient. The modalities for treatment of retinal detachment include laser photocoagulation or vitrectomy combined with intravitreal gas, or silicone oil injection.

Responses to therapy are similar for both CMV gastrointestinal and pulmonary diseases. Complete healing by week 6 of therapy can be demonstrated in CMV gastrointestinal disease. Relapse is common, with a median time to relapse of 9 weeks, although it may be as long as a year in some patients. Response rates of CMV pneumonitis are between 60% and 70%. Relapses have been reported but not consistently enough to justify maintenance therapy.

There are fewer data available regarding response rates for CMV CNS infections. The combination of ganciclovir and foscarnet yielded a 74% response rate in one cohort. Overall, however, the median survival time was only 3 months.

Complications. Numerous case reports have described the sudden onset of decreased visual acuity associated with significant intraocular inflammation in patients with CMV retinitis on HAART. Anterior uveitis, cataracts, vitritis, cystoid macular edema, epiretinal membrane, and disc edema have all been reported. These findings have not been noted in patients without CMV retinitis, so the ocular inflammation observed seems to be related to the presence of CMV infection. The exact mechanism for the development of immune recovery uveitis has not been determined. Initial reports suggested that immune recovery uveitis or vitritis was rare, but subsequent reports suggest that it may occur in over 60% of patients who are HAART responders. Either topical or systemic corticosteroids are helpful in reducing the intraocular inflammation. Anti-CMV therapy neither prevents the development of immune recovery uveitis nor affects the course after its development.

The emergence of resistant virus is a potential risk with the use of prolonged antiviral therapy for CMV retinitis. Ganciclovir-resistant CMV was noted in the clinical setting shortly after ganciclovir became available for the treatment of severe CMV infections. Two mechanisms of resistance to CMV therapy have been demonstrated. Mutation of the CMV UL97 gene can result in resistance to ganciclovir. This gene encodes the kinase that adds the first phosphate to ganciclovir necessary for activation. In most cases, CMV resistant to ganciclovir due to mutations of UL97 will remain susceptible to both foscarnet and cidofovir. Mutations in the CMV DNA polymerase gene can result in resistance to ganciclovir, foscarnet, and cidofovir. CMV resistance testing is not commercially available and is not clinically useful because it cannot be performed rapidly enough to impact on clinical decision making. CMV resistance should be suspected in the setting of refractory disease.

Complications due to adverse events from anti-CMV therapy also need to be considered when making treatment decisions for CMV disease.

When to Refer

Referral to an ophthalmologist experienced in treating CMV retinitis should be made in all patients who are suspected to have CMV retinitis. A baseline funduscopic examination should be performed in all AIDS patients with CD4+ counts less than 100 cells/mm^3. Regular follow up funduscopic examinations should be performed by an ophthalmologist for patients with CD4+ counts less than 50 cells/mm^3.

Referral to an appropriate specialist for biopsy for patients suspected of having CMV gastrointestinal, pulmonary, or CNS disease is also indicated.

Guidelines

The United States Public Health Service (USPHS) and the Infectious Diseases Society of America (IDSA) have published guidelines for the prevention of opportunistic infections in persons infected with HIV. It is recommended that HIV-infected persons who belong to risk groups with low rates of seropositivity for CMV should be tested for antibody to CMV. These groups include patients who have not had male homosexual contact or used injection drugs. HIV-infected patients should be counseled regarding the prevention of exposure to CMV (Table 10-1).

TABLE 10-1
Prevention of Cytomegalovirus Infection

Exposure	Method of prevention
Semen, cervical secretions, or saliva	Latex condoms during sexual contact
HIV-infected parent or child-care provider exposed to children in child-care facilities	Good hygienic practices such as hand washing
HIV-infected child in a child-care facility	Good hygienic practices such as hand washing
HIV-infected persons who are CMV-negative who require a blood transfusion	Administer CMV antibody-negative or leukocyte-reduced cellular blood products in nonemergency situations

The USPHS/IDSA guidelines also recommend that prophylaxis with oral ganciclovir may be considered for HIV-infected subjects with CD4+ counts less than 50 cells/mm^3 who are seropositive for CMV. Ganciclovir-induced neutropenia, anemia, unclear efficacy, lack of proven survival benefit, the risk of developing resistant CMV, and cost should all be considered when deciding whether prophylaxis should be instituted in any individual patient. Neither acyclovir nor valacyclovir is effective in preventing CMV infection and neither should be used for this purpose.

The most important method for prevention of CMV infection is early recognition of disease. Patients must be aware of the symptoms of CMV infection, specifically of retinitis. Regular funduscopic examinations performed by an ophthalmologist are recommended by some experts for patients with CD4+ counts less than 50 cells/mm^3.

The USPHS/IDSA guidelines point out that CMV disease is not curable with the currently available medical treatments and that maintenance therapy following induction is recommended for life. However, they acknowledge that several studies have now shown that maintenance therapy can be safely discontinued in patients with CMV retinitis who have had an increase in their CD4+ counts to greater than 100 to 150 cells/mm^3. Discontinuation of secondary prophylaxis may be considered in patients with sustained (defined as 3 to 6 months) increases in CD4+ counts to greater than 100 to 150 cells/mm^3. They caution that such a decision should be made in consultation with an ophthalmologist and should take into consideration such factors as the magnitude and duration of the CD4+ count response, magnitude and duration of the viral load response, location of the retinal lesion, vision in the contralateral eye, and feasibility with which follow-up examinations can be done. Recurrence of CMV retinitis in patients who have discontinued CMV therapy after response to HAART has occurred with virologic and immunologic failure. All cases of recurrence have occurred when the CD4+ count dropped below 50 cells/mm^3. In this situation, anti-CMV–specific therapy should be resumed before evidence of clinical reactivation occurs because of the risk of systemic involvement and the risk to the contralateral eye.

KEY POINTS

- CMV infections typically occur when CD4+ counts drop below 50 cells/mm^3
- CMV retinitis accounts for approximately 85% of cases of CMV infections in HIV-infected patients
- The diagnosis of CMV retinitis is based solely on clinical findings
- The diagnosis of CMV esophagitis, colitis, and pneumonitis is typically made by biopsy
- Systemic treatment for all CMV infections is recommended
- About 90% of patients with CMV infection not on HAART will initially respond to CMV treatment; relapse rates are high, however

Herpes Simplex
Presentation and Progression

Cause. Herpes simplex type 1 (HSV-1) and type 2 (HSV-2) are both double-stranded DNA viruses. Like the other herpesviruses, HSV-1 and HSV-2 have the unique ability to induce latency with periodic reactivation. The mode of transmission is person to person via infected secretions. After direct inoculation through a mucous membrane, the virus is transported along sensory nerves to the dorsal root ganglia or trigeminal ganglia, where it becomes latent. When reactivation occurs, the virus is transported along sensory nerves to mucocutaneous surfaces, where replication may lead to clinically apparent disease. Both cell-mediated and humoral responses are important for maintaining latency of HSV. Impairment of cell-mediated immunity, as with HIV, leads to higher recurrence rates and severity of disease.

HSV-1 is associated with 70% of orolabial infections and HSV-2 is associated with 70% of genital infections due to HSV. Evidence of prior infection with HSV-1 and HSV-2 is common in the general population. Seroprevalence studies have found that 50% to 70% of adults in the United States have antibodies to HSV-1 and 20% to 30% have antibodies to HSV-2. Seroprevalence rates for HSV-2 are higher among females, blacks, and individuals with a greater number of lifetime sexual partners. There is evidence that seroprevalence rates in individuals with HIV infection are much higher.

Chronic mucocutaneous HSV lesions persisting for more than 1 month are included in the Centers for Disease Control and Prevention (CDC) case definition of AIDS.

Presentation

Mucocutaneous Infections. Mucocutaneous involvement of HSV is the most common manifestation of disease for patients with HIV. Vesiculoulcerative lesions can occur at any site but usually involve the genital and rectal regions. Symptoms usually begin with painful erythematous papules that become vesicular and then rapidly ulcerate. Chronic single or multiple coalescent ulcers are frequently the end result. Ulcers due to HSV are typically superficial and have a scalloped border. Tender lymphadenopathy may also be present. In the vast majority of patients with HIV, the frequency, duration, and severity of HSV recurrences are similar to that reported in immunocompetent hosts. However, evidence of increased incidence and severity of symptoms has been reported in HIV patients with CD4+ counts less than 50 cells/mm³. There is also evidence that the period of viral shedding of HSV is prolonged in patients with HIV. Shedding may also occur in the absence of clinically apparent lesions.

Atypical mucocutaneous lesions of HSV have been described and include necrotizing folliculitis, and hyperkeratotic lesions.

The differential diagnosis of mucocutaneous HSV disease includes varicella-zoster virus (VZV), disseminated CMV, disseminated cryptococcal infection, histoplasmosis, squamous cell carcinoma, and pustular dermatosis.

Herpes Simplex Virus Esophagitis. Similar to CMV, HSV may cause disease throughout the intestinal tract but esophagitis is the most common. HSV esophagitis is typically caused by HSV-1. Incidence is low for patients with AIDS, occurring in only 2.5% of patients with AIDS followed prospectively. HSV is identified as the cause of esophageal symptoms in only 4% to 16% of AIDS cases. Typical symptoms include dysphagia, odynophagia, chest pain, and fever. At the time of diagnosis of herpes esophagitis, only one third of patients typically have evidence of extraesophageal herpes.

On endoscopy, the lesions are predominantly in the distal esophagus (50%) but can be diffuse in almost one third (32%) of patients. Superficial ulcers are typically observed, which may help to distinguish it from CMV where ulcers are often deep.

The differential diagnosis of esophagitis in AIDS patients includes *Candida*, CMV, gastrointestinal reflux disease, lymphoma, and Kaposi's sarcoma. Less commonly it can be caused by infections with *M. tuberculosis* or *M. avium*, histoplasmosis, and cryptosporidia.

Herpes Simplex Virus Proctitis. HSV is the most common cause of nongonococcal proctitis in men who have sex with men and is a frequent site of reactivation among HIV-infected individuals. Symptoms of anorectal pain, constipation, tenesmus, anal pruritus, sacral paresthesias, fever, and inguinal lymphadenopathy have been reported. Perianal ulcerations are observed in 70% of patients who present with HSV proctitis. On sigmoidoscopy, friable mucosa with vesicular or ulcerative lesions may be seen.

Other Presentations. There is no evidence that HSV-associated encephalitis, aseptic meningitis, and ocular keratitis are more common in patients with HIV infection.

Diagnosis

Regardless of the site of infection, confirmation of the diagnosis of HSV infection should be pursued. HSV culture remains the gold standard for diagnosis of HSV infection. Vesicles should be unroofed and a specimen obtained from the base of the ulcer. Newer lesions are more likely to yield positive culture results. After inoculation into tissue culture, cytopathic effect can be observed in 24 to 72 hours. HSV-1 and HSV-2 infections can be distinguished using type-specific monoclonal antibodies.

The Tzanck smear and antigen testing provide more immediate results. For both, the lesion is unroofed and a scraping is taken from the base of the ulcer similar to a culture. The Tzanck smear can be used to demonstrate multinucleated giant cells on Giemsa staining. This method is not specific for HSV, however, since VZV could also give a positive result. Antigen detection can be by one of several methods including direct immunofluorescence, immunoperoxidase staining, or enzyme-linked immunosorbent assays (ELISAs). Sensitivities of these methods in comparison with viral isolation range from 70% to 95%, with specificities of 65% to 90%; the variability is dependent on the adequacy of the specimen.

In PCR, the signal of HSV DNA is amplified, resulting in a much more sensitive HSV detection method compared with detection viral proteins. This technique is available for the diagnosis of both mucocutaneous infection and herpes encephalitis.

Natural History

In vitro studies suggest that HSV can enhance replication of HIV. The impact of active HSV infection on HIV viral load has been evaluated. In one study, 16 subjects were identified with active HSV infection and had pre-outbreak, acute-phase, and post-outbreak plasma samples that could be tested for HIV RNA levels. Plasma viral load increased a median of 3.4-fold during the acute outbreak, and post-outbreak levels remained above pre-outbreak levels in some subjects. This occurred despite treatment of the acute HSV outbreaks with acyclovir followed by chronic suppression. None of the patients in this study were on HAART, so the effect of HSV reactivation on viral load in these patients remains unclear.

Treatment

Methods. The drugs that are currently available for treatment of HSV infections include acyclovir, valacyclovir, famciclovir and foscarnet, cidofovir, and topical therapies.

Acyclovir is a nucleoside analogue that requires phosphorylation by viral thymidine kinase. Two additional phosphorylation steps are carried out by cellular enzymes prior to activation of the drug. Acyclovir is an inhibitor of viral DNA polymerase and acts as a chain terminator. Acyclovir is extremely well tolerated and has few side effects. Side effects that have been reported infrequently include nausea and vomiting, rash, diarrhea, renal toxicity, and CNS side effects. The renal failure due to acyclovir is induced by crystallization of the drug in the renal tubules. It is reversible with cessation of the drug. Rapid infusion of the drug and preexisting renal disease are predisposing factors. Reports of CNS toxicity include encephalopathy and seizures, which have been reported more commonly among the elderly.

Famciclovir is an orally administered prodrug of the antiviral agent penciclovir. Similar to acyclovir, viral thymidine kinase phosphorylates penciclovir to a monophosphate form, which is subsequently converted to penciclovir triphosphate by cellular enzymes. Famciclovir has greater oral bioavailability than acyclovir, allowing for increased dosing intervals compared with acyclovir. Famciclovir use is indicated for treatment of acute herpes zoster (HZ) and treatment of recurrent mucocutaneous HSV in both immunocompetent and HIV-infected patients. The safety and efficacy of famciclovir for HZ in HIV-infected patients have not been established. The side-effect profile of famciclovir is similar to acyclovir.

Valacyclovir is a prodrug of acyclovir that is available in an oral form. After administration, the drug is rapidly absorbed from the gastrointestinal tract and converted to acyclovir. The enhanced bioavailability of valacyclovir leads to serum levels that are equivalent to intravenous dosing of acyclovir. Lower oral doses and increased dosing intervals are possible with valacyclovir in comparison with acyclovir. Thrombotic thrombocytopenic purpura (TTP), hemolytic-uremic syndrome (HUS), and death have occurred in immunosuppressed patients including patients with advanced HIV disease in clinical trials of valacyclovir at a dosage of 8 grams per day. The side effect profile of valacyclovir is otherwise similar to acyclovir. The efficacy of valacyclovir for HSV in HIV-infected patients has not been established.

The role of foscarnet in the treatment of HSV is primarily for acyclovir-resistant strains. Foscarnet remains active against thymidine kinase–deficient HSV and altered strains of HSV, since it does not require phosphorylation to inhibit DNA polymerase.

Cidofovir also has in vitro activity against HSV including acyclovir-resistant strains. Several case reports have described clinical improvement of acyclovir-resistant HSV with intravenous cidofovir. Ease of administration must be weighed against the risks of serious systemic toxicity, however. At the current time, cidofovir should be reserved for patients who fail to respond to acyclovir and foscarnet.

Topical therapy for resistant HSV may also be an option. Both cidofovir gel and foscarnet cream have been evaluated in small clinical trials. The modest benefits of these treatments may be countered by a high incidence of local reactions.

Expected Response. Systemic antiviral drugs can reduce the symptoms and signs of herpes simplex episodes when used to treat primary or recurrent disease or when used as suppressive therapy. Failure of lesions to respond by 10 to 14 days of therapy should increase the suspicion of resistant virus, and alternate therapy should be considered.

Complications. As with CMV, HSV infections due to resistant strains have been demonstrated. In general, infections with these resistant strains occur in AIDS patients whose CD4+ counts have dropped below 100 cells/mm^3. Reduction in viral thymidine kinase activity is one mechanism for resistance of HSV to acyclovir. Other potential mechanisms for resistance include alterations in substrate specificity of either viral thymidine kinase or viral DNA polymerase. In vitro susceptibility testing is possible but not standardized. There is good correlation between in vitro activity and clinical response to therapy. The probability of failure of acyclovir using standard dosing is 95% when an HSV isolate is acyclovir-resistant in vitro.

When to Refer

Referral to an appropriate specialist for biopsy in patients suspected of having atypical mucocutaneous HSV or HSV gastrointestinal disease is indicated.

Guidelines

With regard to herpes simplex, the USPHS/IDSA guidelines for the prevention of opportunistic infections in HIV-infected persons can be easily summarized. It is recommended that HIV-infected persons should use latex condoms during any sexual encounter to reduce the risk of exposure and infection with herpes simplex. Antivirals are not recommended for the use of primary prevention of herpes simplex. Antivirals are also not recommended for the prevention of recurrences unless an individual has either frequent or severe recurrences. Frequent recurrences are typically defined as three or more recurrences in a 6-month time period. Acyclovir, famciclovir, and ganciclovir are all considered appropriate options for suppressive therapy.

KEY POINTS

- Mucocutaneous involvement of HSV is the most common manifestation of disease for patients with HIV
- In the vast majority of patients with HIV, the frequency, duration, and severity of HSV recurrences are similar to that reported in immunocompetent hosts
- There is increased incidence and severity of symptoms in HIV-infected patients with CD4+ counts below 50 cell/mm^3
- HSV is identified as the cause of esophageal symptoms in only 4% to 16% of AIDS cases
- Regardless of the site of infection, confirmation of the diagnosis of HSV infection should be pursued
- HSV culture remains the gold standard for diagnosis of HSV infection

Varicella-Zoster

Presentation and Progression

Cause. Primary infection with VZV usually occurs early in life as chickenpox. Serologic evidence of prior exposure is present in approximately 90% of adults. Following the primary infection, the virus becomes latent in dorsal root and cranial nerve ganglia. VZV reactivation results in virus reaching the skin by transport along sensory neuronal axons, producing the skin lesions and pain that define HZ. An antigen-specific cell-mediated immune response is elicited during the primary exposure to VZV (chickenpox). This immune response may be responsible for maintaining latency of the virus and preventing HZ. Symptomatic reactivation occurs when there is a sufficient decrease in VZV-specific cell-mediated immunity to the point where viral replication can no longer be suppressed. This occurs most commonly in the elderly and in the immunocompromised.

Population-based studies of HZ in the United States have found the overall incidence to be 2.15 cases per 1,000 person-years. Most cases, however, occur in individuals who are greater than 45 to 50 years of age. Estimates of incidence range from 0.5 to 0.7 cases per 1,000 person-years in children less than age 14 to 10 to 14 cases per 1,000 person-years in those over age 75. Reactivation of VZV as HZ is a well-recognized cause of morbidity in the HIV-infected host. It has been described as both an early and a late manifestation of HIV infection. The overall incidence of HZ for HIV-infected patients has been estimated to be 29.4 to 51.1 cases per 1,000 person-years in the pre-HAART era. Whether the incidence and course of HZ have changed in the setting of HAART remains to be seen. The wide use of protease inhibitor therapy has changed the face of HIV infection. Recent studies are confirming the expectation of reduced rates of clinical progression and of opportunistic infections (such as CMV retinitis or *P. carinii* pneumonia) for patients taking these medications. Since the incidence of HZ appears to be increased at all ranges of CD4+ counts, patients may remain at significant risk for HZ despite treatment and benefit from HAART. As patients live longer across all CD4+ counts with HIV there is concern that the incidence of HZ could increase over time. This may depend on when VZV-specific cell-mediated immunity is lost and whether it can be recovered.

Presentation

Varicella. The rash of varicella infection begins as a macular rash that progresses rapidly over hours to papules and then to vesicles with an erythematous base. The development of rash is preceded by a 1- to 2-day prodrome of fevers, myalgias, and headache. Crops of new lesions typically continue to appear for 3 to 4 days. Systemic symptoms of fever, myalgias, and headache are present during this time. Older lesions pustulate, then crust and usually heal without scarring. The most common complication of primary varicella infection in the immunocompetent host is secondary bacterial infection of the skin lesions. Other complications include varicella pneumonia and postinfectious encephalitis. Varicella pneumonia is rare in children but occurs in up to 20% to 30% of adults with primary varicella.

Primary varicella infection does not appear to be a serious problem for most HIV-infected children who develop the disease. Only one in 30 cases of varicella is severe. High rates of HZ have been reported from several cohorts of HIV-infected children. A rate of 467 cases per 1,000 person-years has been reported in children who develop primary varicella when their CD4+ cells are less than 15%. These children were over 15 times more likely to develop HZ compared with children whose CD4+ cells were greater than 15%.

Approximately 95% of HIV-infected adults have antibody to varicella due to prior infection during childhood. Case reports of primary infection with varicella in HIV-infected adults have therefore been rare.

Herpes Zoster. Lesions of HZ typically erupt in one or two adjacent dermatomes. The lesions progress from discrete areas of erythema to grouped vesicles, which pustulate and crust over a period of 7 to 10 days. Dermatomes involved in order of frequency are thoracic (42%), trigeminal (15%), cervical (12%), lumbar (10%), sacral (8%), and lumbar and sacral regions (2%). Presentation is similar in the HIV-infected host in the majority of cases, although atypical lesions, dissemination, complications, and recurrence of zoster are more common.

Nondermatomal atypical lesions occur in 5% of cases of HZ in HIV-infected patients. Atypical lesions that have been described include pox-like ulcerations and hyperkeratotic, verrucous lesions. Both have been described in patients with chronic (more than 4 weeks) lesions. In many of these cases, a prior history of dermatomal zoster and extensive use of acyclovir has been reported. Many of the strains of VZV causing these atypical lesions have been found to be acyclovir-resistant.

Dissemination of HZ occurs in approximately 5% of cases of HZ. The appearance and course of the lesions are similar in most cases to multidermatomal zoster. The CNS is the organ system most commonly involved in cases of dissemination (see below). Hepatitis and pneumonia due to zoster have not been described.

Ocular Lesions. Acute retinal necrosis due to VZV was first recognized in the immunocompetent host but is believed to be a rare occurrence. Soon after the AIDS epidemic began, reports of acute retinal necrosis for patients with AIDS were described.

Symptoms of acute retinal necrosis usually begin as loss of visual acuity and ocular pain. The peripheral retina is usually involved first with focal areas of necrotizing retinitis. Progression usually occurs in a circumferential fashion and is associated with vitritis and symptomatic anterior uveitis. Disease typically begins unilaterally, but subsequent involvement of the contralateral eye develops in one third to one half of cases. Retinal detachment is a common complication, occurring in most patients by 6 months. In most cases of acute retinal necrosis due to VZV in immunocompromised hosts, acute retinal necrosis has followed or has occurred along with HZ ophthalmicus or cutaneous zoster. This association strongly suggests that acute retinal necrosis develops as a result of dissemination of VZV. Untreated, acute retinal necrosis begins to resolve spontaneously in 3 to 4 weeks and usually does not extend to the macula. Retinal detachment is a common complication.

Rapidly progressive herpetic retinal necrosis (RPHRN) is a virulent variant of acute retinal necrosis that has been described in patients with advanced HIV infection.

Central Nervous System Infections. VZV infection of the CNS has also been described in patients with advanced HIV infection. Several different clinicopathologic syndromes of VZV CNS infection have been described including leukoencephalitis, ventriculitis, acute meningomyeloradiculitis, myelitis, cerebral infarcts, and aseptic meningitis. The CNS manifestations probably depend on the severity of the infection and on the different routes of viral spread to the brain and spinal cord. Infection may develop through centripetal neural spread to the brain and spinal cord from VZV trigeminal or spinal ganglionic infection, by hematogenous dissemination, or through CSF pathways.

Diagnosis

HZ can be reliably diagnosed on clinical grounds alone in most cases. In one series, 97% of subjects, in whom there was clinical suspicion of herpes, had laboratory confirmation of VZV infection. The diagnosis of HZ should be confirmed in all patients with atypical lesions, in cases in which there is dissemination, and if acyclovir resistance is suspected.

VZV culture is the gold standard for diagnosis of VZV infection. Vesicles should be unroofed and a specimen obtained from the base of the ulcer. Newer lesions are more likely to yield positive culture results. After inoculation into tissue culture, cytopathic effect can be observed in 3 to 7 days. Due to lability of the virus, culture for VZV is specific but not sensitive.

As with HSV, the Tzanck smear and antigen testing can provide more immediate results. For both, the lesion is unroofed and a scraping is taken from the base of the ulcer similar to a culture. The Tzanck smear can be used to demonstrate multinucleated giant cells on Giemsa staining. This method is not specific for VZV, however, since HSV could also give a positive result. Antigen detection is performed by using direct immunofluorescence and is more sensitive than viral culture. An additional advantage to this method is that it allows discrimination between VZV and HSV, since specific monoclonal antibodies are used for each virus. PCR can also be used as a diagnostic tool but is currently only available as a research tool.

The diagnosis of ocular disease caused by VZV is based on the funduscopic examination and the clinical course and not on diagnostic testing.

The correct diagnosis of VZV infection of the CNS requires a high index of suspicion. In as many as 30% to 40% of cases there is no history of antecedent HZ and in many others the history of HZ precedes the symptoms by months. Diagnosis of CNS infection with VZV is made either by isolation of VZV from viral culture or by PCR analysis of CSF for VZV.

Natural History

In most patients (including immunocompromised hosts), HZ manifests as a painful, cutaneous eruption of vesicular lesions that occurs in a dermatomal distribution. Healing occurs over a period of 2 to 4 weeks. The cutaneous eruption is typically accompanied by significant pain, and in a subset of patients, the pain may persist after healing of the lesions. A variety of other neurologic, ocular, and local complications can develop as described above.

Treatment

Methods. The drugs that are currently available for treatment of VZV infections include acyclovir, valacyclovir, famciclovir, and foscarnet. The mechanisms of action of these drugs have been described above.

Most patients with VZV infection can be treated with oral therapy. Patients with unusually severe disease or disseminated infection should receive intravenous therapy. It should be noted that the concentration of acyclovir required to inhibit replication of VZV is fivefold to tenfold higher than for HSV, so higher doses of antivirals are required for treatment (Table 10-2).

The use of steroids for the treatment of HZ remains controversial. Clinical trials to determine whether steroids are beneficial in preventing postherpetic neuralgia have yielded mixed results. In one study of adults over the age of 50, prednisone decreased the duration of acute neuritis pain and the period of required analgesic treatment. The safety and benefit of steroids in immunosuppressed patients including patients with HIV infection have not been evaluated, and they should be used with caution.

Acyclovir-resistant VZV infections have been well described in patients with HIV infection. Resistance typically occurs in patients with advanced HIV infection who have previously been treated with acyclovir. Thymidine kinase–deficient and altered strains of VZV are generally responsible for acyclovir resistance in these subjects. Acyclovir-resistant strains of VZV are usually cross-resistant to other antivirals that are thymidine kinase–dependent including valacyclovir, famciclovir, and ganciclovir. Data on treatment of acyclovir-resistant strains of VZV are limited, but foscarnet has in vitro activity and has been used successfully in several small case series. Cidofovir also has in vitro activity and may be effective, but at the current time there are no clinical data to support its use.

Expected Response. Placebo-controlled trials of both intravenous and oral acyclovir have demonstrated clinical benefit in healthy and immunocompromised patients with HZ who were treated within 72 hours after onset of disease. Therapy decreases the number of days of new lesion formation, reduces the extent of involvement in the primary dermatome, and diminishes the time to crusting of lesions. Specifically in immunocompromised hosts, studies using acyclovir have shown that progressive disease is slowed and therapy protects against dissemination of VZV.

Complications. Based on pathogenesis, complications of HZ can be divided into two groups, those attributable to local disease and those related to dissemination. Complications from

TABLE 10-2
Treatment of Infections Caused by Varicella-Zoster Virus

Drug	Indication	Dose
Acyclovir (intravenous)	Severe or disseminated VZV infection	10 mg/kg IV q 8 hours for 7 to 10 days
Acyclovir (oral)	HZ	800 mg po 5 times daily for 7 to 10 days
Valacyclovir	HZ	1 g po q 8 hours for 7 to 10 days
Famciclovir	HZ	500 mg po q 8 hours for 7 to 10 days

local disease include prolonged lesions (more than 1 month), superinfection of cutaneous lesions, postherpetic neuralgia, neuropathy, HZ ophthalmicus, and myelitis. Complications arising from dissemination include disseminated cutaneous lesions, CNS involvement, and retinitis. The incidence of complications of HZ in HIV-infected individuals has been evaluated in several studies. Unidermatomal zoster occurs in the vast majority of patients. Multidermatomal lesions were present in 11% of episodes, and disseminated skin lesions were present in 5% of episodes in one series. In 60% of cases there was resolution without complications, 13% had minor complications (such as bacterial superinfection), 13% had postherpetic neuralgia, and 27% had a major complication of zoster.

More serious complications, such as ocular complications, neurologic complications, chronic atypical skin lesions, and postherpetic neuralgia, have been reported in 11% to 40% of cases. Low CD4+ counts below 200 cells/mm^3 are predictive of the development of a complication of HZ.

When to Refer

All patients with disseminated VZV infection or atypical VZV disease should be referred to an HIV specialist for diagnosis and treatment. This includes referral to an experienced ophthalmologist for treatment of acute retinal necrosis and referral to an appropriate specialist for biopsy in patients suspected of having atypical VZV.

Guidelines

The USPHS and IDSA have made recommendations for the prevention of varicella infections in their guidelines for the prevention of opportunistic infections in persons with HIV. Any HIV-infected person without a history of prior infection with VZV should avoid exposure to persons with chickenpox or shingles. Additionally, all household contacts of HIV-infected patients should be vaccinated with live-attenuated VZV vaccine if they have no prior history of chickenpox and are not HIV-infected. The safety and efficacy of the vaccine in patients with HIV have not been established, so no recommendation has been made regarding its use in HIV-infected patients who are susceptible to VZV.

In the event of an exposure to chickenpox or shingles, HIV-infected patients without a history of prior chickenpox should be administered varicella zoster immune globulin within 96 hours of the contact. There are no data regarding the efficacy of acyclovir in the prevention of chickenpox in patients with HIV and no prior history of VZV infection.

There are currently no recommendations for the prevention of HZ or its recurrence in patients with HIV.

KEY POINTS

- Since the incidence of HZ appears to be increased at all ranges of CD4+ counts, HIV-infected patients may remain at significant risk for HZ despite treatment and benefit from HAART
- The lesions of HZ progress from discrete areas of erythema to grouped vesicles, which pustulate and crust over a period of 7 to 10 days
- Presentation is similar in the HIV-infected host in the majority of cases, although atypical lesions, dissemination, complications, and recurrence of HZ are more common
- Many of the strains of VZV causing atypical lesions have been found to be acyclovir-resistant
- Dissemination occurs in approximately 5% of cases of HZ
- HZ can be reliably diagnosed on clinical grounds alone in most cases
- Placebo-controlled trials of both intravenous and oral acyclovir have demonstrated clinical benefit in healthy and immunocompromised patients with HZ who were treated within 72 hours after onset of disease

Epstein-Barr Virus

Presentation and Progression

Cause. Epstein-Barr virus (EBV) is a double-stranded DNA virus that is a member of the herpesvirus family. Humans and nonhuman primates are the only reservoirs for disease. Symptoms of primary infection are dependent on age; children often have subclinical infection, whereas adolescents and adults typically present with infectious mononucleosis. Symptoms and signs of infectious mononucleosis include sore throat, fever, lymphadenopathy, and an atypical lymphocytosis on peripheral smear. Transmission is believed to be from infected oral secretions in patients with primary infection. EBV is capable of infecting only B lymphocytes and epithelial cells of the nasopharynx. It is in these cells that the virus establishes latency replicating with each cell division. The infection appears to be kept in latency by CD8 cytotoxic T lymphocytes. Decreased activity and number of these cells with advanced HIV infection helps to explain the increased occurrence of EBV-related conditions among patients with HIV.

Presentation

Oral Lesions. Oral hairy leukoplakia (OHL) usually presents as adherent, white or gray patches on the lateral margins of the tongue. The patches are usually irregular and form folds and projections that resemble hair. OHL can also occur on the dorsum or ventral side of the tongue and occasionally may occur elsewhere in the oropharynx. Patients are frequently asymptomatic, but soreness or burning of the tongue may occur.

On histologic examination, the lesions consistently show epithelial hyperplasia, hyperparakeratosis, and acanthosis. Swollen and vacuolated cells in the prickle cell layer contain large numbers of EBV particles. Characteristic nuclear changes of OHL can also be helpful in distinguishing it from other diagnoses.

The differential diagnosis of OHL includes *Candida,* smoker's leukoplakia, frictional keratosis, geographic tongue, hyperplastic candidiasis, lichen planus, and squamous cell carcinoma.

Lymphoma. Almost all cases of CNS lymphoma and approximately 50% of cases of non-Hodgkin's lymphoma in patients with AIDS are directly related to EBV. This topic will be further discussed in Chapter 24.

Diagnosis

A presumptive diagnosis of OHL can be made clinically, but a definitive diagnosis can only be made with biopsy and demonstration of replicating EBV.

Natural History

OHL frequently resolves spontaneously without treatment, and is benign and does not lead to malignancy if left untreated. OHL is a sign of significant immunocompromise, however, and is predictive of the rapid onset of AIDS.

Treatment

There is no clinically proven benefit of the treatment of OHL. Since the majority of cases are asymptomatic, it is rare that treatment is warranted. Case reports have suggested a possible role of acyclovir, ganciclovir, and foscarnet. The lesions typically recur immediately after treatment has been discontinued. The harmlessness of the disease, the side effects of the medications, and the risk of antiviral resistance all need to be considered prior to instituting systemic therapy.

Other potential courses of treatment include topical retinoids, topical podophyllin, surgical excision, and cryotherapy. Regardless of the treatment method, the lesions recur as a rule.

When to Refer

There are no clear guidelines as to when suspected OHL should be biopsied to confirm the diagnosis.

KEY POINTS

- OHL usually presents as adherent, white or gray patches on the lateral margins of the tongue
- Patients are frequently asymptomatic, but soreness or burning of the tongue may occur
- The differential diagnosis of OHL includes *Candida,* smoker's leukoplakia, frictional keratosis, geographic tongue, hyperplastic candidiasis, lichen planus, and squamous cell carcinoma
- A presumptive diagnosis of OHL can be made clinically, but a definitive diagnosis can only be made with biopsy and demonstration of replicating EBV
- There is no clinically proven benefit of the treatment of OHL

SUGGESTED READINGS

Cheung TW, Teich SA: Cytomegalovirus infection in patients with HIV infection, *Mt Sinai J Med* 66(2):113-124, 1999.

Drew WL et al: Cytomegalovirus (CMV) resistance in patients with CMV retinitis and AIDS treated with oral or intravenous ganciclovir, *J Infect Dis* 179(6):1352-1355, 1999.

Erlich KS et al: Acyclovir-resistant herpes simplex virus infections in patients with the acquired immunodeficiency syndrome, *N Engl J Med* 320(5):293-296, 1989.

Glesby MJ, Moore RD, Chaisson RE: Clinical spectrum of herpes zoster in adults infected with human immunodeficiency virus, *Clin Infect Dis* 21(2):370-375, 1995.

Holbrook JT et al: Risk factors for advancement of cytomegalovirus retinitis in patients with acquired immunodeficiency syndrome: Studies of Ocular Complications of AIDS Research Group, *Arch Ophthalmol* 118(9):1196-1204, 2000.

Martinez E et al: High incidence of herpes zoster in patients with AIDS soon after therapy with protease inhibitors, *Clin Infect Dis* 27(6):1510-1513, 1998.

Mole L et al: The impact of active herpes simplex virus infection on human immunodeficiency virus load, *J Infect Dis* 76(3):766-770, 1997.

Ormerod LD et al: Rapidly progressive herpetic retinal necrosis: a blinding disease characteristic of advanced AIDS, *Clin Infect Dis* 26(1):34-45; discussion 46-47, 1998.

Roullet E: Opportunistic infections of the central nervous system during HIV-1 infection (emphasis on cytomegalovirus disease), *J Neurol* 246(4):237-243, 1999.

Stewart JA et al: Herpesvirus infections in persons infected with human immunodeficiency virus, *Clin Infect Dis* 21(Suppl 1):S114-S120, 1995.

Triantos D et al: Oral hairy leukoplakia: clinicopathologic features, pathogenesis, diagnosis, and clinical significance *Clin Infect Dis* 25(6):1392-1396, 1997.

Veenstra J et al: Complications of varicella-zoster virus reactivation in HIV-infected homosexual men, *AIDS* 10(4):393-399, 1996.

Whitcup SM: Cytomegalovirus retinitis in the era of highly active antiretroviral therapy, *JAMA* 283(5):653-657, 2000.

Whitley RJ et al: Guidelines for the treatment of cytomegalovirus diseases in patients with AIDS in the era of potent antiretroviral therapy: recommendations of an international panel: International AIDS Society-USA, *Arch Intern Med* 158(9):957-969, 1998.

11 Toxoplasmosis and Other Protozoal Infections

EBBING LAUTENBACH, STUART N. ISAACS

Toxoplasma gondii
Presentation and Progression

Cause. *Toxoplasma gondii* is an intracellular protozoan parasite and a major cause of disease in patients infected with the human immunodeficiency virus (HIV). Primary infection with *T. gondii* is nearly always asymptomatic and leads to chronic infection due to persistence of the organism in its cyst form. In the setting of severe immune dysfunction, there may be reactivation of *T. gondii* cysts to produce active disease.

T. gondii exists in three stages: oocyst, tachyzoite, and tissue cyst. The oocyst, which measures 10×12 μm and is ovoid in shape, is produced by a sexual cycle in the small intestine of infected cats. After excretion, oocysts may remain viable for up to 1½ years in the environment. The oocyst must mature, or sporulate, before it is able to cause infection; this process requires a few days to several weeks, depending on the temperature. Initial infection occurs through ingestion of food products contaminated with oocysts or through ingestion of the tissue cyst in raw or undercooked meat. The tachyzoite, which measures 3×7 μm and has a crescentlike appearance, is the invasive form of the organism and can infect almost any mammalian cell. The tachyzoite lyses the host cell, subsequently infecting adjacent cells, and hematogenous dissemination allows the organism to spread to various other organs. Finally, the tissue cyst, which measures approximately 10 to 200 μm, persists in tissues during the chronic phase of infection. It can be found in nearly any organ but is most commonly located in the brain, myocardium, and skeletal muscle.

T. gondii is found ubiquitously in the environment and is distributed worldwide. Although cats are the definitive host, birds and domestic animals can also serve as reservoirs. Up to 38% of domestic cats and 58% of stray cats are seropositive for *T. gondii* and excrete the organism in their feces for about 3 to 14 days after the initial infection.

The major routes of transmission are oral (from contaminated foods or exposure to infected cat feces) and congenital (in a woman who develops acute infection during pregnancy). There has been no documented human to human transmission.

In humans, seroprevalence increases with age and there may be marked regional variation. In the United States, approximately 10% to 30% of adults are seropositive compared with up to 90% of adults in France. Seroprevalence among HIV-infected patients in the United States is about 10% to 40%, while up to 70% to 90% of HIV-positive patients in some African, Latin American, and Western European countries have evidence of chronic infection.

Reactivation of toxoplasmosis is estimated to occur in 3% to 10% of all HIV-infected patients, with the risk increasing markedly as the CD4+ count drops below 100 cells/mm³.

Of acquired immunodeficiency syndrome (AIDS) patients with a CD4+ count in this range who are seropositive for *T. gondii*, about 20% to 35% will develop active disease.

Presentation
Central Nervous System. The central nervous system (CNS) is the most common site of active *T. gondii* infection in AIDS patients, and symptoms generally occur subacutely over several weeks. The most frequent manifestation of CNS toxoplasmosis is a focal mass lesion, and it is often focal symptoms and signs that predominate on presentation. Common findings include lethargy, weakness, dysarthria, localized headache, hemiparesis, hemiplegia, hemisensory loss, seizures, cerebellar tremor, visual field defects, cranial nerve palsies, and aphasia. Fever is present in fewer than half of patients. Nonfocal signs such as disorientation, confusion, nausea, and vomiting may also predominate, although meningismus is rare. Finally, neuropsychiatric symptoms such as personality changes, agitation, anxiety, and psychosis may be prominent.

Cerebrospinal fluid (CSF) analysis usually reveals between 0 and 40 leukocytes with a mononuclear predominance. Glucose is typically normal, with a normal to mildly elevated protein. The CSF profile is normal in 25% of patients with toxoplasmic encephalitis. Diagnosis is usually made by imaging studies. Computed tomography (CT) scan typically reveals multiple, bilateral, ring-enhancing, focal lesions in 70% to 80% of patients, although magnetic resonance imaging (MRI) is generally more sensitive in identifying lesions. Lesions are most commonly found in the basal ganglia and brain stem, often at the corticomedullary junction. Frontal and parietal lesions are also common.

Although CNS *T. gondii* infection most often presents with focal disease, diffuse toxoplasmic encephalitis may also occur. In this situation, patients present acutely with generalized CNS dysfunction without focal signs, and imaging studies reveal no focal lesions. This presentation of toxoplasmic encephalitis often progresses rapidly to death.

Pulmonary. The lung is the second most common site of active *T. gondii* infection. Disease usually presents with fever, cough, and dyspnea, with rales often noted on examination. Bilateral interstitial infiltrates are the most common radiographic finding, but other patterns, including micronodular infiltrates, nodular densities, cavitary infiltrates, and lobar pneumonia, may be noted. Both the symptoms and radiographic findings often make *T. gondii* pneumonia indistinguishable from *Pneumocystis carinii* pneumonia (PCP).

Although presumptive diagnosis may be made on the basis of suggestive clinical findings with a positive *Toxoplasma* serology, definitive diagnosis requires identification of the organism on lung biopsy or bronchoalveolar lavage (BAL). Extrapulmonary disease is found in half of patients with pulmonary disease, while in one third of cases of extrapulmonary toxoplasmosis there is also evidence of disease in the lungs.

Although treatment appears to improve survival, relapse is common, and it is recommended that suppressive therapy be given after an acute infection. Mortality may be as high as 40% because the diagnosis is often not considered until after the patient's death.

Ocular. *T. gondii* is the second most common retinal infection in AIDS after cytomegalovirus (CMV). Patients commonly present with ocular pain and loss of visual acuity and are noted to have cerebral involvement about 30% of the time. Although retinal biopsies can be performed, diagnosis is typically based on the funduscopic appearance of multiple, often bilateral, indurated, necrotizing retinal lesions with sharp borders. There is often associated vitreal inflammation, with optic nerve involvement noted in about 10% of cases. Compared with CMV, *T. gondii* lesions are nonhemorrhagic and more fluffy and edematous. The response to appropriate therapy is good, with more complete recovery of vision than after treatment for CMV.

Cardiac. *T. gondii* infection of the heart is usually clinically inapparent, often being found only at autopsy. When symptomatic, myocardial involvement may present with cardiomegaly, dysrhythmias, pericarditis, pericardial tamponade, or congestive heart failure. Definitive diagnosis requires endomyocardial biopsy, which reveals focal necrosis with edema and often microabscesses.

Musculoskeletal. Involvement of the muscle with *T. gondii* is seen in about 4% of AIDS patients on autopsy specimens and is usually found as part of disseminated toxoplasma infection. Clinical evidence of involvement, which may be acute or subacute in onset, includes weakness, wasting, myalgias, and high serum creatine kinase levels. Organisms can be seen on biopsy, with intramyocytic cysts demonstrated in all patients in one series. Symptoms usually resolve with appropriate therapy.

Diagnosis

Antibodies to *T. gondii* appear within 1 to 2 weeks of acquisition of the infection, and peak within the first 1 to 2 months. They decrease thereafter, but the rate of decline is variable from person to person. Antibody titers usually persist at some level for life. The problem with the use of serologic tests in HIV is that even in the presence of active *T. gondii* disease, serologic titers may be low in AIDS patients, whereas persons infected in the past may still have high antibody titers despite not having active disease. Approximately 90% to 95% of patients who have toxoplasmic encephalitis have positive serologies.

There are several situations in which some might recommend serologic testing: at the initial visit to determine latent infection; in patients who become eligible for prophylaxis due to a CD4+ count less than 100 cells/mm^3, who are not on trimethoprim-sulfamethoxazole (TMP-SMX) for PCP prophylaxis; and in patients with prior negative or unknown serostatus in whom CNS toxoplasmosis is suspected. However, as discussed, even with negative serology, toxoplasmosis disease can occur in AIDS patients.

Serologic evaluation for determination of prior infection with *T. gondii* can be performed by several methods including enzyme-linked immunosorbent assay (ELISA), which is most widely used; immunofluorescent antibody (IFA) testing, which is easy to perform and economical, but false-negative results may occur when serum titers are low; and the Sabin-Feldman dye test, which is the reference serologic test against which others are measured but is only available in a few laboratories.

Diagnosis of active toxoplasmosis often rests on the evaluation of the response of disease to empiric therapy against this pathogen. The predictive value for toxoplasmic encephalitis in patients with multiple characteristic lesions and a positive serology is estimated to be about 80%. It should be noted that identification of only a single lesion on CT scan makes the diagnosis of CNS lymphoma as likely as toxoplasmosis. Although *T. gondii* is the most common cause of a focal CNS lesion in a patient with AIDS, several other diagnoses must be considered (Table 11-1). Lymphoma, progressive multifocal leukoencephalopathy (PML), tuberculosis, and cryptococcosis should all be considered in the evaluation. Although many of these diagnoses differ with regard to their clinical presentation, CSF findings, and CT images, definitive diagnosis often requires biopsy. Since toxoplasmosis is statistically the most common etiology of a CNS lesion, it is reasonable to treat for toxoplasmosis empirically, given the morbidity associated with brain biopsy. If there is no clinical improvement after 1 week and/or no improvement on CT scan after 2 weeks, further diagnostic evaluation should be undertaken. However, it should be noted that, even in the setting of appropriate therapy, toxoplasmic encephalitis may progress to death. For definitive diagnosis of toxoplasmic encephalitis, the tachyzoite must be identified on biopsy of tissue or fluid.

Although polymerase chain reaction (PCR) identification has been demonstrated to be useful in the detection of *T. gondii* DNA in a variety of tissues and body fluids, false-positive findings are of concern, and therefore this test is not yet recommended. It has also been suggested that comparing *Toxoplasma* antibody levels in the CSF with those in the serum may be helpful in diagnosing CNS toxoplasmosis.

Treatment

Acute Therapy. The treatment of choice for active infection with *T. gondii* is the combination of pyrimethamine and sulfadiazine (Table 11-2). Although this regimen is associated with a clinical response rate of 70% to 95%, 40% of patients discontinue therapy due to side effects of the medications. Alternative regimens include pyrimethamine combined with either clindamycin, clarithromycin, azithromycin, or dapsone. Therapy with any of these combinations should be continued for 6 weeks and subsequently followed by life-long suppressive therapy. Pyrimethamine alters the folic acid cycle and often results in severe dose-related marrow toxicity. The risk of this side effect may be reduced with the concomitant use of leucovorin (folinic acid), which should be added to each of the above regimens. In addition, a blood cell and platelet count should thus be monitored during therapy.

Adjunctive corticosteroid therapy has occasionally been recommended in the treatment of cerebral toxoplasmosis, particularly if significant edema is noted on CT scan. However, this practice has not been shown to decrease mortality and may confuse the diagnostic evaluation because reduction of

TABLE 11-1
Differential Diagnosis of a Focal CNS Lesion in a Patient with AIDS

	Incidence	CD4+ (cells/mm³)	Symptoms	CSF	CT
Toxoplasmosis	3%-10%	<100	Fever <50% Headache Lethargy Confusion Focal signs	0-40 wbc (monos) Normal in 25%	Ring-enhancing Mass effect Multiple Basal ganglia Corticomedullary junction
Lymphoma	2%-5%	<100	Afebrile Headache Lethargy Focal signs	0-100 wbc (monos) Normal in 40%	Enhancing Mass effect Multiple in 40%-60% Periventricular
PML	1%-3%	<200	Afebrile Often alert Gait difficulty	Normal	Nonenhancing No mass effect Multifocal Subcortical white matter
Tuberculosis	0.5%-1%	Any	Febrile Headache Meningeal signs	5-2,000 wbc (monos) Decreased glucose Normal in 5%-10%	Enhancing +/− Mass effect Multiple in 25%-70% Basilar
Cryptococcus	8%-12%	<100	Febrile Headache Nausea	0-100 wbc (monos) Decreased glucose Increased protein Normal in 20% Cryptococcal antigen	Nonenhancing Focal lesions rare (cryptococcoma) Basal ganglia
Others*	Rare				

PML, Progressive multifocal leukoencephalopathy; *rbc*, red blood cell count; *wbc*, white blood cell count; *monos*, mononuclear cells.
Histoplasma, Candida, Aspergillus, cytomegalovirus, varicella-zoster virus, herpes simplex virus, human immunodeficiency virus encephalopathy, *Nocardia, Bartonella henselae, Rhodococcus equi,* Kaposi's sarcoma.

edema may result in clinical improvement despite an incorrect presumptive diagnosis and because steroids may result in some clinical improvement in unsuspected CNS lymphoma.

Since seizures may occur in up to 35% of patients with toxoplasmic encephalitis, antiepileptics have often been given prophylactically. This practice, however, was noted to result in worse outcomes, and thus these agents should only be prescribed in cases in which a seizure has occurred.

In assessing the response to therapy, it should be noted that radiographic resolution lags behind clinical improvement. With appropriate therapy, one generally sees improvement in CNS lesions by CT scan in 2 to 3 weeks, with total resolution often requiring from 1 to 6 months. Peripheral lesions resolve more rapidly than deeper lesions.

Suppressive Therapy. For patients who survive the first episode of cerebral toxoplasmosis, the risk of relapse is approximately 30% to 50%. Thus, after therapy for an active infection is completed, patients should receive suppressive therapy to prevent recurrence. The regimen of choice is the combination of pyrimethamine and sulfadiazine (see Table 11-2). An alternative choice is the combination of pyrimethamine and clindamycin. Other agents that have been used but for which there is little supportive data include dapsone, atovaquone, TMP-SMX), azithromycin, and clarithromycin.

Preventive Therapy. Primary prophylaxis against *T. gondii* infection should be recommended to all HIV-infected patients whose CD4+ count falls below 100 cells/mm³ and who have serologic evidence of past infection (see Table 11-2). First-line prophylaxis is with TMP-SMX, while alternatives include dapsone plus pyrimethamine or atovaquone with or without pyrimethamine. It should be noted that the combinations of pyrimethamine plus dapsone and pyrimethamine plus sulfadiazine are effective prophylaxis against PCP, but the combination of pyrimethamine plus clindamycin is not.

Whether patients receiving suppressive or prophylactic therapy against *T. gondii* may be able to discontinue such therapy as their immune function improves on highly active antiretroviral therapy (HAART) remains an active area of investigation. It appears that patients whose CD4+ counts rise above 100 cells/mm³ with HAART and whose *T. gondii* prophylaxis is discontinued are at low risk for disease. However, the number of patients in whom this has been attempted has been small and is not sufficient to recommend routine discontinuation of prophylaxis. Similarly, although patients who are on suppressive therapy for *T. gondii* disease may be able to safely stop prophylaxis as CD4+ counts increase, there are insufficient data to recommend this at this time.

TABLE 11-2
Treatment and Prophylaxis for Toxoplasmosis

	First-line	Alternative
Acute disease	Pyrimethamine 100-200 mg po load, then 75-100 mg po qd + sulfadiazine 1-1.5 g po q6h + leucovorin 10-20 mg po qd × 3-6 wks	Pyrimethamine + leucovorin (dosed as in first-line therapy) + one of the following: Clindamycin 600 mg po/IV q6h Clarithromycin 1 g po bid Azithromycin 1.2-1.5 g po qd Dapsone 100 mg po qd
Suppressive treatment	Pyrimethamine 25-75 mg po qd + sulfadiazine 500-1,000 mg po qid + leucovorin 10 mg po qd	Pyrimethamine 25-75 mg po qd + clindamycin 300-450 mg po tid + leucovorin 10 mg po qd
Prophylaxis (recommended if CD4+ count ≤100 cells/mm³ and positive *Toxoplasma* serology)	TMP-SMX 1 DS po qd	TMP-SMX 1 SS po qd Dapsone 50 mg po qd + pyrimethamine 50 mg po qwk + leucovorin 25 mg po qwk Dapsone 200 mg/wk + pyrimethamine 75 mg/wk + leucovorin 25 mg/wk Atovaquone 1,500 mg po qd*

TMP-SMX, Trimethoprim-sulfamethoxazole; *DS*, double strength; *SS*, single strength.
*May be used with or without pyrimethamine.

Several steps should be taken to minimize the risk of *T. gondii* exposure in those HIV-infected patients who are seronegative. If the patient owns a cat, litter boxes should be cleaned daily, preferably by someone not HIV-infected. If done by someone HIV-positive, hands should be washed thoroughly afterward. Cats should be kept indoors, should not hunt, and should not be fed raw or undercooked meat. It is, however, not necessary to declaw the cat or test it for toxoplasmosis.

In addition, patients should not eat raw or undercooked meat, and should wash hands after handling raw meat and vegetables. Because of animal-derived fertilizers, they should thoroughly wash fruits and vegetables before eating them raw. Finally, they should wash hands after gardening and/or other contact with soil.

When to Refer

A patient should be referred when clinical presentation is consistent with toxoplasmosis but does not respond to appropriate empiric antimicrobial therapy.

KEY POINTS

- Reactivation of toxoplasmosis will occur in up to 10% of HIV-infected patients
- Toxoplasmosis is the most common cause of a mass lesion in the CNS in HIV-infected patients
- Initial therapy is usually empiric
- Pyrimethamine plus sulfadiazine is treatment of choice

Cryptosporidium
Presentation and Progression

Cause. *Cryptosporidium* is an intracellular parasite initially described in 1907 and first isolated in humans in 1976. Like microsporidia, *Isospora*, and *Cyclospora*, it is a spore-forming protozoan and a common cause of chronic diarrheal illness in HIV-infected patients. Although these four protozoal parasites often have similar clinical presentations, identification of the specific infecting pathogen is of great importance given their different therapeutic options (Tables 11-3 and 11-4).

There are approximately 20 species of *Cryptosporidium* of which *Cryptosporidium parvum* is the major pathogen in humans. *Cryptosporidium* exists in both an oocyst and trophozoite stage. The life cycle of the parasite begins with ingestion of the spherical, 4- to 5-μm-diameter oocyst. The oocyst subsequently excysts in response to digestive enzymes, releasing four sporozoites. The sporozoites undergo both sexual and asexual maturation in the intestine, leading to production of new oocysts, which are then expelled into the environment. On release, oocysts are fully sporulated and infectious; they do not require a period of maturation outside the host. Of note, ingestion of as few as 10 oocysts may result in infection.

Cryptosporidium is found ubiquitously in the environment and has been isolated from humans and other mammals, birds, fish, and reptiles. It is acquired from contaminated drinking water, from recreational water use, from contact with infected animals, or from person to person transmission. It has also been linked to contaminated oysters in which cryp-

TABLE 11-3
Differential Diagnosis of Diarrhea Due to Spore-Forming Organisms

	Cryptosporidium	Microsporidia	Isospora	Cyclospora
Prevalence*	10%-30%	15%-20%	1%-2%	<1%
Size	4-5 µm	1-2 µm	25-33 µm	8-10 µm
Shape	Spherical	Ovoid	Ellipsoid	Spherical
Acid-fast	Yes	No	Yes	Variable
Stool wbc	No	No	No	No
Stool rbc	No	No	No	No
Other tests	IFA or ELISA for stool antigen	Trichrome stain EM of small bowel		PCR?

IFA, Immunofluorescent antibody; *ELISA*, enzyme-linked immunosorbent assay; *EM*, electron microscopy; *PCR*, polymerase chain reaction; *wbc*, white blood cell count; *rbc*, red blood cell count.
*Percentage of diarrhea caused by organism.

tosporidial oocysts may survive for up to 2 months. Many outbreaks have been described, including several linked to municipal water supplies.

The prevalence of *Cryptosporidium* in stool specimens in the general population has been reported to be around 1% to 3% in Europe and North America and 5% to 10% in Asia and Africa. It is the most common cause of chronic diarrhea due to spore-forming organisms in AIDS patients, causing between 10% and 30% of such illnesses. It is the AIDS-defining illness in about 2% of HIV-infected patients and usually occurs at CD4+ counts below 200 cells/mm^3.

Presentation. There is an incubation period of about 7 to 10 days between ingestion of the cryptosporidial oocysts and the onset of symptoms. Onset of symptoms may be acute or subacute, and symptoms consist of diarrhea that is watery and often voluminous, crampy abdominal pain, weight loss, anorexia, nausea, vomiting, malaise, and fatigue. Fever is uncommon. The course of disease is variable and may be intermittent or continuous, and the severity of disease varies markedly from person to person. Volume loss may be severe enough to require hospitalization for rehydration and parenteral nutrition.

Ten percent of patients with diarrhea will also have involvement of the biliary tract. Presentation may be consistent with sclerosing cholangitis or cholecystitis and includes findings such as fever, right upper quadrant abdominal pain, nausea, vomiting, and weight loss. There is often marked elevation of the alkaline phosphatase, with mild elevation of the transaminases. Chronic gallbladder carriage of *Cryptosporidium* may be responsible for the inability to clear the parasite from the gastrointestinal tract.

Cryptosporidium has also been associated with a variety of respiratory complaints including cough, shortness of breath, hoarseness, and wheezing. Although the organism has been isolated from a variety of respiratory samples, its exact role in disease causation remains unclear.

Diagnosis

Diagnosis of *Cryptosporidium* is generally accomplished through examination of the stool. Acid-fast stain reveals the typical spherical, 4- to 5-µm-diameter oocysts. Differentiation of *Cryptosporidium* from other spore-forming protozoal pathogens may be based on several features (see Table 11-3). Its spherical shape helps to distinguish it from microsporidia and *Isospora*. Although *Cyclospora* is also spherical, it is twice as large as *Cryptosporidium*. *Cryptosporidium* is often routinely tested for when a stool examination for ova and parasites is requested, but evaluation for the presence of the other spore-forming protozoa must be specifically requested. Other diagnostic techniques involve IFA or ELISA detection of *Cryptosporidium* antigens in the stool. Diagnostic techniques utilizing PCR methodology remain experimental. The stool is generally without blood or leukocytes.

Although *Cryptosporidium*-associated biliary tract disease may be evaluated with ultrasonography, which often reveals dilated biliary ducts or gallbladder wall thickening, endoscopic retrograde cholangiopancreatography (ERCP), with appropriate sampling of bile, is the diagnostic modality of choice.

Natural History and Treatment

To date, there are no therapies proven effective for *Cryptosporidium*. Paromomycin alone or in combination with azithromycin is the current recommended treatment (see Table 11-4). Alternative therapies include azithromycin and atovaquone. Octreotide, a synthetic analogue of somatostatin, may be useful in reducing stool volume even without effecting a parasitologic cure. HIV-infected patients receiving HAART including a protease inhibitor

TABLE 11-4
Treatment of Diarrhea Caused by Spore-Forming Protozoa

	Initial treatment	Suppressive treatment

Cryptosporidium	*Preferred*
	Paromomycin 500-750 mg po qid × 2-4 wks
	Paromomycin 1 g bid × 2-4 wks
	Paromomycin 1 g bid +
	    azithromycin 600 mg po qd × 2-4 wks
	HAART?
	
	Alternative
	Octreotide 50-500 μg tid SC or IV tid
	Azithromycin 1,200 mg po bid × 1d,
	    then 1,200 mg po qd × 2-4 wks
	Atovaquone 750 mg bid × 2-4 wks
		Preferred
		Paromomycin 500 mg po bid
		
		Alternative
		Azithromycin 600 mg po qd

Microsporidia		
E. bieneusi	No effective therapy	None
E. intestinalis	*Preferred* Albendazole 200-400 mg po bid × 4 wks *Alternative* Metronidazole 500 mg po tid × 4 wks Atovaquone 750 mg po tid × 4 wks HAART?	Albendazole 200 mg po qd

Isospora	*Preferred*
	TMP-SMX 2 DS po bid × 2-4 wks
	    (may also use 1 DS po tid)
	
	Alternative
	Pyrimethamine 25-75 mg po qd +
	    leucovorin 5-10 mg po qd × 4 wks
		Preferred
		TMP-SMX 1-2 DS po qd
		
		Alternative
		Pyrimethamine 25 mg po qd +
		    sulfadoxine 500 mg po qwk +
		    leucovorin 5 mg po qd

Cyclospora	*Preferred* TMP-SMX 1 DS po qid × 10d	*Preferred* TMP-SMX 1 DS po MWF

TMP-SMX, Trimethoprim-sulfamethoxazole; *HAART*, highly active antiretroviral therapy; *DS*, double strength; *MWF*, Monday, Wednesday, Friday.

have been noted to have complete clinical, microbiologic, and histologic responses. Given the high rate of recurrence of this disease in the cases in which there is a response to therapy, suppressive therapy with paromomycin or azithromycin is suggested.

Symptomatic and supportive therapy is of great importance in the treatment of *Cryptosporidium* infections. Volume depletion is often severe and may require hospitalization for rehydration. In addition, nutritional supplementation, usually in the form of total parenteral nutrition, may be required. Antidiarrheal agents including both luminal agents such as kaolin-pectin, bismuth subsalicylate, cholestyramine, and psyllium, as well as antimotility agents such as loperamide, diphenoxylate, tincture of opium, and codeine, may be helpful.

The *Cryptosporidium* oocyst is resistant to many standard disinfectants. Patients should wash hands after fecal contact, handling pets, gardening, or other contact with soil. Patients should be warned not to drink from lakes or rivers and should avoid eating oysters. Water boiled for 1 minute will remove *Cryptosporidium*, and use of a microfilter (less than 1 μm) on all drinking water or bottled water may also reduce the risk in the setting of an outbreak. It is not generally recommended to perform these procedures in non-outbreak settings. Finally, *Cryptosporidium*-infected patients should not work as food handlers.

When to Refer

A patient should be referred when volume loss is severe enough to require hospitalization for rehydration and parenteral nutrition or if fever, nausea, vomiting, or right upper quadrant abdominal pain develops.

KEY POINTS

- Very common cause of chronic diarrhea in HIV-infected patients
- Ingestion of a few organisms can result in infection
- Usually not associated with fever
- Diagnosed by routine ova and parasite stool examination
- No proven effective therapy
- Good hand washing is necessary after fecal contact, handling pets, or gardening or other contact with soil
- Patients should be warned not to drink from lakes or rivers and should avoid eating oysters

Microsporidia

Presentation and Progression

Cause. There are approximately 1,000 species contained in over 100 genera that comprise the organisms referred to as *Microsporidia*. Such organisms were first identified in 1857 and are known to affect a variety of vertebrate and nonvertebrate hosts. Although several genera have been noted to cause disease in humans, the two most commonly associated with disease in HIV-infected patients are *Enterocytozoon bieneusi* and *Encephalitozoon intestinalis* (formerly *Septata intestinalis*).

The life cycle of this small (1- to 2-μm-diameter), spore-forming protozoa begins with ingestion, or possible inhalation, of the spore. Following ingestion, the spore is stimulated by factors such as pH or ionic concentration changes to project a tubular structure through which infective sporoplasm is injected into the host cell. Further multiplication and maturation occur intracellularly within the enterocyte. Many mature spores accumulate in the cell, eventually causing the cell to rupture and release the spores, thereby continuing the cycle.

Epidemiology. Microsporidia are found ubiquitously in the environment and have caused infections worldwide. The species that infect humans are different from those that infect animals, suggesting that infection is spread from person to person.

These organisms rarely cause disease in immunocompetent persons and most often cause disease in HIV-infected patients only at advanced stages (CD4+ counts less than 100 cells/mm^3). Of the two genera that most often cause disease in HIV-positive patients, *E. bieneusi* causes approximately 90% of disease compared with *E. intestinalis*, which causes approximately 10%. Of the spore-forming diarrheal pathogens affecting patients with AIDS, *Microsporidia* is second in frequency only to *Cryptosporidium*, causing approximately 15% to 20% of chronic diarrhea in this population.

Presentation. The most common clinical presentation with infection with either *E. bieneusi* or *E. intestinalis* is chronic watery diarrhea. The diarrheal symptoms are generally of subacute onset, and the volume of diarrhea is less than that seen with *Cryptosporidium*. Associated symptoms include abdominal pain, nausea, vomiting, and weight loss. Fever is uncommon.

E. bieneusi and *E. intestinalis* infections may also involve the biliary tract. The most common presentation in this setting is sclerosing cholangitis caused by progressive and irregular obstruction and dilation of both the intrahepatic and extrahepatic bile ducts. Biliary involvement is manifested clinically by fever, right upper quadrant abdominal pain, nausea, vomiting, and weight loss. Laboratory evaluation reveals a moderately elevated alkaline phosphatase with mild elevation of the transaminases. These organisms may also cause acalculous cholecystitis by infection of the gallbladder wall. Radiographic evaluation often reveals thickening and distension of the gallbladder wall. Most patients with biliary tract findings have concurrent diarrhea. Other organisms to consider in biliary tract disease include CMV, *Cryptosporidium*, and *Isospora*.

Although both organisms have been found in other tissues and fluids, *E. intestinalis* more commonly causes disseminated disease than does *E. bieneusi*. Organisms have been found in many sites including the bronchopulmonary tree, sinuses, muscle, kidney, and liver. The true pathogenicity of these organisms in these sites, however, remains a matter of debate.

Diagnosis

Light microscopic techniques are generally used to identify the organism in various tissues. A modified trichrome stain of stool is used to detect the small spores (1- to 2-μm-diameter), which are the most commonly identified stage of the organism but are often hard to differentiate from bacteria and debris. Electron microscopy of a small bowel biopsy is considered the gold standard. This technique is also frequently used to confirm a diagnosis made initially on light microscopic examination. This technique can also be used to determine the ultrastructural features of the organism, which, in most cases, can distinguish the various genera of *Microsporidia*. Although culture can be used to confirm diagnosis, it is rarely used in clinical practice, and PCR diagnosis is still experimental. Patients with microsporidial intestinal infections do not have blood or leukocytes in their stool. In evaluating symptoms consistent with biliary tract involvement, ultrasonography is often normal and ERCP is the test of choice.

Features useful in differentiating *Microsporidia* from the other spore-forming protozoal infections include its small size, its ovoid shape, and its lack of acid-fast staining (see Table 11-3).

Natural History and Treatment

There are few data from comparative trials to guide therapy (see Table 11-4). Most of the information comes from anecdotal reports and small case series. No treatment has been shown to be effective for infection with *E. bieneusi*. *E. intestinalis* should be treated with albendazole for at least 4 weeks and should thereafter be followed by suppressive therapy with this agent. Possible alternative agents include metronidazole or atovaquone. Of interest, it has been noted that patients on combination antiretroviral therapy including a protease inhibitor have had complete clinical, microbiologic, and histologic responses. As for any of the spore-forming diarrheal pathogens, antidiarrheal agents may be used for symptomatic relief.

When to Refer

A patient should be referred when volume loss is severe enough to require hospitalization for rehydration and par-

TABLE 11-5
Treatment of *Giardia lamblia* and *Entamoeba histolytica*

	Preferred treatment	Alternative
G. lamblia	Metronidazole 250 mg po tid × 5d	Albendazole 400 mg po qd × 5d Quinacrine 100 mg po tid × 5d Tinidazole* 2 g po × 1
E. histolytica	Metronidazole 750 mg po tid × 10d (must be followed by either iodoquinol 650 mg po tid × 3 wks, or paromomycin 500 mg po tid × 7d)	Tinidazole* (diarrhea) 1 g po q12h × 3d Tinidazole* (abscess) 600 mg po bid × 5d (followed by iodoquinol or paromomycin) Tetracycline 250 mg po tid × 10d† Erythromycin 500 mg po qid × 10d†

*Not available in the United States.
†These agents will not eradicate trophozoites in the liver.

enteral nutrition or if fever, nausea, vomiting, or right upper quadrant abdominal pain develops.

KEY POINTS

- Very common cause of chronic diarrhea in HIV-infected patients with CD4+ counts less than 100 cells/mm^3
- Usually not associated with fever
- Due to the small size of the organism, it is difficult to diagnose by routine ova and parasite stool examination unless specifically requested. Definitive diagnosis often made by electron microscopy
- No proven effective therapy

Isospora belli
Presentation and Progression

Cause. *Isospora belli* was first described in 1915. This large (20- to 30-μm-diameter), ellipsoid, spore-forming protozoa exists in both an asexual and sexual phase during its life cycle. After the infectious oocyst is ingested, the organism advances to the small intestine where it sporulates and releases sporozoites. The sporozoites subsequently mature and multiply intracellularly within the enterocyte, eventually encysting again to form oocytes, which are released in the feces.

I. belli infects only humans, whereas other *Isospora* species infect only animals. *Isospora* infection is believed to be due to fecal contamination of food and water. Infections due to this organism occur more commonly in tropical and subtropical climates and are endemic in many parts of Africa, Asia, and South America. In the United States, infection is more commonly found in the Southwest.

Infection with *Isospora* in HIV-positive patients is generally limited to those patients with CD4+ counts below 100 cells/mm^3. Even in this population, infection is uncommon, accounting for just 0.2% of AIDS-defining illnesses, and about 1% to 2% of chronic diarrhea in patients with AIDS.

Presentation. The clinical features of *Isospora* infection include chronic watery diarrhea, abdominal pain, malaise, anorexia, and weight loss. Fever is uncommon. In an immunocompetent person, the diarrhea is generally self-limited. In an HIV-infected patient, the disease is prolonged and occasionally disseminated. The biliary tract is frequently involved. Presentation is characterized by fever, right upper quadrant abdominal pain, epigastric pain, nausea, and vomiting. On laboratory evaluation, the alkaline phosphatase is moderately elevated with mild elevation in the transaminases. Biliary tract involvement with this pathogen causes a progressive and irregular obstruction and dilation of the intrahepatic and extrahepatic bile ducts. In addition, it may also cause acalculous cholecystitis. Other pathogens that may cause similar biliary syndromes include *Microsporidia*, CMV, and *Cryptosporidium*.

Diagnosis

Diagnosis is based on identification of the oocyst in the stool by acid-fast staining. Examination of multiple stool specimens is advisable if initial examination is negative, since the oocytes may be shed intermittently and in small numbers. These organisms can be distinguished from the other spore-forming protozoal pathogens by their large size (20- to 30-μm-diameter), ellipsoid shape, and acid-fast staining properties (see Table 11-3). Stool examination reveals no leukocytes or blood. Evaluation of the biliary tract disease is often normal by ultrasonography and must be evaluated by ERCP.

Natural History and Treatment

TMP-SMX is the drug of choice for *Isospora* infection and should be continued for approximately 2 to 4 weeks (Table 11-5). Since approximately 50% of AIDS patients will relapse about 2 months after therapy is completed, lifetime suppressive therapy with TMP-SMX is recommended. For patients who are unable to tolerate TMP-SMX, the combination of pyrimethamine and sulfadoxine is an alternative.

When to Refer

A patient should be referred when volume loss is severe enough to require hospitalization for rehydration and parenteral nutrition or if fever, vomiting, or right upper quadrant abdominal pain develops.

> **KEY POINTS**

◯ Uncommon cause of chronic diarrhea in HIV-infected patients
◯ Usually not associated with fever
◯ Diagnosed by routine ova and parasite stool examination
◯ Trimethoprim-sulfamethoxazole is the drug of choice

Cyclospora

Presentation and Progression

Cause. *Cyclospora* was first described over 100 years ago, with the earliest identification of its spore-forming protozoa in human stool samples occurring in 1977. The cyclosporan organisms, designated *Cyclospora cayetanensis,* are spherical in shape, measure approximately 8 to 10 µm in diameter, and are somewhat smaller than the *Cyclospora* detected in nonhuman hosts. Although the life cycle is not fully understood, both sexual and asexual development occurs in the human host. Oocysts are not infectious when shed in the stool but require time outside the host for sporulation to occur. The time required for this process remains unclear.

Cyclospora is found worldwide and infects people of all ages. Infection due to this organism has been reported most commonly as outbreaks among immunocompetent persons and has been often linked to contaminated water or food. The first known outbreak occurred in 1990, with increasing numbers of outbreaks, as well as sporadic cases, reported in recent years. There seems to be marked seasonal variation in infection rates, perhaps due to changes in humidity and temperature.

Cyclospora is an uncommon cause of chronic diarrhea in HIV-infected patients, responsible for fewer than 1% of such illnesses in this population.

Presentation. The incubation period for *Cyclospora* is approximately 1 week. Symptoms include the subacute onset of watery diarrhea, crampy abdominal pain, nausea, vomiting, and weight loss. Marked fatigue and anorexia may also occur. Diarrheal symptoms are occasionally preceded by a prodrome of arthralgias and myalgias. Fever is uncommon. In an immunocompetent patient, symptoms are generally self-limited but may last for several weeks. In HIV-infected patients, symptoms are prolonged and more severe. Diarrheal symptoms may occur in a cyclical pattern alternating with constipation. If symptoms resolve, there is a high recurrence rate. Although *Cyclospora* mainly affects the gastrointestinal tract, biliary tract involvement has also been noted.

Diagnosis

Oocysts are shed in abundant numbers in the stool and are variably acid-fast. The organism may also be seen on a wet preparation of the stool. It is unknown whether affected patients shed organisms intermittently as occurs in *Isospora* infection. The stool contains no leukocytes or blood.

Several features are useful in distinguishing *Cyclospora* from other spore-forming protozoal pathogens (see Table 11-3). Its spherical shape helps distinguish it from *Microsporidia* and *Isospora.* Although *Cryptosporidium* is also spherical, *Cyclospora* is approximately twice its size at 8 to 10 µm in diameter. The variable acid-fast staining of *Cyclospora* also helps to distinguish it from the other spore-forming protozoa. PCR-based detection methods are currently in development.

Natural History and Treatment

Preferred therapy for *Cyclospora* infection is TMP-SMX (see Table 11-4). Given the frequency of recurrence of disease after treatment, suppressive therapy with TMP-SMX is recommended. Many agents have been found to be ineffective as possible alternatives to TMP-SMX. Pyrimethamine may be a second-line therapy, although it has not been adequately studied.

When to Refer

A patient should be referred when volume loss is severe enough to require hospitalization for rehydration and parenteral nutrition or if fever, nausea, vomiting, or right upper quadrant abdominal pain develops.

> **KEY POINTS**

◯ Very uncommon cause of chronic diarrhea in HIV-infected patients
◯ Usually not associated with fever
◯ Diagnosed by routine ova and parasite stool examination
◯ Trimethoprim-sulfamethoxazole is the drug of choice

Giardia lamblia

Presentation and Progression

Cause. In addition to the four spore-forming protozoa described above, another enteric parasite that should be considered in the evaluation of an HIV-infected patient with chronic diarrhea is *Giardia lamblia. G. lamblia* is a flagellated protozoan and exists in both a trophozoite and cyst stage. After the infectious cyst is ingested, it sporulates in the stomach to form two trophozoites. These trophozoites then colonize the upper small bowel, where they undergo further maturation and multiplication. The trophozoites subsequently encyst again and are passed into the environment, where they may survive in water for up to several months. As few as 10 to 20 cysts are required to cause infection.

G. lamblia is distributed worldwide and occurs in areas where sanitation is poor. It is the most commonly identified intestinal parasite in the United States. Humans are the main reservoir of *G. lamblia,* but a variety of animals may also carry the parasite.

Infection occurs through ingestion of the cyst, usually following exposure to contaminated water or food. Person to person exposure is also common and occurs most frequently in settings such as day-care centers and long-term care facilities and among sexually active homosexuals. Hikers in wilderness areas are at risk of infection due to contaminated water. Overseas travelers are at risk as well, particularly when visiting areas where the disease is endemic such as Mexico, western South America, Russia, southeast and south Asia, and tropical Africa.

Although giardiasis is more common among male homosexuals, there does not appear to be an association between

G. lamblia infection and HIV seropositivity. *G. lamblia* causes 1% to 2% of chronic diarrhea in HIV-seropositive patients and may occur at any CD4+ count. Although patients with AIDS exhibit impaired immune responses to the organism, they do not appear to develop more severe or prolonged disease.

Presentation. As mentioned earlier it is unclear what leads some persons to become symptomatic while others do not. For those who do have symptoms, the symptoms include chronic watery diarrhea, which may become foul-smelling and greasy; flatulence; abdominal cramps; bloating; nausea; anorexia; malaise; and weight loss. Ten percent may have constipation, while fever develops in about 10% to 15%. Although some acute infections may clear spontaneously, most go on to develop chronic symptoms. If symptoms continue for several weeks, there may be periods of constipation or normal bowel habits alternating with diarrhea. Other reported manifestations of giardiasis include urticaria, reactive arthritis, pancreatitis, and cholecystitis.

Diagnosis

Diagnosis rests on identification of the trophozoite or cyst in the stool. Trophozoites are pear-shaped and measure 9 to 21 μm long and 5 to 15 μm wide. Cysts are smooth and oval-shaped, measuring 8 to 12 μm long and 7 to 10 μm wide. A saline wet mount of fresh liquid stool may demonstrate motile trophozoites. It may take longer than the duration of the incubation period for cysts to begin to appear in the stool. Thus stool examination may be negative at the time of onset of symptoms. Since *G. lamblia* cysts may be excreted intermittently, multiple stool specimens should be examined. Cysts will be identified about 50% to 70% of the time after one stool, and up to more than 90% after three stools. Concurrent antibiotic therapy, antacids, laxatives, and antidiarrheal agents may cause organism distortion or decreased numbers of organisms, thereby decreasing the yield of stool examination. No blood or leukocytes are found in the stool in giardiasis.

G. lamblia antigens may be detected in the stool through IFA or ELISA serologies. These tests are 85% to 95% sensitive and 90% to 100% specific and may be positive early in the disease, when a stool examination might still be negative.

Although the diagnosis of *G. lamblia* infection can nearly always be made with the above tests, in the setting of persistent symptoms with negative stool studies, one may consider performing duodenal sampling with the use of the string test, duodenal aspiration, or duodenal biopsy in order to identify the organism. Other options include testing for systemic anti-*Giardia* antibody, although this is not widely available and generally useful only for seroepidemiologic studies; in vitro culture, which is available only in research settings; PCR detection techniques, which remain experimental; and barium studies, which are abnormal in 20% of patients but are nonspecific.

Treatment

Several agents are available to treat infections with *G. lamblia* (see Table 11-5). Preferred therapy for giardiasis is metronidazole, with alternatives including albendazole and quinacrine. All of these agents are given for a 5-day course of therapy. Although quinacrine has a higher cure rate than metronidazole, 90% to 95% and 85% to 95%, respectively, the latter is preferred given its lower incidence of side effects. Tinidazole, given in a single 2-g dose, is another alternative, providing a 90% cure rate and easier tolerability compared with metronidazole. However, it is not available in the United States.

Asymptomatic cyst passers should be treated, since they may pass the disease to others and may themselves at some point become symptomatic.

When to Refer

A patient should be referred when volume loss is severe enough to require hospitalization for rehydration and parenteral nutrition or if fever, nausea, vomiting, or right upper quadrant abdominal pain develops.

KEY POINTS

◌ *Giardia* causes about 1%-2% of chronic diarrhea in HIV-infected patients
◌ No more common in HIV than in other populations
◌ Stool examination may be negative when symptoms first appear
◌ Metronidazole is treatment of choice

Entamoeba histolytica
Presentation and Progression

Cause. As with *G. lamblia*, infection with *Entamoeba histolytica* must be considered in the differential diagnosis of an HIV-infected patient with chronic diarrhea. *E. histolytica* is an enteric protozoan that may exist in either trophozoite or cyst form. The infectious cycle begins when the cyst is ingested. The organism sporulates in the small intestine to form multiple trophozoites, which then colonize the colon and invade the colonic epithelium. The trophozoites then become encysted in the large bowel, continuing the cycle. Although trophozoites are passed in the stool, they degenerate rapidly on exiting the body. However, the expelled cysts may, depending on environmental conditions, remain viable for weeks to months. The infectivity of *E. histolytica* is demonstrated by the observation that the ingestion of even one cyst can cause infection.

It is estimated that approximately 10% of the global population is infected with *E. histolytica*, with about a 4% prevalence of disease in the United States. Areas in which the disease is common include India, southern and western Africa, the Far East, and South and Central America. *E. histolytica* infection is associated with conditions that predispose to poor hygiene such as lack of indoor plumbing, institutionalization, crowding, and communal living. Underlying conditions that place patients at greater risk for more severe disease or complications include pregnancy, corticosteroid use, malignancy, and malnutrition.

Approximately 1% to 2% of chronic diarrhea in patients infected with HIV is due to this pathogen. Although amebiasis is more commonly found in sexually active homosexual men, there does not seem to be a general association between HIV seropositivity and *E. histolytica* infection. Likewise, there is no evidence that disease due to *E. histolytica* is more severe in patients with HIV infection. However, it has been suggested that *E. histolytica* infection, due to its T cell stimulation, might accelerate HIV replication.

Presentation. After infection with *E. histolytica,* there is an incubation period of approximately 1 to 2 weeks, although the time may be shorter with a larger inoculum of infecting organisms. Up to 90% of infections are asymptomatic. When symptoms do occur, they are usually of gradual onset over 1 to 3 weeks and include diarrhea that is watery, foul-smelling, and bloody; crampy abdominal pain; flatulence; and weight loss. Fever occurs in about one third of patients. The liver may be enlarged and tender to percussion.

E. histolytica infection may be characterized by both intestinal and nonintestinal complications. Intestinal complications include fulminant colitis, intestinal perforation, toxic megacolon, perianal ulceration, and ameboma. Fulminant colitis, in which colonic mucosal ulceration progresses to transmural necrosis of the bowel, is characterized by the rapid onset of severe, bloody diarrhea associated with abdominal pain and fever. It is associated with a mortality rate of greater than 50%. An ameboma is an annular colonic lesion, found most commonly in the cecum and ascending colon, that is indistinguishable from colonic carcinoma. It may also present as an extrahepatic tender palpable mass suggesting a pyogenic abscess. Lesions may be single or multiple and diagnosis must be established by biopsy.

Nonintestinal complications include liver abscess, lung abscess/empyema, pericarditis, and brain abscess. Although liver abscess, the most common of the extraintestinal manifestations of amebiasis, can occur in the presence of colitis, diarrhea is present in only about 30% to 40% of patients, and microscopic examination of stool is usually negative. Pulmonary and cardiac manifestations are usually due to rupture of a liver abscess with erosion through the diaphragm.

Diagnosis

Diagnosis rests primarily on microscopic identification of trophozoites or cysts in the stool. The trophozoite measures approximately 25 µm, while the cyst averages about 12 µm. It is estimated that a single stool specimen identifies only about 33% of infected patients, and thus three specimens should be examined to optimize the yield. Substances that may interfere with stool examination include bismuth, barium, tetracyclines, erythromycin, antacids, and laxatives. Blood is typically found in the stool, while leukocytes may or may not be noted.

Several other diagnostic modalities exist but are not widely available. Culture for *E. histolytica* is more sensitive than stool examination but is not routinely available. PCR identification of parasitic DNA is still experimental. Endoscopy typically reveals punctate, hemorrhagic ulcers located throughout the colon.

Serologic tests are positive only when there is tissue invasion. These tests are valuable when the diagnosis of amebic liver abscess is being considered, in order to help differentiate such lesions from other possibilities including pyogenic abscess, hepatocellular carcinoma, and echinococcal cyst. In a patient with a liver abscess, positive serology is considered diagnostic of *E. histolytica,* since it is positive in about 99% of such patients. However, if a patient presents acutely with a liver abscess, serologies may be negative in the first 7 to 10 days. In this case, the serologies should be repeated in approximately 5 to 7 days.

Although ultrasonography, CT, or MRI may be used to evaluate a liver lesion, none of these modalities is specific in differentiating an amebic liver abscess from a pyogenic abscess or tumor. Aspiration of an amebic abscess will reveal a sterile, odorless, brown or yellow fluid. Microscopy and culture of such fluid are usually negative, since the organisms are predominantly located in the wall of the abscess. Aspiration is usually not attempted, however, given the danger of spillage of contents into the peritoneum.

Natural History

Following infection with *E. histolytica,* there is an incubation period of approximately 1 to 2 weeks, although the time may be shorter with a larger inoculum of infecting organisms. Up to 90% of infections are asymptomatic.

Treatment

The treatment of choice for *E. histolytica* infection is metronidazole (see Table 11-5). To eradicate encysted intraluminal organisms, metronidazole must be followed by therapy with either iodoquinol or paromomycin. An alternative to metronidazole is tinidazole, although this agent is not available in the United States. For less severe colitis in which there is no liver involvement, other alternatives include tetracycline and erythromycin. A liver abscess may take up to 2 years to resolve completely and may increase in size during the early course of therapy.

When to Refer

A patient should be referred when volume loss is severe enough to require hospitalization for rehydration and parenteral nutrition or if fever, nausea, vomiting, or right upper quadrant abdominal pain develops.

KEY POINTS

- Causes about 1%-2% of chronic diarrhea in HIV-infected patients
- No more common in HIV than in other populations
- Serologies useful when tissue invasion (liver abscess) present
- Metronidazole is treatment of choice

SUGGESTED READINGS

Cappell MS, Mikhail N, Ortega A: Toxoplasma myocarditis in AIDS, *Am Heart J* 123:1728-1729, 1992.

Carr A et al: Treatment of HIV-1–associated microsporidiosis and cryptosporidiosis with combination antiretroviral therapy, *Lancet* 351:256-261, 1998.

Cochereau-Massin I et al: Ocular toxoplasmosis in human immunodeficiency virus–infected patients, *Am J Ophthalmol* 114:130-135, 1992.

Druckman DA, Quinn TC: *Entamoeba histolytica* infection in homosexual men. In. Ravdin JI, editor: *Amebiasis: human infection by* Entamoeba histolytica, Edinburgh, 1988, Churchill Livingstone.

Gherardi R et al: Skeletal muscle toxoplasmosis in patients with acquired immunodeficiency syndrome: a clinical and pathological study, *Ann Neurol* 35:535-542, 1992.

Goodgame RW: Understanding intestinal spore-forming protozoa: cryptosporidia, microsporidia, isospora, and cyclospora, *Ann Intern Med* 124:429-441, 1996.

Luft BJ, Remington JS: Toxoplasmic encephalitis in AIDS, *Clin Infect Dis* 155:211-222, 1992.

Petri WA, Ravdin JI: Treatment of homosexual men infected with *Entamoeba histolytica* [letter], *N Engl J Med* 315:393, 1988.

Pomeroy C, Filice GA: Pulmonary toxoplasmosis: A review, *Clin Infect Dis* 14:863-870, 1992.

Ravdin JI: Amebiasis, *Clin Infect Dis* 20:1453-1466, 1995.

Smith PD et al: Intestinal infections in patients with the acquired immunodeficiency syndrome (AIDS): etiology and response to therapy, *Ann Intern Med* 108:328-333, 1988.

Soave R, Herwaldt BL, Relman DA: *Cyclospora, Infect Dis Clin North Am* 12:1-12, 1998.

Wolfe MS: Giardiasis, *Clin Microbiol Rev* 5:93-100, 1992.

12 Bacterial Infections in HIV

ROBERT M. GROSSBERG

Introduction

Much of the focus on infectious complications of human immunodeficiency virus (HIV) infection has been directed toward the opportunistic viruses, fungi, and parasites that rarely cause severe diseases in the immunocompetent host. Bacterial infections, however, are a very common and exceedingly important cause of morbidity and mortality in HIV disease. The progressive loss of CD4+ T-helper lymphocytes that is characteristic of infection with HIV leads to irregularities in B lymphocyte function and impaired antibody production. This deficiency of the humoral immune system is largely responsible for the propensity for bacteria to cause disease in patients infected with HIV. Additionally, the deterioration of the cellular and humoral immune system in the gastrointestinal tract makes this a common site of infection or portal of entry for infection elsewhere. In the advanced stages of HIV infection, granulocytopenia is frequently encountered. Although the immunodeficiency conferred by neutropenia that is commonly seen in HIV infection tends to be less profound than that seen in the oncology setting, this too puts individuals at risk for invasive bacterial infections.

This chapter is divided into sections based on diseases caused by bacteria in HIV infection. Many of the organisms described commonly cause disease in immunocompetent populations, but their prevalence and unique clinical features warrant attention here. The last few sections address bacterial pathogens that are true opportunists in that they rarely cause disease in immunocompetent hosts. Diseases caused by mycobacteria (e.g., tuberculosis and *Mycobacterium avium* complex [MAC]) have been specifically omitted because they are covered elsewhere.

Pneumonia
Presentation and Progression

The lung is the most common site of infection in HIV disease. Pneumonia caused by *Pneumocystis carinii* (PCP) has received most of the emphasis in reviews of pneumonia in HIV infection because the organism was so rarely encountered prior to the AIDS epidemic. Bacterial pneumonias, however, are more common than PCP and can present at any stage of HIV infection. Many of the studies on bacterial pneumonia in patients with HIV infection were completed prior to the introduction of highly active antiretroviral therapy (HAART). As effective anti-HIV therapy has become widely used and the incidence of AIDS has declined, it is likely that the proportion of pneumonias caused by bacteria is increasing.

HIV-infected individuals are at risk for bacterial pneumonias for several reasons. Progressive HIV infection leads to impaired antibody responses to bacterial pathogens, particularly encapsulated organisms. HIV infection also affects the function of neutrophils and alveolar macrophages, making patients more susceptible to invasive disease.

Cause. The microbiologic etiology of bacterial pneumonia is usually not identified, regardless of HIV seropositivity. Treatment therefore is often empiric and requires a fundamental knowledge of the common causes of bacterial pneumonia in HIV infection and the recognition of clues in an individual patient's presentation. By a very large margin, the most common cause of bacterial pneumonia in patients with HIV infection is *Streptococcus pneumoniae*. Although pneumococcal pneumonia is common in the general population, its incidence in HIV-infected individuals is increased 100-fold to 300-fold. Additionally, injecting drug use, a practice common among HIV-infected patients, is an independent risk factor for this type of pneumonia. The distribution of serotypes of *S. pneumoniae* that have been associated with disease in HIV infection is similar to that seen in uninfected populations. The second most common cause of bacterial pneumonia in HIV infection is *Haemophilus influenzae*, with a frequency 100-fold more common than the general population. Most of the disease caused by *H. influenzae* in adults is caused by nontypeable (unencapsulated) strains. Pneumonia caused by *Staphylococcus aureus* is seen disproportionately in HIV-infected patients, although much of this disease is manifest as a complication of tricuspid valve endocarditis, commonly seen in injecting drug users. With very advanced HIV infection, *Pseudomonas aeruginosa* has caused pneumonia with increased frequency. Among the common causes of community-acquired atypical pneumonia, namely *Legionella, Chlamydia pneumoniae,* and *Mycoplasma pneumoniae,* only *Legionella* has been associated with HIV infection. The incidence of pneumonia caused by *Legionella* may be as high as 40 times that seen in the general population.

Presentation. The clinical presentation of bacterial pneumonia in HIV-infected individuals is similar to that seen in uninfected patients. Bacterial pneumonia can occur at any time during the course of HIV disease, but becomes more common as the disease progresses. The most typical presentation includes the acute onset of fever, chills, cough, and sometimes pleuritic chest pain. The cough is usually productive of sputum and may be accompanied by dyspnea. The acuity of presentation often helps distinguish bacterial pneumonia from PCP, whose symptoms frequently evolve over weeks or longer. A more subacute onset of symptoms can be seen with pneumonia caused by *H. influenzae.*

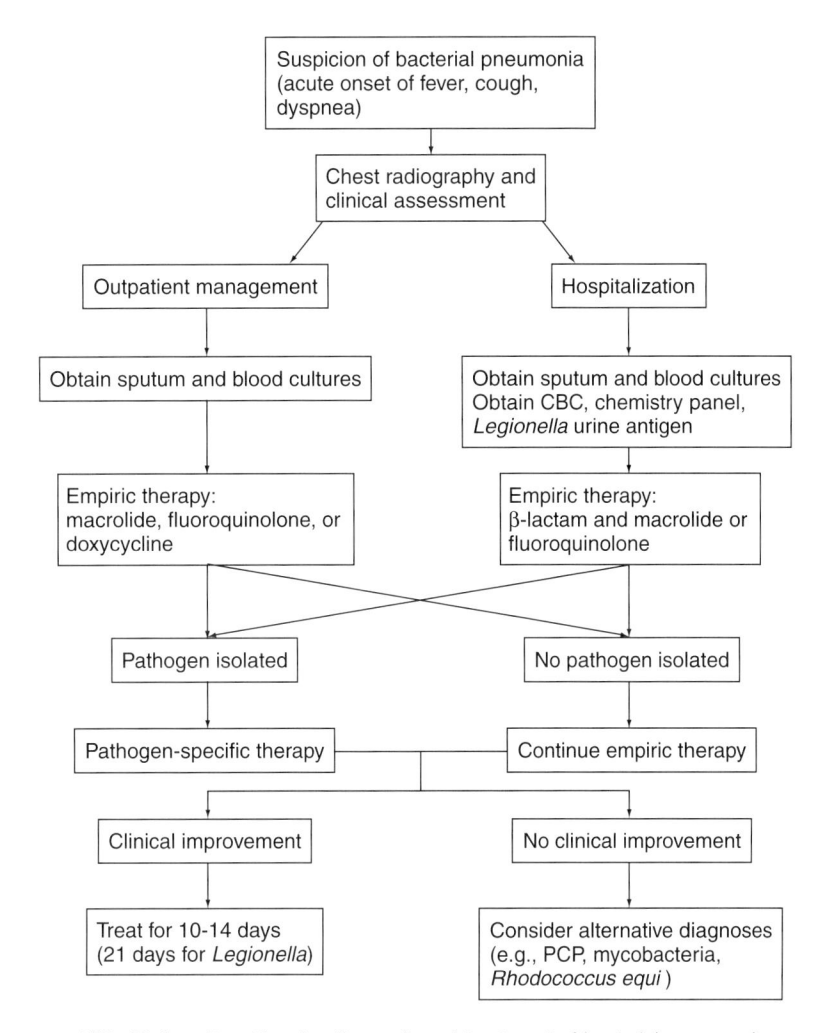

```
                    ┌─────────────────────────┐
                    │ Suspicion of bacterial  │
                    │ pneumonia (acute onset  │
                    │ of fever, cough,        │
                    │ dyspnea)                │
                    └───────────┬─────────────┘
                                │
                    ┌───────────┴─────────────┐
                    │ Chest radiography and   │
                    │ clinical assessment     │
                    └───────────┬─────────────┘
                      ┌─────────┴─────────┐
              ┌───────┴────────┐   ┌──────┴──────────┐
              │ Outpatient     │   │ Hospitalization │
              │ management     │   │                 │
              └───────┬────────┘   └──────┬──────────┘
                      │                   │
              ┌───────┴────────┐   ┌──────┴──────────────────┐
              │ Obtain sputum  │   │ Obtain sputum and blood │
              │ and blood      │   │ cultures                │
              │ cultures       │   │ Obtain CBC, chemistry   │
              │                │   │ panel, Legionella urine │
              │                │   │ antigen                 │
              └───────┬────────┘   └──────┬──────────────────┘
                      │                   │
              ┌───────┴────────┐   ┌──────┴──────────┐
              │ Empiric therapy:│  │ Empiric therapy:│
              │ macrolide,      │  │ β-lactam and    │
              │ fluoroquinolone,│  │ macrolide or    │
              │ or doxycycline  │  │ fluoroquinolone │
              └───────┬────────┘   └──────┬──────────┘
                      │      ╲   ╱        │
                      │        ╳          │
                      │      ╱   ╲        │
              ┌───────┴────────┐   ┌──────┴──────────┐
              │ Pathogen       │   │ No pathogen     │
              │ isolated       │   │ isolated        │
              └───────┬────────┘   └──────┬──────────┘
                      │                   │
              ┌───────┴────────┐   ┌──────┴──────────┐
              │ Pathogen-      ├───┤ Continue        │
              │ specific       │   │ empiric therapy │
              │ therapy        │   │                 │
              └───────┬────────┘   └──────┬──────────┘
                      │                   │
              ┌───────┴────────┐   ┌──────┴──────────┐
              │ Clinical       │   │ No clinical     │
              │ improvement    │   │ improvement     │
              └───────┬────────┘   └──────┬──────────┘
                      │                   │
              ┌───────┴────────┐   ┌──────┴──────────────┐
              │ Treat for      │   │ Consider alternative│
              │ 10-14 days     │   │ diagnoses (e.g.,    │
              │ (21 days for   │   │ PCP, mycobacteria,  │
              │ Legionella)    │   │ Rhodococcus equi)   │
              └────────────────┘   └─────────────────────┘
```

FIG. 12-1 Algorithm for diagnosis and treatment of bacterial pneumonia.

Patients with HIV and bacterial pneumonia can present along a spectrum of severity, ranging from relatively mild symptoms to septic shock. Cavitation and lung necrosis may be seen, but are not more common in HIV-infected patients. In cases of *S. pneumoniae* and *H. influenzae* in particular, the rates of bacteremia accompanying pneumonia are astonishingly high. Between 50% and 70% of cases of pneumococcal pneumonia are complicated by bacteremia compared with 10% to 30% of cases seen in patients without HIV. Despite the extraordinarily high rates of bacteremia, extrapulmonary complications are rare. Septic arthritis, cardiac tamponade, mediastinitis, and brain abscess are all complications of pneumococcal bacteremia that have been reported in HIV-infected individuals.

Diagnosis

The approach to the diagnosis of bacterial pneumonia for patients with HIV infection is similar to that used in uninfected patients. The history should be obtained, with special attention to the onset of symptoms because it may be helpful in distinguishing bacterial pneumonia from PCP, as described above. Attention should also be paid to recent exposure to antimicrobials, because many patients are on prophylaxis for PCP and MAC that may affect the presentation of bacterial pneumonia. Fig. 12-1 summarizes the diagnostic algorithm when bacterial pneumonia is suspected. A chest radiograph should be obtained. Most bacterial pneumonias in HIV-infected individuals appear as lobar or multilobar infiltrates. Interstitial patterns can be seen, and *H. influenzae* should be considered as a possible cause of this presentation. Sputum and blood cultures should be obtained prior to the administration of antimicrobial therapy. Blood cultures are frequently positive in bacterial pneumonia in HIV infection, particularly with *S. pneumoniae*. The finding of an organism in the bloodstream that typically causes pneumonia is diagnostic. Sputum cultures should be transported to the laboratory within 2 hours of collection. Specimens with many inflammatory cells, few epithelial cells, and a predominate morphology of bacteria seen on a Gram's stain are most useful. A sputum culture that grows *H. influenzae*, however, must be interpreted with caution because this organism can colonize the upper airway of healthy individuals. Bronchoscopy is usually unnecessary in the diagnosis of bacterial pneumonia in an HIV-infected patient, unless there is uncertainty in the diagnosis or the patient fails to improve. The diagnosis of pneumonia caused by *Legionella* can often be made by testing for the urinary antigen. This test, however, will detect only *L. pneumophila* serogroup 1,

> **BOX 12-1**
> **Diagnostic Tests for Bacterial Pneumonia**
>
> **ALL PATIENTS**
> Chest radiograph
> Sputum Gram's stain and culture
> Blood cultures
>
> **SELECTED PATIENTS**
> *Legionella* urinary antigen
> Sputum culture for *Legionella*
> CBC, chemistry panel
> Lactate dehydrogenase (LDH) (If elevated, may support the diagnosis of PCP)
> Arterial blood gas
> Induced sputum for acid-fast bacilli (AFB)
> Bronchoscopy
> Thoracentesis

which causes 70% of cases. Culture of sputum or bronchoscopy washings may grow all species of *Legionella,* but these cultures require special media and have a high false-negative rate.

In patients in whom the diagnosis of bacterial pneumonia is not ensured, a diagnostic evaluation for alternative conditions may be undertaken simultaneously. For patients at risk for PCP, bronchoscopy early in the clinical course of disease often proves useful for establishing a definitive diagnosis. Induced sputum or bronchoscopy specimens should be obtained for acid-fast smear and culture in patients in whom there is a suspicion of tuberculosis. Box 12-1 summarizes the diagnostic tests commonly employed in cases of suspected bacterial pneumonia in an HIV-infected patient.

Natural History

Fortunately, the outcome of bacterial pneumonia in HIV infection is usually favorable. The mortality of pneumococcal pneumonia, the most common cause, is between 5% and 10%. This figure is actually lower than the mortality rate in non–HIV-infected patients. As stated above, complications of pneumonia, particularly extrapulmonary complications, are rare. There is, however, a relatively high rate of recurrence of pneumococcal disease in individuals with HIV infection. The recurrence rate is estimated to be between 10% and 15%.

Treatment

The treatment of bacterial pneumonia in HIV-infected individuals is essentially the same as that for the general population. Antimicrobial therapy is usually empiric, at least initially. Consideration should be given to the regional trends in antimicrobial susceptibility for various organisms. Of particular importance are the increasing rates of penicillin resistance in pneumococci seen to varying degrees across the United States. Consideration should also be given to the individual patient's exposure to antimicrobials. The widespread use of co-trimoxazole and azithromycin, for prophylaxis against PCP and MAC, respectively, is somewhat protective against bacterial pneumonias, but may also be contributing to increasing rates of drug-resistant organisms. Pneumococcal resistance to co-trimoxazole is particularly prevalent, and this agent should not be used for this indication.

Choices for the empiric treatment of bacterial pneumonia that does not require hospital admission include doxycycline, macrolides, or fluoroquinolones. In more seriously ill patients, options include fluoroquinolones or an extended-spectrum β-lactam (e.g., ceftriaxone) with or without a macrolide. For patients requiring admission to an intensive care unit, an extended-spectrum β-lactam in combination with either a fluoroquinolone or macrolide is recommended. If a microbiologic diagnosis is made, therapy should be directed at that organism based on antimicrobial susceptibility testing.

A response to antibiotics is usually seen within 48 hours and is similar to that seen in immunocompetent individuals. If the response to therapy is appropriate, the duration of therapy should be approximately 10 to 14 days. The presence of bacteremia with pneumonia does not alter treatment. Pneumonia caused by *Legionella,* however, should be treated for at least 21 days. For patients who fail to respond to antibiotics, microbiologic and susceptibility data should be reviewed if available. If the antimicrobial therapy is appropriate and the patient is still not responding, additional diagnoses (e.g., PCP) should be considered. Despite the favorable response to antimicrobial therapy for bacterial pneumonia in HIV infection, the relapse rate is significantly higher than that seen in the general population.

When to Refer or Hospitalize

Criteria that are used to evaluate the need for hospital admission in cases of community-acquired pneumonia (CAP) can be applied to suspected bacterial pneumonia in HIV infection. Consideration should be given to patients' hemodynamic stability, oxygen saturation, laboratory values, and ability to adhere to an outpatient regimen. In cases in which the diagnosis is uncertain or patients fail to respond to therapy, consultation with an infectious disease specialist is indicated. For patients in whom the diagnosis of PCP is suspected, induced sputum evaluation followed, if necessary, by a bronchoscopy should be strongly considered.

Guidelines

Practice guidelines for the management of CAP are available from a variety of organizations including the Infectious Diseases Society of America (IDSA). These guidelines can be used in the management of suspected bacterial pneumonia in HIV infection with careful consideration given to alternative diagnoses as described above. See the Suggested Readings for more details.

KEY POINTS

- *Streptococcus pneumoniae* is the most common cause of bacterial pneumonia in HIV infection
- Blood cultures and sputum cultures should be obtained in all cases of suspected bacterial pneumonia
- Alternative diagnoses should be considered in patients who fail to respond to antimicrobial therapy

Gastroenteritis

Presentation and Progression

The combination of fever and diarrhea is one of the most common symptom complexes in HIV infection. Many such presentations are caused by enteric bacterial infections. The bowel is the immune system's largest organ. Progressive HIV infection impacts on the ability of the bowel mucosa to form an effective barrier to microorganisms and on the ability of patients to control systemic infection. Thus most causes of bacterial gastroenteritis in HIV infection are similar to those seen in the general population. The prevalence, severity, and risk of relapse, however, deserve special attention.

Cause. *Salmonella* was recognized as an important pathogen in HIV disease from the earliest days of the epidemic. Recurrent *Salmonella* septicemia, in fact, is one of the AIDS-defining illnesses in the Centers for Disease Control and Prevention (CDC) surveillance case definition. There are many subtypes and serotypes of *Salmonella* and they are found in a variety of animal hosts. In humans, the two species isolated most commonly are *S. enteritidis* and *S. typhimurium*. Infection is acquired through ingestion of the organism, typically from undercooked meat, poultry, eggs, or dairy products. Another important source of disease in humans is via contact with certain pets. Reptiles (turtles, lizards, and snakes) may be asymptomatic carriers of *Salmonella,* and young cats and dogs with diarrhea are frequently infected with this organism. The incidence of salmonellosis in HIV-infected individuals is estimated to be 20 to 100 times that seen in the general population.

It is unclear whether HIV infection increases the risk of infection with *Campylobacter* or *Shigella,* but it appears that more severe disease can present in patients with advanced HIV. *C. jejuni* is the most common species to cause illness, although *C. fetus, C. cinaedi,* and *C. fennelliae* have also been reported in HIV-infected patients. The organism is usually acquired from raw or undercooked poultry. Shigellosis is more common in men who have sex with men, but it is not clear what impact HIV has on the acquisition of this disease. These organisms are found only in humans, and the most common species is *S. sonnei.* Most transmission occurs via person to person contact, although this contact may be indirect, such as when an infected food-handler is connected to a food-borne outbreak. Disease transmitted by sexual contact has been associated with *S. flexneri.*

Listeria monocytogenes has also been recognized as a rare, but important, cause of disease in patients with HIV infection. The organism is acquired from contaminated food sources, typically dairy and meat products. Although the organism may cause a gastrointestinal illness, listeriosis manifested by bacteremia and meningitis is the more worrisome presentation. The estimated incidence of listeriosis in the HIV-infected population is over 60 times that of the general population.

Presentation. The clinical presentation of bacterial gastroenteritis is similar, in many ways, to that seen in immunocompetent hosts. Patients typically present with fever; diarrhea, which may be bloody; and abdominal pain or cramping. Bacteremia complicating gastroenteritis is far more prevalent in HIV infection than in the general population. For *Salmonella,* bacteremia is five times more frequent in patients with HIV infection. Particularly with more advanced immunosuppression, salmonellosis commonly presents with bacteremia in the absence of gastrointestinal symptoms. This presentation is typical of typhoid fever caused by *S. typhi,* but as described here can be seen with the nontyphoidal strains of *Salmonella. Salmonella* sepsis is a manifestation of late-stage AIDS. *Campylobacter* and *Shigella* gastroenteritis have presentations that are indistinguishable on clinical grounds. Bacteremia with these organisms is very rare in immunocompetent patients but has been reported in patients with HIV infection. Listeriosis usually is manifest as a febrile illness with bacteremia. Meningitis, if present, may have features of a rhomboencephalitis (cranial nerve abnormalities), in addition to the more classic symptoms of bacterial meningitis.

Diagnosis

If bacterial gastroenteritis is suspected, a microbiologic diagnosis should be sought. A methylene blue stain of stool looking for the presence of white blood cells may be useful in identifying inflammatory conditions but is nonspecific and insensitive. Stool specimens should be sent for bacterial culture. Blood cultures should be obtained in all patients with HIV infection and fever and diarrhea. This is particularly important for identifying *Salmonella* because it is not uncommonly found in blood cultures without being identified in stool.

Infection with *L. monocytogenes* is usually diagnosed by isolation of the organism from blood or cerebrospinal fluid (CSF). Except for the investigation of food-borne outbreaks, stool culture for *Listeria* is generally not performed.

Natural History

Bacterial gastroenteritis in immunocompetent individuals is usually a self-limited illness that in many cases does not require antimicrobial therapy. In patients with HIV infection, however, these diseases are frequently more severe. Bacteremia is common and the sepsis syndrome may occur, especially with salmonellosis.

Salmonella has a propensity for causing metastatic infection with a tropism for endovascular sites. The complications of *Salmonella* infection that have been reported in patients with HIV infection include endocarditis, mycotic aneurysms, lung abscesses, peritonitis, septic arthritis, osteomyelitis, brain abscesses, and meningitis.

Infections with *Campylobacter* have been linked to development of Guillain-Barré syndrome, but this condition does not appear to be more prevalent in the HIV-infected population.

Treatment

Fluid and electrolyte repletion remains of paramount importance in the treatment of bacterial gastroenteritis and in many cases requires intravenous therapy. Because of the increased likelihood of severe disease and bacteremia, antimicrobial treatment of bacterial gastroenteritis in HIV-infected patients is advised. Because of increasing rates of antimicrobial resistance among these pathogens, definitive therapy should be based on susceptibility testing when possible. The best empiric choice for the treatment of bacterial gastroenteritis is a fluoroquinolone (e.g., ciprofloxacin) because of its broad spectrum of activity. Treatment of specific pathogens should be tailored as described below.

While ampicillin and co-trimoxazole are the classic drugs to treat *Salmonella* infections, they have become less effective because of rising resistance. In patients requiring hospitalization, intravenous ceftriaxone followed by oral therapy with ciprofloxacin is a reasonable approach. The optimal duration of therapy is unknown, but chronic suppressive therapy with ciprofloxacin or co-trimoxazole is worthy of consideration, particularly in patients with severe immunosuppression that is unlikely to improve.

Campylobacter and *Shigella* infections should be treated in HIV-infected individuals. As stated above, fluoroquinolones are a good empiric choice while awaiting identification of an organism and susceptibility testing. If *Campylobacter* is isolated, macrolides remain the drug class of choice. Co-trimoxazole is effective in many cases of shigellosis. The optimal duration of therapy is unknown, but prolonged carriage as is seen with *Salmonella* is less common.

The generally accepted treatment of listeriosis is intravenous ampicillin. In severe disease and in the immunocompromised host, gentamicin may be added. For patients intolerant of this regimen, co-trimoxazole is an acceptable alternative. In cases of meningitis, patients should be treated at least 3 weeks, but for bacteremia alone, shorter courses may be as efficacious.

The expected response to the treatment of bacterial gastrointestinal infections is good, with one caveat. There is a significant relapse rate of *Salmonella* infections in patients who do not receive chronic suppressive therapy. Additionally, bacteremia may recur while on treatment for *Salmonella*. The optimal antimicrobial regimen for chronic suppression is unknown, as is the efficacy of this strategy in preventing relapse.

KEY POINTS

- *Salmonella* is the most important enteric bacterial pathogen in HIV infection
- Bacteremia commonly complicates bacterial gastroenteritis in HIV infection
- Prolonged illness and relapse are common
- Chronic suppressive therapy may be indicated for patients with HIV and *Salmonella* infection

Syphilis

Presentation and Progression

The impact of HIV infection on social, political, economic, and medical developments over the past 20 years is rivaled by few diseases in human history. Syphilis, however, has a long history of influence on the course of human events. The interaction of these diseases with one another is an important entity worthy of discussion.

Cause. Syphilis is caused by the spirochete *Treponema pallidum*. Despite its prominent role in human illness for at least the past several hundred years, little clinically applicable information is known about this organism. No widely available culture media support the growth of the organism, and most techniques for detecting the organism have relied on the inoculation of infected material into live tissue (e.g., rabbit testicles). The diagnosis and treatment of syphilis have become well standardized since the introduction of serologic tests and the discovery of penicillin. When syphilis occurs in the setting of HIV infection, these conventions may be challenged and careful interpretation of diagnostic tests and response to therapy is required.

Both antibody responses and cellular immune responses are important for the control of *T. pallidum*. HIV's effect on these two arms of the immune system may alter the course of syphilis in co-infected patients.

Presentation. Syphilis is classified into three stages of disease: primary, secondary, and tertiary. Typical presentation of any of these stages may be altered by coinfection with HIV.

Primary syphilis is characterized by the presence of a painless chancre. This clean-appearing ulcer occurs at the site of inoculation, so typical locations include the penis, labia, and perianal area. It is usually single, but multiple lesions may be seen. The chancre will heal with or without antimicrobial treatment.

Secondary syphilis usually occurs within 2 to 8 weeks of the chancre's appearance. It appears that patients with HIV infection may be more likely to develop secondary syphilis while the chancre is still present. This stage of syphilis is a systemic illness, and fever and constitutional symptoms are common. There are a variety of dermatologic manifestations, but the classic findings include a macular, maculopapular, or pustular rash that begins on the trunk and may involve the palms and soles. Condylomata lata are heaped-up plaques that tend to occur in intertriginous areas, particularly the groin. When similar lesions occur on mucosal surfaces they are known as mucous patches. Other manifestations include patchy alopecia, aseptic meningitis, anterior uveitis, and hepatitis. Anecdotal reports and some case series document severe manifestations of secondary syphilis in patients with HIV infection. These are reports of conditions that have also been seen in the non–HIV-infected population and indeed the pre-HIV era, so it is unclear if the severity of these cases can truly be attributed to concomitant HIV infection.

Tertiary syphilis includes a variety of organ complications that generally occur 10 to 30 years after initial infection, but can occur much sooner in persons coinfected with HIV. Manifestations include cardiovascular syphilis (aortic aneurysms), gummatous syphilis (nodular or mass lesions that can involve virtually any organ), and a variety of manifestations of neurosyphilis that will be described below.

Syphilis can involve the nervous system at any stage of disease and may occur without symptoms or may cause severe debilitating disease. Among the early manifestations of neurosyphilis, patients with secondary syphilis may have an aseptic meningitis. Cranial nerve abnormalities are common in this condition, particularly II, III, VI, VII, and VIII. Meningovascular syphilis occurs months to 10 years after infection and presents with focal neurologic deficits that evolve over days to weeks. These deficits are sometimes accompanied by headaches and psychiatric disturbances. Parenchymatous neurosyphilis (general paresis and tabes dorsalis) presents 10 to 30 years after initial infection. General paresis is a dementing illness that may be indistinguishable from other causes of dementia. Tabes dorsalis is the result of neuronal cell loss in the posterior columns of the spinal cord, resulting in ataxia and loss of proprioceptive sense. Patients may also experience "lightning" or shooting pains. All of these manifestations of neurosyphilis have been

Bacterial Infections in HIV   113

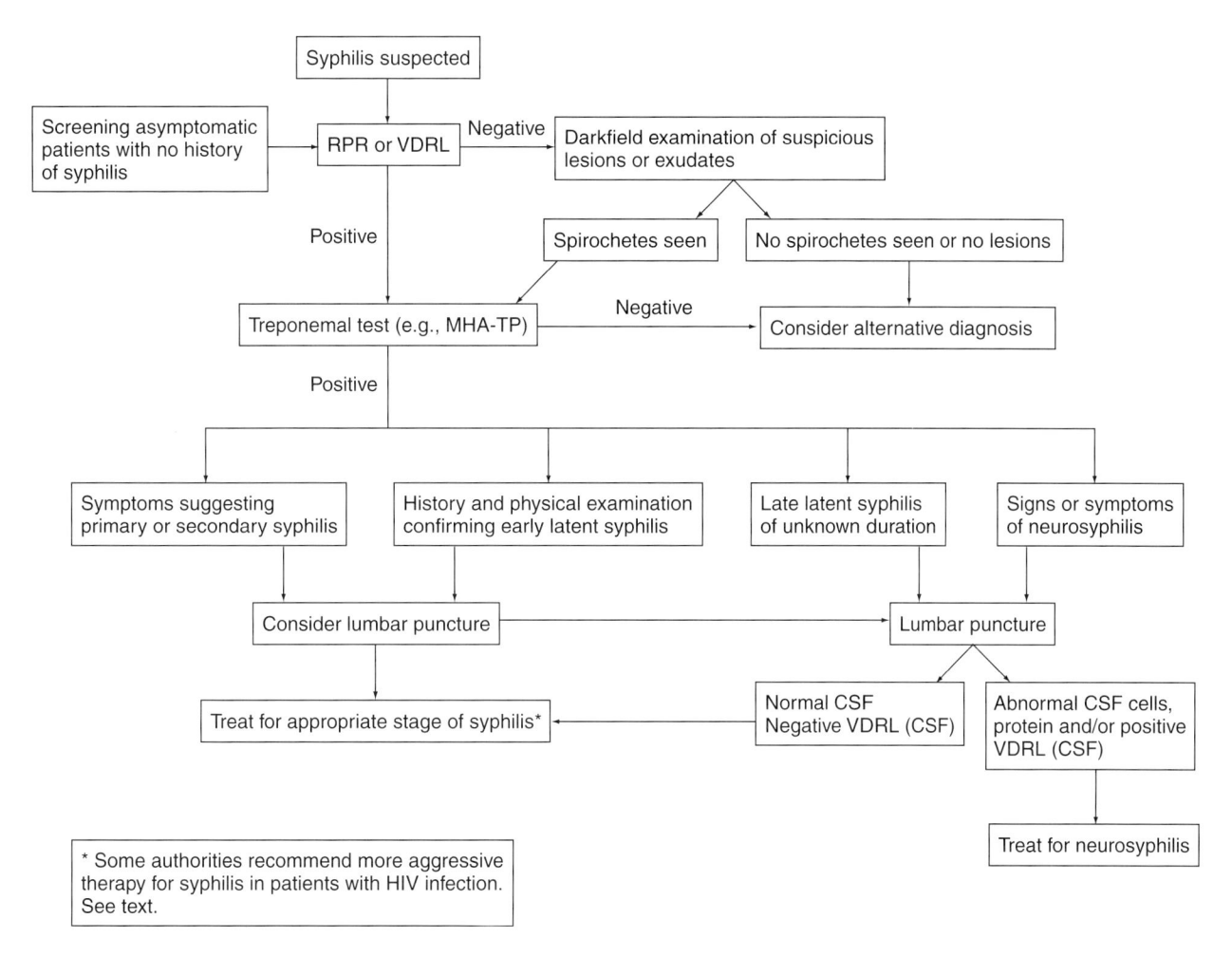

FIG. 12-2 Algorithm for syphilis in HIV-infected individuals.

described in patients with HIV infection, in addition to several unusual presentations. Reliable data are not available, but experience suggests that neurosyphilis, particularly the earlier manifestation, may be more common in the HIV-infected population. The relationship of early manifestations of neurosyphilis to the development of parenchymatous disease is unknown.

Diagnosis

Clinical suspicion for syphilis should be pursued aggressively in patients with HIV infection, and because of relatively high coinfection rates, testing for latent syphilis with a rapid plasma reagin (RPR) test is a standard component of the initial laboratory work-up after the diagnosis of HIV infection is established. Likewise, the diagnosis of syphilis, or any sexually transmitted infection, in a patient with unknown HIV serology should prompt HIV testing. Fig. 12-2 summarizes a diagnostic algorithm for suspected syphilis in patients with HIV infection.

In patients with primary or secondary disease, scrapings of lesions or exudates can be examined for spirochetes by darkfield microscopy. This technique is particularly important when patients present very early in the course of infection because serologic tests are occasionally negative in this setting. Spirochetes are too thin to be seen by Gram's stain and conventional light microscopy.

The serologic tests for syphilis include nontreponemal assays and tests for treponeme-specific antibodies. The RPR and Venereal Disease Research Laboratory (VDRL) tests are nontreponemal tests. These tests detect antibodies against a cardiolipin antigen. Unfortunately the polyclonal gammopathy of HIV infection frequently includes anticardiolipin antibodies, and this may lead to false-positive nontreponemal tests. Most biologically false-positive tests will be of low titers (less than 1:8). All positive nontreponemal tests should be confirmed at least once with a more specific treponemal test such as the microhemagglutination-*T. pallidum* (MHA-TP) or the fluorescent treponemal antibody-absorbed (FTA-abs) test. Only persons who are positive with the treponemal tests are truly positive for syphilis.

Several caveats should be made regarding the interpretation of these tests for patients with HIV infection. As stated above, HIV infection may cause false-positive RPR and VDRL tests, the nontreponemal tests. There are also reports of false-negative serologic tests for syphilis in the presence of HIV infection, as well as evidence that patients with reactive treponemal antibody tests may "serorevert" with progressive immunosuppression. Nonetheless, because of the rarity of these events, and the vast experience using these tests to diagnose syphilis, serologic tests should generally be interpreted the same for patients with or without HIV infection.

Compared with non–HIV-infected patients, patients with HIV infection may be at increased risk for neurologic complications of syphilis. Many authorities advise CSF examinations for all patients diagnosed with syphilis at any stage. The CDC recommends CSF examinations for patients with late latent syphilis (infection over 1 year) or syphilis of unknown duration. Physicians should be aware, however, that many patients with primary or secondary syphilis have abnormalities in their CSF without symptoms. The significance of these findings and treatment implications are unknown. The typical CSF findings of neurosyphilis include a pleocytosis, elevated protein, and a reactive CSF VDRL test. In the presence of neurologic symptoms and a positive serology for syphilis, unless there is an alternative explanation, any one of these CSF features alone may indicate neurosyphilis. There are case reports of patients with symptoms of neurosyphilis and negative CSF VDRL tests, but these are distinctly unusual and the CSF VDRL tests became positive after treatment. Repeated lumbar punctures are required to assess normalization of CSF as an indicator of response to therapy.

Natural History

The natural history of untreated syphilis is variable. Approximately 30% of non–HIV-infected persons will progress to the tertiary stage, whereas many infections will remain latent for life. The impact of HIV infection on the progression of disease is not certain, but defects in humoral and cell-mediated immunity have been reported to lead to a telescoped progression. The classic development of tertiary disease over as long as 30 years may be accelerated for patients with HIV infection. Many authorities believe that neurosyphilis may be more common in HIV infection. Although unusual manifestations have been reported in HIV-infected patients, there is no evidence that these are more common in this setting as opposed to in the general population.

Treatment

The mainstay of the treatment of syphilis remains penicillin. According to the CDC, primary and secondary syphilis can be treated with a single dose of benzathine penicillin 2.4 million units intramuscularly (IM). In patients with HIV infection, there are reports of both chancres and symptoms of secondary syphilis that are slow to resolve following this treatment. Many authorities recommend supplemental antibiotics in the form of additional injections of benzathine penicillin 2.4 million units IM weekly for 2 weeks. Patients with early latent syphilis, that is, latent infection that can be clearly identified as having occurred within 1 year, should be treated the same as those with primary or secondary syphilis. Patients with late latent syphilis or syphilis of unknown duration should receive at least three weekly injections of benzathine penicillin 2.4 million units IM. As stated above, these patients should have CSF examinations to ensure that the treatment employed does not result in the inadequate treatment of neurosyphilis.

Penicillin is likely to be the most efficacious agent in treating syphilis, and every effort should be employed to use it. Skin testing should be considered in patients with a history of an allergic reaction to penicillin. Doxycycline may be used in patients who are allergic to penicillin. The dosage is 100 mg orally twice a day. Patients with primary, secondary, or early latent syphilis should be treated for at least 2 weeks. For late latent syphilis, at least 4 weeks is indicated.

Neurosyphilis should be treated with intravenous penicillin G 18 to 24 million units daily (3 to 4 million units every 4 hours) for 10 to 14 days. Alternative penicillin regimens, which are unproven in patients with coexistent HIV infection, include procaine penicillin 2.4 million units IM daily plus probenecid 500 mg orally four times a day for 10 to 14 days. Although alternative treatment regimens have been employed using doxycycline, ceftriaxone, and other agents, every effort should be made to treat neurosyphilis with penicillin. For patients with an allergy to penicillin, desensitization is preferable to alternative therapy.

The efficacy of these regimens for patients with HIV infection is not well described. There is ample evidence that clinical and serologic relapses occur, and are probably more common than in the general population. For this reason, close follow-up is recommended. Quantitative nontreponemal tests should be repeated on all patients treated for syphilis at 3, 6, 9, 12, and 24 months after therapy, and those without a fourfold decrease in titer at 6 months should be retreated. Lumbar punctures for CSF examination should also be considered in nonresponders. In patients treated for neurosyphilis, CSF examinations should be performed at 6-month intervals until findings have stabilized. CSF VDRL test may not revert to negative, but the white blood cell (WBC) count should normalize. Retreatment is indicated for persistently abnormal CSF after 2 years.

When to Refer

All cases of syphilis should be reported to the local health department. Contact investigations are essential for reducing the spread of disease.

Syphilis in HIV-infected patients should be treated by infectious disease specialists or physicians with experience in this area because of the serious risk and consequences of relapse and the need for close follow-up.

Guidelines

Guidelines for the treatment of syphilis, including individuals with HIV infection, are available from the CDC. For more information see the Suggested Readings.

▶ KEY POINTS

- ⊃ Syphilis diagnosis and treatment should be pursued aggressively in patients with HIV infection
- ⊃ Cerebrospinal fluid examination should be considered for all HIV-infected patients with syphilis and definitely in cases of late latent syphilis or syphilis of unknown duration
- ⊃ Neurologic manifestations of syphilis may be more common in patients with HIV infection
- ⊃ Follow-up serology and follow-up lumbar punctures when indicated are essential in the management of syphilis

Bartonella Infections

Presentation and Progression

Cause. Several clinical syndromes that may complicate HIV infection are attributable to members of the genus *Bartonella*. These are small gram-negative organisms, many of which were formerly classified in the genus *Rochalimaea*. The two species of most importance in humans, and of particular importance in HIV, are *B. henselae* and *B. quintana*. The former is the etiologic agent of cat-scratch disease, a condition commonly seen in immunocompetent hosts. The latter is the cause of trench fever. Either organism can cause disease in HIV infection and generally cause one of two syndromes, bacteremia alone or tissue infection. The bacteremia may result in or be caused by endovascular infection, and occasionally this is seen in non–HIV-infected individuals. The tissue infection may involve the skin or many other sites and is known as bacillary angiomatosis (BA). *Bartonella* infection in the liver or spleen is one of the causes of bacillary peliosis (BP).

Presentation. BA and BP are manifestations of late-stage HIV infection and typically occur when the CD4+ cell count is less than 100 cells/mm^3. These infections are subacute in onset, and in some studies, patients have noted symptoms for over 1 year before coming to medical attention.

The best-described manifestation of BA is that seen in the skin. These lesions have a variable appearance and may be either cutaneous or subcutaneous, and single or multiple. They are most often papular, red lesions with a smooth surface. They may have a vascular appearance and tend to bleed when traumatized. Other presentations are not uncommon and include dry, scaly lesions and subcutaneous nodules. On dark-skinned patients, lesions may appear as nearly black raised papules.

Osteolytic lesions due to BA can occur with or without skin lesions. Similarly, vascular lesions due to *Bartonella* have been reported in the gastrointestinal and respiratory tracts. CNS lesions, bone marrow infection, and lymphadenitis like that seen in cat-scratch disease have also been seen in HIV-infected patients.

Patients with BP usually have fever and abdominal pain. Some will have simultaneous cutaneous lesions, although many will not. Alkaline phosphatase levels tend to be elevated but hepatic transaminase levels are usually normal or only mildly elevated. With splenic involvement, pancytopenia or isolated thrombocytopenia has been seen.

Bacteremia may accompany any of the manifestations of BA or BP, or may occur without tissue disease. The presentation of *Bartonella* bacteremia is similar to that seen in many other febrile illnesses of late-stage HIV infection and includes fever, chills, and weight loss. Endocarditis, although rare, has been seen more commonly in patients without HIV infection, and *B. quintana* has usually been implicated.

Anecdotal reports and several studies have established important epidemiologic links to the development of *Bartonella* infection. Cats are probably the main reservoirs of *B. henselae*, and high-grade bacteremia has been observed in apparently healthy cats. The modes of transmission between cats and from cats to humans are not fully elucidated. Cat fleas are vectors for *B. henselae* and ticks may also have the ability to transmit the organism. There is, however, no association of *B. quintana* and cat contact. The principal vector for *B. quintana* appears to be the human body louse. The finding of *B. quintana* bacteremia in non–HIV-infected homeless men suggests that homelessness may be a risk factor for the acquisition of *B. quintana*.

Diagnosis

The diagnosis of BA is best made by biopsy. Because BA lesions on the skin and elsewhere may resemble many other conditions, most importantly Kaposi's sarcoma, establishing a definitive diagnosis is favored. For BP, a tissue diagnosis may require an excisional biopsy or splenectomy. The causative bacilli can be seen with a modified silver stain (e.g., Warthin-Starry stain) but are not seen on other fungal stains, Gram's stain, or stains for acid-fast bacilli (AFB). Without visualization of the organism, the histopathologic appearance of these lesions may be difficult to distinguish from other vascular or neoplastic lesions.

Even without signs or symptoms of bacteremia, all patients with suspected BA or BP should have blood cultures. *Bartonella* is most likely to be recovered using lysis-centrifugation tubes. This blood culture technique is also preferred for the isolation of mycobacteria. When tissue biopsy is riskier, as with splenic BP, or not possible, the finding of *Bartonella* bacteremia will lend support to a clinical diagnosis. Culture of the organism from tissue specimens is of lower yield.

An indirect immunofluorescent antibody (IFA) is the preferred serologic test for *Bartonella* antibodies. This is often the preferred approach to the diagnosis of cat-scratch disease. Its utility in the diagnosis of BA and BP is less well established, but it may prove useful in monitoring response to therapy.

Identification of *Bartonella* DNA by polymerase chain reaction (PCR) is a technique that is not widely available. Anecdotal reports, however, suggest that it may be of clinical use in cases in which traditional diagnostic tests are not helpful.

Treatment

There are no standardized treatment protocols for the treatment of *Bartonella* infections in patients with HIV. These organisms are sensitive to a variety of antimicrobials in vitro. Most clinical experience has been with either erythromycin (500 mg qid) or doxycycline (100 mg bid). Newer macrolides (azithromycin and clarithromycin) are also effective. For patients with severe disease, such as endocarditis, the addition of rifampin to either erythromycin or doxycycline should be considered. Of note, there have been varying responses to fluoroquinolones, and these agents should not be among the first-line agents considered. Penicillins and first-generation cephalosporins are not active against *Bartonella*.

Response to therapy is usually prompt, and cases of cutaneous BA may resolve within a week after initiating antimicrobials. At the start of therapy, some patients will experience a Jarisch-Herxheimer reaction characterized by a transient fever and exacerbation of symptoms. Because infections with *Bartonella* have the tendency to relapse, prolonged courses of therapy are advisable. For limited BA, at least 2 months of antimicrobials should be administered. For more severe disease, including BP and endocarditis, treatment should be extended to at least 4 months.

The prevention of *Bartonella* infections for patients with HIV has not been systematically studied. Although cat exposure has been associated with the development of BA and BP, many patients report no such exposure. Given the considerable psychologic benefit of pet ownership for many individuals, most authorities do not recommend that patients with HIV infection give away their cats. If new cats are to be acquired, however, mature cats should be favored over kittens. It also may be advisable that a cat be confined to the home and not be allowed outdoors to minimize the chance to acquire the organism. Vigilance for and treatment of louse infestation in susceptible populations may be effective in preventing disease caused by *B. quintana*.

> **KEY POINTS**

- Infections with *Bartonella* are uncommon for patients with CD4+ counts over 100 cells/mm³
- Biopsy is favored for the diagnosis of tissue lesions
- Blood cultures are indicated if *Bartonella* infection is suspected
- Therapeutic options include doxycycline or erythromycin

Rhodococcus equi

Presentation and Progression

Although rare, *Rhodococcus equi* represents an important bacterial pathogen in HIV-infected patients. Long recognized as a pathogen in horses and other farm animals, disease in humans was not reported until 1967.

Rhodococcus is a facultative, intracellular gram-positive coccobacillus. It is aerobic and does not form spores. Because of the presence of mycolic acids in the cell well, this organism stains weakly acid-fast. Transmission to humans probably occurs primarily by inhalation of the organism from soil, where it is frequently found. Up to one third of patients with *Rhodococcus* infection report an exposure to farm soil. Inoculation into the skin through open wounds has also been reported.

Pulmonary disease is the most common site of infection and occurs in the later stages of HIV infection with CD4+ counts typically less than 100 cells/mm³. Common symptoms include fever, chest pain, productive cough, dyspnea, and hemoptysis. Indolent presentations are also seen, characterized by anorexia and weight loss, with symptoms evolving over weeks to months. Findings on chest films are variable but cavitary lesions are typical. Other radiographic presentations include pulmonary infiltrates and pleural effusions.

Bacteremia without pulmonary disease is a less common presentation of *R. equi* infection. Additionally, brain, renal, and pelvic abscesses have all been reported in HIV-infected patients, probably as a consequence of bacteremia.

Diagnosis

The diagnosis of *R. equi* infections is best made by identification of the organism because the clinical presentation is protean and the radiographic findings nonspecific. The finding of cavitary lung disease in a patient with advanced AIDS should raise suspicion for *R. equi*. The differential diagnosis also includes *Nocardia, Pseudomonas, M. kansasii,* and *Aspergillus*. Tuberculosis, another important pulmonary pathogen in HIV, classically does not cause cavitation in the setting of severe immunosuppression. About half of the patients with pulmonary disease have positive blood cultures.

R. equi can be isolated from sputum, bronchoscopy washings, pleural fluid, and tissue specimens. Several caveats are important to mention with regard to identification of this organism. Because of their similar appearance (gram-positive rods), *R. equi* organisms can be mistaken for diphtheroids on a Gram's stain and thus can be mistakenly labeled as normal respiratory flora. Similarly, in blood cultures, they may be mistaken for contaminants. These organisms may also be mistaken for mycobacteria because they stain partially acid-fast. The microbiology laboratory therefore should be notified if there is a clinical suspicion of *R. equi* infection.

The histopathologic appearance of tissue infected with *R. equi* is usually necrotizing granulomatous inflammation with many polymorphonuclear cells. Because of the nonspecific nature of this appearance, identification of the organism is essential for a definitive diagnosis.

Treatment

Antimicrobial therapy for *R. equi* infection should be based on susceptibility testing. In general, this organism is resistant to penicillin and first-generation cephalosporins. A variety of other antimicrobials have been used, but there is no consensus on the optimal regimen for the treatment of *R. equi*. Because of the ability of this organism to develop resistance during therapy, at least two agents should be employed. The combination of vancomycin and imipenem has proved effective in some cases. Macrolides or fluoroquinolones in combination with rifampin have also been used and have the advantage of an oral route of administration.

The duration of therapy should be individualized, but long courses of therapy are usually required. A minimum of 2 months of at least two drugs should be used. In patients with positive cultures for *R. equi* while on therapy, antimicrobial susceptibility testing should be repeated and, if necessary, drug selection adjusted based on the results. Relapses are common and the extent to which prolonged antimicrobial therapy prevents relapses is unknown. Lifelong therapy may be reasonable in some cases.

Surgical interventions for *R. equi* infection have been attempted, but their optimal use is unclear. In a patient with a single cavitary lesion who fails to respond to antimicrobials, surgical resection may be a viable option.

The expected outcome of *R. equi* infection varies with the degree of immunosuppression. Patients with more advanced immunosuppression have a worse prognosis, even with antimicrobial therapy. Relapse after therapy is common. The overall mortality in patients with HIV and *Rhodococcus* infections is in part reflective of the occurrence of this disease in patients with late-stage HIV. In one review, the mortality attributable to *R. equi* infection was 15.4%. In other studies, mortality approached 50%.

> **KEY POINTS**

- *Rhodococcus equi* can cause cavitary pulmonary disease in the late stages of HIV infection
- Diagnosis is made by culturing the organism from the primary site of infection or blood
- Antimicrobial therapy generally requires the use of at least two agents
- Drug resistance may emerge during therapy

SUGGESTED READINGS

Angulo FJ, Swerdlow DL: Bacterial enteric infections in persons infected with human immunodeficiency virus, *Clin Infect Dis* 21(Suppl 1):S84-S93, 1995.

Bartlett JG et al: Practice guidelines for the management of community-acquired pneumonia in adults, *Clin Infect Dis* 31:347-382, 2000. *www.idsociety.org*

Berger BJ, Hussain F, Roistacher K: Bacterial infections in HIV-infected patients, *Infect Dis Clin North Am* 8(2):449-465, 1994.

Capdevila JA et al: *Rhodococcus equi* pneumonia in patients infected with the human immunodeficiency virus: report of 2 cases and review of the literature, *Scand J Infect Dis* 29:535-541, 1997.

Donisi A et al: *Rhodococcus equi* infection in HIV-infected patients, *AIDS* 10:359-362, 1996.

Hirschtick RE et al: Bacterial pneumonia in persons infected with the human immunodeficiency virus, *N Engl J Med* 333:845-851, 1995.

Hutchinson CM et al: Altered clinical presentation of early syphilis in patients with human immunodeficiency virus, *Ann Intern Med* 121:94-99, 1994.

Malone JL et al: Syphilis and neurosyphilis in a human immunodeficiency virus type-1 seropositive population: evidence for frequent serologic relapse after therapy, *Am J Med* 99:55-62, 1995.

Musher DM, Hamill RJ, Baughn RE: Effect of human immunodeficiency virus infection on the course of syphilis and on the response to treatment, *Ann Intern Med* 113:872-881, 1990.

Regnery RL, Childs JE, Koehler JE: Infections associated with Bartonella species in persons infected with human immunodeficiency virus, *Clin Infect Dis* 21(Suppl 1):S94-S98, 1995.

1998 Guidelines for treatment of sexually transmitted diseases, *MMWR* 47(RR-1):1-111, 1998. *www.cdc.gov*

Section 2 **Symptoms and Signs Indicative of Progressive Infection**

13 Skin Manifestations of HIV Infection

YVETTE E. APPIAH, PAUL R. GROSS

Introduction

The majority of people infected with the human immunodeficiency virus (HIV) will develop one or more skin diseases before or after diagnosis of HIV. Samet et al reported that in their case series of 95 HIV-infected patients presenting for initial primary care at Boston City Hospital, 86% of these patients had one or more skin manifestations. Dermatologic diseases are frequently the presenting sign of HIV disease. Specifically, skin diseases such as severe seborrheic dermatitis, oral candidiasis, secondary syphilis, and Kaposi's sarcoma (KS) are clues to the need for serologic testing for HIV (Box 13-1). Thus heightened awareness of all physicians to the presentations of such skin diseases impacts the diagnosis, management, and prognosis of HIV-infected individuals. Barton et al found "no appreciable difference in the spectrum or prevalence of dermatologic disease in HIV-infected women versus HIV-infected men," with minor exceptions such as the lower incidence of KS, oral hairy leukoplakia (OHL), and onychomycosis in women.

Skin diseases are more frequent with declining immune function and thus advancing HIV disease. Kaplan et al reported that although 64% of patients with HIV as a group had one or more cutaneous disorders, 87% of those with CD4+ T lymphocyte counts less than 100 cells/mm³ were affected. Some dermatologic complications of HIV disease fulfill the criteria for the diagnosis of acquired immunodeficiency syndrome (AIDS) (Box 13-2). In fact, some of these disorders are considered diagnostic of HIV infection, whereas others are similar to those seen in the general population, although more severe and often presenting with deviations from the typical morphology.

Since the advent of highly active antiretroviral therapy (HAART) in 1997, the prognosis of HIV disease has dramatically improved. By improving the CD4+ cell count and decreasing viral load to undetectable levels, these drugs have reduced the incidence of certain dermatologic manifestations of HIV disease. Although not specifically reported, the incidence of cutaneous deep fungal and parasitic infections has probably followed the downward trend observed in systemic disease. There have been reports of stabilization, improvement, and even remission of KS after initiation of HAART in patients not receiving specific treatment for KS. These opportunistic diseases adversely affect prognosis and thus survival of HIV disease, such that keeping them at bay has a positive impact on the war against HIV disease. Unfortunately, since HAART is not available in most of the developing nations, the profile for dermatologic diseases in those countries now differs from that of developed countries.

Skin diseases in the HIV population tend to have a more severe and more chronic presentation than in the general population. Many HIV-infected individuals already live in fear of social rejection once their HIV status is disclosed. The added stigma of a very visible skin disease has a profound impact on the psyche. Not surprisingly, HIV-infected individuals with skin diseases suffer from emotional distresses, leading to social introversion. The importance of prompt dermatologic evaluation and diagnosis in the HIV-infected population cannot be overemphasized. Successful treatment of a dermatologic problem may reaffirm social validation and significantly improve the quality of life.

The cutaneous disorders associated with HIV disease can be categorized into three major groups: infections, inflammatory diseases, and neoplasms. The atypical presentation of cutaneous disorders, especially infectious disorders, in HIV-infected individuals cannot be stressed enough because this may sometimes lead the physician astray. In HIV disease, an infectious etiology should be considered in the differential diagnosis of every rash. Skin biopsies, tissue, and wound cultures can help clarify the pathologic process. This is especially true if a seemingly straightforward diagnosis fails to respond to therapy or worsens despite appropriate therapy.

When to Refer

Since much of dermatology relies on an experienced eye, most of the diseases encountered may be difficult to diagnose based solely on clinical presentation. In general, a high clinical index of suspicion is required to accurately diagnose various conditions. In addition, despite a significant amount of certainty on the part of the physician, certain dermatologic-specific technical procedures such as skin biopsy are often necessary to confirm the diagnosis or rule out other entities. Particularly in immunocompromised states, atypical presentations are frequently encountered, even in common dermatoses. With the danger of missing impending fatal diagnoses such as infections and malignant conditions, it is imperative that patients undergo fast and accurate diagnoses so that the correct and most effective methods of treatment can be employed. Thus any chronic rash that is unremitting or recurrent despite adequate standard treatment should be referred to a dermatologist

BOX 13-1
Mucocutaneous Disorders as Indications for HIV Serotesting

HIGHLY INDICATIVE OF HIV INFECTION
Exanthem of acute retroviral syndrome
Proximal subungual onychomycosis
Chronic herpetic ulcers
Oral hairy leukoplakia
Kaposi's sarcoma
Eosinophilic folliculitis
Multiple facial molluscum contagiosum

STRONGLY ASSOCIATED WITH HIV INFECTION
Any sexually transmitted disease
Herpes zoster
Signs of injecting drug use
Candidiasis: oropharyngeal or recurrent vulvovaginal

MAY BE ASSOCIATED WITH HIV INFECTION
Generalized lymphadenopathy
Seborrheic dermatitis (extensive, refractory to therapy)
Aphthous ulcers (recurrent, refractory to therapy)

From Johnson RA: Cutaneous manifestations of human immunodeficiency virus disease. In: *Fitzpatrick's dermatology in general medicine,* vol II, ed 51h, New York, 1999, McGraw-Hill, pp 2505-2538.

BOX 13-2
Dermatologic Conditions Diagnostic of AIDS

WITH OR WITHOUT LABORATORY EVIDENCE OF HIV INFECTION
Kaposi's sarcoma in a patient under age 60
Herpes simplex virus infection characterized by a mucocutaneous ulcer that persists longer than 1 month
Cutaneous cryptococcosis

WITH LABORATORY EVIDENCE OF HIV INFECTION
Kaposi's sarcoma at any age
Coccidioidomycosis or histoplasmosis of the skin

From Berger TG, Obuch ML, Goldschmidt RH: Dermatologic manifestations of HIV infection, *Am Fam Physician* 4(6):1729-1742, 1990.

for further evaluation. In addition, any unclear acute dermatoses should also be referred for the appropriate diagnostic evaluation.

Primary Infection
Presentation and Progression

Approximately 80% of cases of primary HIV infection are symptomatic. The incubation period ranges from 3 to 6 weeks. Exposure is followed by an acute febrile illness that signifies the acute retroviral syndrome (ARS).

Symptoms of ARS include fever, rigors, lethargy, malaise, sore throat, anorexia, myalgia, arthralgia, headache, stiff neck, photophobia, nausea, diarrhea, and abdominal cramps. About 75% of patients will have cutaneous findings. The typical exanthem is characterized by erythematous macules and papules on the trunk and extremities, sometimes involving the palms and soles. Mucous membrane involvement is manifested as genital and/or oropharyngeal ulcers. The rash typically lasts for 4 to 5 days with complete resolution. Patients are highly infectious at this stage. Patients with ARS seem to have a higher risk of developing AIDS than asymptomatic converters and thus have a significantly poorer prognosis.

Diagnosis

Seroconversion does not occur until approximately 6 weeks after the acute illness, and 95% of individuals will have antibodies to HIV 6 months after primary infection.

Treatment

Prompt institution of antiretroviral drugs, specifically HAART, can reduce viral loads and alter the prognosis of HIV infection.

Infections

Various infectious agents can cause dermatologic conditions including bacteria, virus, mycobacteria, and fungi. Although some of the infections seen in dermatology may be limited to the skin (herpes simplex virus [HSV], molluscum contagiosum [MC] virus, and superficial fungi), many of them tend to cause other organ disease (deep fungal, bacterial, and bacillary angiomatosis).

Viral Infections
Herpes Simplex Virus

Presentation and Progression. The two types of HSV, HSV-I and HSV-II, are common causes of infections in the HIV population. Grouped vesicles on an erythematous base progress to deep painful ulcerations involving the orofacial, genital, and perianal areas. In the HIV-infected individual, these ulcerations tend to be chronic and severe in nature (Fig. 13-1). HSV is also a common cause of chronic digital ulceration also known as herpetic whitlow. Secondary bacterial infection with *Staphylococcus aureus* is a frequent complication of HSV infections.

Diagnosis. Diagnosis of HSV is confirmed by Tzanck smear (Fig. 13-2), a fluorescent antibody test, or viral culture.

Treatment. Treatment is with oral or intravenous acyclovir. Famciclovir and valacyclovir are also effective. IV acyclovir is recommended for severe infection. Acyclovir-resistant HSV can develop in profoundly immunosuppressed patients with CD4+ counts less than 50 cells/mm^3. Alternative treatment for this subset of patients is trisodium phosphonoformate (foscarnet). HSV is a chronic and recurrent infection; thus chronic suppression with oral acyclovir is recommended once the ulcers have healed. Dissemination of herpes simplex is uncommon, even in severely immunosuppressed AIDS patients, but can occur.

KEY POINTS

- Grouped vesicles on an erythematous base
- May be acute or chronic
- Treat with acyclovir, famciclovir, or valacyclovir

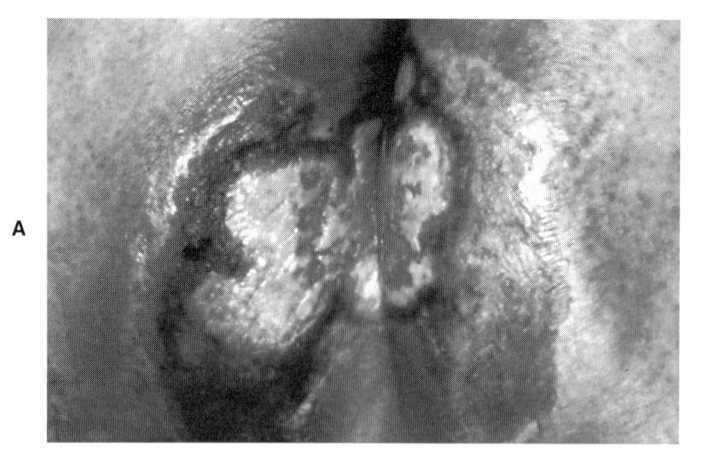

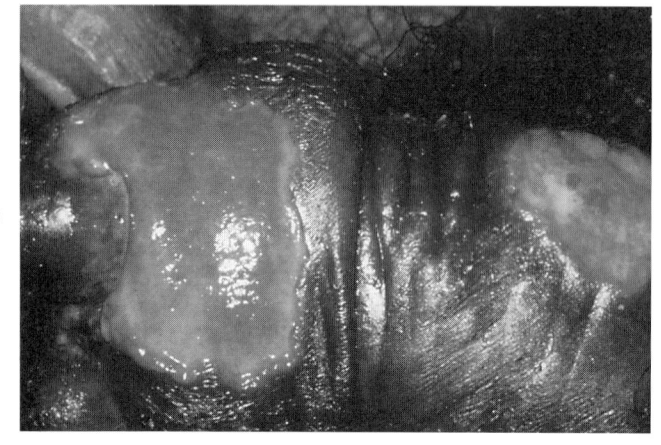

FIG. 13-1 **A,** Chronic herpes simplex. **B,** Chronic herpes simplex virus ulcer.

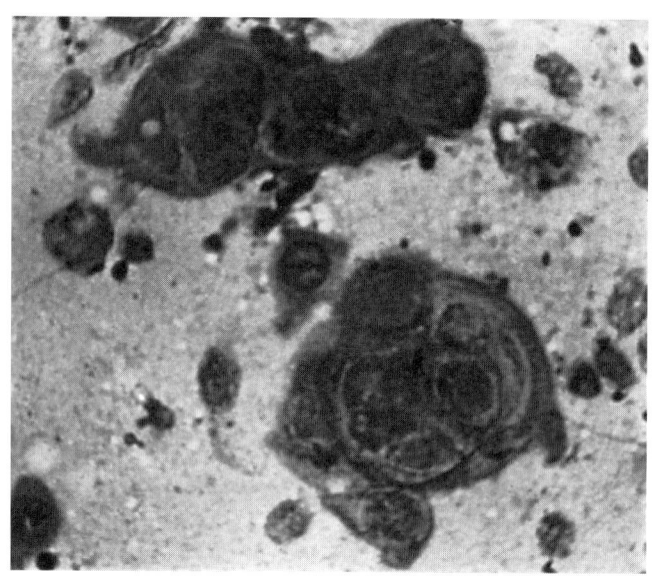

FIG. 13-2 Tzanck smear.

Herpes Zoster
Presentation and Progression. Also known as shingles, herpes zoster may develop in patients with asymptomatic HIV infection, signaling HIV infection. The incidence is seven times greater than in the general population.

The classic eruption is a vesicular rash in a dermatomal distribution respecting the midline; however, atypical dissemination, recurrent attacks, or severe postherpetic neuralgia may occur. Patients with HIV and herpes zoster usually have CD4+ counts less than 400 cells/mm^3. Blindness and cerebral infarction secondary to herpes zoster vasculitis (involving the ophthalmic branch of the trigeminal nerve) have been reported in HIV-infected patients. An ophthalmologic evaluation should be obtained in every patient with lesions clinically involving the ophthalmic branch of the trigeminal nerve.

Diagnosis. Diagnosis is by the same methods used for HSV. The varicella-zoster virus grows more slowly than HSV cultures, taking 7 to 10 days.

Treatment. For localized lesions, the disease responds to acyclovir 800 mg orally five times daily for 7 to 10 days, valacyclovir 1 g orally three times daily for 7 to 10 days, or famciclovir 500 mg orally three times daily for 7 days. Intravenous acyclovir is used for severe or disseminated disease. As with HSV disease, acyclovir-resistant herpes zoster may be treated successfully with foscarnet.

KEY POINTS
- Erythema, vesicles, pain or itching in dermatomal distribution
- Need ophthalmologic evaluation if involves ophthalmic branch of the trigeminal nerve
- Postherpetic neuralgia can be difficult to manage

Molluscum Contagiosum
Presentation and Progression. MC is another common cutaneous viral infection in HIV-infected patients. The virus is a double-stranded DNA virus of the poxvirus family. MC is usually seen in healthy children. The number and extent of the lesions in HIV-infected individuals tend to correlate with the degree of immunosuppression. The appearance of extensive MC lesions in an adult should prompt the clinician to rule out underlying HIV infection. Genital MC is considered a sexually transmitted disease; therefore any patient with these lesions must be carefully evaluated for other sexually transmitted diseases, specifically syphilis.

The typical clinical presentation is of multiple, centrally umbilicated, flesh-colored papules occurring on the face, axillae, groin, or buttocks.

Diagnosis. Diagnosis is usually clinical with the aid of a light source. Shining a light on the side of a papule will produce illumination with an opaque center. Lesions may sometimes be atypical, resembling deep fungal infections. In these instances, a biopsy may be needed to confirm the diagnosis. The differential diagnosis of MC-like lesions in an HIV-infected patient includes cryptococcosis, histoplasmosis, coccidioidomycosis, and penicilliosis.

Treatment. Treatment of MC lesions in HIV is often difficult, with complete resolution of the lesions being almost impossible. Recurrence is inevitable until CD4+ counts increase. Various physical and chemical destructive methods such as curettage, liquid nitrogen cryotherapy, trichloroacetic acid, and podophyllum resin are all reasonable options for treatment. Topical tretinoin in addition to any one of the above methods is effective in reducing recurrent facial lesions. Immunomodulation with imiquimod, an interferon-inducing agent, is also effective.

> **KEY POINTS**

- Centrally umbilicated flesh-colored papules with central core
- Multiple lesions should prompt evaluation for HIV in any adult
- Rule out cryptococcosis in HIV patient

Warts

Presentation and Progression. The many serotypes of the human papillomavirus (HPV) are the cause of warts. HPV 16 and 18, the most common serotypes known to increase the risk of transformation into squamous cell cancer, are even more common in HIV-infected patients. This risk of dysplastic changes and carcinoma is typical for genital warts, especially those occurring at cellular transformation zones such as the cervix or rectum. Periodic pelvic examinations with Papanicolaou tests for women and rectal examinations for men are recommended. When perianal warts are present, sigmoidoscopic examination should be performed to rule out internal lesions and the occurrence of HPV-induced neoplasia.

The morphology of warts is no different in the HIV-infected population than in the general population. However, they tend to be larger, more extensive, refractory to conventional therapy, and more frequently recurrent. Nongenital warts (verrucae) frequently occur on the hands, soles, and face and may be verrucous or filiform in presentation. Warts in the anogenital region, known as condylomata acuminata, are more common in homosexual and bisexual men. Clinically, the lesions vary from flesh-colored flat-topped papules to verrucous papules. Whereas anogenital condylomata are tan to brown in color, oropharyngeal HPV lesions are pink or white in color and may be extensive, with the potential for malignant transformation.

Diagnosis. Although diagnosis of verrucae and condylomata tends to be by clinical appearance, biopsy of anogenital warts is recommended for large and recurrent lesions due to the high prevalence of squamous cell carcinoma.

Treatment. Treatment of verrucae vulgaris and condylomata acuminata varies with the degree of immunodeficiency. In early HIV disease, lesions respond to usual modalities such as cryotherapy, trichloroacetic acid, and podophyllum resin. Topical tretinoin and imiquimod are worth considering for refractive lesions. Intralesional interferon, bleomycin, and 5-fluorouracil are newer options with reported success; however, these should be done by a physician experienced in these treatments.

> **KEY POINTS**

- HPV types 16 and 18 are carcinogenic—risk of transformation into squamous cell cancer
- If perianal involvement, rule out internal warts—high rate of malignant transformation

Cytomegalovirus

Presentation and Progression. Cytomegalovirus (CMV) infection is the most common viral pathogen in advanced HIV disease (CD4+ counts less than 50 cells/mm^3), causing retinitis, gastrointestinal involvement, and central nervous system disease. Specific CMV-induced skin lesions have not been identified in HIV-infected patients. However, perianal ulcers can develop by direct extension of gastrointestinal disease. Purpuric macules of the lower extremities associated with leukocytoclastic vasculitis have been reported as a manifestation of CMV infection. These lesions respond to ganciclovir or foscarnet.

> **KEY POINTS**

- No specific skin lesions
- Perianal ulcers from gastrointestinal extension

Oral Hairy Leukoplakia

Presentation and Progression. Chronic Epstein-Barr virus (EBV) infection of epithelial cells is the cause of OHL. It occurs in about 25% of HIV-infected individuals. Once diagnosed with OHL, HIV-infected patients have a 48% probability of developing AIDS in 16 months and 83% by 31 months.

On examination, lesions are white, hyperplastic, verrucous white to grayish-white plaques on the lateral tongue. Unlike candidal infection of the oral cavity, the main differential diagnosis, these lesions cannot be rubbed off and do not respond to antifungal treatment.

Treatment. Typically this is an asymptomatic condition and does not require treatment. In the event of dysphagia or discomfort, lesions can be treated with oral acyclovir, zidovudine, topical tretinoin, or podophyllum resin.

> **KEY POINTS**

- Caused by EBV infection
- White plaques on lateral tongue—do not rub off
- Resistant to antifungal therapy

Bacterial Infections

Staphylococcal Infections

Presentation and Progression. *S. aureus* is the most common cutaneous bacterial pathogen in HIV-infected individuals. Infection may manifest primarily as folliculitis, furuncles, impetigo, or cellulitis. It may also cause secondary infection of any cutaneous disorder with open lesions. A folliculitis represents a superficial infection of a hair follicle, whereas a furuncle is a deeper infection of a hair follicle. The two forms of impetigo are bullous and nonbullous. Lesions of impetigo commonly arise on the skin of the face and extremities usually after trauma. AIDS patients are common nasal carriers of *S. aureus,* explaining its prevalence and recurrence in this population.

The lesions of folliculitis are erythematous follicular-based papules or pustules commonly on the face, trunk, groin, and buttocks. A furuncle is a fluctuant, tender, red folliculocentric nodule that may drain pus with rupture. Both folli-

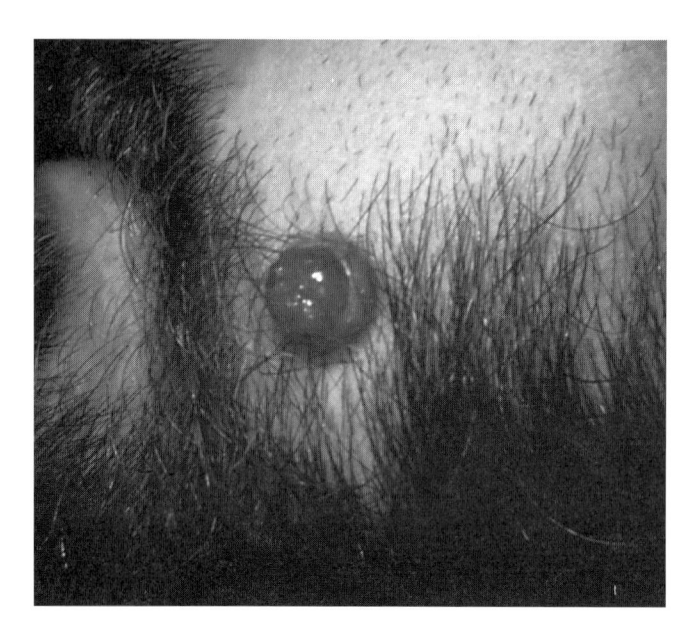

FIG. 13-3 Bacillary angiomatosis.

culitis and furuncles can occur on any hair-bearing region of the skin but are common on the face, axillae, and buttocks. Nonbullous impetigo is typically a honey-colored crusted papule or plaque. Bullous impetigo starts as vesicles that rapidly progress to flaccid bullae containing clear yellow fluid. Cellulitis presents as an enlarging erythematous patch with increased warmth.

Diagnosis. Bacterial culture complements clinical presentation, and bacterial culture of the nares confirms colonization.

Treatment. Therapy is with systemic penicillinase-resistant penicillins or cephalosporins. Cellulitis, associated with systemic signs such as fever, requires intravenous antibiotics. Chronic nasal colonization with *S. aureus* can be treated with topical Bactroban ointment to the nostrils, twice a day, for a minimum of 10 days.

KEY POINTS

- Most common pathogen in HIV
- Honey-colored encrusted papules, patches
- HIV-infected patients frequently nasal carriers of *Staphylococcus,* so culture
- Bactroban ointment bid × 10 days if positive
- Treat with IV antibiotics if any systemic signs

Bacillary Angiomatosis

Presentation and Progression. The gram-negative rods of *Bartonella quintana* cause the vascular disorder bacillary angiomatosis. Cats are a reservoir for this organism, and spread to humans is by cat scratch or bite. Infection with *Bartonella* may also involve internal organs including the brain, liver, spleen, and bones.

Bacillary angiomatosis presents as red to purple, vascular papules and nodules, sometimes with a hyperkeratotic surface (Fig. 13-3). Another clinical variant may occur in the form of dome-shaped subcutaneous masses without the characteristic red or purple color change. The most important differential diagnosis to consider in HIV-infected patients is KS, but these papules and nodules may be easily confused with pyogenic granulomas. Biopsy can usually differentiate between these conditions.

Diagnosis. Organisms can be identified by silver stain after skin biopsy. This condition may be fatal if not promptly treated with appropriate antibiotics, namely erythromycin or doxycycline for 3 to 4 weeks.

KEY POINTS

- Cats are reservoir
- Purplish papules or nodules
- Rule out Kaposi's sarcoma
- Fatal if not treated promptly

Mycobacterial Infections

Presentation and Progression. With the advent of the HIV virus, there has been a worldwide increase in the prevalence of tuberculosis, yet cutaneous tuberculosis remains rare. The clinical spectrum of cutaneous tuberculosis varies widely from disseminated papules and necrotic plaques to lymphadenitis and draining abscesses. Skin involvement can occur via direct extension of underlying infection as in lymphadenitis and scrofuloderma; primary infection of the skin as in lupus vulgaris; or hematogenous spread as in acute miliary tuberculosis and metastatic disease, which form abscesses.

Mycobacterium avium complex (MAC) is a frequent infection (CD4+ count less than 50 cells/mm^3), and again cutaneous involvement is uncommon. Lesions present as papules, nodules, pustules, abscesses, or ulcerations. Ulcerations adjacent to abscesses and lymphadenitis associated with MAC have been reported. The presence of MAC in a skin biopsy specimen can be incidental.

M. fortuitum and *M. haemophilum* are atypical mycobacteria recently recognized as important pathogens in HIV disease. *M. fortuitum* infection manifests as subcutaneous nodules with necrosis, especially in HIV-infected intravenous drug users. Cutaneous *M. haemophilum* infection ranges from ulcerative painful papules to erythema and swelling and abscess formation. Response to antimycobacterial agents is variable, and recurrences are common despite multidrug antibiotic therapy.

KEY POINTS

- Lymphadenitis and draining abscesses clinically
- Cultures may take up to several weeks
- Biopsy with appropriate stains quicker

Syphilis

Presentation and Progression. Genital ulcer disease, especially primary syphilis, increases the risk and likelihood of HIV infection. In patients with syphilis and HIV infection, a range of unusual features has been reported. Some patients with HIV and syphilis experience an altered course of either disease. Inability of the patient to mount an adequate immune response to *Treponema pallidum,* the causative organism of syphilis, is the likely reason for the variable clinical manifestations seen in these patients. HIV-infected patients with syphilis present in the secondary stage of syphilis more often than do non–HIV-infected patients. In some cases, progression from the primary stage to the tertiary stage can occur in a matter of months. In addition, late recurrence, recurrent neurosyphilis, or recrudescent cutaneous secondary syphilis may occur despite standard antibiotic therapy.

The classic presentation of secondary syphilis is a generalized papulosquamous eruption consisting of erythematous, well-demarcated, flattened plaques covered with scales involving the palms and soles and the mucous membranes. Alternatively, patients may present with pustular and ulcerative lesions. Malignant secondary syphilis presents with widespread papulopustules and vesicles that progress to ulcers covered by thick necrotic crust (Fig. 13-4). This eruption typically involves the face and scalp and is associated with fever, malaise, and arthralgias. Itching of lesions may be a complaint in this presentation. Oral and genital ulcers are not uncommon in this variant.

Diagnosis. There have been reports of patients with HIV and syphilis who have been seronegative with all standard tests for syphilis, but spirochetes can be found in tissue with special stains specific for *T. pallidum*. In some cases, the seronegative result is an artifact, and serum dilution past the prozone level may be needed. In other cases, no antibody is present. In instances when serologic tests remain negative despite strong clinical suspicion, alternative tests such as biopsy of lesions, darkfield examination, and direct fluorescent antibody staining of lesion material should be used. Neurosyphilis should always be considered in the differential diagnosis of neurologic disease in HIV-infected persons. Needless to say, lumbar puncture should be performed with appropriate cerebrospinal fluid (CSF) evaluations on all HIV-infected patients with neurologic symptoms and diagnosed or suspected to have syphilis.

Treatment. According to the 1998 guidelines of the Centers for Disease Control and Prevention (CDC), no treatment regimens have been shown to be more effective in preventing neurosyphilis in HIV-infected individuals when compared with the recommended regimens for HIV-negative individuals. In primary or secondary syphilis, patients should be treated with 2.4 million units IM of benzathine penicillin G in a single dose. Some experts recommend three weekly doses of benzathine penicillin G of 2.4 million units each. Nonpregnant patients who are allergic to penicillin may be treated with doxycycline 100 mg orally twice a day for 2 weeks or tetracycline 500 mg orally four times a day for 2 weeks. Pregnant patients who are allergic to penicillin should undergo desensitization and be treated with penicillin since tetracycline and doxycycline are not used in pregnancy. Patients with positive CSF tests for syphilis by lumbar puncture should be treated as in neurosyphilis—aqueous crystalline penicillin G 3 to 4 million units intravenously every 4 hours for 10 to 14 days.

Since treatment failure can occur, patients should be followed closely with serologic and clinical evaluations every 3 months for 1 year and then at 24 months. If a patient is considered to have failed treatment, CSF examination to rule out neurosyphilis and then retreatment with three weekly doses of 2.4 million units each of benzathine penicillin G is recommended.

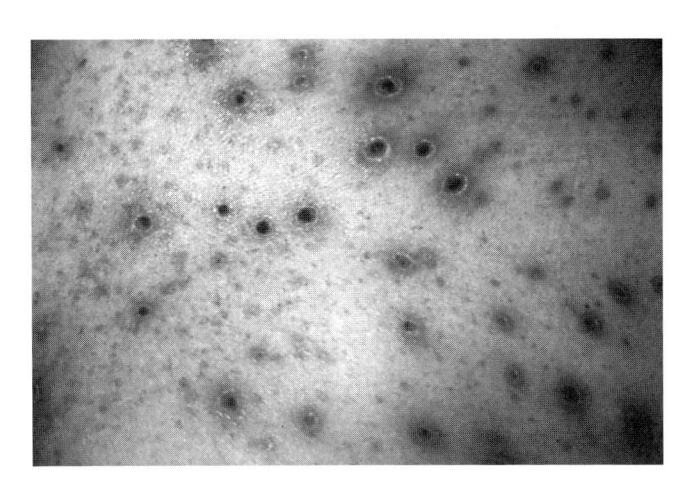

FIG. 13-4 Papulonecrotic secondary syphilis.

KEY POINTS

- *Treponema pallidum* is causative agent
- False seronegativity may occur
- Palms and soles frequently involved

Fungal Infections
Candidal Infection

Presentation and Progression. In 10% of patients with HIV, oral candidiasis (thrush) may be the first manifestation of HIV infection. This usually occurs when CD4+ counts are less than 400 cells/mm^3. Oral candidiasis is the most common fungal infection in HIV-infected patients. The oral mucosa is the most common site; however, it may extend to the esophagus and/or tracheobronchial tree. Esophageal candidiasis is an AIDS-defining illness, occurring with advanced disease (CD4+ count less than 100 cells/mm^3).

Oropharyngeal candidiasis is usually asymptomatic. Rarely, patients may complain of soreness or burning in the mouth or altered taste sense when eating. There are four recognized clinical patterns of oropharyngeal candidiasis: atrophic, pseudomembranous, hyperplastic, and as an angular cheilitis. The pseudomembranous form is most common and presents as removable, white, cottage cheese–like patches on the oral mucosa. Atrophic candidiasis appears as erythematous patches on the soft and hard palate, with depapillation of the dorsal tongue presenting as a smooth, red glossal surface. The hyperplastic type is a thick white confluent coating on the dorsum of the tongue. Angular cheilitis (perlèche) presents as painful, erythematous fissures at the oral commissures. Intertriginous areas (axillary, groin, and inframammary) are also common sites for candidiasis. They present as beefy, red, desquamating patches with satellite erythematous pustules or papules.

Treatment. Although oropharyngeal candidiasis is asymptomatic, if left untreated it may progress to involve the esophagus, causing significant discomfort and morbidity. Therefore treatment is recommended to at least improve the quality of life of the patient. Therapy with antifungals may be systemic or topical, keeping in mind the risk of resistance with continued usage. Whether topical or systemic agents are employed

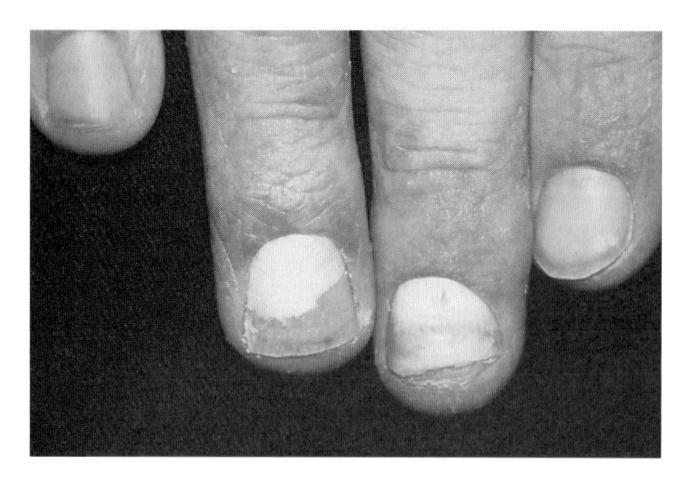

FIG. 13-5 Proximal subungual onychomycosis.

depends on the physician and the patient. Topical agents such as nystatin suspension and amphotericin B solution may be used as initial treatment, with planned prophylaxis once the condition resolves. Compliance is an important issue when using topical agents because although these are effective, they require usage multiple times daily. Systemic agents on the other hand usually only require once-daily dosage.

Esophageal involvement should be treated with systemic agents such as fluconazole or itraconazole to reduce the risk of relapses once therapy is discontinued. Lack of a clinical response should prompt endoscopic evaluation with biopsy and cultures to rule out other pathogens such as CMV or azole resistance. Resistance to fluconazole and itraconazole is treated with amphotericin B.

Candidal intertrigo responds to antifungal creams, although oral antifungal therapy may be needed in severe disease.

KEY POINTS

- Most common fungal infection in HIV
- Esophageal candidiasis is an AIDS-defining illness
- May be atrophic, pseudomembranous, or hyperplastic variant

Dermatophyte Infections

Presentation and Progression. Samet et al found dermatophytosis to be the most common skin manifestation among 82 HIV-infected patients at the beginning of medical treatment for HIV. *Trichophyton rubrum* causes the majority of all the dermatophyte infections in the HIV-infected patient. The HIV-infected patient is susceptible to repeated dermatophyte infection, and the severity of the infection is increased in this population. Although it may occur on any site, it is most common on the feet, with interdigital maceration; hands; and groin.

Most dermatophyte infections present as annular, erythematous scaling patches, sometimes with central clearing and heaped-up edges that enlarge without treatment. Atypical presentations can mimic seborrheic dermatitis (e.g., tinea faciei). The clinical presentation is usually well-demarcated, erythematous patches with scaling, sometimes with significant hyperkeratosis. Secondary bacterial infection is a common complication of dermatophyte infection in the HIV-infected patient.

Proximal subungual onychomycosis is a classic nail sign of HIV infection and represents 90% of onychomycosis in patients with AIDS (Fig. 13-5). Patients can also develop a chalky white involvement of the outer nail plate known as superficial white onychomycosis, an infection rarely seen in immunocompetent hosts.

Treatment. Treatment is usually with topical antifungal agents, except in extensive disease when oral antifungals are employed. Onychomycosis, however, does not respond to topical treatment and requires systemic therapy, with itraconazole or terbinafine being most effective.

KEY POINTS

- Most common skin manifestation in HIV
- *Trichophyton rubrum* causes majority of infections
- Any scaly skin lesion—potassium hydroxide (KOH) to rule out dermatophyte
- Proximal subungual onychomycosis is a classic nail sign of HIV
- Onychomycosis does not respond to topical therapy—needs systemic therapy

Pityrosporum Infection

Presentation and Progression. *Pityrosporum ovale* is a lipophilic yeast that can cause folliculitis or tinea versicolor. It has also been implicated as the causative organism in seborrheic dermatitis.

Clinically, tinea versicolor presents as small annular hypopigmented or hyperpigmented scaly patches of the upper trunk, upper back, neck, or face and responds to topical or oral ketoconazole or other azoles. Prophylaxis with ketoconazole shampoo prevents a recurrence. Seborrheic dermatitis (see below) may look like tinea versicolor, although it typically presents as erythematous, greasy yellow scaling in the nasolabial folds, eyebrows, eyelashes, inner ears, chest, scalp, and pubic area.

Diagnosis. Potassium hydroxide applied to scale on a glass slide easily shows numerous spores with admixed short, septate hyphae and confirms clinical suspicion.

Treatment. Therapy consists of topical azole cream in combination with a short course of low-potency topical steroid. Pruritic, perifollicular papules and pustules on the upper trunk and proximal upper extremities characterize *Pityrosporum* folliculitis. It also responds to oral azole drugs.

KEY POINTS

- Annular, hypopigmented or hyperpigmented, minimally scaly macules
- Prophylaxis with ketoconazole shampoo prevents recurrence

Cryptococcosis

Presentation and Progression. *Cryptococcus neoformans* is found in soil and bird droppings. It is acquired via the respiratory route, with subsequent hematogenous spread to the skin, meninges, and other organs. It is the second most common fungal opportunistic infection in the HIV-infected patient, occurring in 5% to 10% of AIDS patients. Disseminated cryptococcosis is the most common cause of fatal fungal infections in this population. Cutaneous lesions are seen in 5% to 20% of patients with disseminated disease, usually occurring in advanced HIV disease (CD4+ count less than 50 cells/mm^3). The presence of cutaneous lesions without systemic infection is extremely rare. Skin lesions may appear 2 to 6 weeks before any signs of systemic infection, typically of the central nervous system presenting as meningitis. For this reason, lumbar puncture and chest roentgenogram are required in any patient with cutaneous cryptococcosis.

Cutaneous cryptococcosis most commonly occurs on the head and neck, especially on the face, as skin-colored or pink papules or nodules with central umbilication, ranging from a solitary lesion to as many as 100 lesions (Fig. 13-6). Since they frequently resemble MC lesions, the possibility of cryptococcosis must be entertained in any HIV-infected patient with molluscum-like lesions. Diagnosis can be made by touch preparation, culture, or skin biopsy of a representative lesion, with confirmation by a serum cryptococcal antigen. Other presentations of cutaneous lesions include pustules, cellulitis, ulceration, subcutaneous abscesses, and vegetating plaques.

Diagnosis. Since the clinical presentation of cryptococcosis is variable and may be confusing, skin biopsy of lesions is advisable for histologic evaluation with special stains and for tissue culture. India ink staining of lesional skin scraping can also be used to demonstrate encapsulated and budding yeast forms.

Treatment. Amphotericin B is the treatment of choice with addition of 5-flucytosine, which allows the use of lower doses of amphotericin B. Unfortunately, 5-flucytosine causes bone marrow suppression and may not be a viable option in HIV-infected patients. Cutaneous lesions respond to therapy in 2 to 4 weeks, but relapses are common. Oral fluconazole or itraconazole is used as lifelong maintenance therapy.

KEY POINTS

- Caused by *Cryptococcus neoformans*
- Disseminated cryptococcosis is the most common cause of fatal fungal infections in HIV
- Any cutaneous lesions require lumbar puncture and chest x-ray
- Clinically, may resemble molluscum contagiosum

Histoplasmosis

Presentation and Progression. *Histoplasma capsulatum* is endemic in the central and eastern United States and Africa. About 10% of patients with AIDS and disseminated histoplasmosis have cutaneous involvement.

Skin lesions have a variable presentation, sometimes in a single patient. They include molluscum-like lesions, papulonecrotic lesions, erythematous macules, folliculitis, ulcers, pustules, and acneiform lesions. The most common site is the face, especially the nasal vestibule, and oral ulcerative lesions

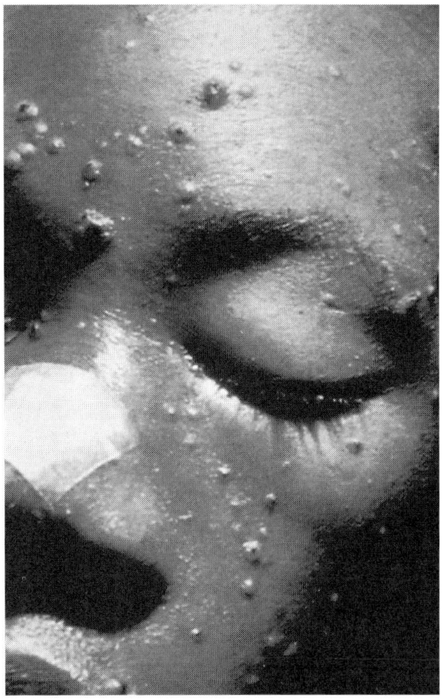

FIG. 13-6 Cutaneous cryptococcosis.

are common. Hepatosplenomegaly and lymphadenopathy are common signs of disseminated histoplasmosis.

Diagnosis. Diagnosis can be made by skin biopsy for histologic evaluation and tissue culture.

Treatment. Amphotericin B is used as induction therapy followed by oral therapy for 8 weeks. Since recurrences are common, itraconazole or fluconazole is used as maintenance therapy for 1 year or longer.

KEY POINTS

- Variable presentation
- Face is a common area, especially the nasal vestibule and oral cavity

Coccidioidomycosis

Presentation and Progression. *Coccidioides immitis* is found only in the southwestern United States, Mexico, and South and Central America. In HIV-infected hosts with disseminated disease, cutaneous lesions can occur.

Skin findings consist of papules that progress to pustules, nodules, or plaques, with eventual development of abscesses, draining sinus tracts, ulcerations, and cellulitis.

Diagnosis. Diagnosis is by lesional biopsy with tissue culture.
Treatment. Amphotericin B is the mainstay of therapy.

KEY POINTS

- *Coccidioides immitis* is cause
- Pustules, nodules, abscesses, draining sinus tracts, and ulcerations can all occur

Sporotrichosis

Presentation and Progression. Sporotrichosis is acquired by cutaneous inoculation, with extension to other organs such as the liver, spleen, lung, joints, intestine, and meninges in AIDS patients.

Cutaneous lesions are chronic ulcerative papules and nodules that may be crusted, eroded, or hyperkeratotic. Lesions tend to occur along the lymphatics. In HIV-infected patients, lesions are often disseminated, sparing the oral cavity. Ocular infection may occur. Septic arthritis is common.

Diagnosis. Lesional biopsy aids in identification of organisms.
Treatment. Treatment is with amphotericin B or itraconazole.

KEY POINTS

- *Sporothrix schenckii*
- Skin lesions occurring along lymphatic spread
- Often disseminated in HIV
- Septic arthritis is common

Infestations
Scabies

Presentation and Progression. *Sarcoptes scabiei* in HIV infection can present as typical papules and burrows of the finger webs, wrists, and genitalia, and periumbilically. This variant usually responds to classic therapy. Exuberant reactions to overwhelming infection can cause bullous lesions or hyperkeratotic lesions, as in crusted (Norwegian) scabies. Crusted scabies is defined as the presence of hyperkeratotic, crusted papules and plaques of the trunk, palms, soles, and extensor surfaces associated with intense pruritus. Scabies should be considered in the differential diagnosis of pruritus in any HIV-infected patient. *Staphylococcus* frequently complicates scabies with impetiginization, and even sepsis can occur.

Diagnosis. Diagnosis is by scraping the crusted surface off a lesion onto a glass slide and identifying the mites under the microscope. Numerous mites are easily identified in crusted scabies.

Treatment. Treatment of scabies is usually with topical lindane. The mechanism of action of lindane is by immobilizing the mite by paralysis. Due to the risk of neurotoxicity in infants and children, it must be used with caution. Failure to respond to lindane seems to be related to high mite burden, immunosuppression, and central nervous system disease. Topical permethrin is an alternate and effective first-line agent. 10% sulfur ointment is safe to use in pregnant women with scabies. Treatment with any of the above topicals may require multiple applications for weeks or months and must be done properly to avoid reinfection. Topical agents are applied from head to toes, including under the fingernails. Household members should be treated also, and clothing and linens should be washed thoroughly in hot water. Oral ivermectin has been reported to be effective in scabies, with relatively minor side effects.

KEY POINTS

- Extremely pruritic papules
- Look for burrows of finger webs, wrists, and genitalia, and periumbilically
- Crusted (Norwegian) scabies common in HIV
- Always consider scabies in differential diagnosis of pruritus in HIV

Inflammatory Conditions
Pruritus

Presentation and Progression. Pruritus is a very common complaint from HIV-infected individuals that tends to be very debilitating. The etiology of pruritus may be difficult to elucidate. The most common reason for itching is dry skin, but the differential diagnosis includes a possible drug reaction, scabies infestations, insect bites, eosinophilic folliculitis, atopic dermatitis, dermatographism, and metabolic disease.

Primary lesions may or may not be present, depending on the cause of pruritus. Secondary lesions are almost always present in the form of excoriated papules and lichenification due to rubbing and scratching. These lesions are frequently superinfected with *Staphylococcus*.

Diagnosis. A detailed history and careful physical examination are crucial to identifying the etiology of pruritus.

Treatment. Pruritus is resolved by treating the underlying disease. Antihistamines, menthol lotions, low- to mid-potency topical steroids, and ultraviolet B (UVB) light are effective for symptomatic relief.

KEY POINTS

- Need detailed history and physical examination to elucidate underlying etiology
- Differential diagnosis includes drug reaction, scabies infestation, insect bites, and eosinophilic folliculitis
- Treat the underlying disease to resolve pruritus

Xerosis/Ichthyosis

Dry skin is very common in HIV disease and can be quite severe. It may be associated with intense pruritus. In its severe form, fissuring and oozing are present. Acquired ichthyosis typically resembles large, fishlike scales starting on the extensor surfaces of the lower extremities and then becoming generalized. Thick emollients and keratolytics are the mainstay of therapy, combined with antihistamines in the presence of pruritus.

Psoriasis Vulgaris

Presentation and Progression. Psoriasis is an inflammatory disorder of the skin. The etiology of this disease is unknown. Various theories implicating infectious, environmental, and genetic factors have been postulated. Psoriasis is frequently precipitated by infections such as *Streptococcus* and HIV. HIV-infected individuals with psoriasis experience more frequent flares and more extensive disease that may be refractory to therapy. Psoriatic arthritis, often associated with HLA-B27, is usually progressive, leading to crippling deformities with poor response to traditional therapies.

The different presentations of psoriasis include (1) patch/plaque psoriasis, which involves erythematous patches or plaques with silvery white scale located on the trunk, extremities, elbows, or knees. The scalp is involved with similar lesions. This type is usually symmetric and is the most common type (Fig. 13-7); (2) guttate psoriasis, which presents as several small, annular, scaly, erythematous macules, the size of water drops. This type usually follows an acute infection such as streptococcal pharyngitis; (3) pustular psoriasis (von Zumbusch's type), which is a severe and sometimes fatal form of psoriasis. Patients typically have a prior history of psoriasis and psoriatic arthritis. It is characterized by sudden onset of lakes of pus periungually, on the palms, and in preexisting psoriatic plaques, followed by generalized erythema and pustules associated with fever; (4) erythrodermic psoriasis, in which erythroderma may be a presenting sign or a complication of psoriasis. This is associated with fever, chills, and electrolyte imbalance; and (5) inverse psoriasis, in which psoriasis involves folds, recesses, and the intertriginous areas of the body (i.e., the axillae, groin, inframammary folds, intergluteal crease, and navel). Chronic large plaque psoriasis is the more common type seen in the HIV-infected population and it worsens with declining immune status. Progression to pustular or erythrodermic disease is not uncommon.

Manifestation of nail involvement includes nail pitting, oil drop sign (reddish brown foci beneath the nail plate), and subungual hyperkeratotic debris. Extensive nail involvement may be confused with fungal infections, since the two conditions frequently co-exist in these patients.

Diagnosis. Psoriasis has a characteristic clinical appearance; however, atypical presentations can occur. Biopsy of a lesion in such cases aids in diagnosis.

Treatment. Management of psoriasis in the general population frequently involves immunosuppressive therapy such as methotrexate and cyclosporine, which have all been used with success. Needless to say, immunosuppression is an undesirable effect in the HIV-infected individual and caution must be exercised when using these agents. Extra care must be taken with methotrexate in an HIV-positive patient, since death has been reported. Topical steroids, topical calcipotriene, or topical retinoids can be effective in limited disease. Ultraviolet radiation with UVB or Psoralen ultraviolet A (PUVA) is also safe and effective. Acitretin, an oral retinoid, may be helpful, but must not be employed in women of reproductive age due to its teratogenic effects.

KEY POINTS

- HIV disease can precipitate psoriasis
- Psoriatic arthritis can be debilitating
- In plaques with thick silvery scale, removal of scale shows pinpoint bleeding (Auspitz sign)
- Large plaque type of psoriasis is more common in HIV but can progress to pustular psoriasis or erythroderma

Reiter's Syndrome

Presentation and Progression. The classic triad of this disorder is severe arthritis, urethritis, and conjunctivitis, although only one or two of these manifestations are usually present.

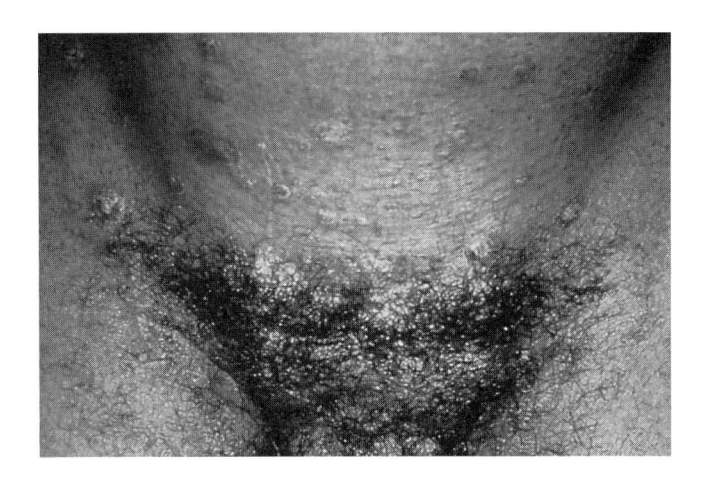

FIG. 13-7 Psoriasis vulgaris.

The severity of Reiter's syndrome is increased in HIV-infected patients. It is considered a reactive condition to infectious agents of the gastrointestinal (*Shigella, Salmonella, Yersinia, Campylobacter*) or genitourinary (*Chlamydia trachomatis*) tracts.

Keratoderma blennorrhagicum, the most common cutaneous manifestation, presents as erythematous-based, hyperkeratotic, yellow papules and plaques, pustules, or vesicles on the hands and feet, extensor surfaces of the extremities, and scalp. Shallow erosions and vesicles on the glans penis also occur. Plaque-type psoriasis, arthritis, and keratoderma blennorrhagicum may represent an overlap between psoriasis and Reiter's syndrome.

Treatment. Therapeutic options are similar to those employed in treating psoriasis.

KEY POINTS

- Triad of severe arthritis, urethritis, and conjunctivitis
- Reactive condition to infectious agents of gastrointestinal and genitourinary tracts
- May closely resemble or overlap psoriasis

Seborrheic Dermatitis

Presentation and Progression. Seborrheic dermatitis, a common dermatosis of the general population, is even more common in the HIV-infected population. It also tends to be more severe and more extensive, with an acute onset or worsening of previously limited disease. *P. ovale* has been implicated as the causative organism in seborrheic dermatitis but this remains controversial.

Erythematous, yellow, greasy scaling plaques are found in the hair-bearing areas (i.e., the scalp, eyebrows, nasolabial folds, beard, mustache, and chest area) (Fig. 13-8). Plaques on the scalp may be encrusted with thick scale. It can also occur in the groin and axillae. Pruritus is mild if present. The severity of the disease increases with advanced HIV disease.

Treatment. Standard therapies including topical ketoconazole, low- to mid-potency topical steroid preparations, coal tar

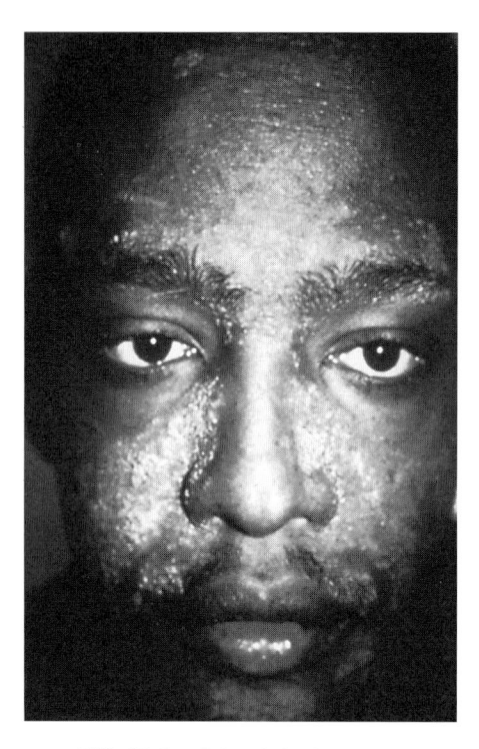

FIG. 13-8 Seborrheic dermatitis.

shampoos, salicylic acid shampoos, zinc pyrithione shampoos, and sulfur shampoos are all effective.

KEY POINTS

- May be presenting sign in advanced HIV disease
- Erythematous, yellow, greasy scaling plaques of hair-bearing regions

Photosensitivity

Presentation and Progression. Photosensitivity can be a presentation of HIV disease. Various types of reactions can occur including lichenoid (pruritic, violaceous to hyperpigmented papules and plaques), acute or chronic eczematous (lichenified, erythematous, scaly plaques), and sunburnlike eruptions of the sun-exposed areas.

Photoallergic drug reactions typically are of the eczematous or lichenoid type. They may be due to either oral medication or topical applications of chemicals. More commonly, phototoxic drug reactions usually manifest as an exaggerated sunburn. The most common culprit drugs are sulfonamides and nonsteroidal antiinflammatory drugs.

Chronic actinic dermatitis is a rare idiopathic photosensitizing disorder. It is defined as a chronic photodermatitis with no identified exposure to photosensitizers that usually lasts months or years. It occurs most commonly in dark-skinned, older men with CD4+ counts less than 200 cells/mm^3. Patients present with an eczematous dermatitis in the sun-exposed areas of the body. As with other eczematous dermatitis, *S. aureus* superinfection is common. Treatment is only by removing the inciting agent, in this case, UV light. Sunscreens and sun protective clothing are helpful. Topical or systemic steroids are needed to resolve the eczematous dermatitis.

KEY POINTS

- Photodistributed rash—spares photoprotected areas of face and neck
- Photosensitivity can be presentation of HIV disease
- Sulfonamides and nonsteroidal antiinflammatory drugs are common causes of photoallergic drug reactions

Porphyria Cutanea Tarda

Presentation and Progression. Porphyria cutanea tarda (PCT) is caused by a defect in the activity of uroporphyrinogen decarboxylase, a hepatic enzyme involved in the heme biosynthesis pathway. This condition may be acquired or inherited. An excess of porphyrins leads to photosensitivity because porphyrins absorb radiation in the Soret band (400 to 410) of the light spectrum. There is a high association with hepatitis C, which is sometimes a coexisting infection of HIV patients. Factors known to trigger this condition include sunlight, alcohol, estrogens, and hepatotoxic medications.

PCT is characterized by blisters and erosions on sun-exposed areas (face, dorsa of hands, and forearms), increased skin fragility, hypertrichosis, and hyperpigmentation. Later, scarring, milia, and sclerodermatous changes are seen in these areas.

Diagnosis. Urine and stool specimens are examined for increased levels of porphyrins. Skin biopsy with direct immunofluorescence can also identify PCT.

Treatment. Management includes antimalarials, phlebotomy, and avoidance of triggering factors.

KEY POINTS

- Defect in heme biosynthesis pathway
- Blisters and erosions on sun-exposed areas, hypertrichosis, and increased skin fragility
- High association with hepatitis C—common coexisting infection in HIV disease
- Sunlight, alcohol, estrogen, and hepatotoxic medications trigger PCT

Eosinophilic Folliculitis

Presentation and Progression. Eosinophilic folliculitis is a chronic, intensely pruritic condition involving the face, upper trunk above the nipple line, and upper extremities. It is associated with HIV infection. The severity of the disease increases with advancing HIV disease and usually occurs in patients with declining CD4+ counts (less than 200 cells/mm^3). A similar disease, eosinophilic pustular dermatosis, occurs in non–HIV-infected Japanese males and was first described by Ofuji. The cause of eosinophilic folliculitis is unknown. An infectious etiology is suspected but so far not confirmed.

Characteristically, the lesions are pink to red, edematous follicular papules and sometimes pustules. Itching may be very debilitating and may interfere with sleep. As a result of chronic scratching and rubbing, secondary changes such as excoriations, lichenification, and superinfection with *S. aureus* are common. Peripheral eosinophilia and elevated serum IgE levels are seen.

Diagnosis. Culture of pustules is usually unyielding unless the lesions are superinfected. Diagnosis is by clinical suspicion and biopsy of an early lesion. On histology, numerous eosinophils are identified infiltrating the follicular epithelium.
Treatment. Treatment presents a difficult challenge. Therapy includes high-potency topical steroids, antihistamines for itching, and permethrin. Ultraviolet radiation (UVR) has been used with good results but is usually reserved as a last resort. UVR has been shown to activate and increase proliferation of HIV in vitro, but no effect on CD4+ cell count or viral load has been demonstrated. Prednisone with a quick taper over 2 to 3 weeks is also effective, although a second course may be required because discontinuation may cause symptoms to recur. Oral itraconazole, oral ketoconazole and metronidazole (250 mg tid), and oral isotretinoin have been used with variable success.

KEY POINTS

- Intensely pruritic and edematous follicular papules or pustules
- Peripheral eosinophilia can be present
- Treatment can be frustratingly difficult

Drug Reactions

Presentation and Progression. Drug reactions in the HIV-infected population are common. They can be erythematous maculopapular exanthems, morbilliform eruptions, erythema multiforme–like, Stevens-Johnson syndrome, or even toxic epidermal necrolysis (TEN). Trimethoprim-sulfamethoxazole is a common culprit because of its use in prophylaxis of *Pneumocystis carinii* and toxoplasmosis. Severe bullous eruptions to sulfa drugs may be seen in HIV-infected patients. Cross-reactions to dapsone in patients who are sulfa-allergic, although uncommon, have been reported. Antiretroviral medications can also cause cutaneous reactions. Zidovudine (AZT) causes hyperpigmented longitudinal bands in the nail plates, appearing within 4 to 8 weeks of initiation of therapy. Hyperpigmented macules of the mucous membranes can occur with AZT. Indinavir and lamivudine have caused reactions such as pyogenic granuloma of the nail bed or periungual region (Fig. 13-9). Foscarnet causes a fixed drug eruption, with ulcerations in the groin region, particularly of the penis. This reaction is thought to be due to high concentrations of the urinary metabolites of foscarnet, and thus hyperhydration may reduce the risk of ulcers. A fixed drug eruption is a localized drug reaction occurring in the same focus on every exposure

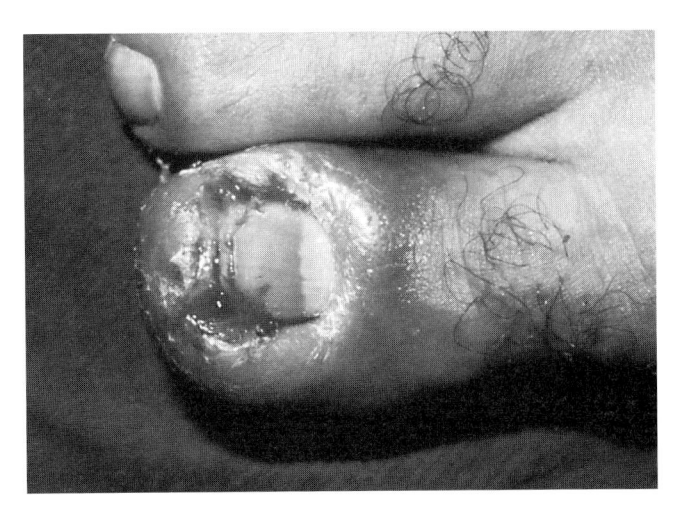

FIG. 13-9 Indinavir-induced pyogenic granuloma.

to the offending medication. Any patient with a suspected drug reaction needs a detailed history of all medications, including over-the-counter medications. Careful physical examination, especially of the mucous membranes, is important to rule out Stevens-Johnson syndrome. A positive Nikolsky's sign (pressure on normal skin leading to blister formation) is a clue to impending TEN.

KEY POINTS

- Trimethoprim-sulfamethoxazole—severe bullous eruptions can occur in HIV-infected patients
- Zidovudine—hyperpigmented longitudinal bands in the nail plates, hyperpigmented macules of mucous membranes
- Indinavir and lamivudine—pyogenic granuloma of the nail bed or periungual region
- Foscarnet—ulcerations in the groin region

Neoplasms
Kaposi's Sarcoma

Presentation and Progression. The cause of KS, although unknown, is suspected to be infectious. Human herpesvirus 8 has been recovered from tumors of both HIV-related and non–HIV-related KS. Different subtypes exist: classical KS, which occurs in elderly men of Mediterranean or Eastern European descent; endemic African KS, found in adults and children in central Africa; and epidemic KS in homosexual and bisexual males with HIV disease. KS is the most common malignant tumor in AIDS patients. It tends to be more aggressive and disseminated than the other types of KS.

Lesions start as asymptomatic, violaceous macules, papules, or nodules that later coalesce into plaques, often along the cleavage planes of the skin (Fig. 13-10, *A*). Initially, they may resemble bruises, insect bites, or benign nevi. Lesions increase in size and number over time if left untreated. They may begin in the oral mucosa and may even be the presenting sign of HIV (Fig. 13-10, *B*). With advancing disease, tumors become ulcerated and secondarily infected. Internal organs may be involved in KS, although it is usually asymptomatic. Rarely, gastrointestinal involvement may be manifested by hemorrhage, requiring intervention. Lymphatic obstruction with tumor can lead to massive limb edema.

Diagnosis. Biopsy must be undertaken to confirm diagnosis of KS, since it may resemble bacillary angiomatosis in the nodular stage.

Treatment. Treatment of KS can be local or systemic depending on the extent of disease and the severity of underlying HIV infection. Local modalities include radiation therapy, intralesional chemotherapy, and cryotherapy. Most of these local methods are used for cosmetic

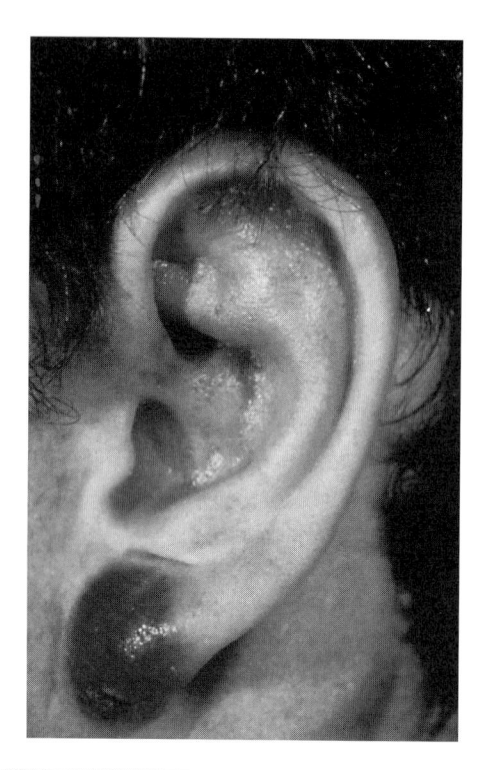

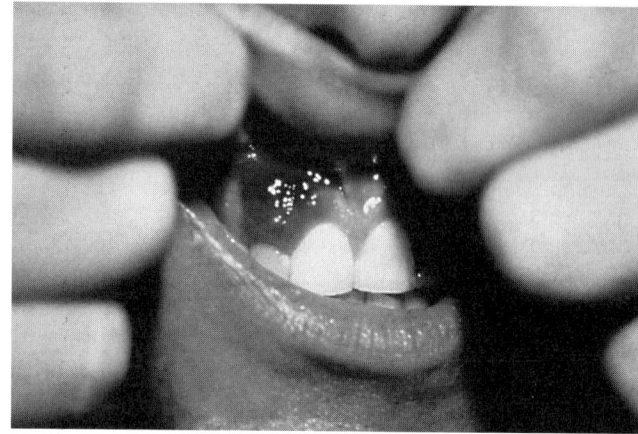

FIG. 13-10 **A**, Kaposi's sarcoma. **B**, Oral Kaposi's sarcoma.

improvement of limited disease. Radiation therapy may also be used as a systemic therapy. It is useful for control of bulky disease and for treatment of ulcerative lesions of the oral mucosa and lower extremity lesions complicated by edema. Chemotherapeutic agents such as the vincalkaloids, bleomycin, etoposide, doxorubicin, and interferon-α are administered systemically for aggressive and extensive disease and involvement of internal organs. The combination of doxorubicin, bleomycin, and vincristine is the first-line therapy for visceral involvement. Other newer effective cytotoxic agents include liposomal anthracyclines, paclitaxel, and vinorelbine. KS is rarely the cause of death in HIV disease; therefore the risks and benefits of any treatment must be analyzed.

Skin Cancer

Presentation and Progression. The incidence of nonmelanoma skin cancer may be increased in HIV disease. The risk factors for squamous cell carcinoma (SCC) and basal cell carcinoma (BCC) appear to be the same as in the general population: fair skin and excessive sun exposure. The difference between BCC and SCC in the HIV-infected individual is mainly in location and stage of HIV disease. SCCs occur on the head and neck and BCCs are commonly found on the trunk. SCCs are more common than BCCs in advanced HIV disease. As noted above, oncogenic strains of HPV can lead to the development of genital, perianal, and rectal SCCs in immunosuppressed individuals.

Nonmelanoma skin cancer in HIV disease is no different in appearance than in the general population but can be more aggressive. BCCs occur as pink, pearly, and telangiectatic papules or plaques with rolled borders. They may be superficially ulcerated or bleed spontaneously. Superficial BCCs are usually red, scaly plaques without telangiectasias. SCCs on the other hand are usually red, scaly, and ulcerated plaques with or without a hyperkeratotic crust. Any longstanding nonhealing ulcer should be biopsied to rule out BCC or SCC.

Treatment. Electrodesiccation and curettage, surgical excision, or Mohs' micrographic surgery is employed for the treatment of nonmelanoma skin cancer, depending on the type, size, location, or depth of the lesion. Frequent follow-up is recommended.

Malignant Melanoma. It is unclear if the risk of malignant melanoma is increased in HIV disease, although malignant melanoma has been seen in HIV-infected individuals. Malignant melanoma may have a worse prognosis in HIV disease.

Lymphoma. There is an increased incidence of lymphoma in HIV disease. Non-Hodgkin's lymphoma occurs more commonly than Hodgkin's disease and is usually of B cell lineage. It tends to present at an advanced stage, with nodal and extranodal manifestations. Epidermotropic T cell lymphoma has been described in HIV disease. Clinically, patients can present with eczematous patches, plaques, or frank tumors as in mycosis fungoides. Erythroderma with Sézary syndrome can also occur.

▶ KEY POINTS

- Human herpesvirus 8 is consistently isolated from KS tumors
- Violaceous macules, papules, or nodules
- May be presenting sign of HIV
- Biopsy needed to confirm and rule out bacillary angiomatosis

▶ KEY POINTS

- Longstanding nonhealing ulcers should be biopsied to rule out malignancy
- Large or resistant wart may be a sign of malignant transformation
- The differential diagnosis of erythroderma includes cutaneous T cell lymphoma

SUGGESTED READINGS

Barton JC, Buchness MR: Nongenital dermatologic disease in HIV-infected women, *J Am Acad Dermatol* 40:938-948, 1999.

Berger TG, Obuch ML, Goldschmidt RH: Dermatologic manifestations of HIV infection, *Am Fam Physician* 4(6):1729-1742, 1990.

Centers for Disease Control and Prevention: 1998 Guidelines for treatment of sexually transmitted diseases, *MMWR* 47(No. RR-l): 28-40, 1998.

Chouela et al: Equivalent therapeutic efficacy and safety of ivermectin and lindane in the treatment of human scabies, *Arch Dermatol* 135:651-655, 1999.

Cockerell CJ: Cutaneous manifestations of HIV infection other than Kaposi's sarcoma: clinical and histologic aspects, *J Am Acad Dermatol* 22:1260-1269, 1990.

Costner M, Cockerell CJ: The changing spectrum of the cutaneous manifestations of HIV disease, *Arch Dermatol* 134:1290-1292, 1998.

Dover JS, Johnson RA: Cutaneous manifestations of human immunodeficiency virus infection: Part I, *Arch Dermatol* 127: 1383-1391, 1991.

Greenspan D et al: Relation of oral hairy leukoplakia to infection with the human immunodeficiency virus and the risk of developing AIDS, *J Infect Dis* 155:475, 1987.

Holtzer CD et al: Cross-reactivity in HIV-infected patients switched from trimethoprim-sulfamethoxazole to dapsone, *Pharmacotherapy* 18(4):831-835, 1998.

Johnson RA: Cutaneous manifestations of human immunodeficiency virus disease, *Fitzpatrick's dermatology in general medicine*, vol II, ed 51h, New York, 1999, McGraw-Hill, pp 2505-2538.

Kaplan MH et al: Dermatologic findings and manifestations of acquired immunodeficiency syndrome, *J Am Acad Dermatol* 16:485-506, 1987.

Maurer TA et al: Cutaneous squamous cell carcinoma in human immunodeficiency virus-infected patients: a study of epidemiologic risk factors, human papillomavirus, and p53 expression, *Arch Dermatol* 133:577-583, 1997.

Myskowski PL, Ahkami R: Dermatologic complications of HIV infections, *Med Clin North Am* 80(No. 6):1415-1434, 1996.

Nasti G et al: A risk and benefit assessment of treatment for AIDS-related Kaposi's sarcoma, *Drug Saf* 20(5):403-425, 1999.

Samet JH et al: Dermatologic manifestations in HIV-infected patients: a primary care perspective, *Mayo Clin Proc* 74:658-660, 1999.

Zalla MJ, Su WPD, Fransway AF: Dermatologic manifestations of human immunodeficiency virus infection, *Mayo Clin Proc* 67: 1089-1108, 1992.

14 Oral Manifestations of HIV Infection

MICHAEL GLICK, PETER BERTHOLD

Introduction

Different oral lesions and conditions have been associated with human immunodeficiency virus (HIV) infection since the first description of HIV disease (HIVD). Although many of the different HIV-associated lesions are commonly found in persons with HIV infection, none is unique to HIVD or directly caused by HIV. Rather, all lesions and conditions observed in HIV-infected individuals are idiopathic, are associated with immunosuppression, are side effects from specific medications, or are associated with systemic opportunistic infections. Several factors influence the incidence and the prevalence rates of specific oral lesions. These factors include diverse types of treatment and prophylactic approaches in different care facilities and/or the variable geographic distribution of specific pathogens, such as histoplasmosis in the central United States.

There is a strong association between the immune status of a patient and the development of certain oral lesions. Consequently, these oral lesions are utilized as clinical markers for the degree of immunosuppression and disease progression.

Oral Examination

Oral lesions are readily available for examination. Most are assessable with only a good light source, a tongue blade, and a mouth mirror. Furthermore, very little training is needed to differentiate between normal findings and more common oral abnormalities.

As with other clinical descriptions, oral lesions have distinct characteristics, which are depicted as the number of lesions, location, size, color, texture, duration, and symptomatology. Furthermore, a differential diagnosis can also be elucidated by a lesion's response to specific therapies. Differentiation between ulcerative disorders and conditions can be used to illustrate the importance of these characteristics.

The most common cause of single ulcers is trauma, whereas multiple ulcers may suggest a viral etiology. Some lesions have a predilection for specific locations in the oral cavity. Whereas aphthous ulcers are more commonly found on less keratinized mucosa, such as the buccal mucosa, ventral surface of the tongue, and inner aspects of the lips, herpes simplex virus (HSV)-associated lesions are mostly found on more keratinized mucosa, such as the hard palate, and gingiva. Large lesions may represent major aphthous ulcers, whereas these types of lesions are uncommon with HSV infections among immunocompetent patients. Minor aphthous ulcerations are usually surrounded by an erythematous halo, but this characteristic may be missing in a neutropenic-induced ulceration. Chronic HSV lesions sometimes present with a deep base surrounded by a slightly elevated white border, whereas acute lesions are shallow, with nonraised borders. Aphthous ulcers usually resolve spontaneously within 5 to 10 days, whereas neoplasia should be suspected in ulcerations present for longer than 3 weeks. Pain is a common complaint associated with almost all ulcers, but may be missing in ulcers associated with a granulomatous disease such as tuberculosis. HSV ulcers usually respond favorably to acyclovir therapy, while antiviral medications will not resolve aphthous ulcerations. It is important to realize that classic signs and symptoms found in immunocompetent persons vary greatly in immunosuppressed individuals. Although this makes it more difficult to establish a clinical diagnosis, lesions associated with immunosuppression are usually more severe and can be more readily distinguished from normal mucosa.

Several different systems have been proposed to characterize and classify oral lesions in HIVD. In this chapter, lesions will be described according to etiology (Table 14-1). A table summarizing oral ulcerations has also been included to aid in establishing differential diagnoses for a specific oral manifestation (Table 14-2).

Xerostomia
Presentation and Progression

Dry mouth, or xerostomia, is a frequent complaint among HIV-infected individuals. Although the feeling of a dry mouth is very subjective, hyposalivation is a measurable entity. The reduced salivary flow in this patient population most commonly results from side effects from medications. Several antiretroviral medications, including zidovudine, didanosine (ddI), foscarnet, and, to various degrees, all of the protease inhibitors, are associated with patient complaints of oral dryness. Other medications, including antianxiety agents, antihistamines, anticholinergics, antihypertensives, decongestants, diuretics, narcotic analgesics such as meperidine, and tricyclic antidepressants, have been implicated in causing reduced salivary flow. Furthermore, HIV-infected individuals may also present with diminished salivary flow due to HIV-associated salivary gland disease. The parotid glands are often affected, which manifests as unilateral or bilateral enlargement. Minor salivary gland dysfunction, sometimes caused by viral infections such as cytomegalovirus (CMV), may also contribute to oral dryness. Radiation therapy to the head and neck region, which includes salivary glands within the mantle, can also induce xerostomia.

TABLE 14-1
Guide to Oral Manifestations

Lesion	Clinical appearance	Treatment	Significance
LOCAL FUNGAL INFECTIONS			
Erythematous (atrophic) candidiasis	Red macular patches found on mucosal surfaces; depapillated areas may appear on the dorsal surface of the tongue	Topical antifungal medications	Associated with early stages of HIVD
Pseudomembranous (thrush) candidiasis	Yellowish-white removable plaques found on any oral surface	Topical antifungal medications for patients with CD4+ cell counts above 150-200 cells/mm^3 Systemic antifungal medications for patients with CD4+ cell counts below 150-200 cells/mm^3	Associated with initial and progressive immune deterioration and HIVD progression
Hyperplastic (chronic) candidiasis	Longstanding nonremovable, confluent, white-yellowish plaques that may be stained by food	Oral or intravenous antifungal medications	Associated with severe immune deterioration
Angular cheilitis	Red radiating fissures or linear ulcers at commissures of the mouth; sometimes covered with a pseudomembrane	Topical antifungal medications	Can be detected during all stages of HIVD
DISSEMINATED FUNGAL INFECTIONS			
Cryptococcosis	Ulceration	Intravenous antifungal medications Usually amphotericin B	Sign of disseminated disease
Histoplasmosis	Ulceration	Intravenous antifungal medications Usually amphotericin B	Sign of disseminated disease
Geotrichosis	Ulcer covered with a pseudomembrane	Intravenous antifungal medications Usually amphotericin B	Sign of disseminated disease
Aspergillosis	Ulceration	Intravenous antifungal medications Usually amphotericin B	Sign of disseminated disease
VIRAL INFECTIONS			
Herpes simplex virus	*Intraoral:* solitary, multiple or confluent vesicles on keratinized mucosa *Perioral:* single or multiple vesicles or ulcers with crusting on the vermilion portion of the lip	Oral acyclovir	Increased frequency and increased severity during progression of HIVD. Resistance to acyclovir more common during severe immune deterioration and with HSV-2
Cytomegalovirus	Nonspecific nonhealing large painful ulceration(s) on any oral mucosal surface	Most resolve spontaneously; treatment, if necessary, is with ganciclovir	Associated with CD4+ counts below 100 cells/mm^3; may be an early indication of disseminated CMV infection
Oral hairy leukoplakia	Vertically corrugated, slightly elevated, white surface alterations; usually on lateral or ventral margins of the tongue, but can also be found on buccal mucosa and floor of the mouth	Treatment rarely required; if necessary, oral acyclovir	Early marker for immunosuppression when CD4+ cell counts drop below 300 cells/mm^3; more common among MSM
Human papillomavirus	White or pink nodules with a cauliflower-like surface; commonly found on the anterior part of the oral cavity	Surgical excision Intralesional injections with interferon	May be more common in patients on HAART

Continued

TABLE 14-1—cont'd
Guide to Oral Manifestations

Lesion	Clinical appearance	Treatment	Significance
VIRAL INFECTIONS—CONT'D			
Kaposi's sarcoma	Red, bluish, or purplish macular or nodular lesion most commonly found on the hard and soft palate; some lesions may be associated with ulcerations	Radiation therapy or intralesion injections with vinblastine or sodium tetradecyl sulfate	Represents an AIDS diagnosis; oral lesions may be the first sign of this neoplasm; associated with CD4+ cell counts below 200 cells/mm³; more common in MSM
BACTERIAL INFECTIONS			
Bacillary epithelioid angiomatosis	Bluish red macular to nodular lesion with a similar clinical appearance to Kaposi's sarcoma	Systemic erythromycin	Associated with severe immune deterioration
Necrotizing ulcerative periodontitis	Rapidly progressive non-self-healing loss of periodontal attachment and bone; associated with deep-seated pain and spontaneous bleeding	Scaling, metronidazole or tetracycline, and an antibacterial mouth rinse	Associated with severe immunosuppression, with CD4+ cell counts below 100 cells/mm³; more common in MSM
Linear gingival erythema	Erythematous gingival marginal band that may extend into the attached mucosa	Scaling, metronidazole or tetracycline, and an antibacterial mouth rinse	Associated with increased immunosuppression
Syphilis	Ulcerations, mucous patches, or gummas	Intramuscular injections of penicillin	Lesions are very contagious
NONSPECIFIC LESIONS			
Hyperpigmentation	Blue, red macular lesions on any mucosal surface	Not indicated	May be an early sign of adrenal insufficiency or secondary to medications
Minor aphthous ulcer	Self-healing, shallow, often recurrent ulceration; more common on nonkeratinized mucosa; will sometimes lack the characteristic surrounding red halo	Symptomatic relief Topical corticosteroids may be instituted	Not more commonly found in HIV-infected patients
Major aphthous ulcer	Large (>10 mm), painful, nonhealing, deep-seated, often recurrent ulcerations without an associated etiologic pathogen	Topical, mouth rinse, or oral corticosteroid therapy	Associated with severe immunosuppression, with CD4+ cell counts below 100 cells/mm³
Necrotizing stomatitis	Rapid localized destruction of alveolar bone accompanied by necrosis of overlying tissues; initially not necessarily painful	Topical or oral metronidazole or tetracycline Topical, mouth rinse, or oral corticosteroid therapy Protect lesion with a mouthguard	Associated with severe immunosuppression, with CD4+ cell counts below 100 cells/mm³
NEOPLASMS			
Non-Hodgkin's lymphoma	Ulcerative or exophytic lesions on any mucosal surface	Surgical excision, multiple drug chemotherapy in conjunction with radiation therapy	Found in a younger age bracket among HIV-infected individuals than among non-HIV-infected individuals
Squamous cell carcinoma	Ulcerative, exophytic, red and white lesion more commonly found on the posterior part of the tongue and the floor of the mouth	Surgical excision, multiple drug chemotherapy in conjunction with radiation therapy	Found in a younger age bracket among HIV-infected individuals than among non-HIV-infected individuals

MSM, Men who have sex with men; *HAART*, highly active antiretroviral therapy.

TABLE 14-2
Conditions and Etiologies Associated with Ulcerations in the Oral Cavity

	Ulcers strongly associated with HIV infection	Ulcers suggestive of HIV infection	Ulcers observed in, but not specifically suggestive of, HIV infection	Ulcers not reported, but that can occur, in persons with HIV infection
Infections				
Bacterial	Necrotizing stomatitis, necrotizing ulcerative gingivitis, necrotizing ulcerative periodontitis	*Mycobacterium avium, M. tuberculosis, Treponema pallidum*	*Enterobacter cloacae, Escherichia coli, Klebsiella pneumoniae*	
Viral	CMV, HIV (primary)	HSV-1, HSV-2, VZV		
Fungal	Aspergillosis, cryptococcosis, histoplasmosis, atrophic candidiasis, hyperplastic candidiasis	Angular cheilitis		
Neoplasms	Kaposi's sarcoma, non-Hodgkin's lymphoma		Squamous cell carcinoma	
Idiopathic origin	Major aphthous ulcer		Minor aphthous ulcers, herpetiform ulcers	
Drug-induced	Zidovudine, foscarnet, interferon, ganciclovir, dideoxycytidine, protease inhibitors			
Systemic diseases and conditions other than HIV			Behçet's syndrome, Reiter's syndrome, neutropenia	
Hematinic deficiencies				Iron deficiency, folate deficiency, vitamin B_{12} deficiency
Immune dysregulation				Antibody-dependent cellular cytotoxicity, T cell dysfunction
Not otherwise defined				Genetic, hypersensitivity, stress and menses, trauma, cessation of smoking

CMV, Cytomegalovirus; *HSV,* herpes simplex virus; *VZV,* varicella-zoster virus.

Decreased salivary flow enhances the growth of candidal infections in the oral cavity, may contribute to abrasions of the oral mucosa when patients are dissolving antifungal troches, increases the risk of caries and periodontal disease, and may reduce patients' ability to chew and swallow.

Treatment

Relief from oral dryness can be accomplished by various measures (Box 14-1). Encouraging the patient to continuously sip water during the day, or suck on crushed ice, will reduce the discomfort but obviously not rectify the cause of the dryness. The use of humidifiers at night and application of Vaseline to the lips will also reduce discomfort. Commercial artificial saliva substitutes may need to be instituted to achieve temporary relief from severe dryness. Many of these formulations can be purchased over the counter without a prescription. Patients should also minimize the use of liquids containing caffeine or alcohol, since these compounds act as diuretics.

Conservative therapy for stimulation of salivary flow includes chewing sugarless gum or sucking on sugarless can-

> **BOX 14-1**
> **Treatment of Reduced Salivary Flow**
>
> **REDUCTION OF DISCOMFORT**
> Frequent sipping of water
> Sucking on crushed ice
> Saliva substitutes
> Nightly use of humidifiers
> Coating lips with Vaseline
>
> **AVOIDANCE OF COMMONLY USED SALIVARY-REDUCING COMPOUNDS**
> Restrict caffeine intake
> Reduce alcohol intake
> Avoid alcohol-containing mouth rinses
>
> **SALIVA STIMULATION**
> Chewing of sugarless gum or sugarless candies
> Pilocarpine HCl (Salagen) tablets (5 to 7.5 mg tid)
> Pilocarpine HCl solution (1 mg/ml) (5 ml tid)
> Bethanechol (Urecholine) tablets (25 mg three to five times daily)

dies. The use of pilocarpine and bethanechol to stimulate salivary flow can also be employed. A low starting dose should be gradually increased to achieve an individual therapeutic beneficial response without causing unwanted effects, which include excessive sweating and cardiovascular symptoms.

Discontinuation or change of xerostomia-inducing drugs may sometimes be a viable option prior to instituting treatment for this condition.

Viral Infections

Human Immunodeficiency Virus

Oral manifestations associated with acute HIV infection are not uncommon. Nonspecific oral ulcerations, accompanied by sore throat, exudative pharyngitis, and oral candidiasis, may be signs of the acute seroconversion syndrome. These signs and symptoms disappear after the acute phase.

Herpes Virus Infections

Presentation and Progression. Both HSV infection type 1 (HSV-1) and type 2 (HSV-2) can cause oral ulcerations. Although clinically indistinguishable, HSV-1 infections are more commonly found in the oral cavity, whereas HSV-2 infections are traditionally associated with genital lesions. However, oral ulcerations due to HSV-2 are associated with a higher recurrence rate than HSV-1.

HSV manifests as single or coalescent, localized or generalized vesicles on intraoral surfaces and/or on the lips. These vesicles rapidly rupture and are usually not appreciated, leaving an underlying ulcer. The ulcers are often small, oval, irregular, and shallow, with a diameter of 2 to 4 mm. Coalescent lesions in immunocompromised patients form large ulcers that can be hemorrhagic and covered by a yellowish pseudomembrane. Chronic ulcers present for more than 3 weeks may be surrounded by a raised, white border.

In the immunocompetent individual, ulcers usually occur on more keratinized epithelium. However, this tendency is not necessarily observed in the immunocompromised individual where herpetic lesions may present on any intraoral surface.

In such individuals, labial lesions may not be confined within the vermilion border, but extend beyond the lips on to the surrounding skin.

HSV-associated lesions can be extremely painful and may make eating, swallowing, and speaking very difficult. This may lead to dehydration, weight loss, and restricted oral intake of medications.

The healing time of HSV ulcers in the immunocompromised individual is longer than the usual 7 to 10 days. The lesions may be misdiagnosed as recurrent aphthous lesions or CMV-associated ulcers. It is important to make a correct diagnosis, since treatment, prognosis, and prophylaxis options differ.

Diagnosis. A definitive diagnosis is generally established by viral culture of the ulcers. Cytologic staining for multinucleated giant cells or biopsy for detecting the occurrence of viral intranuclear inclusions can also be diagnostic. Intraoral HSV-associated ulcers can occur in persons with a normal immune system. However, frequently occurring or large confluent lesions may suggest advanced stages of HIVD.

Treatment. Treatment with 800 mg of acyclovir five times per day or valacyclovir 500 mg bid until the lesions heal should be initiated to reduce the severity of the lesions in the immunocompromised host.

Cytomegalovirus

Presentation and Progression. Oral manifestations of CMV infection indicate severe immunosuppression. CD4+ cell counts are generally less than 100 cells/mm^3. CMV-associated lesions are nonspecific, large ulcerations primarily located on less keratinized tissue. The ulcers may be shallow or deep with an eroded base. These painful lesions are usually more than 5 mm in diameter and heal poorly.

Diagnosis. Differential diagnoses include recurrent aphthous ulcers and HSV lesions. A diagnosis requires a biopsy demonstrating perivascular inflammation and large central basophilic intranuclear inclusions of CMV. An oral diagnosis of CMV necessitates further evaluation to rule out ophthalmologic or other CMV-associated problems.

Treatment. Oral ulcerations can be treated with ganciclovir. The best prevention is a response to antiretroviral therapy.

Epstein-Barr Virus

Presentation and Progression. Oral hairy leukoplakia (OHL) was first described in HIV-infected males and was initially thought to be an HIV-specific lesion. However, OHL has since been described in other immunosuppressed cohorts, and even in immunocompetent individuals. Still, the presence of this lesion necessitates an HIV test in an individual with an unknown HIV status, since the incidence of OHL in persons with HIV far outnumbers the incidence of this lesion in any other patient category.

The lesion commonly occurs on the lateral borders of the tongue as white, vertical, hyperkeratotic striae that cannot be wiped off. It is asymptomatic, and patients are often not aware of its existence. The lesion may occasionally be observed on other intraoral surfaces, also as white patches. OHL is caused by the Epstein-Barr virus (EBV).

Diagnosis. The differential diagnosis of OHL includes hyperplastic, or chronic, candidiasis. Interestingly, *Candida albicans* is present in more than 50% of OHL lesions. A diagnosis of

OHL is often accompanied by immunosuppression. Studies have shown that although OHL is present in all phases of HIVD, it is most commonly found in patients with CD4+ cell counts below 200 cells/mm^3.

Treatment. Treatment is rarely necessary. It is usually only instituted when the patient is complaining of impaired masticatory function or for aesthetic reasons, since the lesion is painless and has not been reported to be transmissible. Antiviral therapy with 800 mg of acyclovir orally five times daily is effective and will usually eradicate the lesion within 14 days. Recurrence is common, and prophylactic therapy with 800 mg of acyclovir daily may be necessary. Other treatments are also available, including topical application of 25% podophyllum resin.

Varicella-Zoster Virus

Shingles is not an uncommon occurrence during the progression of HIV disease. Although intraoral lesions have been described, they are not common. Varicella-zoster virus (VZV)-associated lesions resemble HSV-associated ulcers but present unilaterally and are usually larger. An association between intraoral VZV infection and immune status of HIV-infected individuals has not been established.

Human Herpesvirus 8

Presentation and Progression. Recent reports have implicated a novel herpesvirus, human herpesvirus 8 (HHV-8), as the etiologic pathogen for Kaposi's sarcoma (KS). Over 90% of intraoral KS lesions are found on the hard and soft palates, with the gingiva as the second most common location. The lesions usually present as red or purple to blue macules or nodules. During the early macular stages, lesions are mostly asymptomatic, but larger lesions may interfere with normal oral functions and become painful due to trauma or secondary ulcerations. Lesions close to the gingival margin will sometimes impair patients' ability to floss and brush their teeth. Inability to perform proper oral hygiene for long periods of time may result in periodontal disease. Large lesions may also impact on patients' ability to eat, speak, and swallow.

Oral KS usually presents when patients' CD4+ cell counts drop below 100 cells/mm^3. However, lesions have been found during all stages of HIV disease. Extrapalatal lesions and the change from a macular to a nodular stage are associated with a worse prognosis. As with cutaneous lesions, oral KS is more commonly found in patients who acquired HIV through homosexual sex and in patients with increased episodes of sexually transmitted diseases.

Diagnosis. The macular lesions may resemble physiologic pigmentation. A differential diagnosis should include both bacillary angiomatosis and lymphoma. A biopsy is necessary for a definitive diagnosis.

Treatment. Available therapies do not cure the disease but merely reduce the size and number of lesions. Radiation and surgical intervention are the most common treatment modalities. Isolated smaller lesions may be treated by direct injection into the lesion with a chemotherapeutic agent such as vinblastine sulfate (0.1 mg/mm^2) or sodium tetradecyl sulfate (0.1 mg/mm^2). Local treatments are successful but may not be long lasting. The most effective therapy is improving immune function by treatment of the underlying HIV infection. KS can go into complete remission with control of HIV infection.

Human Papillomavirus

Presentation and Progression. Since the introduction of protease inhibitors, there has been a reported increase in the prevalence of oral human papillomavirus (HPV) infections among HIV-infected patients. Multiple lesions often cover large areas of the oral cavity. Although nontraumatized lesions are asymptomatic, they often interfere with chewing and may even be disfiguring. The lesions can be found on all oral mucosal surfaces but seem to have a predilection for inside the lips and the gingiva. The reason for the increase in prevalence and severity is not clear.

Several different clinical forms of oral HPV have been described. They are traditionally described as hyperplastic, papillomatous, or verrucous. Oral squamous cell papillomas present as solitary or multiple, exophytic, pedunculated papules with a cauliflower-like or pebbled surface. Condylomata acuminata are small white to pink nodules, also with a pebbled or cauliflower-like surface. Verruca vulgaris, or the common wart, may present as a firm sessile, exophytic, whitish lesion. This lesion has a hyperkeratinized superficial epithelium, with slight invagination of the center of the lesion. Focal epithelial hyperplasia, or Heck's disease, presents as smooth, pebbled, or cauliflower-like, large, solitary or multiple, whitish, hyperplastic nodular areas.

Diagnosis. Differential diagnoses for HPV include fibromas, which are usually caused by trauma. No association has been reported between HPV and immune status.

Treatment. Various treatment modalities are being utilized with mixed success. They include surgical removal with a scalpel, laser ablation, cryotherapy, topical application of keratinolytic agents, and intralesional injections of antiviral agents. Topical application of 25% podophyllum resin may reduce the size of a lesion and can be used for smaller size lesions. Larger lesions can be treated with intralesional injections accompanied by subcutaneous injections of interferon-α. The intralesional injections are administered once or twice weekly with 1,000,000 IU per cm^2 of lesion, while the subcutaneous injections of 3,000,000 IU are given two or three times weekly. Although the recurrence rate is rather high, eradication of lesions can usually be accomplished with a combination of treatments over time.

Fungal Infections: Candidiasis

Intraoral candidiasis is the most common oral manifestation of immunosuppression. It is not in itself pathognomonic for HIV disease, but oral candidiasis may be an early sign of infection and a marker for advanced disease. A tentative diagnosis based on the clinical appearance of the lesion should be verified by a potassium hydroxide preparation of an oral scraping. Four different clinical presentations of oral candidiasis have been described: pseudomembranous, erythematous, and hyperplastic candidiasis, and angular cheilitis.

Pseudomembranous and Erythematous Candidiasis

Presentation and Progression. Pseudomembranous candidiasis, also commonly known as thrush, manifests as white or yellowish, single or confluent plaques that can easily be rubbed off from the oral mucosa. The plaques are found on all oral surfaces and may leave an erythematous or even bleeding surface if mechanically removed. Patients are often not aware of the condition, but in severe situations eating and swallowing can become painful and may prevent a normal nutritional intake. Pseudomembranous candidiasis is indicative of immunosuppression, with CD4+ cell counts usually below 200 cells/mm³.

Erythematous, or atrophic, candidiasis manifests as red or atrophic patches affecting all oral mucosal surfaces, but with a predilection for the tongue and hard palate. When the dorsum of the tongue is affected, the infection manifests as areas of depapillation. Erythematous *Candida* infections may exist alone or in combination with the pseudomembranous form. The involved areas often appear without a distinct border, making it difficult to account for the extension of the lesion. Although usually asymptomatic, longstanding lesions may be accompanied by a burning sensation. The lesions may be seen in the earliest stages of immunosuppression, but have been found throughout the course of HIV disease.

Treatment. Treatment of both pseudomembranous and erythematous oral candidiasis is similar and usually very effective. Topical therapy with troches or mouth rinses is usually beneficial for patients with CD4+ cell counts above 150 to 200 cells/mm³. For patients with a more impaired immune response, systemic medications are indicated. The choice of medication is dependent on various factors. Some of the topical preparations need to be used five times daily. For patients who are not homebound or bedridden it is more convenient to carry around troches than mouth rinses. However, reduced salivary flow may cause difficulties with medications that need to dissolve in the mouth. The choice of systemic medication is dependent on such factors as concomitant medications, liver function status, and patient compliance.

Topical medications include nystatin oral pastille, one or two pastilles dissolved slowly four to five times a day; clotrimazole oral troche, 10 mg, one troche dissolved five times a day; and nystatin oral suspension. The high sugar content in topical antifungal preparations predisposes patients to caries. Nystatin formulations contain sucrose, which is more cariogenic than dextrose, found in clotrimazole preparations. Patients undergoing long-term therapy with topical agents should be instructed in improved oral hygiene, and daily fluoride rinses should be recommended. Topical formulations with low sugar content include vaginal preparations such as clotrimazole vaginal troche that are dissolved in the mouth, and nystatin vaginal troche 100,000 units, one troche dissolved in the mouth three times a day.

For systemic antifungal therapy for oral candidiasis, the most commonly used medications are fluconazole, one or two 100-mg tablets daily; ketoconazole, one or two 200-mg tablets taken daily with food; or itraconazole, 2 ml (20 mg) daily. Oral candidiasis has a high recurrence rate, and secondary prophylaxis may sometimes be required.

Hyperplastic Candidiasis

Presentation and Progression. Hyperplastic, or chronic, candidiasis is relatively uncommon and is mainly found in severely debilitated patients with severe immunosuppression and oral dryness. Many patients with this condition will also have, or be at high risk for developing, esophageal candidiasis. Hyperplastic oral candidiasis manifests as white or discolored plaques that may be solitary or confluent but, in contrast to pseudomembranous candidiasis, cannot be wiped off the mucosa. Patients may complain of a burning sensation and describe a feeling of having a large piece of cotton in their mouths. The lesion is found on all oral surfaces, but most commonly on the hard and soft palate.

The chronic type may be misdiagnosed as a leukoplakia, and when located on the tongue, it may be mistaken for OHL. Although the clinical presentation of this lesion is virtually pathognomonic, the presence of hyphae and blastospores, seen on smears examined with potassium hydroxide or Gram's stain, will confirm the diagnosis.

Treatment. Treatment for hyperplastic candidiasis consists of systemic antifungal medications, which may include intravenous formulations.

Angular Cheilitis

Presentation and Progression. Angular cheilitis, or perlèche, presents as radiating red fissures, sometimes with a pseudomembranous coverage, from the corners of the mouth. This condition is not pathognomonic for HIV disease and is commonly seen in older individuals wearing ill fitting complete dentures. It is often found in conjunction with xerostomia and may worsen during cold weather.

Treatment. Angular cheilitis is treated with application of a topical antifungal such as clotrimazole ointment 1%, miconazole ointment 2%, ketoconazole cream 2%, or nystatin ointment four times a day for 2 weeks. The addition of an antibacterial ointment is beneficial to treat accompanying bacterial superinfections.

Bacterial Infections: Periodontal Disease

Periodontal disease is a common condition in both HIV-positive and HIV-negative individuals. However, HIV-infected persons may exhibit a faster progressing type of conventional chronic periodontal disease in which younger adults present with periodontal conditions more similar to what is expected in older patients. Acute, rapidly progressive periodontal conditions may be early signs of immunosuppression and HIV infection. Studies have shown a correlation between aggressive periodontal conditions in HIV-infected individuals and progressive deterioration of individuals' immune status. Interestingly, although different periodontal conditions in the HIV-infected individual are related to the person's immune status, they are not associated with a change in the microbiota. There are three forms of periodontal conditions that have been associated with HIV disease: linear gingival erythema (LGE), necrotizing ulcerative gingivitis (NUG), and necrotizing ulcerative periodontitis (NUP).

Linear Gingival Erythema

Presentation and Progression. LGE is described as an atypical gingivitis that is recognized by its fiery 2- to 3-mm red band at the gingival margin, with an equal distribution around the teeth. The redness is disproportional to the plaque accumulation, the more common cause of gingivitis, along the margin. There is no ulceration, no increased pocket depth with periodontal attachment loss, and no bleeding on probing. Punctuated or diffuse erythema is sometimes seen on the attached gingiva toward the alveolar mucosa. The condition is not necessarily painful. LGE is not strongly associated with HIV disease.

Diagnosis. The differential diagnosis includes a localized effect secondary to dry mucosa associated with open mouth breathing, localized candidiasis, oral lichen planus, mucous membrane pemphigoid, hypersensitivity reactions manifesting as plasma cell gingivitis, *Geotrichum candidum* infection, and thrombocytopenia. It has been speculated that this condition may be caused by a subgingival *Candida* infection.

Treatment. Treatment is empiric, with standard dental scaling and root planing. This treatment alone has rather limited effect. The use of chlorhexidine gluconate (0.12%) mouth rinses twice daily for up to 3 months may result in a significant improvement. The patient should swish with 15 ml of the solution for about 30 seconds and then expectorate. Addition of topical antifungal medications may also be beneficial. Careful oral hygiene is imperative. The primary health care provider should refer the patient to an oral health care provider for scaling and root planing procedures.

Necrotizing Ulcerative Gingivitis and Necrotizing Ulcerative Periodontitis

Presentation and Progression. NUG and NUP are severe periodontal disorders caused by bacteria. These two entities may represent different stages of the same disease. NUG is limited to the gingiva with no associated periodontal attachment loss, whereas NUP involves loss of periodontal attachment and severe destruction of the surrounding alveolar mucosa. These conditions range from initial lesions with limited necrosis at the top of the papillae to a situation that involves the entire attached gingiva accompanied by tooth mobility and bone sequestering. Patients with NUP often complain of severe deep-seated jaw pain, spontaneous bleeding from the gingiva, and, in longstanding cases, tooth mobility. Fetor ex ore, or halitosis, is a common and characteristic symptom. If untreated, NUP may progress, with 1- to 2-mm soft and hard tissue destruction per week. This condition has been associated with severe immunosuppression and CD4+ cell counts below 100 cells/mm^3.

Diagnosis. There are few differential diagnoses. These include bullous lesions of benign mucous membrane pemphigoid, erythema multiforme exudativum, and acute forms of leukemia.

Treatment. Treatment for both NUG and NUP is effective and consists of tissue debridement and antibiotic therapy with metronidazole (250 to 500 mg) or tetracycline (250 to 500 mg) four times a day for a week. Pain is relieved and the healing starts relatively quickly. Because of the high risk of secondary *Candida* infection, an antifungal medication should be prescribed at the same time. A twice-a-day mouth rinse with a chlorhexidine gluconate (0.12%) is recommended as maintenance therapy. The patient should swish with 15 ml of the solution for about 30 seconds and then expectorate.

Conditions with Nonspecific Etiology
Necrotizing Stomatitis

Presentation and Progression. Necrotizing stomatitis is a rapidly progressive localized ulceration causing necrosis of soft tissue overlying bone. The lesions may be very painful, prohibiting eating, speech, and swallowing. Necrotizing stomatitis presents in stages of severe immunosuppression with CD4+ cell counts below 100 cells/mm^3.

Diagnosis. A differential diagnosis is an aggressive form of aphthous ulcer. It has also been hypothesized that necrotizing stomatitis is an extensive type of NUP.

Treatment. The necrotic areas should be carefully debrided with a curet. If possible, a stent should be constructed to cover the affected area, protect it from trauma, and allow topical application of medication. Treatment consists of application of topical glucocorticosteroids, such as clobetasol or fluocinonide gel, or dexamethasone elixir mouth rinse 0.5 mg/5 ml for 10 to 14 days. In severe and resistant cases, systemic steroid formulations, such as prednisone up to 15 mg four times per day for 1 week, can be used. The patient should also rinse with 15 ml chlorhexidine gluconate (0.12%) twice a day. Addition of a systemic antibiotic, such as metronidazole or tetracycline, prevents bacterial superinfection and promotes healing.

Aphthous Ulcers

Presentation and Progression. Recurrent aphthous ulcers (RAU) typically present as 2 to 5 mm in diameter small ulcers on less keratinized tissue in the oral cavity, such as inside the lips, floor of the mouth, or buccal mucosa, and resolve spontaneously within 5 to 7 days. These minor RAU (MiRAU) are characterized by their tendency to recur, often at the same site, and are usually associated with the onset of stressful situations. They are mildly painful and heal without scarring. These minor ulcers are not uncommon among the general population and can easily be misdiagnosed as recurrent herpesvirus infections. An analgesic mouth rinse, such as 2% to 4% viscous lidocaine solution for swish and expectoration, can be prescribed to reduce the oral discomfort. This symptomatic treatment will increase the patient's ability to eat, chew, and swallow.

Major RAU (MjRAU) are more than 10 mm in diameter and crater formed, with a deep eroded base. They persist for more than 3 weeks and often heal with scarring. Large ulcers can severely impair the patient's ability to eat, speak, and swallow. No clear etiology has been established, but stress, vitamin deficiency, diet, hormonal changes, trauma, and immune dysfunction have all been suggested.

For patients with HIVD, MjRAU has been associated with severe immunosuppression, with CD4+ cell counts below 100 cells/mm^3.

Treatment. Resolution of MjRAU is essential in order to enable masticatory function and reduce intraoral pain. Systemic or topical glucocorticosteroids can be given as initial therapy. Prednisone 20 mg tablets three or four times daily for 7 days is suggested as systemic therapy. As a topical rinse, dexamethasone elixir 0.5 mg/5 ml four times per day for 7 days can be used. Often an antibiotic and an antifungal medication may be prescribed to prevent superimposed infections. A topical analgesic may enable the patient to eat and apply other prescribed medications.

Resistance to glucocorticosteroids may be present, and alternative therapies may have to be implemented. Thalidomide has been used to treat both oral and esophageal ulcerations with some success. The dosage of thalidomide is 100 to 200 mg per day. Adverse events among patients receiving thalidomide include somnolence, rash, and peripheral sensory neuropathy. Thalidomide should not be given to women with the potential for becoming pregnant.

Neoplasms

Oral squamous cell carcinoma (SCC) and oral non-Hodgkin's lymphoma (NHL) present in the HIV-infected population at an earlier age than in noninfected individuals. No increased incidence of these oral neoplasms has been documented. The prognosis for patients with oral NHL is not good, since death usually ensues within 4 to 10 months of a diagnosis.

Hyperpigmentation

Hyperpigmentation is found on any oral mucosal surface. Macular hyperpigmented areas are usually associated with various medications, but may also be an early sign of adrenal insufficiency.

SUGGESTED READINGS

Agency for Healthcare Research and Quality: Management of dental patients who are HIV positive. Summary, Evidence Report/Technology Assessment: Number 37. AHRQ Publication No. 01-E041, March 2001, Agency for Healthcare Research and Quality, Rockville, MD. *http://www.ahrq.gov/clinic/denthivsum.htm*

Barr CE, Glick M: Diagnosis and management of oral and cutaneous lesions in HIV-1 disease, *Oral Maxillo Surg Clin North Am* 1:25, 1998.

Chapple ILC, Hamburger J: The significance of oral health in HIV disease, *Sex Transm Dis* 76:236, 2000.

EC Clearing House on Oral Problems Related to HIV Infection and WHO Collaborating Centre on Oral Manifestations of the Human Immunodeficiency Virus: Classification and diagnostic criteria of oral lesions in HIV infection, *J Oral Pathol Med* 22:289, 1993.

Glick M et al: Oral manifestations associated with HIV disease as markers for immune suppression and AIDS, *Oral Surg Oral Med Oral Pathol* 77:344, 1994.

Glick M et al: Necrotizing ulcerative periodontitis: a marker for immune deterioration and a predictor for the diagnosis of AIDS, *J Periodontol* 65:393, 1994.

Glick M: *Dental management of patients with HIV,* Chicago, 1994, Quintessence Publishing.

Greenspan D et al: Effect of highly active antiretroviral therapy on frequency of oral warts, *Lancet* 357:1411, 2001.

Greenspan JS: Sentinels and signposts: the epidemiology and significance of oral manifestations of HIV disease, *Oral Dis* 3:S13, 1997.

Greenspan JS, Greenspan D: *Oral manifestations of HIV infection,* Chicago, 1995, Quintessence Publishing.

Kademani D, Glick M: Oral ulcerations in individuals infected with human immunodeficiency virus: clinical presentations, diagnosis, management, and relevance to disease progression, *Quint International* 29:523, 1998.

Patton LL: Sensitivity, specificity, and positive predictive value of oral opportunistic infections in adults with HIV/AIDS as markers of immune suppression and viral burden, *Oral Surg Oral Med Oral Pathol Oral Radiol Endod* 90:182, 2000.

Patton LL et al: Changing prevalence of oral manifestations of human immunodeficiency virus in the era of protease inhibitor therapy, *Oral Surg Oral Med Oral Pathol Oral Radiol Endod* 89:299, 2000.

Sifri R et al: Oral health care issues in HIV disease: developing a core curriculum for primary care physicians, *J Am Board Fam Pract* 11:434, 1998.

Silverman S Jr: *Color atlas of oral manifestations of AIDS,* ed 2, St Louis, 1996, Mosby.

http://www.hivdent.org

http://www.critpath.org/daac/

15 Ocular Complications of AIDS

STEPHEN M. GOLDMAN

Introduction

Ocular manifestations of HIV disease are myriad and can affect the ocular adnexa and all layers of the globe itself. The ocular adnexal structures include the lids, orbit, and lacrimal gland. The globe is segregated into the anterior segment, which includes the conjunctiva, sclera, cornea, anterior chamber, iris, and crystalline lens. The posterior segment includes the ciliary body, vitreous humor, sensory retina, choroid, posterior sclera, and optic nerve. The diseases that affect the eye range from inflammatory, such as dry eye syndrome and uveitis, to neoplastic, as well as many opportunistic infections. These infections include molluscum contagiosum, herpes simplex, varicella-zoster, cytomegalovirus (CMV), *Toxoplasma gondii, Treponema pallidum, Pneumocystis carinii*, and various fungal infections.

Adnexal and Anterior Segment Complications
Noninfectious
Keratoconjunctivitis Sicca

Presentation and Progression. The tear film is a trilaminar fluid layer consisting of oil, aqueous, and mucinous layers. If any of the layers are abnormal, patients develop a dry eye. Extreme dry eye conditions occur rarely in the general population but are very common in HIV-infected patients. The syndrome can produce symptoms of burning pain and a sticky ocular surface. Because of the decreased aqueous layer, mucus often clumps, leaving strands in the conjunctival cul-de-sac, or the mucus strands attach to the cornea as filaments, leading to a severe foreign body sensation. Since the quality of vision is dependent on the mirrorlike surface of the cornea, patients with an aqueous deficit will have blurred and fluctuating vision. These symptoms are exacerbated by preexisting lid abnormalities such as blepharitis, a common disease that interferes with the oily layer of the tear film. Finally, a severe dry eye leads to a breakdown in the corneal integrity, predisposing the patient to corneal infections.

Diagnosis. Keratoconjunctivitis sicca is a syndrome that occurs when the aqueous production decreases to a point where the Schirmer's test strip wets to less than 10 mm after a 5-minute period. When the dry eye is combined with a dry mouth and arthritis, Sjögren's syndrome is diagnosed. Other causes include hypovitaminosis A secondary to malnutrition or malabsorption, radiation exposure to the lacrimal gland, and age-related decrease in lacrimal function.

Treatment. The treatment of severe dry eyes includes intensive lubrication with artificial tears, lubricating ointments, and, if symptomatically severe, permanent punctal occlusion. If filaments are present on the ocular surface, application of mucolytics such as 5% acetylcysteine (Mucosil, Dey Laboratories) can help reduce the associated foreign body pain. Of equal importance is the treatment of underlying conditions with vitamin A supplementation, warm compresses and eyelid scrubs for blepharitis, and the avoidance of dry smoky or windy environments. In recalcitrant cases, moisture chambers on protective glasses or tarsorrhaphy can be employed.

When to Refer. Patients who have recalcitrant symptoms that do not respond to intensive lubrication may require surgical interventions to reduce tear evaporation. These patients are at risk for severe vision loss and could potentially lose their eye from corneal perforations.

▶ KEY POINTS

- Extremely common in all HIV-infected patients
- In mild cases use artificial tears; in severe cases use preservative-free drops

Uveitis

Presentation and Progression. Mild to severe bouts of anterior and posterior segment inflammation can occur with or without an infectious etiology. The noninfectious type of iridocyclitis (uveitis) is associated with the administration of medications or with the restoration of the patient's immune system, or can be a direct result of HIV infection. The onset of the uveitis is often heralded by an increase in the number of floaters, conjunctival injection, pain, blurred vision, and photophobia.

Uveitis associated with the administration of rifabutin (Mycobutin, Pharmacia & Upjohn Co.) used for the treatment or prophylaxis of *Mycobacterium avium* complex (MAC) infections has been documented in patients with or without the acquired immunodeficiency syndrome (AIDS) virus. The uveitis is a dose-related phenomenon and appears with higher dosing schedules. Immunosuppressed patients commonly receive multiple drugs, each of which can interfere with the hepatic metabolism of rifabutin, potentially leading to higher than expected drug levels. The higher drug concentration may be the cause of the increased incidence of rifabutin-induced uveitis seen in AIDS patients. The onset of the uveitis can occur several weeks to many months after the start of therapy. When the inflammation is gradual in onset and is mild, the symptoms are minimal and the uveitis will be diagnosed at a routine eye examination. In its more severe presentation, the uveitis onset can occur rapidly in as short a time as several hours, leading to severe panophthalmitis. These patients will have a dense vitritis and an anterior uveitis with hypopyon. This type of presentation mimics acute bacterial endophthalmitis and must be treated as infectious.

Another medication that has been associated with a drug-induced uveitis is the nucleoside analogue cidofovir used to combat CMV. The iritis is found whether the cidofovir is administered intravenously or via intravitreal injections. Onset can occur after the first dose or later in the course of treatment. The uveitis is characterized by a mild nongranulomatous anterior chamber cell and flare reaction. There is an absence of keratoprecipitates and posterior synechiae. Because the reaction is mild, it may be entirely asymptomatic or associated with the typical complaints of redness, floaters, and photophobia. Patients on chronic cidofovir therapy require serial anterior segment biomicroscopic evaluations to screen for the asymptomatic uveitis. Topical steroid drops are used to treat the iritis but are difficult to taper while on continued cidofovir therapy.

Diagnosis. After a diagnostic anterior chamber paracentesis and a vitreous biopsy are performed, intravitreal and, at times, intravenous antibiotics are administered. Once the inflammation has been judged noninfectious, high-dose parenteral steroids and topical steroids will lead to a rapid resolution of the inflammation. The inflammation will return with the tapering of the steroids unless the dose of the rifabutin is reduced or is stopped.

Direct infection with the HIV virus has been implicated as a rare cause of both anterior and posterior segment inflammation without the presence of opportunistic infectious organisms or medications known to cause ocular inflammation. These patients have a nongranulomatous anterior reaction with variable vitreous cells. The inflammation responds minimally to topical or regional steroid administration. The patient's uveitis responds to the administration of zidovudine (AZT).

As the treatment of immunosuppression has improved immune function of HIV-infected individuals, as measured by increasing CD4+ counts and the decrease in HIV viral messenger RNA loads, a new cause of uveitis has been described. This noninfectious, non–drug-induced cause of uveitis has been termed immune recovery vitritis. These patients commonly had low CD4+ counts and developed CMV retinitis. The retinitis was treated with appropriate anti-CMV medications and developed inactive retinal scars typical of healed CMV. Subsequently these patients were placed on highly active antiretroviral therapy (HAART) and responded with an improved cellular immunity. After the improvement in immune function, patients with this new syndrome develop a moderate vitreous cellular reaction, with only minimal anterior chamber cells. These patients complain more of blurring of vision and of floaters and less of pain, photophobia, or conjunctival injection. Associated with the vitritis are cystoid macular edema, epiretinal membrane formation, and hyperemia of the optic nerve.

Treatment. The treatment of any anterior inflammatory condition begins with treating the underlying cause. The first-line medical treatment is topical steroids. The frequency of the drops can be titrated to the severity of inflammation. In severe cases that are resistant to frequent topical drops, parenteral steroids can then be added to the drops.

When to Refer. Any patient presenting with symptoms of new floaters, a red eye, and photophobia needs a slit lamp examination to rule out iridocyclitis.

KEY POINTS

⊃ Must rule out infectious etiology
⊃ Generally rare in the HIV-infected population
⊃ Symptoms include photophobia, redness, and new floaters
⊃ Steroids, both topical and parenteral, are often needed to control the inflammation
⊃ May need to withdraw inciting medication

Ocular Hypotension

Presentation and Progression. The average intraocular pressure when measured via Goldmann's applanation tonometry is 16 mm Hg, with a standard deviation of 2.5 mm Hg. Certain ocular conditions can lead to ocular hypotony including iritis, ipsilateral carotid vascular disease, CMV retinitis, intravitreal cidofovir injections, and rhegmatogenous retinal detachments.

The intraocular pressure is also consistently lower when patients have none of these conditions but are simply immunodeficient. This decrease is directly related to the CD4+ count. The cause is unknown but may be related to intraocular hemodynamics, which in turn directly impacts on the ciliary body's vascular supply, or may be a direct effect of the HIV virus on the site of aqueous production in the ciliary body. The decrease in intraocular pressure in these patients does not cause visual loss or seem to predispose to other ocular complications such as hypotensive macular edema.

KEY POINTS

⊃ Generally asymptomatic
⊃ Can only be diagnosed by tonometry

Kaposi's Sarcoma

Presentation and Progression. Kaposi's sarcoma is the most common neoplasm in patients with immunosuppression. It is a mesenchymal tumor that appears as a dark blue or deep purple plaque or nodule when found on the eyelids. When it involves the conjunctiva, the tumor can be flat or nodular, with the color ranging from bright red to deep violet. The typical patient will complain of cosmetic changes to the eyelid. If the tumor enlarges or affects the eyelid margins, mild surface pain may occur secondary to corneal drying. Similar complaints also occur when the tumor is located solely in the conjunctiva.

Diagnosis. The lesion is composed of multiple vascular channels. The channels vary in size and shape. There are prominent atypical spindle cells and endothelial cells interspersed with the vascular channels. The amount of spindle cells and thickness of the tumor increase with the length of time the tumor is present. Because of their color and location, the conjunctival tumors mimic chronic subconjunctival hemorrhages or a cavernous hemangioma. The lesions in the eyelid can appear similar to chalazions, pyogenic granulomas, melanomas, or metastatic tumors.

Treatment. Kaposi's sarcoma is usually an indolent tumor in patients with normal immunity. Patients with AIDS have tumors that are more aggressive locally but are still relatively slow growing. It has been treated successfully with local excision, chemotherapy, interferon alfa-2a, and radiation therapy. Recurrence tends to happen when there is increased spindle cell and endothelial cell density found in the larger and more advanced tumors. There also can be spontaneous regression when a patient's immune status partially recovers with HAART.

When to Refer. Patients with a chronic lid lesion that does not respond to local compresses or a subconjunctival hemorrhage that persists beyond 3 weeks should be evaluated by an ophthalmologist.

KEY POINTS

- Affects both the eyelid and conjunctiva
- Often can masquerade as chronic chalazion or a subconjunctival hemorrhage

Infectious
Molluscum Contagiosum

Presentation, Progression, and Diagnosis. Molluscum contagiosum virus is the causative organism of molluscum contagiosum, a common cutaneous infection that can affect the eyelids of immunosuppressed patients. The molluscum virus is a DNA virus that belongs to the poxvirus family. It is estimated to affect up to 18% of HIV-infected patients. The cutaneous lesions consist of single or multiple dome-shaped umbilicated papules. The central crater contains infected cells that are necrotic and appear sebumlike in consistency. The white cheeselike material can be expressed from the crater. Histologic evaluation of the papules reveals infected keratocytes, which contain intracytoplasmic inclusion bodies. The papules are highly contagious and will spread locally and may appear nearly confluent in severe cases. The lesions are generally small in size but can grow larger than the normal size of several millimeters with increasing immunosuppression. When the papules are found on the eyelids, they cause a chronic follicular conjunctivitis, which can result in a refractory red eye. Although it is generally a cutaneous infection, there are case reports of conjunctival and corneal lesions. These are generally solitary and small in size and are associated with cutaneous lesions in the periocular region.

Treatment. Treatment response among patients who are HIV-infected is variable and recurrence is common. The treatment of molluscum contagiosum is generally localized to the individual lesions and includes curettage of the central crater, excision, cryotherapy, and electrodesiccation. There are case reports of response to cidofovir (Vistide, Gilead Sciences). The best treatment is the recovery of the patient's own immune function with antiretroviral therapy, which causes the spontaneous resolution of molluscum contagiosum. The lesions shrink in size and number and have an associated inflammatory response during the healing phase. The skin often has residual scarring at the site of the healed molluscum.

When to Refer. Referral to an ophthalmologist or a dermatologist should occur when patients present with a chronic periocular rash.

KEY POINTS

- Affects up to 20% of HIV-infected patients
- May cause a chronic red eye
- The pox spread locally and are treated locally

Herpes Zoster Ophthalmicus

Presentation and Progression. Herpes zoster ophthalmicus is caused by the reactivation of the varicella-zoster virus that has been latent in the trigeminal nerve after a primary chickenpox infection. The dermatitis obeys the facial midline and stays within the V1 and/or the V2 facial distribution. Patients at risk include the elderly, those under emotional or physical stress, or those with excessive sun exposure. These patients all are relatively immunosuppressed. Patients who are HIV-infected are at significantly higher risk for the development of herpes zoster ophthalmicus than the general population. The herpes zoster dermatitis found in patients with AIDS is more aggressive, has an increased number of vesicles, lasts longer, and is frequently recurrent.

Diagnosis. The typical herpes zoster dermatomal lesions are preceded by pain often described as burning or tingling in nature. As the dermatitis progresses the skin becomes erythematous and swollen. Later, a vesicular eruption occurs, which involutes, crusts, and forms large eschars. New eruptions are mixed with older lesions in various stages of healing. The Hutchinson's sign occurs when a vesicle is found on the side of the nose, indicating involvement of the nasociliary branch of the maxillary division of the trigeminal nerve. This sign places the patient at higher risk for intraocular complications. In HIV-infected patients the acute rash tends to last longer and is more likely to be polydermatomal.

Natural History. Once the acute lesions resolve, the skin can be thinned, hypopigmented, and atrophic, leaving the patient's face disfigured. The patient may develop chronic postherpetic neuralgia, which lasts months to years and ranges from a mild tingling sensation to severe burning. Because both herpes simplex 1 and herpes simplex 2 can also cause herpetic viral cutaneous eruptions, the herpes zoster virus–induced exanthema can be differentiated from these by the rash appearance. Herpes simplex infections appear as small white vesicles on an erythematous base. These lesions do not strictly obey dermatomal patterns as seen in zoster. In disseminated herpes zoster, the rash can cross the mid-line and make differentiation difficult.

The anterior segment complications are myriad and often severe. The conjunctiva can develop mild papillary injection with secondary tearing. The cornea develops positive-staining dendrites that lack the terminal bulbs seen with herpes simplex keratitis. Herpes zoster keratitis leads to corneal denervation and the development of an anesthetic or neurotrophic cornea. The corneal epithelium requires innervation to remain healthy and intact. The denervated epithelial cells tend to slough, leading to painful erosions. These erosions are very difficult to heal and put the eye at high risk for permanent loss of vision from infection or neovascularization. The corneal endothelium can become coated with large mutton fat keratoprecipitates. The keratoprecipitates are aggregations of lymphocytes that range in color from a creamy tan to brown.

When the keratoprecipitates are dense, the loss of corneal clarity leads the patient to complain of blurred vision. The keratoprecipitates are a sign of granulomatous iridocyclitis. The iritis is often recalcitrant to treatment and frequently recurs. The recurrences can either be early in treatment or months after the zoster has resolved. The iris often shows postherpetic sectorial atrophy. The atrophic areas are lighter in color, react poorly to light, and have pigmented epithelium defects, causing transillumination defects. Intraocular pressure elevations can occur with or without anterior segment inflammation. The intraocular pressure spikes are often asymptomatic and without treatment lead to glaucomatous optic atrophy. Cataract formation is a late and relatively uncommon finding. Posterior segment involvement includes acute retinal necrosis, varicella-zoster retinitis, and progressive outer retinal necrosis (PORN) syndromes. The optic nerve can rarely develop herpes zoster–mediated optic neuropathy.

Treatment. There are several effective oral medications available to treat herpes zoster. Acyclovir, famciclovir (Famvir, SmithKline Beecham Pharmaceuticals), and valacyclovir (Valtrex, Glaxo Wellcome Inc.) are all effective medications for most cases. When the patient has been on prophylactic acyclovir treatment, there is an increased risk of resistant disease. These patients should be treated with intravenous acyclovir or foscarnet (Foscavir, Astra Pharmaceuticals) initially. This can be followed with prolonged oral treatment with either valacyclovir or famciclovir. Because of the risk of recurrence, the patient should remain on long-term oral maintenance therapy.

KEY POINTS

⊃ Generally follows dermatomal patterns
⊃ Intraocular complications can be subtle but have devastating consequences

Herpes Simplex Keratitis

Presentation and Progression. Herpes simplex keratitis is more commonly caused by the herpes simplex virus type 1 than by the herpes simplex virus type 2 genotype. This is not an uncommon disease in patients both with and without immunosuppression, with similar rates of infection in both groups. It is a common cause of blindness secondary to corneal scarring throughout the world. Patients' complaints range from a minimal foreign body irritation to severe pain and loss of vision. The eye is variably red and has a watery discharge. The epithelial disease is often recurrent, since the virus becomes latent in the ciliary ganglion or the cornea only to reappear at a later date. The recurrence rate and severity of the keratitis are greater in immunocompromised patients, and the location is in the peripheral cornea rather than in the central cornea. Untreated epithelial herpes simplex keratitis eventually causes loss of vision, with a pronounced loss of corneal clarity.

The second type of keratitis is stromal keratitis. This appears as a diffuse edematous corneal haze, often without epithelial involvement. As the stromal disease progresses, deep neovascularization occurs. Biomicroscopic evaluation of the corneal scarring reveals both deep neovascularization (interstitial keratitis) and diffuse stromal haze. It is the stromal variant that leads to severe permanent loss of vision. Fortunately, the rate of stromal keratitis is decreased compared with patients with an intact immune system.

Diagnosis. There are several corneal diseases caused by herpes simplex. Isolated epithelial herpes simplex virus keratitis appears as the negative type of fluorescein-staining corneal dendrites (erosions located below the corneal epithelium that stain well) associated with terminal bulbs. Untreated, the dendrites can expand and coalesce into a larger geographic ulceration. These ulcerations predispose the cornea to bacterial superinfection. The initial epithelial type of keratitis can be preceded by prior primary herpetic conjunctivitis.

Treatment. Treatment of the epithelial infection consists of frequent administration of topical antiviral drops or epithelial debridement. The most commonly used antiviral is trifluridine (Viroptic, Glaxo Wellcome Inc.), a pyrimidine nucleoside that interferes with viral DNA synthesis. It is used topically nine times per day initially and is tapered to clinical responsiveness. The drug must be kept refrigerated to maintain potency. Other topical medications less commonly utilized are vidarabine monohydrate (Vira-A, Parke-Davis) and idoxuridine (Herplex, Allergan Pharmaceutical). Utilization of long-term oral acyclovir for quicker resolution and reduction of recurrences is an option to help prevent the loss of vision associated with recurrent disease. Topical acyclovir is not available in the United States but can be tried in resistant cases.

When to Refer. If a dendritic lesion persists or becomes unresponsive to therapy, corneal scraping may become necessary.

KEY POINTS

⊃ The corneal staining pattern is dendritic
⊃ Recurrent infection can lead to corneal blindness
⊃ May require chronic oral suppressive therapy

Varicella-Zoster Keratitis

Presentation and Progression. Varicella-zoster virus can also cause a corneal epitheliopathy. It most commonly occurs when patients have a recent or, less commonly, distant past history of zosteriform dermatitis or primary varicella infection. On casual examination, the dendrite formation of the infected cornea appears similar to the typical ones found in herpes simplex infections. Unlike herpes simplex keratitis, the slit lamp examination reveals a corneal staining pattern in varicella-zoster keratitis that is positive in nature (elevated from the corneal surface).

Diagnosis. The dendrites stain preferentially with rose Bengal solution (Rosets, Akorn Inc.), as opposed to the typical herpetic dendrites, which stain better with fluorescein sodium (Flour-I-Strips, Wyeth-Ayerst Laboratories). The dendrites appear grayish-white in color and are not associated with terminal bulb formation.

Natural History. As the keratitis progresses the anterior corneal stroma becomes hazy and begins to obscure the view of the anterior chamber. The lesions cause a foreign body–like pain and/or a burning sensation that is often severe and difficult to treat. Intraocular complications can occur, including granulomatous iridocyclitis and severe glaucoma.

Treatment. These dendrites have two separate etiologies. The more common variant occurs when mucus and devitalized epithelial cells adhere to the corneal surface. This type of dendrite responds to intensive lubrication, antimucolytic therapy, and topical steroids. The other etiology is secondary to swollen epithelial cells that are actively infected with the varicella-zoster virus. This etiology is more difficult to treat and requires topical antiviral therapy, often requiring combination therapy including topical trifluridine and an oral agent such as acyclovir or famciclovir. This variant is more likely to become chronic or recur quickly without long-term maintenance therapy. These complications are hard to treat and often recur years after the initial attack.

When to Refer. Because of the often severe complications associated with this type of keratitis, all patients with suspected herpes zoster keratitis need ophthalmologic evaluation.

KEY POINTS

- Causes foreign body sensation
- Frequently recurs
- Needs intensive lubrication

Microsporidia Keratitis

Presentation and Progression. Microsporidia are small obligate intracellular protozoan parasites that are an uncommon cause of infection in the cornea. Two species of microsporidia have been implicated as corneal pathogens in immunosuppressed patients: *Encephalitozoon cuniculi* and *E. hellem*. Each species causes a similar constellation of anterior segment changes. Microsporidia cause a diffuse superficial punctate epithelial keratitis that stains with fluorescein and appears similar to a severe dry eye. The keratitis progresses to involve the entire surface of the cornea. The disease may be unilateral initially but often involves both eyes with time. Patients' complaints are similar to other ocular surface diseases. Pain, especially of a foreign body sensation, is associated with redness, tearing, and photophobia. If the corneal punctate epithelial keratopathy is significant, then a loss of visual acuity also can be a presenting complaint.

Diagnosis. The fluorescein pattern can be subtle, especially when the entire corneal surface is involved, with a coarse punctate staining pattern. This is best evaluated with the aid of a slit lamp biomicroscopy. There is variable conjunctival injection, with both papillary and follicular reactions present. Preauricular and submandibular lymph nodes may be present. Evaluation and treatment are difficult, since the organism is difficult to culture, and may require a corneal scraping or biopsy for a definitive diagnosis. Gram's staining of corneal or conjunctival biopsy reveals gram-positive small oval intracytoplasmic spores located in the cytoplasm of epithelial cells.

Treatment. There is no definitive treatment for microsporidial corneal infections. Palliative treatment with intensive topical lubrication can give short-term relief of the symptoms, as in a dry-eyed patient. Various drug regimens have been utilized, including itraconazole (Sporanox, Janssen Pharmaceutica Inc.), fumagillin (Fumidil B, Mid-Continent Agrimarketing), oral albendazole (Albenza, SmithKline Beecham Pharmaceuticals), and propamidine isethionate (Brolene), with variable results.

When to Refer. Patients complaining of a dry eye syndrome who do not respond to topical lubrication should be evaluated in an ophthalmology setting.

KEY POINTS

- Very difficult to treat
- Palliative treatment only
- Use intensive lubrication

Corneal Ulcers

Presentation and Progression. Bacterial corneal ulcers do not appear to have an increased incidence in patients with poor cellular immunity. Common corneal pathogens such as the gram-positive *Staphylococcus epidermidis*, *Staphylococcus aureus*, α-hemolytic streptococci, and the gram-negative *Pseudomonas aeruginosa* are still the predominant bacteria found in HIV-infected patients. Opportunistic infections such as *Candida albicans* and uncommon bacterial ocular pathogens such as *Capnocytophaga* species, as well as rare viral corneal infections such CMV, occur with much greater frequency and severity than found in the normal population.

Diagnosis. Infectious corneal ulcers clinically appear similar in both immunosuppressed and immunocompetent patients. The lesions are white, with a hazy edge. There is an overlying epithelial ulceration that may be smaller than the stromal infiltrate and will stain intensely with topical fluorescein. The stroma has a halo of surrounding inflammatory cells that gives the involved cornea a ground-glass appearance. If the infectious organism is fungal, the main ulcer may have small satellite ulcers or infiltrates extending from the edge of the primary focus of infection. The eye is generally painful, erythematous, often with a ciliary flush pattern, photophobic, and tearing. There is an absence of associated preauricular adenopathy, as opposed to the enlarged lymph nodes seen with viral infections.

Natural History. Most corneal ulcers will respond to intensive topical antibiotics. As the ulcer heals, the patient's pain and photophobia will quickly resolve. If the ulcer is central, a corneal scar may form. Any loss of vision will be dependent on the size and location of the scar.

If the ulcer progresses while on treatment, progressive corneal thinning and possible perforation can occur. Severe loss of vision often follows corneal thinning because of either irregular astigmatism or corneal pannus formation.

Treatment. Prior to empiric treatment, the ulcer and conjunctiva should be cultured for definitive diagnosis. Aggressive corneal scraping used to culture the infection also helps to debride the infection and unroof the ulcer, which allows antibiotics better access to the site of infection. Broad-spectrum topical fortified antibiotic drops, often an aminoglycoside and cephalosporin, are applied frequently as the mainstay of treatment. The regimen is then tailored, based on the organism cultured and its antibiotic sensitivity profile. Bacterial infections usually respond well when on appropriate drug regimen. The patient should also use topical cycloplegic drops to help reduce photophobia induced by ciliary muscle spasm.

When the clinical response is poor, a polymicrobial infection may be present with a rare organism such as *Acanthamoeba* or a fungus. *C. albicans* and other even less common fungal corneal ulcers are treated after topical debridement, with a dilute solution of amphotericin B (Fungizone, Apothecon) or natamycin (Natacyn, Alcon Laboratories). Intravenous antiinfectives are generally not effective in corneal infections.

When to Refer. Patients who complain of photophobia, loss of vision, and chronic tearing, and who have corneal staining with fluorescein, should be evaluated in an ophthalmologic setting.

KEY POINTS

- All ulcers need culturing
- Initially treat with broad-spectrum topical antibiotics
- If the ulcer responds poorly, think fungal

Posterior Segment Complications

Noninfectious

AIDS Retinopathy

Presentation and Progression. Microvascular changes in the retina are the most common ophthalmic manifestation of the AIDS virus. Cotton-wool spots, retinal hemorrhages, and microaneurysm formation reflect the disruption of the normal retinal vascular architecture. These changes can occur individually or, more commonly, together. When they occur in the absence of other systemic or opportunistic diseases, the fundus picture is referred to as AIDS retinopathy.

Microaneurysms are tiny outpouchings of the small retinal arterioles. They appear as tiny red dots when viewed with the direct ophthalmoscope and are found in up to 100% of AIDS patients when evaluated with fluorescein angiography. The microaneurysm can leak fluid and protein, leading to exudate formation. The exudate extends in a centrifugal manner from the central microaneurysm and is referred to as a circinate exudate, reflecting its circular appearance. The microaneurysm can also leak blood, causing retinal hemorrhages. The presence of the exudates and hemorrhages indicates a breach of the blood-retinal barrier.

Cotton-wool spots are another very common ophthalmic manifestation of the AIDS virus and are found in up to 50% of patients when evaluated by direct ophthalmoscopy. The cotton-wool spots are small microinfarctions of the retinal nerve fiber layer and are nonspecific in nature. The cotton-wool spots histologically are composed of cytoid bodies, which are the swollen axons of retinal ganglion cells found in the nerve fiber layer. Clinically they appear as small, irregular-shaped patches that are a bright white and unchanging in size. The edges of the cotton-wool spots are indistinct. They are located in the posterior pole of the retina and surrounding the optic nerve and will obscure underlying blood vessels. The spots will slowly fade in 6 to 10 weeks without any treatment. After the spots fade, the retina resumes its normal coloration but will be subtly thinner and will develop a dulling of its normal reflectiveness. Although generally asymptomatic, cotton-wool spots occasionally produce a small scotoma that can be particularly annoying when located close to fixation.

Retinal hemorrhages can occur both deep in the retina and near the inner surface. Hemorrhages in the plexiform layer (deep) assume a dot or blot configuration. Those in the inner retina (superficial) conform to the striations of the nerve fiber layer and appear flame-shaped. The more superficial hemorrhages will obscure any underlying blood vessels. Roth's spots, the white-centered hemorrhages described as occurring in subacute bacterial endocarditis, leukemia, and diabetes, can also occur in AIDS retinopathy without signifying a septic embolus.

Diagnosis. The retinal microvasculopathy found in AIDS patients is nonspecific in nature, with a wide differential diagnosis associated with each type of vasculopathy. Diseases that commonly cause cotton-wool spots and retinal hemorrhages in the normal patient population include diabetes mellitus, hypertension, severe anemia, and various collagen vascular diseases, especially systemic lupus erythematosus. Early in their course, opportunistic infections such as CMV retinitis, syphilitic chorioretinitis, and early fungal chorioretinitis can mimic AIDS vasculopathy. They also must be excluded before the diagnosis is finalized. Because the majority of opportunistic infections will progress over several weeks while the AIDS vasculopathy usually is stationary, serial examinations and photographs of suspicious lesions can be helpful in determining the etiology of the vascular changes.

Treatment. AIDS microvasculopathy is generally self-limited and is rarely symptomatic. There is no treatment indicated unless retinal edema threatens the macula. The edema can be treated by applying laser photocoagulation burns to cauterize the leaking blood vessels in a manner similar to that utilized to treat diabetic retinopathy.

When to Refer. This is a self-limiting disease and rarely causes significant vision loss. Patients need only reassurance that their eye findings are common and self-limiting. Cotton-wool spots that progressively enlarge over time may actually be CMV retinitis. These patients need ophthalmic evaluation.

KEY POINTS

- Very common
- Rarely sight threatening
- If progresses, rule out CMV retinitis

Papilledema

Presentation and Progression. Papilledema, or optic nerve edema, is caused by intracranial hypertension. The increase in intracranial pressure can be caused by an intracranial mass lesion, systemic malignant hypertension, and infectious meningitis, or it can be idiopathic. Patients with papilledema rarely complain of visual symptoms or of ocular pain. Vision loss is rare until the swelling has become chronic, causing the late development of optic atrophy. The papilledema is often found fortuitously or during the work-up of other medical conditions.

Diagnosis. The optic nerve head appears swollen and hyperemic, and has blurred margins. There is peripapillary nerve fiber layer edema and obscuration of the origin of the large retinal blood vessels. The large central veins lack spontaneous venous pulsations, which are also absent in up to 20% of the normal population.

In immunosuppressed patients, the medical evaluation must rule out intracranial opportunistic infections. Cryptococcal meningitis and intracranial toxoplasmosis are the more frequently found infectious causes of papilledema. Lymphomas, metastatic tumors, and primary central nervous system (CNS) tumors account for the majority of neoplastic causes of papilledema. Systemic hypertension and idiopathic intracranial hypertension are rare causes of papilledema in AIDS patients.

The differential diagnosis of optic nerve edema includes infectious or inflammatory optic neuropathy, drusen of the optic nerve, diabetic papillopathy, and anterior ischemic optic neuritis. These conditions share elevation of the optic nerve head but can be differentiated by their associated symptoms of pain, by loss of vision, and by signs including the absence of hyperemia or the presence of an afferent pupillary defect. The usual visual field defect found with acute papilledema is enlargement of the blind spot. In contrast, patients with inflammatory optic neuropathies have nerve fiber layer defects that can appear as altitudinal and arcuate visual field defects.

Natural History. When the underlying condition is treated, few if any permanent sequelae will occur. If the papilledema becomes chronic, optic atrophy will occur. The patient's vision will slowly decrease. The visual fields will progress from normal or only an enlarged blind spot to nerve fiber defects and progressive constriction. These changes will become permanent over time.

Treatment. The treatment of papilledema is treatment of the underlying cause. Once the etiology has been diagnosed and treated, the edema will slowly resolve over several days to weeks. Once the edema resolves, the visual field defects may reverse, and there is often little permanent visual loss. If the papilledema is longstanding, the optic nerve may become atrophic, with permanent bilateral vision loss. The visual field loss is often of severe constriction, with preservation of the central field yielding good central visual acuity.

KEY POINTS

⊃ Must rule out malignant hypertension, mass, or infectious causes
⊃ Usually asymptomatic
⊃ Visual defects resolve with early treatment

Optic Nerve Atrophy

Presentation and Progression. Optic nerve atrophy in immunosuppressed patients is either primary or secondary to an extraocular cause. The patient with optic nerve atrophy will have a decrease in visual acuity, red color desaturation, dyschromatopsia, decrease in night vision, and variable visual field loss. If the atrophy is asymmetric, there may be an afferent pupillary defect.

Diagnosis. Optic nerve atrophy appears as global or sectorial optic nerve pallor. The nerve head is flat, and in severe cases appears chalk white.

Natural History. The cause of primary optic nerve atrophy in HIV-infected patients is unknown. Possible causes include direct infection by the HIV virus, decrease in the blood supply to the optic nerve, and nutritional deficiency. Infectious etiologies of optic neuritis include viral infections including varicella-zoster virus, herpes simplex virus, and CMV. Syphilis and fungal infections with *Cryptococcus neoformans* are also a major cause of optic neuritis in immunosuppressed patients.

Treatment. After the appropriate treatment of the underlying infection, any residual optic nerve damage is irreversible. If there is an inflammatory component to the neuritis and the infection has been adequately treated, a careful trial of systemic steroids can be utilized in an attempt to decrease the ultimate vision loss.

KEY POINTS

⊃ Treat underlying cause, if any
⊃ Most cases are idiopathic
⊃ Vision loss can vary and is generally permanent

Infectious

Herpesvirus-Associated Retinitis. The herpes family of viruses causes the vast majority of opportunistic retinal infections. The subtypes that have been implicated in ocular diseases include CMV, herpes simplex virus, and varicella-zoster virus. The viruses are similar in their genetic composition, but the spectrum of diseases they cause is varied, with some overlap in rare cases. The appearance and clinical behavior of each virus can also differ as the level of immunosuppression increases.

Cytomegalovirus Retinitis

Presentation and Progression. CMV is a hematogenously disseminated virus of the Herpesviridae family. It is a double-stranded DNA virus that causes the most common intraocular infection. CMV retinitis is an AIDS-defining diagnosis. CMV causes a full-thickness coagulative necrosis of the retina, leading to a slowly expanding scotoma that, left untreated, will ultimately lead to irreversible loss of retinal tissue and total blindness. CMV is generally found in patients who are profoundly immunodeficient. It is rarely a cause of retinitis when a patient's CD4+ T cell count is above 200 cells/mm^3 and is more commonly found in those patients whose CD4+ T cell counts have fallen below 50 cells/mm^3. A poorer ultimate visual prognosis and higher mortality are associated with positive CMV blood cultures at the time of diagnosis, especially when the blood cultures remain positive after treatment has begun. Prior to the use of HAART, the incidence of CMV retinitis was as high as 45% in HIV-infected patients at the time of their death. Since the advent of HAART, and the partial reconstitution of patients' immune function, the incidence of newly diagnosed CMV retinitis has fallen dramatically.

The retinal areas that are initially infected are perivascular. As the CMV proliferates, it infects adjacent cells, spreading centrifugally from the original site. The infected regions can be present anywhere in the retina and, if the presenting lesion is in the retinal periphery, are not easily seen on direct ophthalmoscopic examination and may be entirely asymptomatic. These lesions can occur unilaterally or bilaterally. Patients' symptoms often include new, changed, or more numerous floaters, photopsias, and scotomas; dimming sight; and blurred vision. They rarely complain of pain, redness, discharge, or photophobia.

Histologic evaluation of infected retinas reveals full-thickness coagulative necrosis of the retina, as well as of the retinal pigment epithelium (RPE), leaving the tissue severely disorganized. There is acute and chronic granulomatous inflammation present in the retina, RPE, and eventually choroid.

The infected cells have an "owl's eye" appearance secondary to intranuclear viral inclusion bodies surrounded by a clear zone. The enlargement of the cells caused by the intranuclear and intracytoplasmic inclusion bodies is the origin of the name, CMV.

Diagnosis. The initial areas of retinitis most often appear as a patch of granular whitened retina that obscures small-caliber underlying blood vessels. The patches can be solitary or multifocal. If the patch is small, it appears similar to a small cotton-wool spot. Unlike a typical cotton-wool spot, which is a microinfarction of the nerve fiber layer that will fade over time, the CMV patch will enlarge at the rate of 500 to 750 μm per week. As the viral retinitis spreads, it develops areas containing dot/blot and flame-shaped hemorrhages. When the retinitis is in the central retina, there is intense white to grayish-white retinal opacification along the entire leading edge or border of the infected area. This is referred to as a "brush fire" border. In cases in which the retinitis originates in the retinal periphery, it is subtler in appearance and may look like grouped small white dots. As the infection spreads, the active leading border remains slightly thickened and white, while the necrotic retina trailing the leading edge loses its white color as it thins and atrophies. The leading edge may have small white satellite lesions preceding the more obvious border, interspersed with normal-appearing retina. The atrophic retina is mottled in appearance, with areas of hyperpigmentation and hypopigmentation. In patients with light retinal pigmentation the atrophic areas are difficult to detect on casual examination. The blood vessels in the atrophic areas often become narrowed and sclerotic and can have a white perivascular sheathing, especially vessels located near the posterior pole. In disseminated cases the retinal vascular tree is heavily sheathed, an appearance referred to as frosted angiitis. There is little to no overlying vitreous reaction, leaving an excellent view of the posterior pole. The anterior chamber will occasionally develop a mild nongranulomatous reaction. When the reaction does occur, fine stellate precipitates can collect on the corneal endothelium. The keratoprecipitates are generally heaviest in the periphery, do not always resolve after the iritis has been adequately treated, and appear to yellow with time. These inflammatory aggregations are best seen with a slit lamp examination.

Natural History. Once a diagnosis of CMV retinitis has been made, careful retinal drawings or, preferably, fundus photography is performed during the initial ophthalmologic examination. These are used to establish a baseline for the area of necrosis. Subsequent eye examinations are then compared with the photographs to determine if the virus has stopped spreading, comparing location of the leading borders in relation to blood vessels and other landmarks documented on prior examinations. Careful monthly evaluations and serial photography are needed to determine if the retinitis has reactivated. Breakthrough retinitis can be difficult to diagnose because the retinitis is often less impressive while on treatment and tends to creep along without the dramatic retinal whitening and its associated hemorrhages that are seen in primary infections. At times the border appears to advance when compared with blood vessel landmarks, without any apparent activity other than pigment changes seen as the retina atrophies.

When there are large areas of atrophic retina, the thinned retina is prone to develop holes, or breaks, that lead to rhegmatogenous retinal detachments. The detachment rate increases with more peripherally located disease and with larger areas of necrosis. Laser photocoagulation has been successfully used to treat macula-attached retinal detachments by walling off the necrotic retina from the remainder of the viable retina. When the macula is detached, the repair is more difficult to perform. The repair may require multiple intraocular surgical procedures including vitrectomy with or without scleral buckling, and the use of silicone oil to tamponade the friable retina against the choroid. Unlike retinal detachment repairs in immunocompetent patients, the silicone oil must remain in the vitreous cavity indefinitely in most AIDS patients or the detachment can recur. Although sight preserving, the oil will shift the refractive state of the eye in the hyperopic direction, necessitating the use of contact lenses. Other complications of silicone oil usage include premature posterior subcapsular cataracts, glaucoma, corneal decompensation, and oil-induced optic atrophy. Many of these complications require additional surgical procedures to help maintain useful vision.

Treatment. The treatment of CMV retinitis can be administered intravenously, orally, or locally via repeated intravitreal injection or a surgically implanted reservoir device (Table 15-1). Induction therapy is generally with intravenous administration of ganciclovir (Cytovene, Roche Laboratories) or foscarnet twice daily for 2 weeks. Cidofovir is an alternative that is given only once weekly for 2 weeks. Because of cidofovir's nephrotoxicity it is also given with extensive intravenous hydration and with probenecid. Valganciclovir, an oral alternative, has also been used for induction. Whatever the induction therapy, long-term maintenance therapy (suppression) is required as long as the CD4+ cell count remains low. When the count stays above 100 to 150 cells/mm^3 for 3 to 6 months most authorities feel comfortable in discontinuing the suppressive treatment. An alternative route of administration for either ganciclovir or foscarnet is repeated intravitreal injection. This is rarely used for long-term maintenance because of the risk of infection, vitreal hemorrhage, and retinal detachment, and because of the difficulty in patient compliance with follow-up. Cidofovir, although very effective in the treatment of CMV via intravitreal injections, has a very narrow therapeutic window and is less commonly used intravitreally than ganciclovir or foscarnet. A long-term intraocular depot device called a Vitrasert, containing an 8-month supply of ganciclovir, is another alternative that can be used instead of daily intravenous maintenance. The small depot device consists of a semipermeable membrane made of polyvinyl alcohol and ethylvinyl alcohol surrounding a pellet of ganciclovir. This depot device allows for the controlled delivery of 1 μg per hour of ganciclovir directly into the vitreous cavity. The steady release of ganciclovir theoretically might prevent drug resistance from emerging because the drug trough, seen with an intermittent intravenous dosing schedule, is avoided. The Vitrasert should be replaced regularly to prevent breakthrough retinitis as the depot's supply of ganciclovir is exhausted. A drawback to isolated local therapy is the absence of prophylaxis to the fellow eye and other extraocular sites afforded by systemic treatment. This can be ameliorated by the concomitant use of oral ganciclovir in addition to the Vitrasert.

If drug resistance emerges, allowing the CMV to reactivate, reinduction with the same medication followed by higher maintenance dosing can be tried as the initial treatment

TABLE 15-1
Treatment for Cytomegalovirus Retinitis

Medication	Routes of administration	Mechanism of action	Dosing schedule	Systemic side effects
Ganciclovir	Intravenous, oral	Acyclic Nucleoside antiviral inhibits viral DNA polymerase	5 mg/kg bid induction; 5 mg/kg daily maintenance	Reversible bone marrow toxicity
	Intravitreal		0.1 ml of 2 mg/ml concentration solution weekly	Lack of extraocular protection
	Vitrasert			Lack of extraocular protection Needs replacement
Foscarnet	Intravenous	Inhibits viral DNA polymerase	90 mg/kg bid induction 90-120 mg/kg maintenance	Hypocalcemia, hypophosphatemia and hyperphosphatemia, renal failure
	Intravitreal		1,200 μg weekly	
Cidofovir	Intravenous	Nucleotide analogue inhibits viral DNA polymerase	5 mg/kg cidofovir for 2 weeks induction, with 2 g probenecid 3 hr prior to infusion and 1 g 2 hr after; then every 2 weeks as maintenance	Nephrotoxicity, bone marrow suppression
Fomivirsen	Intravitreal	RNA antisense	330 μg biweekly as induction, then monthly for maintenance	Iritis, vitritis

strategy. If the CMV does not respond to the reinduction dosing, a different medication is substituted. When a patient's CMV retinitis is resistant to individual medications, a trial of combination therapy with ganciclovir and foscarnet can be employed. This is limited in cases when cross-resistance between drugs is encountered, especially between ganciclovir and cidofovir.

Fomivirsen is the initial drug of a novel class of anti-CMV drugs, the anti-sense RNA inhibitors, and is an alternative to ganciclovir, foscarnet, and cidofovir. Fomivirsen is solely administered intravitreally. The dosing schedule of one injection every 2 weeks as an induction period followed by an injection only monthly makes local therapy with this drug less burdensome for the patient.

After the initial diagnosis, monthly follow-up visits and treatment with fundus photography are necessary to detect treatment failures or breakthrough retinitis. It is common for minimal progression to occur as an infected retina that appeared normal at the initial examination becomes clinically infected. This initial progression is not a sign of drug resistance and should not be cause for reinduction with the same drug or changing to a second drug. If on later examinations additional retina is lost, the drug regimen should be reevaluated. Most patients will have a breakthrough of active retinitis within 3 months and subsequent breakthroughs at shorter intervals. Options include reinduction with a higher maintenance dosage or switching to a second-line medication. A short trial of intravitreal injected ganciclovir or foscarnet can, by increasing the local drug level, help differentiate between suboptimal dosing and true drug resistance as the cause of the reactivation.

If a patient's immune function responds well to HAART and the CD4+ T cell count rises 100 cells/mm³ over its prior baseline level and maintains this higher level for 3 consecutive months, the surveillance visit interval can be lengthened. As mentioned above, withdrawal of therapy is a potential option with improved immune status. The increase in CD4+ T cell should be sustained and the CMV retinitis quiescent for at least 3 months prior to any attempt at treatment reduction. These patients must be followed closely to detect immune system regression and CMV reactivation before the loss of additional retina occurs. If the retinitis threatens the macula or the optic nerve or involves the remaining eye of a one-eyed patient, great caution must be exercised before treatment is withdrawn.

When to Refer. Patients will require regular ophthalmic examinations to evaluate treatment efficacy and breakthroughs. In addition, the complexity and toxicity of the treatment options make referral to a specialist skilled in the use of these drugs mandatory.

KEY POINTS

- Early CMV appears similar to cotton-wool spots
- May be unifocal or multifocal
- Occurs with severe immunodeficiency

Acute Retinal Necrosis

Presentation and Progression. Varicella-zoster and herpes simplex viruses each can cause several types of viral retinitis. The most commonly encountered infection is acute retinal necrosis, which can be either unilateral (ARN) or bilateral (BARN) and can occur either simultaneously or sequentially. It can occur rarely in a patient who is immunocompromised and is more common when a patient's immune system is intact. Patients will complain of blurred vision, floaters, and, when there is significant anterior uveitis present, variable pain and photophobia. If the patient's immune system can muster an inflammatory response, an anterior granulomatous or nongranulomatous iridocyclitis often occurs.

Diagnosis. The initial presenting lesions appear in the peripheral retina as multifocal areas of full-thickness retinal necrosis that coalesce to form diffuse, ever-enlarging, white, edematous plaques. These patches then progress in a very rapid fashion posteriorly toward the macula. There is a variable amount of overlying vitritis, which is inversely proportional to the level of immunosuppression and can be severe, when the patient is immunocompetent. The necrotic retina appears whitened, as in CMV retinitis, but the advancing border lacks the granular appearance of CMV and can be obscured by the overlying cellular reaction. There is significantly less hemorrhaging present in the area of retinitis. An occlusive vasculitis of the arterioles and venules both in the retina and the choroid leaves the blood vessels with an early inflammatory sheathing and later narrowing. As the leading edge of the infection progresses toward the macula, the trailing retina atrophies and thins. The thinned retina is prone to retinal tears and detachments. If treatment is not instituted quickly, the entire retina can be lost to infection in only 1 or 2 weeks. Even with prompt treatment there is a high incidence of retinal detachment and permanent loss of vision.

Treatment. Successful treatment of acute retinal necrosis depends on prompt diagnosis and the administration of high-dose intravenous acyclovir. The initial dosing is generally started at 10 mg/kg and is adjusted based on clinical response. Once clinical efficacy has been demonstrated, prolonged oral acyclovir or valacyclovir is used to prevent recurrent disease. The patient must be aware of the danger of reactivation of the retinitis even on oral therapy, especially during the first 6 weeks of maintenance treatment. If reactivation does occur, resumption of intravenous therapy is necessary, often at a higher dose, to prevent total vision loss.

When to Refer. Because the retinitis progresses rapidly, urgent diagnosis and institution of the appropriate antiviral treatment are essential.

KEY POINTS

- Rapidly progressive
- Needs lifelong treatment
- High risk of retinal detachment

Varicella-Zoster Retinitis

Presentation and Progression. Varicella-zoster retinitis appears similar ophthalmoscopically to acute retinal necrosis, but the initial focus of infection is located in the macular region and is found predominantly in patients with AIDS. Due to the central location of retinitis, severe vision loss occurs early in the disease, even with prompt treatment. Patients at risk often have a recent history of cutaneous herpes zoster. The zoster does not have to be present in the typical V1 or V2 dermatomal distribution of herpes zoster ophthalmicus.

Diagnosis. The lesions can be either multifocal or solitary and will progress very rapidly. They appear deep in the retina and lack the typical overlying vitritis seen with acute retinal necrosis. The obliterative vasculitis is also absent early in the course of varicella-zoster retinitis, whereas severe arteriolitis is associated with acute retinal necrosis. Later, as the disease continues its progression, all layers of the retina will opacify and thicken. The thickened necrotic retina can give the appearance of a "cherry red spot" similar to that seen in a central retinal artery occlusion. Retinal detachment, as a late complication, is less commonly seen than with acute retinal necrosis but still can occur within several months of the diagnosis. The infection spreads peripherally rather than centrally, although it progresses very quickly. The optic nerve is commonly affected, appearing either pale or hyperemic initially, then later white and atrophic.

Natural History. Patients with varicella-zoster retinitis complain of loss of central vision. The loss is rapid and is not associated with pain, photophobia, or redness. The lack of pain is because of the relative sparing of the anterior segment of the eye.

Treatment. Treatment of the varicella-zoster virus–induced retinitis yields variable visual outcomes that are generally poor. Many different treatment regimens have been tried, including the use of intravenous acyclovir, ganciclovir, and foscarnet. The drugs have been used alone or in various combinations. Steroids, given to decrease inflammation, are not effective, since they will further reduce already-compromised cellular immunity of HIV-infected patients. Despite chemotherapeutic intervention to control the retinitis and various surgical procedures to repair the commonly found retinal detachments, the ultimate visual prognosis is grim, with progression to no light perception in as many as 70% of involved eyes.

Progressive Outer Retinal Necrosis

Presentation and Progression. A second variant of herpetic virus–associated retinal necrosis is PORN, which can be either unilateral or, more commonly, bilateral. As with varicella-zoster retinitis, there is often a temporal relationship with a recent bout of zoster dermatitis. The onset of the PORN also has been reported to follow the onset of varicella-zoster virus–induced optic neuritis.

Diagnosis and Natural History. This type of progressive retinitis is initially limited to the outer retinal layers and lacks the inflammatory response seen with the full-thickness variants. The presenting lesions are white, patchy, and multifocal. The patches are located in the peripheral and midperipheral retina, while initially sparing the central retina. The opacities become confluent with time and then spread centrally. The borders of each lesion lack the granular appearance typical of CMV retinitis. The optic nerve can appear hyperemic and swollen during the acute phase and later white and atrophic in end-stage disease. The retinal vasculature is spared, and there is little to no vitreous inflammation and only occasional anterior segment inflammation. Later in the course of PORN, the blood vessels atrophy and the retinitis becomes full-thickness and ultimately atrophies. The severely atrophic retina is thinned and may contain multiple holes. Late complications include severe vision loss down to a level of no light perception. There is a high incidence of retinal detachment, with all the typical difficulties in repair as seen with CMV retinitis.

Treatment. As with varicella-zoster retinitis, the treatment of PORN has yielded less than satisfactory visual results. The same medications used in varicella-zoster retinitis have been used, with the similar poor visual outcomes. This may be because of a delay in diagnosis and treatment in a peripheral retinal presentation, as well as poor viral response in the presence of extremely suppressed immune function. An additional theory as to why there may be a poor viral response relates to the issue of prior subtherapeutic dosages of acyclovir used for maintenance in patients with a history of dermatomal zoster. The prolonged use of acyclovir may predispose these patients to develop resistant strains of varicella-zoster.

KEY POINTS

⊃ Early peripheral retinal involvement
⊃ Little overlying inflammation
⊃ Poor visual prognosis

Toxoplasmosis

Presentation and Progression. Toxoplasmosis is caused by *T. gondii,* an intracellular protozoan that is one of the most common opportunistic organisms infecting the CNS in immunocompromised patients and is the leading cause of retinal infections in immunocompetent patients. However, when compared with virus-associated retinopathies, it is a relatively uncommon cause of ocular disease in patients with AIDS. The disease is transmitted congenitally from an infected mother to her fetus or via ingestion of the encysted form of *T. gondii.* Active disease is derived when the cysts release the trophozoite form. In immunocompromised patients acute ocular disease can be from reactivation of latent infection or from newly acquired infection. Because of the severe vitreous inflammation, patients complain of a large increase in vitreous floaters. As the inflammation builds, visual acuity decreases, often to very low levels. Severe photophobia and redness accompany the vision loss.

The differential diagnosis of toxoplasmosis retinochoroiditis includes CMV, acute retinal necrosis, PORN, syphilitic retinitis, and branch arterial occlusion. There have been case reports of simultaneous infection with CMV and toxoplasmosis. Tissue is rarely available for evaluation. Serologic testing is generally nondiagnostic. The definitive diagnosis is made by the clinical response to treatment.

Diagnosis. Primary ocular infections appear similar to satellite lesions and can be very large in size. The retinal lesion may have associated retinal vascular sheathing. There are few, if any, retinal hemorrhages located in the area of necrosis. Less common presentations have been reported with either the inner retina or outer retina preferentially involved or with small punctate outer retinal lesions. The retinitis is often associated with a variable amount of overlying vitreous infiltration. There is less or no vitreous reaction when the infection is limited to the outer retina or when the patient's immune status cannot mount a satisfactory response to the trophozoites. On direct ophthalmoscopic examination, the view of the posterior pole is often blurred because of the vitritis. The "headlight in the fog" sign occurs when the white retinal lesion is almost entirely obscured by an intense vitritis. A spillover anterior chamber iridocyclitis commonly occurs. It can appear either granulomatous or nongranulomatous when evaluated by biomicroscopy.

Natural History. Congenitally acquired toxoplasmosis often leaves an isolated scar in the macula region of the retina but can be associated with additional lesions in the central, midperipheral, and peripheral retina of either eye. Active toxoplasmosis begins when the trophozoite stage of *T. gondii* is released from the inactive cyst form, causing a reactivation of the retinitis at the edge of the scar. The satellite lesion appears as an edematous tan to creamy white area jutting into the normal retina from the edge of the atrophic scar. The satellite lesion can vary in size and will continue to enlarge if not adequately treated in immunocompromised patients. The atrophic retina appears as full-thickness scar with loss of the choroid, leaving a clear view of the sclera centrally. There is variable hyperpigmentation of the border, leaving a sharp demarcation line between normal retina and the scar. The scar is variable in size but is often round in shape.

Treatment. When patients have an intact immune system, the decision to treat toxoplasmosis depends on the location of the lesion and the severity of the vision loss. Treatment is indicated when the macula or the optic nerve is threatened or if the vision is severely affected. Peripheral lesions can be observed without treatment without symptomatic loss of vision. Patients with a compromised immune system require treatment for all lesions to prevent progressive involvement of the entire retina.

The treatment of toxoplasmosis in both immunocompetent and immunocompromised patients is similar. A combination of pyrimethamine and a sulfonamide, usually sulfadiazine, is usually employed as first line therapy. Other medications used include clindamycin, tetracycline, and trimethoprim-sulfamethoxazole. If there is a threat to the macula or a severe vitritis, a short course of oral steroids can be administered concomitantly. Steroids are less commonly needed in immunocompromised patients, whose inflammatory response is already diminished. None of these therapies will cure the patient of all the encapsulated cysts. Lifelong maintenance therapy is utilized to prevent recurrent retinochoroiditis. Finally, because toxoplasmosis in the AIDS patient is more likely to be a new infection rather than a reactivation, a systemic evaluation for other foci of infection is mandatory.

When to Refer. Patients who present with vision loss and photophobia or a large increase in floaters should have a dilated fundus examination by an ophthalmologist.

KEY POINTS

⊃ Patients have a rapid increase in vitreous floaters
⊃ Severe loss of vision
⊃ Can be a primary infection or a reactivation of latent disease

Syphilitic Retinitis

Presentation and Progression. *T. pallidum* is a spirochete that causes ocular infections that clinically mimic many different types of ophthalmic diseases. It can affect all parts of the anterior and posterior segments of the eye. In immunosuppressed patients, syphilis presents with disseminated inflammation including anterior uveitis, vitritis, optic neuritis, and retinitis. Syphilis tends to be more aggressive, with a higher likelihood of retinitis and neurosyphilis with lowered immunity. Patients often present with painful loss of vision and photophobia. The etiology of the pain can be either an anterior uveitis or a retrobulbar optic neuritis. The pain ranges from moderate to severe in intensity. The loss of vision can also have multiple causes, including vitritis, retinitis, or optic neuritis.

Diagnosis. The diagnosis of ocular syphilitic manifestations requires a high degree of suspicion and is based on appropriate positive serologic titers. A positive rapid plasma reagin (RPR) when combined with either a confirmatory positive microhemagglutination-*T. pallidum* (MHA-TP) or fluorescent treponemal antibody-absorbed (FTA-abs) test is indicative of *T. pallidum* infection. It is common for ocular manifestations of syphilis to have accompanying mucocutaneous lesions characteristic of secondary syphilis.

Natural History. Syphilitic-induced uveitis is generally granulomatous in nature, with precipitates often coating the cornea and the adhesions forming between the iris and lens (posterior synechiae). The uveitis is associated with mild papillary conjunctivitis, often with a ciliary flush pattern. When the anterior segment is severely inflamed, the intraocular pressure can rise, causing uveitic glaucoma. This type of inflammation appears very similar to that seen with sarcoidosis, tuberculosis, and Wegener's granulomatosis. When the iritis is mild, the keratoprecipitates are minimal to absent and the inflammation appears nongranulomatous. The pupil in untreated patients becomes constricted and unreactive to direct illumination but remains reactive to accommodation, which is the Argyll Robertson pupil. The retinitis initially appears as a pale yellow area of deep retinal necrosis. The blood vessels are sheathed with an inflammatory exudate. The necrotic retina can be associated with exudates in the macular area. Because of the radial alignment of the nerve fiber layer, the exudates often form a macular star pattern. A cellular reaction, possibly severe, may develop in the vitreous body. If the optic nerve head is involved, indicating a neuroretinitis, it may become edematous and erythematous, resembling papilledema, but it may also appear normal if the process is retrobulbar. After treatment, the involved retina will assume a "salt and pepper" appearance and the optic nerve will become atrophic and pale.

Treatment. Patients are treated with a neurosyphilis drug regimen. High-dose intravenous aqueous penicillin G is the drug of choice. In penicillin-allergic patients some experts desensitize to penicillin and others use doxycycline. Treatment is for 10 to 14 days. Posttreatment surveillance RPR titers should be evaluated every 3 months to ensure adequate drug response.

KEY POINTS

⊃ Can mimic many other ocular diseases
⊃ Can affect all portions of the eye

Mycobacterium avium *Complex*

Presentation and Progression. MAC is a common systemic bacterial infection in patients with AIDS but it is a very rare intraocular pathogen. It causes a choroiditis characterized by small whitish-yellow lesions. The lesions can either be multifocal or appear as a solitary, slightly raised nodule.

Diagnosis and Natural History. The plaques slowly enlarge over time and do not have an overlying vitritis. Histologic evaluation of the nodules reveals them to be choroidal or retinal granulomas. The lesions will involute with systemic treatment of the atypical mycobacterial infection and will leave an area of retinal depigmentation overlying the affected choroid.

Treatment. The treatment of MAC-induced choroiditis is similar to other treatments for disseminated MAC infections. Clarithromycin or azithromycin plus ethambutol are the basic drugs. Occasionally others are added. The treatment is long term and, in the absence of immune system reconstitution, requires chronic maintenance therapy.

KEY POINTS

⊃ Minimal symptoms
⊃ Needs long-term systemic treatment

Pneumocystis carinii

Presentation and Progression. *P. carinii* is the most common opportunistic infection in patients with AIDS and is often the AIDS-defining diagnosis. The lung is the most common site of *P. carinii* infection. It rarely causes intraocular disease.

Those at risk for *P. carinii* choroiditis are severely immunocompromised patients with a prior history of *P. carinii* pneumonia infection and low CD4+ T cell counts who are taking monthly inhaled pentamidine prophylaxis or are not on any antipneumocystis treatment. Patients on systemic prophylaxis appear to be less at risk. Patients generally are without visual complaints and only occasionally complain of mild distortions to their vision.

Diagnosis. The clinical appearance of the choroiditis is of solitary or, more commonly, multiple round, golden-yellow to yellow-white irregular plaques. The plaques are slightly elevated and are of variable size. The retina often appears normal, but it may have pigment epithelial mottling.

Natural History. When the infection is chronic, the lesions calcify and may have scant associated hemorrhages. Once the choroidal infection is treated, the lesions involute and leave a pigmented scar.

Treatment. Because ocular *P. carinii* is a sign of disseminated systemic disease, the treatment is also systemic with trimethoprim-sulfamethoxazole, intravenous pentamidine isethionate, or dapsone/trimethoprim. The plaques respond slowly to treatment, leaving behind variable pigmentary disturbances of the retina. Once treated, the patient will need prolonged systemic oral medications because of the high recurrence rate with inhaled pentamidine prophylaxis alone. Although it is likely that immune reconstitution would eliminate the need for chronic treatment, there is not enough experience with this rare infection to recommend this.

KEY POINTS

⊃ Slowly enlarging asymptomatic yellow retinal plaques
⊃ Associated with inhaled pentamidine
⊃ Requires prolonged systemic treatment

Fungal Chorioretinitis

Presentation and Progression. *C. albicans, Histoplasma capsulatum, Aspergillus fumigatus, Fusarium* species, *Sporothrix schenckii, Bipolaris hawaiiensis,* and *C. neoformans* have all been rarely implicated as a cause of fungal endophthalmitis. *C. albicans* is the most common intraocular fungal pathogen. This can be seen in both immunocompetent and immunosuppressed patients and is generally related to an infected intravenous catheter. In most fungal endophthalmitis, the fungi spread via a hematogenous route and are a sign of disseminated disease. A second route of infection is possible in cryptococcal meningitis. When the fungi track along the subarachnoid space, they then can follow along the path of the optic nerve into the posterior segment of the eye.

Patients will complain of blurred vision, scotomas, and distorted vision early in the infection, with increasingly severe vision loss as the fungi spread. They may also complain of an increased number of floaters or photophobia with increasing vitreous cellular reaction.

Diagnosis. The anterior segment is variably injected, with mild to moderate anterior cellular reaction. Precipitates are found on the endothelium of the cornea. The retinal lesions are pale yellow to creamy white and appear initially in the outer layers of the retina. As the infection progresses, the entire thickness of the retina will become involved. The borders appear distinct with cryptococcosis and histoplasmosis, but are fluffy with candidal infections. There is minimal retinal hemorrhaging and a variable amount of vitritis, which can range from nearly absent to severe. After treatment, a well-circumscribed chorioretinal scar forms.

Natural History. Light microscopic evaluation reveals yeast cells in the choroid. They are located in the perivascular spaces and in the lumens of choroidal blood vessels. A similar pattern is seen in the retina. The yeast cells are phagocytized by macrophages and are seen with an associated lymphocytic infiltrate.

Treatment. Treatment with intravenous and intravitreal amphotericin B for prolonged periods may be combined with a diagnostic and/or therapeutic vitrectomy. Prolonged posttreatment prophylaxis is generally necessary to prevent a relapse.

KEY POINTS

⊃ Initial symptoms of increased floaters, late vision loss
⊃ May be associated with conjunctivitis
⊃ May need both intravitreal and intravenous treatment

SUGGESTED READINGS

Clinical vs photographic assessment of treatment of cytomegalovirus retinitis. Foscarnet-Ganciclovir Cytomegalovirus Retinitis Trial Report 8. Studies of Ocular Complications of AIDS Research Group, AIDS Clinical Trials Group, *Arch Ophthalmol* 114(7): 848-855, 1996.

Cochereau-Massin I et al: Ocular toxoplasmosis in human immunodeficiency virus–infected patients, *Am J Ophthalmol* 114(2): 130-135, 1992.

Jabs DA et al: Discontinuing anticytomegalovirus therapy in patients with immune reconstitution after combination antiretroviral therapy, *Am J Ophthalmol* 126(6):817-822, 1998.

Karavellas MP et al: Immune recovery vitritis associated with inactive cytomegalovirus retinitis: a new syndrome, *Arch Ophthalmol* 116(2):169-175, 1998.

Kuppermann BD et al: Clinical and histopathologic study of varicella zoster virus retinitis in patients with the acquired immunodeficiency syndrome, *Am J Ophthalmol* 118(5):589-600, 1994.

Kuppermann BD et al: Correlation between CD4+ counts and prevalence of cytomegalovirus retinitis and human immunodeficiency virus–related noninfectious retinal vasculopathy in patients with acquired immunodeficiency syndrome, *Am J Ophthalmol* 115(5):575-582, 1993.

McLeish WM et al: The ocular manifestations of syphilis in the human immunodeficiency virus type 1–infected host, *Ophthalmology* 97(2):196-203, 1990.

Moorthy RS et al: Management of varicella-zoster virus retinitis in AIDS, *Br J Ophthalmol* 81(3):189-194, 1997.

Parenteral cidofovir for cytomegalovirus retinitis in patients with AIDS: the HPMPC peripheral cytomegalovirus retinitis trial. A randomized, controlled trial. Studies of Ocular Complications of AIDS Research Group in Collaboration with the AIDS Clinical Trials Group, *Ann Intern Med* 126(4):264-274, 1997.

Passo MS, Rosenbaum JT: Ocular syphilis in patients with human immunodeficiency virus infection, *Am J Ophthalmol* 106(1): 1-6, 1988.

16 Renal Disease in HIV

K. ADU NTOSO

Introduction

Renal disease was recognized very early in the human immunodeficiency virus (HIV) and acquired immunodeficiency syndrome (AIDS) epidemic. This chapter will discuss the various renal manifestations of HIV infection. Primary renal syndromes, as well as secondary renal syndromes associated with systemic complications of HIV infection or HIV therapy, will be reviewed. The variety of electrolyte disorders seen in HIV-infected patients will also be discussed.

HIV-Associated Nephropathy
Presentation and Progression

Cause. Renal disease was noted early in the recognition of the AIDS epidemic, before the availability of HIV serologic testing. A syndrome characterized by heavy proteinuria and renal failure, with rapid progression to end-stage renal disease (ESRD), was reported by two separate investigators in 1984. When kidney biopsy was performed, pathology was consistent with focal segmental glomerulosclerosis (FSGS). The syndrome, as initially reported, was seen in intravenous drug (IVD) users or homosexuals with advanced AIDS. Renal and patient prognoses were uniformly poor. Terminal renal failure occurred within a few weeks of presentation and was uniformly fatal even with dialysis. In ensuing years, with the availability of HIV testing, it became recognized that HIV-associated nephropathy (HIVAN) was associated with various stages of HIV infection, from asymptomatic to advanced. The clinical disease, epidemiology, and pathologic entity have been further characterized. Although there remains no definitive therapy for the renal disease, the uniformly poor prognoses associated with the earlier reports have been tempered by more favorable reports.

Pathogenesis. The pathogenesis of HIVAN has not been established. Factors explored include primary HIV infection of renal glomerular and tubular cells. In experimental HIVAN, abnormalities in cell proliferation, apoptosis (programmed cell death), dedifferentiation of podocyte, and extracellular matrix deposition have all been suggested as consequences of a primary epithelial or mesangial cell injury. Immune dysregulation secondary to HIV infection may play a role in facilitating tissue injury by release of proinflammatory cytokines.

Induction of HIVAN in transgenic mice provides near conclusive proof that HIVAN is related to viral genome and not to an epiprocess such as IVD use. In these mice HIV-1 envelope and regulatory genome is expressed in renal epithelial cells without infectious virus. Such expression seems to be responsible for initiating the pathogenetic process in transgenic mice. A normal kidney transplanted into a transgenic HIV-1–infected mouse does not develop HIVAN. However, a transgenic HIV-1–infected kidney transplanted into a normal non–HIV-infected mouse develops HIVAN. HIV viral genome has been detected in human renal tissue in patients with HIVAN. It is, however, not conclusively established whether the expression in renal epithelial cells represents direct infection or passive presence.

Genetic factors also play a significant role in the pathogenesis of HIVAN. The near restriction of HIVAN to blacks suggests genetic differences in the response of the kidney as a whole, or specific renal cells to infection, viral gene products, or immune response factors. Similar genetic modification of disease is seen in Caucasians with homozygous deletion mutation of CCR5 HIV-1 coreceptor who are resistant to HIV infection. CCR5 is found only in Caucasians.

Lastly, the role of cofactors such as other concomitant viral or environmental factors has not been excluded.

Route of HIV Acquisition. Almost one half of the cases of HIVAN in the United States are seen in patients with IVD-associated HIV infection. Whether IVD use is a susceptibility factor or merely represents a coassociation has not been fully settled. The available evidence in adults, and in children with perinatal HIV acquisition, suggests that IVD use is not a pathogenic factor. Instead IVD use represents a common route of HIV acquisition in population at risk for HIVAN. In France, heterosexual transmission is the most common route of HIV infection in black patients of Central African origin who have HIVAN. In Italy, no HIVAN was seen in 26 white patients in spite of 75% IVD use. That IVD use is not a pathogenic factor is further suggested by results of studies that have induced HIVAN in transgenic mice.

Stage of HIV. HIVAN has been seen in all stages of HIV infection. With revision of criteria for AIDS, later reports have associated HIVAN with late HIV infection, generally in patients with CD4+ levels less than 250 cells/mm^3 or AIDS. In one series almost three fourths of patients had stage IV disease.

Pathology. Pathologically, characteristic glomerular and tubulointerstitial changes are seen that in combination give a pathognomonic appearance. The glomeruli show features of collapsing FSGS. However, there is marked glomerular capillary collapse, a result of marked glomerular basement membrane retraction. There is marked hypertrophy and hyperplasia of epithelial cells, with increased mitotic activity and protein resorption droplets in cytoplasm. In areas of capillary collapse, virtually little to no increase in mesangial matrix is seen. The interstitium shows marked tubular degeneration and atrophy, as well as edema, fibrosis, and inflammatory changes. The tubules show microcystic changes with eosinophilic proteinaceous casts. Immunofluorescence shows staining for immunoglobulin M (IgM), C3, and occasional C1 in the mesangium.

Electron microscopy shows nonspecific foot process fusion, and epithelial cell separation from retracted basement membrane. Pathognomonic tubuloreticular inclusions are seen in glomerular and vascular endothelial cells. They may also be seen occasionally in infiltrating lymphocytes and in visceral epithelial cells. These have been termed "interferon footprints" because of similarity to inclusions seen in lymphocytes exposed to interferon-α in vitro or in patients with systemic lupus erythematosus (SLE) nephritis.

Presentation

Epidemiology. Very early in the reports of HIVAN it was recognized that African-American IVD users were predominantly affected in reports from Brooklyn and Miami. The syndrome was rare in homosexual Caucasian AIDS patients in San Francisco. Given the similarity of the pathologic entity, FSGS, to previously described IVD-related heroin nephropathy (HAN), HIVAN was believed to be a manifestation of IVD-related AIDS. However, distinctive pathologic findings, disparate clinical picture, and delineation of the epidemiologic characteristics have shown it to be a separate entity.

From numerous centers in the United States, as well as several reports worldwide, the syndrome has been noted nearly exclusively in blacks. In the United States it is a major cause of ESRD in young African-American males, and is the third leading cause of ESRD in African-Americans between ages 20 and 64. Over the period of 1991 to 1996, an annual 30% increase in incidence was noted, and it accounted for 10% of all new cases of ESRD per year in African-Americans.

HIVAN is seen in about 10% of HIV-infected patients. The prevalence of clinical HIVAN varies in different reports, depending on racial composition. In reports with predominantly black patients, prevalence figures vary from 10% to 15%. In autopsy series including all racial groups, a 2% to 7.5% overall prevalence is noted, while a 12% prevalence has been noted in blacks. In various reviews, 90% of patients with HIVAN were black.

The near absence of HIVAN in non-black racial groups has been confirmed in several other worldwide reports. In a total of 255 non-blacks from Germany, Italy, and Thailand, no HIVAN was seen, while in France 97% of patients with HIVAN were of black race. Rarely, it is seen in HIV-infected Hispanics. When HIVAN is seen in Caucasians it is usually mild, with nonnephrotic proteinuria and mild renal insufficiency. The reason for the near-racial restriction of HIVAN and the more severe disease in blacks is not explained, but genetic factors obviously play a role.

Clinical Presentation. Proteinuria and renal insufficiency are hallmarks of HIVAN. Proteinuria is usually in nephrotic range (2.5 g/24 h), although lower levels may be seen. Mean level of proteinuria in one report was 6.6 g/24 h. Renal insufficiency is characteristic. In earlier reports, rapid progression to terminal renal failure was the rule. Recently, different stages of renal failure have been noted on presentation. Hypoalbuminemia is universal, with average serum albumin levels 2.2 or below. In spite of severe hypoalbuminemia, edema is sur-

---

BOX 16-1
Summary of Diagnostic Points

African-American
Heavy proteinuria with or without renal insufficiency
Absence of hypertension
Absence of edema
Benign urine sediment

---

prisingly uncommon in several reports. This may be related to the presence of hypergammaglobulinemia and increase in total plasma proteins. In contrast to the high incidence of hypertension in non-HIV glomerulopathies, hypertension is notably infrequent in HIVAN, even with advanced renal failure. Associated hypovolemia may partly explain this low frequency of hypertension. Hypercholesterolemia is notably uncommon, in contrast to its high incidence in non–HIV-infected nephrotic patients.

Urinalysis reveals heavy proteinuria, with frequent presence of renal tubular epithelial cells. Microcysts formed from aggregates of renal tubular epithelial cells may be seen. Renal ultrasound characteristically shows enlarged kidneys with marked echogenicity. The enlarged kidneys on ultrasound may be related to the presence of microcystic changes on pathology. Even when renal function is end stage, the kidneys remain large.

Atypical Presentation. Occasionally, non-nephrotic proteinuria may be the presenting sign of HIVAN. In the rare Caucasian with HIVAN, proteinuria and clinical renal disease are usually mild.

Case. A 32-year-old African-American male has had known HIV for 5 years. The patient has been prescribed antiretroviral therapy but has been poorly compliant. There is history of *Pneumocystis carinii* pneumonia (PCP). The last CD4+ cell count was 100 cells/mm^3. He is seen in the office for routine follow-up. Blood pressure is 120/60 and heart rate is 90. There is no edema on examination. The lungs are clear, the cardiac examination is unremarkable, and he has no hepatosplenomegaly. Urinalysis reveals 3+ albuminuria, and there are no abnormalities on microscopy. Serum creatinine is 2.0 mg/dl, blood urea nitrogen (BUN) is 40 mg/dl, and hemoglobin (Hgb) is 10 g/dl.

This African-American patient presents with abnormalities highly suggestive of HIVAN. The relatively normal blood pressure in the face of significant renal insufficiency, and associated heavy proteinuria, strongly suggests underlying HIVAN. Urine protein and creatinine clearance should be quantitated with a 24-hour collection. If this is inconvenient, a timed 2-hour collection could be substituted. In the absence of major contraindications such as bleeding diathesis, coagulopathy, moderate thrombocytopenia, or other severe complicating illness, a kidney biopsy should be considered. Others may suggest, however, that an empiric diagnosis of HIVAN could be made without subjecting the patient to risks of biopsy. Such an argument is made with the supposition that the results of kidney biopsy will not alter the management. However, others suggest that the results of such a biopsy may help to direct specific therapy, as well as help to better define potential prognostic indicators. See Box 16-1 for a summary of diagnostic points.

Natural History

In the early phase of the HIV epidemic, HIVAN was associated with renal failure within a few weeks of presentation and was uniformly fatal, even with dialysis. Advanced AIDS syndromes contributed to death. In recent years the availability of immunomodulating therapy and highly active antiretroviral therapy (HAART) has altered the dismal prognosis of HIVAN. Mild presumed HIVAN may exist in some African-American patients. In patients with progressive disease, survival on dialysis has improved with appropriate management of HIV infection and associated illnesses.

Complications

In the United States HIVAN is a major cause of ESRD in young African-American males, and is the third leading cause of ESRD in African-Americans between ages 20 and 64. Associated proteinuria may contribute significantly to hypoalbuminemia. Susceptibility to infections may be further increased. As noted, overt nephrotic syndrome is uncommon.

Treatment

Earlier reports suggested a uniformly dismal prognosis in HIVAN, with either rapid progression to ESRD or death from advanced HIV disease. There was also initial concern about use of immunosuppressive agents in patients with HIV/AIDS. Moreover, the underlying glomerular disorder, FSGS, was thought to respond poorly, if at all, to immunosuppressive agents, even in patients without HIV disease. For these reasons, no treatment was offered in patients with HIVAN. Subsequently, anecdotal and rare controlled studies have suggested potential benefit of immunosuppressives or other therapy in HIVAN. Treatments tried include antiretroviral therapy, corticosteroid, cyclosporine, and nonspecific therapy with angiotensin converting enzyme (ACE) inhibitors.

Several retrospective reports and nonrandomized studies have shown that zidovudine decreased the progression of renal disease in patients with renal involvement. It is possible that current and future more aggressive antiretroviral therapy may have significant impact on progression or incidence of HIVAN.

Anecdotal and few clinical trials have reported potential benefit to prolonged corticosteroid therapy, including improvement or remission in nephrotic syndrome, serum creatinine, or stabilization of renal pathology in HIVAN. Uncontrolled reports in pediatric patients showed remission of nephrotic syndrome on cyclosporine. ACE inhibitors have shown some promise in a few case studies, with decrease in proteinuria and slowing of progression to ESRD. The benefits of ACE inhibitors may be multifactorial and include improvement in intraglomerular hemodynamics, inhibition of growth factor synthesis, and effect on protease inhibition and possibly on cytokine function.

More controlled studies will be needed to assess response of HIVAN to immunosuppressives and ACE inhibitors.

When to Refer

Nephrologic consultation should be considered in an African-American HIV-infected patient with greater than a 1+ persistent albuminuria, and/or serum creatinine greater than 1.5 in a susceptible individual. Note that if there is significant weight loss and cachexia, even lower serum creatinine may indicate moderate renal insufficiency.

KEY POINTS

- HIVAN is seen almost exclusively in HIV-infected blacks
- Heavy albuminuria and progressive renal disease are typical
- It is usually associated with advanced HIV disease
- It is a major cause of ESRD in blacks
- Treatment is currently not very well defined, although a few patients may respond to immunosuppressive therapy.

End-Stage Renal Disease and HIV

The population of HIV-infected patients on chronic dialysis is growing. This includes patients with HIV-related renal diseases, as well as those with other primary renal disorders who have coincidental HIV infection.

Dialysis modalities offered include hemodialysis (HD) and peritoneal dialysis (PD). PD was initially preferred in order to minimize risk of HIV transmission with HD. However, such patient-to-patient HIV transmission has not been documented in HD centers in the United States, in spite of growing numbers of HIV-infected patients on HD. In other parts of the world, however, patient-to-patient transmission has been well documented. Reasons for these were related to failure to observe strict infection control protocols in the HD units. Patient isolation or use of dedicated HD machines is not required if standard HD protocols are followed. There have been few reports of patient-to-staff transmission.

In patients on PD, rare reports suggested increase in bacterial peritonitis rate. Overall, however, comparable rates of bacterial peritonitis have been noted in several reports. HIV virus is present in PD effluent.

Finally, data on kidney transplantation in patients with known HIV disease are sparse. The few available reports suggested increased complications and mortality. Therefore chronic dialysis is preferred to transplantation. HIV virus has been transmitted through transplantation from both living and cadaveric donors.

Immune Complex Glomerulonephritis

A complete discussion on immunopathogenesis of immune complexes in renal disease is beyond the scope of this chapter. In brief, viral infections may trigger formation of antibodies that react with viral proteins. In addition, new nonviral or abnormal viral proteins may be synthesized. These may induce new antibody formation. Circulating immune complexes are formed that may deposit in kidneys.

Alternatively, previously formed circulating antibody may interact with viral antigens fixed in renal tissue, or with native or new antigen expressed in response to viral infection. There is ample evidence of expression of HIV genome in glomerular and renal epithelial cells. Such expression has been noted in patients with and without overt renal disease. Whether it represents infection or passive trapping of HIV viral antigens is under investigation. Similarly, the stimulus that triggers renal pathology in patients who develop renal disease is a subject of intense study. Lastly, drugs, other viral or bacterial infections, and malignancy could all trigger immune complex–mediated renal disease in HIV-infected patients.

Immune complex renal syndromes seen in HIV renal disease are listed in Box 16-2.

Although pathology is overlapping, hepatitis C–associated renal disease has been classified separately because of a markedly different prognosis compared with similar disease in non–HIV-infected patients. Similarly, hepatitis C–associated immune complex renal disease has a much worse prognosis than non–hepatitis C–associated disease in HIV-infected patients. In a selected HIV-infected population undergoing kidney biopsy, immune complex glomerulonephritis (GN) was seen in about one third of 40 patients. p40 or gp 120 HIV viral antigen-antibody complexes were noted in patients in whom detailed studies were done.

IgA Glomerulonephritis

IgA nephropathy is increasingly being reported in association with HIV disease. The exact incidence of IgA nephropathy is uncertain. Autopsy of 116 HIV-infected patients from France showed about 8% with diffuse mesangial IgA deposits.

Pathology

Biopsy shows IgA deposits in the mesangium with various degrees of mesangial proliferation. Occasionally crescentic IgA nephropathy may be seen. Some investigators have reported HIV antigen–IgA immune deposits.

Presentation and Progression

Unlike HIVAN, the majority of patients are white and homosexual. However, it is seen in HIV-infected blacks as well, in much higher frequency than seen in non–HIV-infected blacks. Clinical renal disease is usually milder compared with HIVAN. Proteinuria, microscopic or gross hematuria, and mild renal insufficiency are characteristically seen.

Diagnosis

Typically a Caucasian presents with mild proteinuria, mild renal insufficiency, and microscopic or gross hematuria.

Natural History

The course is usually benign compared with HIVAN.

Treatment

There is no defined therapy, but captopril may improve proteinuria. Steroids and fish oil have been tried in non-HIV IgA GN.

Membranoproliferative Glomerulonephritis

Presentation and Progression

Cause. Membranoproliferative GN (MPGN) is the most common form of GN when HIVAN is excluded. Increased association with hepatitis C, as well as hepatitis B, coinfection is noted. In patients with positive hepatitis C antibody, MPGN has been reported in association with cryoglobulinemia and hypocomplementemia.

Presentation. Heavy proteinuria, moderate renal insufficiency, hematuria, and hypertension are characteristic. Urinalysis reveals various degrees of activity including granular and cellular casts.

BOX 16-2
Immune Complex Glomerulonephritis in HIV

NON–HEPATITIS C–ASSOCIATED
IGA nephropathy with or without Henoch-Schönlein purpura
Diffuse proliferative glomerulonephritis
Membranoproliferative glomerulonephritis
Membranous glomerulonephropathy
Lupus-like nephritis
Diffuse mesangial hypercellularity in children
Minimal change disease—mostly in children

HEPATITIS C–ASSOCIATED, WITH OR WITHOUT CRYOGLOBULINEMIA
Membranoproliferative glomerulonephritis
Membranous glomerulopathy
Mesangioproliferative glomerulonephritis
Collapsing glomerulopathy with immune deposits
Mixed essential cryoglobulinemia

Diagnosis

Typically a patient presents with heavy proteinuria, hypertension, moderate renal insufficiency, microscopic hematuria with cellular and granular casts, and a low serum complement.

Natural History

Renal disease is usually severe and rapidly progressive.

Treatment

Modalities tried in non-HIV MPGN include Persantine and aspirin. Results have not been uniformly encouraging. Steroids have not been useful in non-HIV MPGN.

Lupus-Like Nephritis

Low-titer antinuclear antibodies (ANA) without anti-DNA or hypocomplementemia are seen in some HIV-infected patients. There are rare reports of higher titer ANA with anti-DNA and hypocomplementemia in patients with renal disease and a clinical picture consistent with SLE. It has been seen mostly in children, although several adults have been reported. All World Health Organization stages of lupus nephritis have been observed.

Hepatitis C–Associated Immune Complex Glomerulonephritis

Presentation and Progression

Cause and Pathology. In patients with IVD use and HIV, there is a relatively high coinfection rate of hepatitis C. There are several reports of immune complex glomerular diseases associated with acute renal failure (ARF). Kidney biopsy has revealed a variety of immune complex GN, with MPGN (type I and type III) predominating. Other findings include mesangioproliferative GN and atypical membranous glomerulopathy.

Presentation. The majority of patients in the United States have been African-American. Clinical findings include heavy proteinuria and severe renal failure. In contrast to HIVAN, hypertension, edema, and microscopic hematuria are frequent findings. Hepatitis B surface antibody is frequent, indicating past infection. Cryoglobulinemia and hypocomplementemia are common, but typical findings of mixed essential cryoglobulinemia are infrequent on examination.

Diagnosis

The typical patient is African-American, presenting with heavy proteinuria, hypertension, edema, and microscopic hematuria, with or without other sediment abnormalities. Hepatitis C antibody and hepatitis C RNA polymerase titer should be obtained, in addition to serum cryoglobulins and complement levels.

Kidney biopsy is necessary to define specific pathology. However, it is not certain that the results of the biopsy will alter management.

Natural History

In patients who are HIV-infected and who have hepatitis C–associated cryoglobulinemic glomerulopathy, advanced renal failure on presentation or rapid progression to ESRD is the rule. This disease tends to be milder in those patients not infected with HIV.

Treatment

In the few patients who received interferon-α therapy, no benefit was seen.

When to Refer

A patient should be referred when there is elevated serum creatinine and/or proteinuria with evidence of hepatitis C coinfection.

KEY POINTS

- Hepatitis C–associated cryoglobulinemia is not infrequent in HIV disease
- Renal disease is more severe than non–HIV-associated mixed cryoglobulinemia
- HIV-infected blacks predominate
- No effective therapy is currently available, although data on use of interferon and ribavirin are not available.

Mixed Essential Cryoglobulinemia
Presentation and Progression

Cause. Essential mixed cryoglobulinemia has been largely associated with hepatitis C infection in non–HIV-infected patients. A large number of hepatitis C–coinfected HIV-infected patients have circulating cryoglobulins. A recent report has suggested a possible association of mixed cryoglobulinemic disease in HIV-infected patients without hepatitis C coinfection. In 89 patients with HIV infection from Greece, 24 (27%) had mixed cryoglobulins. Only six (25%) of these 24 patients had evidence of hepatitis C coinfection. All 24 cryoglobulinemic patients had HIV antibodies in cryoprecipitates. In addition, four of the six hepatitis C–coinfected patients had hepatitis C antibody in the cryoprecipitate.

Presentation. Clinical disease consistent with typical mixed essential cryoglobulinemia was seen in nine patients. This included purpura, arthralgia, and mononeuritis multiplex. Two patients, one with and the other without hepatitis C, had proteinuria with hypertension. MPGN was found on biopsy in the hepatitis C–positive patient.

This report suggests possible direct HIV-associated cryoglobulinemia with potential for systemic and renal disease.

Diagnosis

In a patient presenting with purpura, polyarthralgia, and systemic findings suggestive of vasculitis, serum cryoglobulins and hepatitis C antibody would strongly suggest essential mixed cryoglobulinemia. Serum complement levels are frequently low. Skin biopsy usually shows nonspecific small vessel vasculitis. If significant renal insufficiency exists, kidney biopsy may be indicated.

Natural History

There are limited data available on the natural history of HIV-associated mixed cryoglobulinemia.

Treatment

In non-HIV essential mixed cryoglobulinemia, interferon and ribavirin therapy has been used. Although this may arrest progression of disease, the recurrence rate is high with discontinuation of therapy. There are limited data on use of interferon and ribavirin in HIV disease. In earlier reports, use of interferon was ineffective. No specific guidelines exist.

When to Refer

Presence of purpura and arthralgia in an HIV-infected patient should prompt evaluation for cryoglobulinemia, even if there is no hepatitis C coinfection.

KEY POINTS

- Cryoglobulinemia may be associated with HIV infection, even in absence of hepatitis C coinfection

Thrombotic Microangiopathy Syndromes in HIV
Presentation and Progression

Cause. The occurrence of thrombotic microangiopathy (TMA) in AIDS has been known since initial reports in 1984, prior to the availability of HIV serotesting. Since then, numerous reports have noted the association between HIV infection and the TMA syndromes, thrombotic thrombocytopenic purpura (TTP) and hemolytic-uremic syndrome (HUS).

In retrospective testing of sera in patients who had TTP/HUS in Miami and San Francisco institutions, 14% and 16% of patients, respectively, were noted to have HIV infection. In two New York City institutions, almost 40% of TTP/HUS patients were noted retrospectively to be HIV-positive. In contrast, in Baltimore only 3% of 62 patients with TTP/HUS over a similar time period were HIV-positive.

In patients with known HIV, TTP/HUS has been reported in about 0.6% to 3%. In patients with ARF and HIV disease, one report from France reported almost 30% of 92 patients had HUS. In a central London HIV unit, 12% of 17 patients undergoing renal biopsy had HUS. These reports may represent highly selective populations. The true incidence figures of TTP/HUS in HIV-infected patients in general and as a cause of renal disease are unclear. However, as implied by these reports, HIV is a significant factor in TTP/HUS.

A predilection for white patients, similar to non–HIV-associated TTP/HUS, has been noted. However, racial background was not always stated in all reports. In contrast to non-HIV TTP/HUS, almost 85% of HIV-associated TTP/HUS cases are men. Whether this represents the difference in prevalence of HIV infection in men and women in the population reported, or a real male predisposition, has not been determined.

Some reports suggested that TTP/HUS was seen in late HIV disease. However, earlier reviews indicated that almost 50% of cases were seen prior to overt AIDS. Overall, two thirds of cases had stage B or C HIV disease at the time of TTP/HUS. In one fourth of patients, TTP/HUS was the presenting manifestation of HIV disease. The prevalence of TTP/HUS is about 5.9% in HIV-infected patients with CDC stage III disease, but only 0.22% in those with stage I to II disease. IVD use or homosexuality was the risk factor for HIV infection in the majority of patients. It has been suggested that TTP/HUS be added to the international AIDS classification.

Pathogenesis. Similar to idiopathic non-HIV TTP/HUS, endothelial cell injury and dysfunction with cytokine activation underlie the disease process. Whether the association of HIV with TMA represents a direct viral causative role or a predisposition in the presence of other causative factors is uncertain. Possible pathogenic factors in HIV TTP/HUS are noted in Box 16-3. In one report only cytomegalovirus (CMV) infection appeared to have significant association in 16 HIV-infected patients with TMA. HIV-associated TTP/HUS has rarely been associated with use of cyclosporine or with pregnancy.

Presentation. Clinical and laboratory abnormalities are indistinguishable from non–HIV-associated TTP/HUS. In patients with HUS, microangiopathic hemolytic anemia and renal failure may dominate, whereas in TTP, thrombocytopenia, neurologic abnormalities, and renal failure, which is usually mild, may complete the pentad of findings, along with fever and microangiopathy. A majority of patients have apparent mild renal failure. However, low muscle mass in many patients may imply more severe renal disease than apparent from serum creatinine value. Severe renal failure with oliguria requiring dialysis occurs in some patients.

In patients with HUS, diarrhea was common. In some patients, enterotoxigenic *Escherichia coli* 0157:H7 was isolated.

Diagnosis

The diagnosis of TTP/HUS syndrome is usually made on clinical grounds. The presence of combinations of pentad of fever, thrombocytopenia, renal insufficiency, neurologic abnormalities, and microangiopathic hemolytic anemia suggests TTP. In HUS, fever and neurologic abnormalities may be milder or absent, while renal disease, with hypertension, is very severe.

Natural History

Prognosis is dependent on stage of HIV disease. In HIV-infected patients without AIDS, plasmapheresis with or without steroid therapy was associated with about 10% acute mortality, similar to non–HIV-infected patients. However, in AIDS patients, prognosis of TTP/HUS was grim, with very high mortality even in the absence of infections or malignancies.

BOX 16-3
Possible Pathogenic Factors in HIV-Associated TTP/HUS

DIRECT HIV VIRUS INFECTION OF ENDOTHELIAL CELLS

OTHER INFECTIONS
Cytomegalovirus

Opportunistic Infections
Mycobacterium avium
Cryptosporidiosis
Microsporidiosis
Herpes simplex virus

Stool Pathogens
Escherichia coli 0157:H7
Shigella Type 1
Salmonella
Streptococcus pneumoniae

DRUGS
Chemotherapeutic
Bleomycin
Mitomycin

Antiviral Agents
Acyclovir
Ganciclovir
Foscarnet

MALIGNANCY
Kaposi's sarcoma

Treatment

Therapy for HIV-associated TTP/HUS is similar to that for non–HIV-associated disease. Plasmapheresis with fresh frozen plasma, steroids, and antiplatelet agents have all been employed. In severe cases, vincristine, prostacyclin, and IV gamma globulin have been used. Infectious complications of such aggressive immunosuppressive therapy were high.

When to Refer

Thrombocytopenia, in association with combinations of renal failure, neurologic symptoms and signs, or fever, should prompt appropriate early and immediate referral for evaluation.

Immediate referral and initiation of plasmapheresis therapy are essential. Mortality is very high with delay in treatment initiation.

KEY POINTS

- HIV infection is a significant cause of TTP/HUS in some geographic areas
- Acute mortality is similar to non–HIV-associated TTP/HUS. However, overall prognosis is much worse in HIV-associated disease

> **BOX 16-4**
> **Causes of Acute Renal Failure or Azotemia in HIV-Infected Patients**
>
> **PSEUDOACUTE RENAL FAILURE**
> **Inhibition of Tubular Creatinine Secretion**
> Trimethoprim (in trimethoprim-sulfamethoxazole or trimethoprim-dapsone)
> Pyrimethamine
>
> **PRERENAL FACTORS**
> **Hypovolemia**
>
> **Hypotension**
> GI losses, poor po intake, acute blood loss, sepsis, third spacing
>
> **INTRINSIC RENAL FACTORS**
> **Acute Tubular Necrosis**
> Severe shock (sepsis, hypovolemia, acute bleeding, acute myocardial infarction)
> Iodinated contrast agents
> Drugs
> Rhabdomyolysis
>
> **Acute Interstitial Nephritis**
> Drug-induced allergic interstitial nephritis
> Acute plasmacytic interstitial nephritis
>
> **Tubulointerstitial Disease**
> Drugs
>
> **Hemodynamic—in Setting of Poor Renal Perfusion**
> Nonsteroidal antiinflammatory agents
>   Cox-2 inhibitors
>   ACE inhibitors
> Angiotensin II receptor blockers
>
> **Other**
> Acute glomerulonephritis
> Thrombotic thrombocytopenic purpura/hemolytic-uremic syndrome
>
> **POSTRENAL FACTORS—OBSTRUCTIVE**
> **Ureteral Obstruction**
> Malignancies
>   Kaposi's sarcoma
>   Lymphomas
> Crystals and/or stones
>   Drugs: indinavir, acyclovir, sulfadiazine
>   Uric acid in tumor lysis syndrome

Acute Renal Failure and Other Renal Abnormalities

The frequency of ARF in hospitalized HIV-infected patients has been variable but is significantly higher than in non–HIV-infected patients. Incidences of 3% and 4% were noted in 750 and 1,635 HIV-infected patients, respectively, in the early 1980s. These figures were not much higher than ARF in non–HIV-infected hospitalized patients. In contrast, later reports have shown much higher incidence figures. ARF was noted in 20% of 449 AIDS patients in New York in the mid 1980s, and more recently a 30% incidence was reported in 431 patients in Houston. The high incidence in later reports appears to coincide with the use of more potent and combination medications with high nephrotoxic potential, as well as with increased frequency of septicemia because drug therapy has prolonged survival.

Presentation and Progression

The differential diagnosis of ARF in HIV is listed in Box 16-4. It is similar to causes in non- HIV ARF, albeit with different relative frequency of the various etiologies.

Inhibition of creatinine secretion in the renal tubule may elevate serum creatinine without a true change in glomerular filtration rate (or renal function.) Trimethoprim (TMP) (used in TMP-sulfamethoxazole [SMX] or TMP/dapsone) inhibits creatinine secretion. Similarly, pyrimethamine may raise serum creatinine. The same effect may be seen with use of cimetidine.

When patients with HIVAN and immune complex glomerular disease are excluded, hypovolemia accounts for close to three fourths or higher of true ARF in hospitalized HIV-infected patients. The frequent presence of gastrointestinal (GI) losses with diarrhea, vomiting, poor oral intake secondary to anorexia, and rare reports of renal salt wasting all predispose to hypovolemia. Hypoalbuminemia, which is quite common, further compromises intravascular volume. Acute blood loss from GI or surgical procedures adds to intravascular depletion. In patients with hypovolemia, use of nonsteroidal antiinflammatory drugs (NSAIDs) may precipitate a hemodynamic ARF that may mimic and occasionally progress to acute tubular necrosis (ATN).

ATN, seen in up to one third or higher of HIV-infected patients with ARF, is largely related to sepsis or nephrotoxic agents. In patients without overt AIDS, drug-associated nephrotoxic ATN predominates. Drugs most frequently associated with renal failure in HIV patients are foscarnet, pentamidine, and amphotericin B. Although true ARF is relatively uncommon with use of TMP-SMX, the relatively high frequency of use and high dosage in HIV-infected patients increase the incidence of ARF associated with the drug. Rhabdomyolysis, possibly drug-related, may cause ATN in some patients.

Acute interstitial nephritis may be seen in association with drug interactions. TMP-SMX and phenytoin are two of several drugs that may cause acute interstitial nephritis in HIV-infected patients. A rare syndrome of acute interstitial plasmacytic nephritis with proteinuria and renal insufficiency has been reported. Diagnosis by biopsy is essential because of excellent response to steroid therapy. Cidofovir may be associated with renal failure in about 12% of patients receiving the drug. Proteinuria and proximal tubular dysfunction are the hallmarks. Pathologically interstitial cellular infiltration is seen.

Non–drug-related interstitial nephritis may be seen in as many as 10% of patients. When associated with symptoms and signs of Sjögren's syndrome, the term diffuse infiltrative lymphocytosis syndrome has been applied. Rarely with severe hypoalbuminemia and fluid overload, severe renal interstitial edema may cause acute renal failure, so-called nephrosarca. This responds to effective diuresis.

TABLE 16-1
Drugs Associated with Intratubular Crystallization

Drugs	Appearance of crystals
Indinavir	Needle-shaped birefringent
Acyclovir	Needle-shaped birefringent
Sulfadiazine	"Shocks of wheat"
Sulfamethoxazole (metabolite)	
High-dose ciprofloxacin	Needle-shaped

BOX 16-5
Drugs Associated with Hyperkalemia in HIV

Trimethoprim (in trimethoprim-sulfamethoxazole or with dapsone)
Pentamidine
Ketoconazole
Rifampin—rare

Obstructive causes of ARF may be related to extra renal obstruction from malignancy, including lymphomas, or intratubular obstruction secondary to crystallization of drugs. See Table 16-1 for a list of drugs that can cause crystallization. Acyclovir, indinavir, and sulfadiazine are drugs that may cause ARF secondary to crystallization. In very large doses the metabolite of SMX (in TMP-SMX) may crystallize in acidic urine and rarely cause ARF. About 20% of patients receiving indinavir may develop crystalluria, 8% may present with clinical symptoms including flank pain or dysuria, and 3% will have kidney stones. Interstitial nephritis with pyuria may be seen. ARF may be seen in about 7% of patients on sulfadiazine. Urine alkalinization (to pH 7.15) increases the solubility of sulfadiazine twentyfold. A Lignin test, with addition of 10% hydrochloric acid to a drop of urine, may yield a positive result, with yellowish-orange color seen. Lastly, in patients on chemotherapy, methotrexate may precipitate in tubules. In patients with bulky lymphomas, acute uric acid nephropathy may be seen with chemotherapy. Box 16-5 summarizes classes of potential nephrotoxic drugs used in HIV.

Diagnosis

The urinalysis is frequently useful in distinguishing prerenal, ATN, acute interstitial nephritis, or crystal-induced acute renal failure from the glomerular or microangiopathic syndromes. Proteinuria is minimal to absent in the nonglomerular causes. In prerenal causes, the urine sediment is usually unremarkable, with absence of cellular elements or casts. However, in the presence of severe hypovolemia, granular casts may be seen. Fractional excretion of sodium is below 1%, except in patients on diuretics or with renal salt wasting. In ATN various degrees of granular casts are seen, although not invariably. In sepsis-, aminoglycoside-, or rhabdomyolysis-induced ATN, numerous granular casts may be seen. The fractional excretion of sodium is high, over 2%, but may be low in radiocontrast or rhabdomyolysis-induced ATN, or in any state of preexisting high sodium retention. In the absence of urinary tract infection, pyuria, particularly in association with rash, fever, eosinophilia, or eosinophiluria, suggests allergic interstitial nephritis. Needle-shaped crystals are seen with acyclovir, indinavir, or rarely with high dose ciprofloxacin, although the latter is not associated with renal failure. Characteristic "shocks of wheat" crystals in acidic urine suggest sulfadiazine crystalluria.

Natural History

The prognosis of ARF depends on the cause and comorbid factors. Overall, ARF significantly impacts on mortality in all hospitalized patients, particularly in HIV-infected patients. Prerenal ARF will correct if the underlying derangement is corrected. ATN is usually self-limited. However, recovery is highly dependent on stability of and correction of comorbid factors, such as sepsis and hypovolemia. Acute interstitial nephritis generally shows improvement with or without steroids. However, unlike ATN recovery, it is not always predictable, even when offending agents are stopped and comorbid factors are corrected. Residual renal impairment is frequent. Cidofovir ARF is frequently irreversible if not recognized early. Crystal-induced ARF may resolve if it is recognized early and if appropriate management is instituted.

Treatment

Prerenal causes of ARF require correction of intravascular volume and restoration of effective organ perfusion. ATN requires no specific therapy other than removal or treatment of causative factors, if possible. Severe allergic interstitial nephritis may require short-term corticosteroid therapy, although the benefit of this has not been proved in controlled trial. Offending drugs should be discontinued, if possible. As noted, diffuse infiltrative lymphocytosis syndrome responds well to corticosteroids. Corticosteroids have not proved effective in the few cases of cidofovir reported (and personal observation). High-saline intravenous fluid with forced diuresis should be instituted in crystal-induced ARF. In acute tumor lysis syndrome, the addition of alkali-forced diuresis may offer additional benefit to saline diuresis. It must be emphasized, however, that these measures are far more superior as preventive rather than therapeutic measures. Allopurinol should be started at least 24 hours prior to initiation of chemotherapy, along with forced saline and alkali diuresis in patients with bulky lymphomas.

Management of ARF includes correcting hypovolemia and discontinuing offending drugs, if possible. Attention to fluid and electrolyte changes and appropriate management of electrolyte abnormalities, particularly hyperkalemia, are essential during the period of ARF. This is particularly important in patients who are oliguric. Appropriate use of bicarbonate preparations to correct acidosis and sodium polystyrene sulfonate (Kayexalate) for hyperkalemia may be needed. If severe hyperkalemia or fluid overload occurs, short-term dialysis may be indicated.

When to Refer
Any significant elevation in BUN and/or creatinine should prompt search for causative factors and discontinuation or correction of such factors. Referral to a nephrologist is indicated if renal function does not improve with initial management.

KEY POINTS

- Acute renal failure is quite frequent in patients with HIV/AIDS
- It carries high morbidity and mortality
- Prevent hypovolemia
- Minimize nephrotoxic medications and/or agents whenever possible

Renal Implications of Antiretroviral Drugs

Recently the class of drugs in treatment of various stages of HIV infection has included the nucleoside reverse transcriptase inhibitors (NRTI) (zidovudine [AZT, ZDV], didanosine [ddI], stavudine [d4T], lamivudine [3TC], abacavir), the non-nucleoside reverse transcriptase inhibitors (NNRTI) (nevirapine, delavirdine, efavirenz), and the protease inhibitors (PI) (indinavir, ritonavir, saquinavir, nelfinavir).

Nucleoside Reverse Transcriptase Inhibitors

As a class, with the exception of zidovudine, the NRTIs have high renal excretion. They have limited, if any, direct nephrotoxicity. Lactic acidosis may be seen. A severe hypersensitivity syndrome characterized by shock and multiorgan failure may be seen with abacavir. Dose adjustment is necessary for all in the setting of renal failure.

Non-Nucleoside Reverse Transcriptase Inhibitors

The NNRTIs have little native drug excretion in urine, and no renal toxicity has been reported. No dosage adjustment is necessary in renal failure. Metabolism is by cytochrome P450 system.

Protease Inhibitors

All PIs are cytochrome P450–metabolized, with little or no renal excretion of active drug, except indinavir, which has less than 20% renal excretion. Except for indinavir crystalluria, the class has limited renal toxicity. Ritonavir may increase creatine phosphokinase (CPK) and uric acid level. Isolated cases of ritonavir-associated renal failure have been reported.

The class as a whole significantly increases the level of simvastatin and lovastatin. Therefore concomitant use of 3-hydroxy-3-methylglutaryl coenzyme A (HMG-CoA) reductase inhibitors with these drugs should be avoided.

See Tables 16-2 and 16-3 for side effects of various HIV drugs.

Electrolyte Abnormalities in HIV

Electrolyte and acid-base abnormalities are very common in HIV-infected patients. Renal insufficiency, renal tubular abnormalities related to either HIV infection or effects of therapy, GI losses, endocrine abnormalities, and infectious complications all contribute to the myriad of electrolyte disturbances seen.

Hyponatremia

Presentation and Progression. Hyponatremia is one of the most frequent electrolyte abnormalities seen in HIV-infected patients. It is seen in about one third to one half of AIDS patients. It occurs as a result of absolute or relative increase in free water intake in the setting of abnormal renal water excretion brought about by underlying conditions. As in non–HIV-infected patients, hyponatremia may be associated with hypovolemic, euvolemic, or hypervolemic states, although the latter situation is exceedingly rare in HIV-infected patients.

Hypovolemic states account for almost 90% of hyponatremia in AIDS patients. GI losses, with diarrhea and vomiting, cause loss of salt and water. Replacement with water and increased renal water retention cause dilution of plasma, with resultant hyponatremia. Renal salt wasting may cause hypovolemic hyponatremia. This may be seen in patients with tubulointerstitial disease or central nervous system (CNS) disease such as tuberculous meningitis, or rarely in association with drugs such as TMP-SMX or capreomycin. Poor solute intake and increased antidiuretic hormone (ADH) release in response to hypovolemia compromise renal water excretion. Large amounts of hypotonic fluids given with IV medications contribute significantly to hyponatremia. This is typically seen with TMP-SMX and amphotericin B, both of which require dilution in dextrose water.

Euvolemic hyponatremia accounts for about 10% of hyponatremia in AIDS. Inappropriate ADH secretion related to pulmonary infections or intracerebral diseases including infections and tumors account for the tendency to hyponatremia in these patients. The syndrome has rarely been seen in disseminated herpes zoster. Adrenal cortical insufficiency secondary to HIV infection or drugs such as ketoconazole is not an infrequent cause of hyponatremia. In patients with adrenal insufficiency, hyponatremia is more prevalent than hyperkalemia. Hypothyroidism should be excluded, although it is not frequent with HIV infection. Hypervolemic hyponatremia, seen in association with cirrhosis with ascites, nephrotic syndrome, or congestive heart failure, is unusual.

Diagnosis

Case 1. A 35-year-old male with HIV has had chronic diarrhea and anorexia. He has 10-lb weight loss in 1 month. Intake consists of soda and juices. He is admitted for evaluation. He has stopped all his medications. On examination the blood pressure is 90/50, heart rate 100, respiratory rate 20, and temperature 98.9° F. Neck veins are flat, lungs clear, cardiac examination with S_1, S_2, and abdomen nontender. There is no edema. Serum sodium is 120, potassium 2.9, chloride 95, and carbon dioxide 14. Blood glucose is 90, BUN 30, and creatinine 1.2. Spot urine sodium is 5meq/l and osmolarity 500 mosm/l.

The normal blood glucose excludes hyponatremia associated with hypertonicity from high serum glucose. The clinical examination suggests hypovolemia, supported by mild azotemia and low urinary sodium excretion. Therefore the patient has hypovolemic, hypotonic hyponatremia. Urine osmolarity is elevated, in response to increased ADH level. The increased ADH level is a result of hypovolemia.

TABLE 16-2
Urine Color Changes with Some HIV Drugs

Drug	Urine color
Rifampin	Orange-brown
Rifabutin	Orange-brown
Clofazimine	Reddish-brown

TABLE 16-3
Rare Renal Syndromes Seen with Drugs in HIV

Drug	Effect
Itraconazole	Reversible nephrotic syndrome Urinary frequency Hypokalemia
Rifampin	Proteinuria Urinary light chain excretion Glycosuria Nephrogenic diabetes insipidus Renal potassium wasting Hyponatremia/hyperkalemia 2° to adrenal crisis
Dapsone	Nephrotic syndrome
Zidovudine	? Type B lactic acidosis

Case 2. A 40-year-old male with known HIV is admitted to the hospital with increasing respiratory distress. He has had 2 days of fever. Appetite has been poor, but he denies nausea, vomiting, or diarrhea. He has not been taking any medications at home. Temperature is 102° F, blood pressure 105/70, heart rate 112, and respiratory rate 30. He is in moderate respiratory distress. Neck veins are not distended, lungs are clear, cardiac examination reveals S_1, S_2, abdomen is nontender, and there is no edema. The sodium is 133, potassium 3.6, chloride 100, carbon dioxide 21, blood glucose 115, BUN 14, creatinine 1.1, Hgb 14.5, and white blood cell count 6.0. Chest x-ray reveals diffuse bilateral interstitial infiltrate consistent with PCP. TMP-SMX in D_5W is begun. Five days into hospitalization the sodium is 122, potassium 5.5, chloride 86, carbon dioxide 27, BUN 17, and creatinine 1.4. He is euvolemic on examination. Spot urine sodium is 50, and osmolarity 900.

This patient has acute pneumonia. On initial evaluation there is evidence of mild hypovolemia. The initial mild hyponatremia may be partly from hypovolemia. Serum sodium worsens, associated with TMP-SMX in dextrose administration. At a time when the patient is euvolemic, the urine osmolarity is markedly elevated. This represents inappropriate ADH activity. The patient likely has syndrome of inappropriate ADH (SIADH), likely induced by PCP. Administration of hypotonic fluid worsened hyponatremia.

Natural History. In retrospective analysis, mortality in HIV-infected patients with hyponatremia is significantly increased, almost twofold in some reports compared with patients without hyponatremia. Two separate reports noted 70% versus 30% and 36.5% versus 19.7% mortality in hyponatremic versus normonatremic patients, respectively. Most of this was related to high incidence of opportunistic infections. In prospective evaluation, short-term mortality was 30% in hyponatremic AIDS patients.

Treatment. Management of hyponatremia involves correction of underlying volume depletion with liberal salt intake, with intravenous saline, and by limiting excessive free water administration. Treatment of underlying pulmonary and CNS conditions may improve SIADH and control hyponatremia.

In mild cases, limiting excessive intravenous hypotonic fluids is usually sufficient to maintain plasma sodium at a stable level of 125 to 135. In moderate hyponatremia, intake of oral fluids needs to be limited. This is usually difficult to balance in patients who need improved oral nutrition with supplements.

In case 1 above, treatment would involve cautious volume repletion with isotonic saline. In case 2 above, treatment is to restrict hypotonic fluids. Note that in setting of SIADH, hyponatremia could worsen, even with isotonic saline administration. In such a setting, a loop diuretic administered with isotonic saline will help correct hyponatremia.

Patients with severe or symptomatic hyponatremia may require 3% saline, with all the precautions to avoid rapid correction. Cortisol replacement is beneficial in patients with adrenal insufficiency.

When to Refer. If mild to moderate hyponatremia fails to respond to initial management, appropriate referral should be made. Moderate to severe hyponatremia, with a plasma sodium of 125 or less, should perhaps be referred for nephrologic consultation.

KEY POINTS

- Hyponatremia is very frequent in the HIV-infected population
- Potentially correctable factors, namely hypovolemia, account for the majority of cases
- It is associated with high morbidity and mortality, perhaps because of comorbid factors

Potassium Disorders

Hypokalemia. Hypokalemia occurs in almost 20% of AIDS patients and is usually related to lower GI losses. Renal potassium wasting may also be seen with a variety of drugs including amphotericin B. Hypokalemia has rarely been associated with didanosine, foscarnet, rifampin, itraconazole, and capreomycin. Rarely hyperaldosteronism has been suggested.

Control of diarrhea and replacement of potassium by oral route are needed. In drug-induced renal potassium wasting states, large doses of potassium replacement may be required.

Hyperkalemia. Although less common than hypokalemia, hyperkalemia is potentially more life threatening. It is related either to decreased renal potassium excretion, adrenal insufficiency, impaired transcellular potassium redistribution, or combinations of these.

Decreased renal potassium excretion may be related to underlying renal disease or drugs. Advanced renal failure from HIVAN, immune complex GN, ARF, or tubulointerstitial disease may all impair renal potassium excretion. Drugs implicated with hyperkalemia in HIV-infected patients include TMP (in TMP-SMX or with dapsone), pentamidine, ketoconazole, and rarely rifampin (see Box 16-5). TMP has structural similarities to amiloride and triamterene, potassium-sparing diuretics that act by inhibiting sodium reabsorption, and hence potassium secretion, in the distal tubule. TMP has been shown to similarly inhibit potassium secretion at distal tubule sites. Almost three fourths of AIDS patients receiving high dose TMP-SMX develop some degree of hyperkalemia, with severe levels seen in about 10%. TMP-associated hyperkalemia is seen within a few days of initiating therapy, typically peaking in 7 to 10 days. Hyperkalemia resolves over a few days after TMP-SMX is stopped. A twofold increase in frequency of hyperkalemia is seen when TMP is combined with dapsone compared with SMX. This may be related to higher plasma levels of TMP secondary to inhibition of TMP metabolism by dapsone. Hyperkalemia with distal renal tubular acidosis has also been reported with TMP.

Pentamidine-associated hyperkalemia is seen in about 25% of patients on the drug. It is usually seen in association with renal failure caused by the drug and typically occurs after more than 7 days of treatment. With renal failure, almost 90% of patients may have hyperkalemia. Decreased distal potassium secretion is seen. Ketoconazole inhibits adrenal steroid synthesis and may unmask adrenal insufficiency, leading to hyperkalemia. Rifampin may precipitate adrenal crisis in patients with decreased adrenal function by increasing hepatic cortisol metabolism.

Adrenal insufficiency, increasingly recognized in AIDS, may cause hyperkalemia. Some 2% of 447 HIV-infected patients with CD4+ cell counts less than 200 cells/mm^3 had adrenal insufficiency. In one report, 22% of 74 patients with AIDS and clinical abnormalities suggestive of adrenal insufficiency had the diagnosis confirmed.

Isolated hypoaldosteronism is being increasingly recognized as a cause of hyperkalemia in patients with HIV/AIDS. Both hyporeninemic and hyperreninemic forms of isolated hypoaldosteronism have been reported in HIV-infected patients. In hypoaldosterone states, hyperkalemia may be related to decreased renal potassium excretion as well as decreased transcellular shift of potassium. Drugs such as NSAIDs, ACE inhibitors, and heparin may cause hyperkalemia by effects on aldosterone synthesis and/or action.

Even in patients without baseline overt hyperkalemia, it has been suggested that impaired cellular potassium uptake may exist, in association with impaired aldosterone response, in HIV-infected patients compared with normal controls. This abnormality caused acute hyperkalemia during challenge in HIV but not in normal controls.

Treatment. Management of hyperkalemia in AIDS patients includes discontinuing offending medications when possible. This usually leads to resolution of hyperkalemia. ACE inhibitors and NSAIDs should be avoided in susceptible individuals. In patients with borderline hypoaldosteronism, even subcutaneous heparin may precipitate hyperkalemia by inhibiting aldosterone synthesis. If alternative drugs are not available, measures to counter potassium retention should be instituted, including high sodium diet and avoidance of hypovolemia. Use of Kayexalate for moderate hyperkalemia is indicated.

In life-threatening hyperkalemia initial therapy with calcium gluconate, insulin/$D_{50}W$, sodium, and bicarbonate may be required, prior to Kayexalate and/or dialysis.

When to Refer. Any significant tendency to hyperkalemia should be referred for appropriate initial evaluation because of potential risks.

KEY POINTS

- Hyperkalemia is not infrequent in patients with HIV/AIDS
- It is frequently drug-related
- Adrenal insufficiency or isolated mineralocorticoid deficiency should be excluded

Divalent Cations
Calcium

Hypocalcemia is generally associated with hypoalbuminemia, drug therapy, or enteropathy. It is seen in close to 20% of patients with AIDS. Drugs implicated in hypocalcemia, either directly or indirectly, include foscarnet, pentamidine, didanosine, and amphotericin B.

Foscarnet is associated with decreased ionized calcium in almost 20% of patients on the drug. It complexes with calcium without change in protein binding. Total serum calcium remains unchanged. The drug may also cause hypomagnesemia with associated hypocalcemia. Hypomagnesemia, as a result of renal magnesium wasting from amphotericin B, pentamidine, capreomycin, and aminoglycosides, may cause hypocalcemia by inhibition of parathyroid hormone release and action.

Vitamin D malabsorption as a result of immune enteropathy has been suggested as a cause of hypocalcemia in a large number of AIDS patients. Rarely, HIV-associated myositis and pancreatitis have been associated with hypocalcemia.

Hypercalcemia is uncommon, seen in about 3% of AIDS patients. It is usually associated with granulomatous diseases, lymphomas, disseminated CMV infection, and human T cell leukemia/lymphoma virus (HTLV)-1 infection. Foscarnet therapy has also been associated with hypercalcemia.

Magnesium

Hypomagnesemia is generally associated with renal magnesium wasting from drugs such as amphotericin B, pentamidine, capreomycin, and aminoglycosides, as well as poor intake and chronic diarrhea. Foscarnet may cause hypomagnesemia by unknown mechanism. Didanosine preparation contains high concentrations of magnesium (as well as sodium), and care should be exercised in patients with advanced renal insufficiency to avoid hypermagnesemia. Magnesium salts may be given orally for replacement. Care should be taken to avoid worsening or precipitating diarrhea.

Phosphorus

Hyperphosphatemia or hypophosphatemia may be seen with foscarnet. Etiology is unclear but it has been suggested that foscarnet deposition in bone may cause phosphorus release and hyperphosphatemia. Hypophosphatemia may also be seen with malnutrition in AIDS patients.

Uric Acid

Abnormalities in uric acid are seen commonly in AIDS patients. Hypouricemia is seen in about one fourth of AIDS patients. It is associated with opportunistic infections—*Mycobacterium avium* complex (MAC) and CMV infections most commonly. Abnormalities in uric acid transport in the kidney contribute to hypouricemia. Fractional excretion of uric acid is elevated in spite of evidence of central hypovolemia. Rifampin increases uric acid excretion. Hypouricemia is associated with increased mortality during follow-up.

Hyperuricemia is associated with use of certain drugs including pyrazinamide (40% to 50%), ethambutol, ritonavir, and didanosine. Didanosine is a purine drug and is metabolized to uric acid. Pyrazinamide inhibits renal tubular secretion of uric acid. Less hyperuricemia is seen when pyrazinamide is combined with rifampin because of opposing effects on tubular secretion of uric acid.

Acidosis

In presence of sepsis, shock, hypovolemia, or hypoxia, type A lactic acidosis is common. A very rare syndrome of type B lactic acidosis has been seen in a few patients without obvious underlying cause. Mitochondrial dysfunction has been suggested, possibly related to zidovudine. However, not all patients were on zidovudine. Thiamine deficiency has been suggested as a possible cause in some patients.

Abacavir may be associated with a severe idiosyncratic hypersensitivity reaction, with hypotension, shock syndrome, acidosis, and death.

Rarely diabetic ketoacidosis may be seen in association with pentamidine-associated pancreatitis. A variety of drugs, including amphotericin B, pentamidine, and rarely TMP-SMX, may be associated with renal tubular acidosis.

SUGGESTED READINGS

Bourgoigne JJ: Renal complications of human immunodeficiency virus type 1, *Kidney Int* 37:1571-1584, 1990.

Burns JS: Hemolytic uremic syndrome and thrombotic thrombocytopenic purpura associated with HIV infection. In Kimmel PL, Burns JS, Stein JH, editors: *Renal and urologic aspects of HIV infection,* New York, 1995, Churchill Livingstone, pp 111-133.

D'Agati V, Appel GB: HIV infection and the kidney, *J Am Soc Nephrol* 8:138-152, 1997.

Kimmel P, Phillips TM, Ferreira-Centeno A: HIV-associated immune-mediated renal disease, *Kidney Int* 44:1327-1340, 1993.

Klotman PE: HIV-associated nephropathy, *Kidney Int* 56:1161-1176, 1999.

Peraldi MN: Acute renal failure in the course of HIV infection: a single-institution retrospective study of ninety-two patients and sixty renal biopsies, *Nephrol Dial Transplant* 14:1578-1585, 1999.

Perazella MA, Brown E: Electrolyte and acid-base disorders associated with AIDS: an etiologic review, *J Gen Intern Med* 9:232-236, 1994.

Rao TKS: Acute renal failure syndromes in human immunodeficiency virus infection, *Semin Nephrol* 18:378-395, 1998.

Rao TKS: Management of the HIV-infected patient, Part I, *Med Clin North Am* 6:1437-1451, 1996.

Rao TKS: Renal complications in HIV disease, *Med Clin North Am* 80:1437-1451, 1996.

17 Central Nervous System Complications

CHARLES R. CANTOR, LEO McCLUSKEY

Introduction

Neurologic involvement is common in human immunodeficiency virus (HIV) infection. Clinically symptomatic neurologic complications of HIV are present in greater than 50% of infected individuals. Postmortem studies suggest an even higher prevalence, with as many as 90% of patients demonstrating HIV-related neuropathologic changes. Although neurologic involvement tends to become more common as the disease state progresses, 10% to 20% of patients with HIV infection may present with neurologic symptoms.

Any level of the neuraxis can be clinically affected in HIV infection (Box 17-1). Symptoms may be due to the direct effects of the virus or due to the immunosuppressed state. Like other lentiviruses, HIV is considered neurotropic: it has been detected in the brain, spinal cord, cerebrospinal fluid (CSF), and peripheral nerve. Immunosuppression predisposes patients to a variety of illnesses and neoplasms affecting the nervous system. In addition, HIV-infected individuals are also at risk for toxic, metabolic, vascular, and nutritional disorders that may present with neurologic symptoms.

This chapter examines both the direct effects of HIV on the nervous system and those illnesses that are related to immunosuppression. Among the disorders directly caused by HIV infection, aseptic meningitis, HIV dementia, and HIV-related myelopathy, neuropathy, and myopathy will be discussed. Also, the neurologic complications of the opportunistic infections and neoplastic disorders commonly associated with the immunosuppressed state will be reviewed. Finally, those complications of therapy for HIV infection that can mimic neurologic disease will be considered. In keeping with the traditional emphasis on localization in neurologic diagnosis, we will focus separately on the central and peripheral nervous system manifestations of the disorders presented.

Approach to the Patient

Careful history-taking and physical examination are essential tools in the assessment of the HIV-infected patient suspected of having neurologic disease. The neurologic examination typically does not provide a specific diagnosis, but is instead designed to localize dysfunction to the central or peripheral nervous systems, or to muscle. Symptoms of headache, dysequilibrium, confusion, or visual disturbance, particularly in association with focal or lateralized signs, suggest central nervous system (CNS) disease. In the absence of localizing signs, mental status changes may also represent toxic or metabolic encephalopathy. Cranial neuropathies imply a lesion in the subarachnoid space (i.e., a meningeal process). Weakness and sensory loss may have either central or peripheral etiologies, and the pattern of dysfunction (e.g., distal, proximal, lateralized) as well as associated signs of increased or decreased deep tendon reflexes can assist with localization. A differential diagnosis can then be formulated on the basis of the time course of symptoms and the presumed site of the lesion. The phase of HIV infection, as indicated by the CD4+ count, can also be helpful in determining diagnostic considerations. Further testing, including imaging studies, CSF examination, electromyography, and occasionally biopsy, may be necessary to establish the specific diagnosis. Because of the risk of intracranial mass lesion in this population, computed tomography (CT) or magnetic resonance imaging (MRI) should typically be performed before lumbar puncture. It should be emphasized that more than one HIV-related illness can produce neurologic symptoms in the same patient, and several levels of the neuraxis can be affected simultaneously.

Primary HIV-Related Central Nervous System Disorders
Aseptic Meningitis

Presentation and Progression. Both acute and chronic meningitis have been described as a direct consequence of HIV infection. Acute aseptic meningitis or meningoencephalitis with symptoms of headache, nuchal rigidity, photophobia, and confusion can occur 3 to 6 weeks following primary HIV infection, typically preceding seroconversion by several weeks. As with other viral meningitides, there may be associated systemic symptoms of fever, nausea, arthralgia, maculopapular rash, lymphadenopathy, and general malaise. Rarely, generalized seizures or cranial neuropathies may occur as well.

Diagnosis. CSF examination demonstrates a mononuclear pleocytosis (usually less than 200 cells/mm^3), with moderately elevated protein (usually less than 100 mg/dl) and normal glucose. HIV seropositivity may not be noted until several weeks after the resolution of the clinical syndrome.

Treatment. The treatment of viral meningitis is directed at amelioration of symptoms; the condition itself is generally self-limited, although a subset of patients may develop chronic headaches.

Chronic Meningitis

Chronic meningitis manifested by a mild mononuclear pleocytosis and mildly increased CSF protein is commonly found in asymptomatic HIV-infected individuals, and evidence of

BOX 17-1
Neurologic Complications of HIV Infection

DISORDERS PRODUCING DIFFUSE AND FOCAL BRAIN DYSFUNCTION
HIV-associated dementia
HIV-related acute and chronic aseptic meningitis
Progressive multifocal leukoencephalopathy
Viral encephalitis
Toxoplasmosis
Neoplasm, especially lymphoma
Syphilis
Cryptococcal meningitis
Tuberculosis
Cerebrovascular disease

DISORDERS PRODUCING SPINAL CORD DYSFUNCTION
Vacuolar myelopathy
B_{12} deficiency
Tuberculosis
Syphilis
Toxoplasmosis
Lymphoma
Cytomegalovirus
Herpes zoster

DISORDERS PRODUCING NERVE ROOT DYSFUNCTION
Cytomegalovirus
Lymphoma
Herpes zoster
Syphilis (tabes dorsalis)

DISORDERS PRODUCING PERIPHERAL NERVE DYSFUNCTION
Motor neuronopathy
Acute and chronic inflammatory demyelinating polyneuropathy
Mononeuropathy multiplex
Sensory-motor polyneuropathy
Nucleoside analogue–induced neuropathy

DISORDERS PRODUCING DYSFUNCTION OF MUSCLE
Polymyositis
Nemaline rod myopathy
Zidovudine-related myopathy
HIV-wasting syndrome

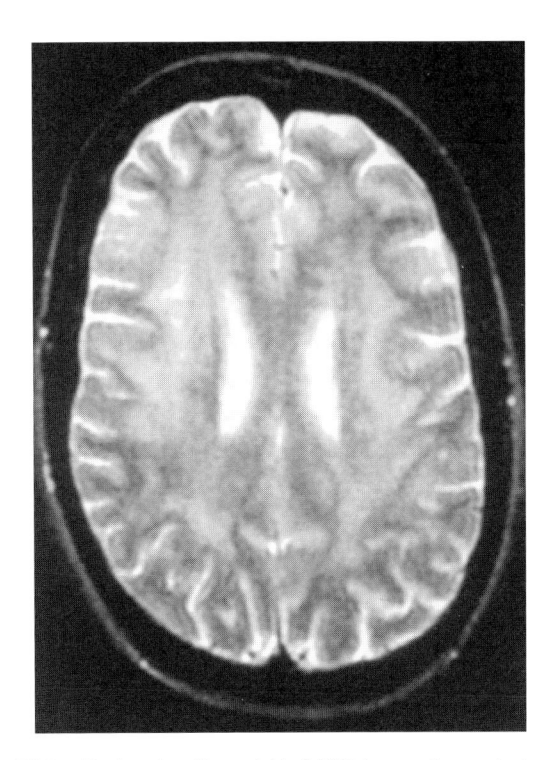

FIG. 17-1 Proton density–weighted MRI image demonstrates mild atrophy and diffuse deep white matter abnormalities in HIV-associated dementia.

chronic meningeal inflammation has been noted on postmortem examination as well. The clinical significance of these findings is unclear.

▶ KEY POINTS

- May be acute or chronic
- Etiologies include viral, bacterial, and fungal
- Typical symptoms include headache, nuchal rigidity, confusion, fever
- Acute aseptic meningitis in HIV infection may occur with seroconversion
- Chronic asymptomatic meningeal inflammation is common
- Common causes of meningitis in the HIV-infected population include syphilis, *Cryptococcus,* tuberculosis, and lymphoma

Dementia

Presentation and Progression. Cognitive impairment is a well-recognized complication of HIV infection. A number of terms have been employed to refer to the dementia associated with the acquired immunodeficiency syndrome (AIDS), including HIV-associated dementia, HIV encephalopathy, AIDS dementia complex, and HIV-associated major cognitive/motor disorder. Neuropathologic findings in this condition demonstrate atrophy, demyelination, gliosis, and perivascular inflammation in cerebral white matter. The HIV virus itself has been identified in multinucleated giant cells, microglia, and a number of subcortical structures.

HIV-associated dementia is characterized by deficits in concentration and memory, apathy, lack of insight, and psychomotor retardation. There are often associated motor deficits including clumsiness of fine motor movements, slowing of gait, and dysequilibrium. Affected individuals may appear mildly parkinsonian or depressed. Rarely, seizures may occur. Both the severity of symptoms and the rate of progression are variable.

Current estimates of the prevalence of HIV-associated dementia among AIDS patients range from 30% to 60%, with an approximately 7% annual incidence. The risk of dementia increases as the disease progresses, but in as many as 3% of adult patients it may represent the presenting symptom of AIDS. The issue of whether or not asymptomatic HIV-infected individuals have mild degrees of cognitive impairment has not yet been settled.

Diagnosis. Brain-imaging studies in individuals with HIV-associated dementia typically show both cortical and subcortical atrophy, with patchy nonspecific abnormalities of white matter (Fig. 17-1). CSF findings, including mononuclear pleocytosis and elevated protein, are nondiagnostic. No specific CSF markers for HIV-associated dementia have been identified, although β_2-microglobulin is commonly elevated. The utility of imaging (preferably MRI) and lumbar puncture in reaching a diagnosis of HIV-associated dementia is therefore to exclude the presence of other more readily treatable disorders. All patients should also be screened with the usual laboratory studies employed in the assessment of dementia, including syphilis serology, B_{12}, folate, and tests of renal, liver, and thyroid function. The presence of reversible metabolic abnormalities does not, of course, exclude the possibility of coexisting HIV-associated dementia.

Treatment. Patients in whom HIV-associated dementia is suspected should be treated with antiretroviral therapy; the role of protease inhibitors and other agents remains unclear.

KEY POINTS

- Deficits in memory and concentration
- Psychomotor retardation
- Minor motor signs may be present
- Focal signs typically absent
- Reversible causes of dementia should be excluded

Myelopathy

Presentation and Progression. Although an acute, self-limited myelitis can occur at the time of seroconversion, spinal cord dysfunction due to the HIV virus is most frequently seen in advanced stages of infection. HIV-associated myelopathy, called vacuolar myelopathy on the basis of pathologic findings, is a common autopsy finding, and may be clinically evident in as many as 27% of HIV-infected patients. Autopsy studies reveal spongy degeneration of the spinal cord, with vacuolar change and demyelination of the dorsal and lateral columns. As in HIV-associated dementia, multinucleated giant cells and microglial nodules are found, and the virus itself has been detected in macrophages.

In its most severe form, vacuolar myelopathy produces progressive bilateral leg weakness, spasticity with hyperreflexia, sensory loss affecting posterior column function (vibration and proprioception), and incontinence. In earlier or milder cases, patients may simply demonstrate hyperreflexia and extensor plantar responses.

Diagnosis. In the HIV-infected patient who presents with signs of progressive myelopathy, imaging of the cord should be obtained to rule out neoplasm, abscess, and other structural lesions. B_{12} deficiency, tuberculosis, syphilis, and other infectious etiologies including type I human T cell lymphotropic virus (HTLV-I) should be excluded. The spinal fluid formula in vacuolar myelopathy is nonspecific.

Treatment. The spasticity caused by vacuolar myelopathy can be treated symptomatically with baclofen or other antispasticity agents, but the underlying degeneration of the spinal cord is irreversible.

KEY POINTS

- Hyperreflexia and extensor plantar responses are early findings
- Later symptoms include spastic paraparesis and posterior column sensory loss
- Vacuolar degeneration of the cord is due to the HIV virus itself and is untreatable
- Other causes of myelopathy including structural lesions (neoplasm, abscess) and infection (syphilis, tuberculosis, cytomegalovirus, herpes simplex virus, toxoplasmosis) should be excluded

Primary HIV-Related Peripheral Nervous System Disorders

Disorders of Motor Neurons

Presentation and Progression. It remains controversial whether HIV directly produces a disorder of the motor neurons or anterior horn cells. Individual cases of HIV-positive patients, without lymphoma, who have developed a progressive clinical syndrome compatible with progressive lower motor neuron cell loss, have been reported. Syndromes resembling amyotrophic lateral sclerosis (ALS) have also been reported. Limited pathology has been described that is not clearly identical to the degenerative form of the disease. These patients have all presented with progressive atrophy and weakness involving the limbs and cranial muscles. Fasciculations have been noted. In the ALS-like syndromes, upper motor neuron signs of spasticity and increased reflexes with extensor plantar responses have been observed.

Diagnosis. The neurologic examination of an HIV-infected patient presenting with a motor neuron disorder demonstrates lower motor neuron dysfunction (atrophy, weakness, fasciculations) and/or upper motor neuron dysfunction (spasticity, slowed rapid movements, increased deep tendon reflexes) in one or more body segments (cranial, cervical, thoracic, lumbosacral). The examination is equally notable for the absence of sensory loss, cognitive dysfunction, sphincter incompetence, or involuntary movements. Neuroimaging of involved segments demonstrates no structural cause while examination of the CSF reveals no evidence of an infectious (e.g., tuberculosis, *Cryptococcus*) or neoplastic process. Electromyography demonstrates the presence of an active multisegmental lower motor neuron process. Motor nerve conduction study reveals preservation of motor conduction velocity and the absence of conduction block. Sensory nerve conduction should reflect relative sparing of sensory axons.

Treatment. No specific treatment is available. Although riluzole, a glutamate release inhibitor, slows the progression in non–HIV-related sporadic and familial ALS, this has not been demonstrated in the few ALS-like disorders reported in HIV. Supportive care centers on symptomatic treatment of limb, bulbar, and respiratory weakness.

Acute Neuropathy

Presentation and Progression. HIV-infected patients may develop acute inflammatory demyelinating polyradiculoneuropathy (AIDP), also known as Guillain-Barré syndrome. The clinical presentation in HIV-positive patients is indistinguishable from that which occurs in HIV-negative individuals. The disorder is often preceded by an acute infection, which may include recent HIV exposure, cytomegalovirus (CMV), or other viral illness. Patients may seroconvert to HIV-positive status during their course.

Weakness, preceded by paresthesias in 50%, evolves progressively over days to a 4-week period (average nadir in 9 days) in a largely symmetric pattern in both proximal and distal muscles of the limbs, cranial muscles (70%), and respiratory muscles. Respiratory muscle involvement may result in progressive neuromuscular respiratory failure, requiring mechanical ventilation. Weakness of pharyngeal and laryngeal muscles may produce dysphagia and dysarthria, as well as produce a risk of aspiration. Extraocular muscle weakness occurs rarely in overlap with the predominantly sensory disorder known as Miller-Fisher syndrome, characterized by ataxia, ophthalmoplegia, and areflexia. Autonomic symptoms including hypertension, hypotension, cardiac dysrhythmias, ileus, and urinary retention may occur. Examination demonstrates an areflexic paralysis, with a less notable accompanying loss of sensation.

Diagnosis. Electromyography and nerve conduction studies demonstrate a disturbance of motor and sensory conduction consistent with a multifocal process predominantly affecting myelin. At times, features more consistent with axonal loss or mixed features of demyelination and axonal loss occur. CSF demonstrates elevated protein with normal glucose. A CSF mononuclear pleocytosis occurs commonly in HIV-related AIDP. This is an uncommon feature in non–HIV-related AIDP.

Treatment. Patients with suspected AIDP should be hospitalized. Treatment includes intravenous immunoglobulin or plasmapheresis, as well as supportive measures. Severely affected patients with respiratory insufficiency and/or dysautonomia require intensive care. Outcome is generally good and is not dissimilar to that enjoyed by non–HIV-related AIDP patients.

Mononeuropathy Multiplex

Presentation and Progression. AIDS patients, usually with CD4+ counts higher than 200 cells/mm^3, are at risk for the development of necrotizing vasculitis of peripheral nerve. Onset may be abrupt or subacute. With involvement of large- and medium-sized arterioles, multiple mononeuropathies and confluent multiple mononeuropathies may occur, producing lower extremity greater than upper extremity weakness, distal greater than proximal weakness, sensory loss, and pain in the distribution of the nerve(s) affected. With involvement of smaller arterioles, multiple, asymmetric, or largely symmetric distal cutaneous neuropathies may occur, producing distal sensory loss.

Diagnosis. Electromyography and nerve conduction studies demonstrate evidence of multiple, asymmetric axonal loss mononeuropathies.

Treatment. Treatment with corticosteroids or other immunosuppressants may be indicated, although the syndrome may improve without treatment.

Chronic Neuropathy

Chronic Inflammatory Demyelinating Polyneuropathy

Presentation and Progression. HIV-positive patients may develop chronic inflammatory demyelinating polyneuropathy (CIDP). The clinical and laboratory features are indistinguishable from the CIDP that occurs in non–HIV-infected patients. The disorder usually produces distal greater than proximal, motor greater than sensory symptoms that are largely symmetric. Variants, however, do occur in which sensory symptoms or asymmetric symptoms predominate. Motor weakness occurs in both proximal and distal muscles. Sensory loss is usually distal and is present in the legs more than in the arms. Reflexes are reduced to absent.

The clinical course is variable. It may take a chronic, progressive form, which evolves over months to years and can reach a plateau, or it may have an acute onset, with progression beyond the 4 weeks that is characteristic of AIDP. It may have a relapsing course.

Diagnosis. Electromyography and nerve conduction studies demonstrate a disturbance of motor and sensory conduction consistent with a multifocal process predominantly affecting myelin, similar to that noted in AIDP. CSF examination demonstrates elevated protein with normal glucose. As in HIV-associated AIDP, a mononuclear pleocytosis may occur. This is atypical in non–HIV-related CIDP.

Treatment. Treatment includes use of corticosteroids, intravenous immune globulin (IVIG), plasmapheresis, cyclosporine, azathioprine, and methotrexate.

Sensory-Motor Axonal Polyneuropathy

Presentation and Progression. Patients with AIDS are at risk for developing a distal, length-dependent, sensory-predominant axonal polyneuropathy. Onset is usually heralded by the development of symmetric, distal, lower extremity dysesthesia and pain. Over the course of the ensuing months to years the symptoms gradually ascend from the feet to the calves and then to the thighs. When the sensory symptoms have reached the level of the mid-thigh, similar symptoms may begin in the fingers. In like fashion, the upper extremity symptoms may ascend as well.

Diagnosis. Electromyography and nerve conduction studies demonstrate evidence of a disturbance of motor and sensory conduction consistent with a symmetric axon loss polyneuropathy. Screening laboratory studies for unrelated causes of polyneuropathy are normal. If the patient is taking nucleoside analogues, an iatrogenic, drug-related neuropathy should be considered as a possible contributing factor (see below.)

Treatment. Neuropathic pain and painful paresthesias can be managed with the use of agents such as gabapentin, carbamazepine, lamotrigine, diphenylhydantoin, or tricyclic antidepressants. At times, opiates are necessary for pain relief. If appropriate, offending medication(s) can be withdrawn.

KEY POINTS

- Acute, progressive symmetric sensory and motor deficits suggest the Guillain-Barré syndrome (acute inflammatory demyelinating polyneuropathy) or CMV radiculitis
- Acute asymmetric motor and sensory deficits in a peripheral nerve distribution suggest mononeuropathy multiplex caused by a vasculitis
- Chronic sensory and motor deficits in a stocking-glove distribution may be due to HIV infection itself, or to the use of nucleoside analogues

Myopathy: Polymyositis

Presentation and Progression. In HIV-infected patients, usually without AIDS, a syndrome identical to non–HIV-related polymyositis may develop. Progressive, symmetric, proximal greater than distal weakness develops in the lower greater than upper extremities. Selective areas of weakness include the posterior neck muscles, with production of "head drop"; pharyngeal muscles, with development of dysphagia; and quadriceps, with development of proximal leg weakness. Myalgia may occur. HIV-related polymyositis may resemble other myopathies

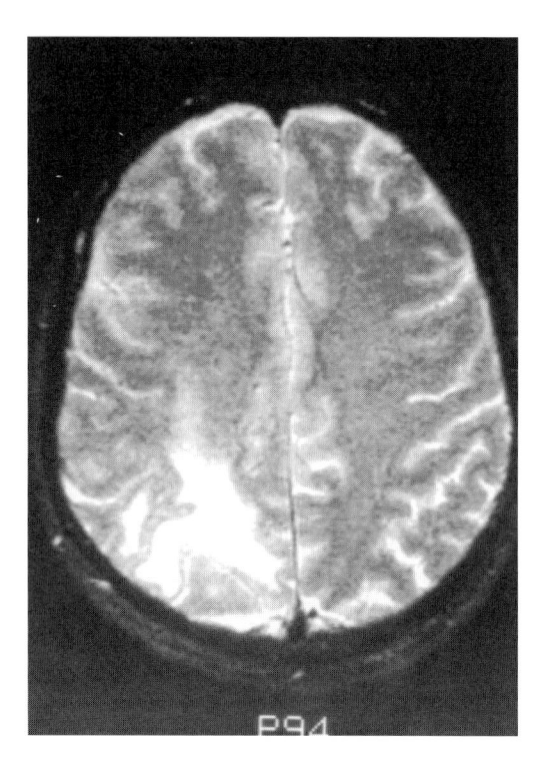

FIG. 17-2 Proton density–weighted MRI image shows nonenhancing right parietal lesion involving both superficial and deep white matter, which is characteristic of progressive multifocal leukoencephalopathy.

including nemaline rod myopathy, zidovudine (AZT)-related myopathy, or HIV wasting syndrome. Distinguishing among these entities is likely to require muscle biopsy.

Diagnosis. In polymyositis, serum creatine phosphokinase (CK) may be 3 to 30 times normal. Electromyography may demonstrate evidence of an irritative myopathy. Muscle biopsy demonstrates myopathy with variation in muscle fiber size, necrosis with muscle cell phagocytosis, regeneration of muscle cells, perivascular and endomysial inflammatory infiltration, and a mild increase in endomysial connective tissue. Biopsy in nemaline rod myopathy shows rodlike cytoplasmic structures in type I greater than type II muscle fibers. Muscle fiber necrosis is present, with sparse inflammation. Biopsy in HIV wasting syndrome is nonspecific.

Treatment. Treatment with corticosteroids is indicated for polymyositis. Drug-induced myopathy is treated with withdrawal of the offending medication. No treatment is available for the other forms of myopathy described.

KEY POINTS

- Progressive, sometimes painful, proximal greater than distal weakness without sensory loss is the hallmark of myopathy
- Causes of myopathy in the HIV-infected population include polymyositis, intramuscular abscess, lymphomatous infiltration of muscle, and HIV wasting syndrome
- Zidovudine can produce a reversible myositis clinically indistinguishable from polymyositis

Central Nervous System Disorders Related to Immunosuppression

Progressive Multifocal Leukoencephalopathy

Presentation and Progression. As its name implies, progressive multifocal leukoencephalopathy (PML) is an illness characterized pathologically by a progressive and diffuse demyelination of subcortical white matter. It is the result of activation of latent infection with the JC virus, a group B papovavirus with a predilection for oligodendrocytes. Prior to the AIDS epidemic, it was most commonly observed in the setting of lymphoproliferative disorders or in patients on immunosuppressive drugs. PML may occur in as many as 5% of adult patients with AIDS and may represent its initial manifestation.

PML presents with a variety of symptoms and signs, depending on which areas of the brain have been affected. Commonly seen are hemiparesis, confusion, visual disturbances, and aphasia, developing over days to weeks. Headache has also been described.

Diagnosis. Neuroimaging demonstrates multifocal or confluent white matter abnormalities, hypodense on CT and hyperintense on T2-weighted MRI, without enhancement or mass effect (Fig. 17-2). Although lesions are typically present in both hemispheres, they tend to be asymmetric. The CSF is normal or shows the sterile mononuclear pleocytosis commonly encountered in HIV infection. Occasionally brain biopsy is necessary, but the diagnosis is typically made on the basis of clinical findings.

Treatment. Both cytosine arabinoside and interferon-α have been used to treat PML, but there is no definitive therapy, and the survival from time of diagnosis is generally 3 to 6 months. Longer survival and remission have occasionally been reported.

Complications of Herpesvirus Infections

Cytomegalovirus

Presentation and Progression. CMV encephalitis is a late complication of HIV infection, typically seen in patients whose CD4+ counts are less than 100 cells/mm³. Although autopsy studies suggest that 25% to 40% of AIDS patients are infected with CMV, this is not always clinically apparent. CMV encephalitis may be difficult to distinguish from HIV-associated dementia. Features that may be helpful in the diagnosis include a history of CMV retinitis, hepatitis, or pneumonitis, or hyponatremia due to adrenal insufficiency. The presentation is often subacute rather than chronic as in HIV-associated dementia, and there are sometimes associated cranial neuropathies or brainstem findings. CMV infection can also cause myelitis and radiculitis as discussed under peripheral nerve disorders.

Diagnosis. A CSF CMV polymerase chain reaction (PCR) may be positive, but otherwise MRI and CSF findings are nonspecific. Treatment with ganciclovir or foscarnet may be helpful.

Herpes Simplex

Presentation and Progression. Herpes simplex virus-1 (HSV-1) causes an acute encephalitis that occurs with approximately equal frequency in AIDS patients and in the general population. Because of the affinity of the virus for the inferior frontal and temporal lobes, infected individuals often present with disturbances of behavior and memory, as well as with changes in level of consciousness that may evolve over several days. Headache, fever, and seizures are common, but the typical oral lesions of HSV-1 are generally not associated with the encephalitis.

Diagnosis. The diagnosis of HSV encephalitis is supported by brain imaging studies, which demonstrate frontotemporal lesions, sometimes hemorrhagic, and by characteristic, although nonspecific, periodic frontotemporal discharges on electroencephalogram. Definitive diagnosis depends on brain biopsy, but CSF PCR is both sensitive and specific. The general CSF profile is nonspecific. It may demonstrate a lymphocytic pleocytosis, with increased protein, decreased glucose, and occasional red cells, but it can be normal early in the disorder.

Treatment. Treatment with acyclovir should be instituted when HSV encephalitis is suspected, without waiting for the results of confirmatory studies. Use of acyclovir is unlikely to produce significant adverse effects, whereas untreated HSV can be catastrophic.

Herpes Zoster Encephalitis

Presentation and Progression. Varicella-zoster virus (VZV) can cause acute encephalitis, often in association with ophthalmic zoster; however, the characteristic rash may have resolved weeks prior to presentation, or in rare instances may never have occurred. Ophthalmic zoster is sometimes also complicated by CNS vasculitis with hemiplegia. Both HSV and VZV have been implicated as a cause of myelitis. (The peripheral manifestations of herpes zoster are discussed further below.)

Diagnosis. In the absence of the characteristic zoster rash, diagnosis can be difficult. CSF examination may demonstrate increased protein, but there are no specific findings.

Treatment. Acyclovir, famciclovir, or valacyclovir is indicated in the treatment of varicella-zoster encephalitis.

KEY POINTS

- Acute confusional states can be seen in the setting of meningitis or systemic infection
- Metabolic abnormalities, particularly azotemia, hypoxemia, hypercalcemia, and elevated ammonia, need to be excluded
- Acute encephalitis may be due to herpes simplex or herpes zoster
- Subacute or chronic encephalopathy is associated with cytomegalovirus, progressive multifocal leukoencephalopathy, syphilis, and HIV-associated dementia

Toxoplasmosis

Presentation and Progression. Latent infection with the protozoan parasite *Toxoplasma gondii* is widespread in adults. In the AIDS population, infection frequently becomes activated, and toxoplasmosis is recognized as the most common cause of intracranial mass lesion in these patients. Pathologic examination reveals focal areas of necrosis and inflammation and the tachyzoite form of the organism. Individuals typically have symptoms and signs of hemiparesis, brainstem or cerebellar dysfunction, or confusion, often following prodromal fever or malaise. The basal ganglia are a common site of in-

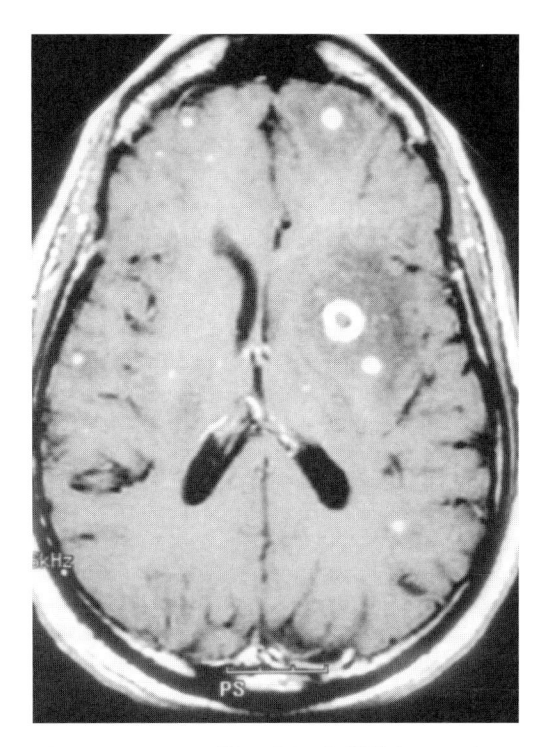

FIG. 17-3 Post-contrast T1-weighted MRI image demonstrates multiple ring-enhancing lesions typical of toxoplasmosis.

fection presenting as a choreiform movement disorder. The cerebral hemispheres also are commonly involved. Toxoplasmosis can occasionally produce a progressive paraparesis due to spinal cord involvement.

Diagnosis. Single or multiple lesions in the brain or spinal cord can be visualized on MRI scan, associated with edema and mass effect. Such lesions generally enhance with the administration of contrast dye (Fig. 17-3). Lumbar puncture may not be safe in the setting of mass lesions, and in any case the CSF formula is nonspecific. Serologic studies are similarly unreliable in making the diagnosis in the immunosuppressed state.

Treatment. Treatment for HIV-infected patients with intracranial mass lesions typically consists of an empiric trial of toxoplasmosis therapy with sulfadiazine and pyrimethamine. Supplemental folinic acid is given to prevent marrow suppression.

The brain should be re-imaged approximately 2 weeks after treatment is begun to determine if there has been radiographic regression of the lesion(s). If so, treatment should continue for a total of 6 weeks, to be followed by maintenance therapy at lower doses or with trimethoprim-sulfamethoxazole. If there is no response to empiric therapy, the major differential consideration is primary CNS lymphoma (discussed below.) Since CNS lymphoma is sensitive to corticosteroids, they should be avoided if possible during the first 2 weeks of treatment to allow accurate interpretation of the patient's response. Other potential etiologies of intracranial masses include bacterial, fungal, tuberculous, and syphilitic lesions. Biopsy should be considered to establish a diagnosis when there is no response to toxoplasmosis therapy or if early decompression of the lesion(s) is indicated to prevent herniation. In suspected spinal cord involvement, empiric therapy with sulfadiazine and pyrimethamine is again recommended before any invasive procedures are undertaken.

Cryptococcosis

Presentation and Progression. *C. neoformans* is encapsulated yeast that is widely disseminated in nature. It is a common cause of fungal meningitis in AIDS patients and is also occasionally associated with mass lesions of the CNS. Estimates of its incidence in AIDS range from 6% to 13%. Patients may present with typical symptoms of meningitis, including headache, photophobia, fever, nausea and vomiting, confusion, and nuchal rigidity, or they may present in subacute fashion with mild headache or fever alone. Cranial neuropathies, including optic neuropathies, can occur. Pathology demonstrates chronic basilar meningitis, with nodular studding of the meninges. The organism occasionally invades the brain parenchyma and produces focal neurologic signs of hemiparesis or brainstem dysfunction due to the presence of a cryptococcoma, a collection of budding yeast. Smaller cystic lesions may also be found in the cortex at autopsy. Other less frequent causes of fungal meningitis in AIDS include histoplasmosis, *Candida,* coccidioidomycosis, aspergillosis, and mucormycosis. The latter two infections can also be responsible for parenchymal lesions, with associated vasculitis.

Diagnosis. The diagnosis is usually established with a positive CSF cryptococcal antigen. Lumbar puncture also typically demonstrates an elevated opening pressure, elevated protein, and mononuclear pleocytosis. CSF glucose may be reduced. Imaging studies are often unremarkable, unless the clinical picture is complicated by the presence of hydrocephalus or a cryptococcoma.

Treatment. Cryptococcal meningitis is treated with intravenous amphotericin B, followed by oral fluconazole, which, at a reduced dose, is continued as prophylactic therapy.

Syphilis

Presentation and Progression. *Treponema pallidum* infection is common in the HIV-infected population, and patients with AIDS may have a more rapid onset of the neurologic complications of syphilis. Following treponemal invasion of the CNS, a syphilitic meningitis ensues, which may be asymptomatic and detectable only by CSF examination or which may present with headache, cranial neuropathies (affecting, in particular, cranial nerves II, VII, and VIII), seizures, and other manifestations of meningeal irritation. Although typically delayed for several years, meningovascular syphilis may also develop at this stage of infection, characterized by an inflammatory reaction in vessel walls that can lead to thrombotic occlusion. In the setting of HIV infection there may also be a shorter latency to parenchymal neurosyphilis in the form of dementia, tabes dorsalis, or intracerebral gumma.

Syphilitic dementia (general paresis) is characterized by progressive cognitive deterioration that in its later stages may be accompanied by tremor, myoclonus, abnormal pupillary responses, and neuropsychiatric symptoms. A gumma, or syphilitic granuloma, behaves like other mass lesions, with variable symptoms depending upon its location. Tabes dorsalis is discussed later in the chapter.

Diagnosis. Patients infected with HIV should be routinely screened for syphilis with the microhemagglutination *T. pallidum* (MHA-TP) or fluorescent treponemal antibody-absorbed (FTA-abs) test, which are both more sensitive and more specific than the commonly used rapid plasma reagin (RPR) test. Patients with positive serology should undergo lumbar puncture to determine if there is a positive CSF Venereal Disease Research Laboratory (VDRL) test. Even if the VDRL test is negative, treatment should be considered when there is a mononuclear pleocytosis, elevated protein, and symptoms consistent with the diagnosis.

Treatment. Neurosyphilis is treated with high-dose intravenous aqueous penicillin at a dose of 2 to 4 million units every 4 hours for 10 to 14 days. Treatment for neurosyphilis may be less effective in HIV-infected individuals than in normal individuals, and follow-up CSF examinations should be performed at 6-month intervals.

Mycobacterial Infection

Presentation and Progression. Both *Mycobacterium tuberculosis* and *M. avium* occur commonly in the AIDS population. The manifestations of CNS tuberculosis include meningitis, tuberculoma (encapsulated caseating granuloma), or more acute abscess of both the brain and spinal cord. Mass lesions may be single or multiple and, depending on size and location, may or may not produce focal deficits. Tuberculous meningitis generally presents subacutely with malaise, headache, and low-grade fever, which progress to symptoms of more fulminant meningitis with confusion, seizures, and focal signs over several weeks. Because of a thick exudate at the base of the brain, cranial neuropathies (particularly involving cranial nerves III, IV, and VI) are common. Vasculitis, producing both thrombotic and hemorrhagic strokes, and CSF block, producing hydrocephalus, are potential complications. Untreated patients die within weeks to months. The prognosis in treated patients depends on when in the course of the illness treatment is begun.

Diagnosis. The diagnosis of tuberculous meningitis is ultimately dependent on the demonstration of the organism in the CSF. A positive smear for acid-fast bacilli may require repeated lumbar punctures; newer methods include PCR and a rapid culture technique. Other CSF findings of mononuclear pleocytosis (50 to 500 cells/mm^3), elevated protein (typically 100 to 500 mg/dl or higher), and low glucose are characteristic but nonspecific. A mixture of neutrophils and lymphocytes may be seen early in the course. A positive skin tuberculin test or other evidence of systemic infection may initially suggest the diagnosis. Diagnosis of tuberculous mass lesions is made with CT or MRI scan.

Treatment. Treatment of both tuberculous meningitis and focal lesions employs a multidrug regimen with isoniazid (INH), rifampin, ethambutol, and pyrazinamide. Pyridoxine should be administered with INH to prevent neuropathy. Some authors advocate the use of corticosteroids in the treatment of edema or raised intracranial pressure. If tuberculomas do not respond to medication, surgical excision may be necessary. MAI also causes mass lesions, detectable on imaging studies, which may be resistant to treatment.

Neoplastic Disease

The most common neoplasm of the brain in the AIDS population is primary CNS lymphoma. Other primary CNS tumors including gliomas have been reported in HIV-infected patients.

Kaposi's sarcoma rarely metastasizes to the brain, but may produce enhancing lesions at the cortical-subcortical junction.

Lymphoma

Presentation and Progression. CNS lymphoma may occur in as many as 5% of patients, the majority of whom have advanced disease. B-cell lymphoma is the most frequent type. Patients may present with progressive cognitive deficits or acute confusion, headache, seizures, cranial neuropathies, and other focal neurologic findings. Papilledema may reflect increased intracranial pressure or direct optic nerve involvement. The most common sites include the cortex, basal ganglia, corpus callosum (with the potential for bihemispheric spread), and periventricular region. Single or multiple lesions may be present. Metastatic lymphoma can also invade the CNS, producing cranial neuropathies, radiculopathies, and paraspinal lesions, which can encroach on the cord through the intervertebral foramina and cause myelopathy.

Diagnosis. Brain imaging studies demonstrate variably enhancing mass lesions or more diffuse parenchymal infiltration. Both the symptoms and the radiographic findings of primary CNS lymphoma may be difficult to distinguish from toxoplasmosis, the most common intracranial mass lesion in AIDS. In the case of significant mass effect and threatened herniation, craniotomy for decompression with open biopsy for diagnosis may be necessary. In the majority of cases of intracranial mass lesion, however, empiric treatment for toxoplasmosis is recommended first, as discussed above. If there is no radiographic evidence of improvement within 2 to 3 weeks, then stereotactic biopsy should be considered to confirm the diagnosis of lymphoma. Thallium-201 SPECT has also recently proven useful in identifying primary CNS lymphoma.

Treatment. The mainstay of treatment has been whole brain irradiation, although these tumors are also steroid-responsive, and methotrexate has been used successfully in the non-AIDS population.

KEY POINTS

- Typically present with focal or lateralized evidence of CNS dysfunction including hemiparesis, hemisensory symptoms, brainstem signs, dyskinesias, and disturbances of vision, equilibrium, and gait
- Should be evaluated with contrast-enhanced MRI scan
- Major differential diagnostic considerations include CNS lymphoma, toxoplasmosis, cytomegalovirus, cryptococcoma, and tuberculoma
- Empiric treatment for toxoplasmosis is recommended, followed by radiographic reassessment and biopsy if the lesion has not regressed
- Biopsy is also indicated if there is significant mass effect with incipient herniation

Cerebrovascular Disease

Presentation and Progression. Both ischemic and hemorrhagic stroke can be seen in HIV-infected individuals. Stroke should be considered in the differential diagnosis of any focal CNS deficit that presents acutely. In addition to the standard vascular risk factors found in any population, specific risk factors for stroke in patients with AIDS include bacterial and nonbacterial endocarditis, meningovascular syphilis, and other causes of infectious vasculitis.

Diagnosis. The clinical impression of stroke can be confirmed with neuroimaging studies. Hemorrhagic stroke is immediately evident on CT scan of the brain. Nonhemorrhagic stroke can be visualized acutely on diffusion-weighted MRI scan, but may not be visible on CT or non–diffusion-weighted MRI scan until approximately 24 hours after the event.

Treatment. Acute treatment of stroke and prevention of further strokes depend on elucidation of the underlying mechanism of cerebral ischemia. A detailed discussion of this topic is beyond the scope of the current chapter.

Peripheral Neurologic Complications of HIV Infection Related to Immunosuppression

Cytomegalovirus

Presentation and Progression. Patients with AIDS, usually with CD4+ counts less than 100 cells/mm^3, are at risk for developing CMV radiculitis involving the lumbar and sacral roots (the cauda equina). Pathologic examination of the roots demonstrates endoneurial neutrophil infiltration with giant cells and typical CMV inclusions.

The rate of progression varies from acute to subacute, evolving over days to weeks. Heralded by back and radiating leg pain, urinary bladder symptoms soon follow, indicating dysfunction of the sacral roots S2-S4. Eventually, a progressive, predominantly motor, and often asymmetric polyradiculopathy results in severe bilateral lower extremity weakness, which can progress to paraplegia. Sensory loss in a polyradicular pattern also occurs, but is overshadowed by the motor loss. Uncommonly, cervical roots and even cranial nerves can be involved in an ascending pattern of weakness. Patients, usually with CD4+ counts less than 100 cells/mm^3, may also develop a rapidly progressive vasculitic mononeuropathy multiplex syndrome in association with infection with CMV.

Diagnosis. In CMV radiculitis, the CSF demonstrates a marked pleocytosis, with a predominance of polymorphonuclear cells, low sugar, and high protein. MRI imaging of the lumbosacral spine with and without contrast may demonstrate root enhancement (Fig. 17-4). There may be evidence of a systemic infection, with CMV demonstrable in the retina, blood, and/or urine. In the case of mononeuropathy multiplex, electromyography and nerve conduction studies demonstrate evidence of multiple, asymmetric axonal loss mononeuropathies. Nerve biopsy demonstrates endoneurial neutrophilic inflammation, giant cells with CMV inclusions, and CMV immunoreactivity in the nerve.

Treatment. Early treatment with ganciclovir, foscarnet, or cidofovir is recommended in both conditions. However, the results of therapy are often disappointing, and the patient is left with a substantial neurologic deficit.

Herpes Zoster

Presentation and Progression. HIV with AIDS places patients at risk for reactivation of latent infection of one or more dorsal sensory ganglia by varicella-zoster. The process begins with a deep, aching, and burning dermatomal pain in the distribution of the affected cranial nerves or spinal roots. Dysesthesias

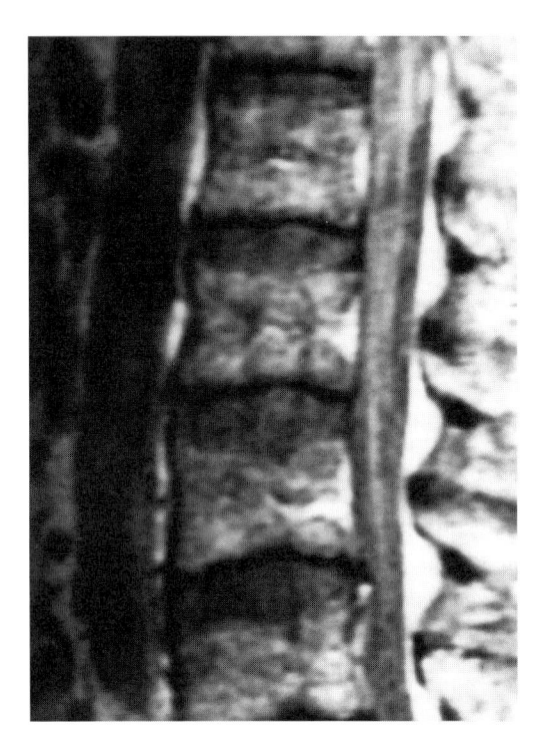

FIG.17-4 Multiple nerve roots of cauda equina enhance in this postcontrast T1-weighted MRI image of CMV radiculitis.

occur in the same distribution. The most commonly involved areas are the face (trigeminal), thoracic, and cervical region. Examination demonstrates sensory loss and often hyperesthesia within the involved dermatome(s). Segmental reflexes served by the involved roots may be lost or reduced. Severe pain is followed within 1 to 3 weeks by a mucocutaneous vesicular rash in the affected dermatome(s). In some patients, segmental motor weakness in the same distribution as the pain and sensory loss can occur, signifying involvement of the associated motor root or anterior horn cells. This occurs particularly in cervical and lumbar segments. The development of facial weakness is referred to as the Ramsay Hunt syndrome. Partial or complete recovery occurs. Postherpetic pain, however, can persist for months.

Diagnosis. Diagnosis is commonly made on the basis of the typical vesicular eruption. CSF examination may demonstrate a pleocytosis, mild increase in protein, normal glucose, and perhaps a positive culture or positive PCR for varicella-zoster.

Treatment. Treatment with the antiviral agents valacyclovir, famciclovir, or acyclovir can be initiated <72 hours after the onset of the rash. Pain is treated with various agents including analgesics, anticonvulsants, tricyclic antidepressants, topical anesthetics, and capsaicin cream.

Syphilis

Presentation and Progression. Patients with HIV and coexistent untreated or inadequately treated syphilis are at risk for the development of tertiary manifestations of syphilis. In tabes dorsalis, chronic meningeal/arachnoid infection and inflammation result in fibrosis and loss of axons in the posterior (sensory) roots and loss of cells within the dorsal root ganglia. The process does not affect the motor neurons or anterior (motor) roots. This occurs predominantly in the lumbosacral region.

Distal sensory loss in the legs and significant imbalance and gait instability occur because of sensory ataxia resulting from the loss of large sensory axons responsible for position and vibration sense. Impotence and bladder dysfunction also occur because of loss of small axons serving autonomic function. Loss of the small sensory axons responsible for pain sensation results in repeated distal limb and joint injury without pain, resulting in painless foot and leg ulcers as well as painless joint injury (Charcot's joints). Involvement of the small sensory axons also results in sudden exacerbations of pain, often referred to as "lightning pain." Other regions of sensory loss referred to as Hitzig zones do not follow a lumbosacral pattern but may include areas of sensory loss involving the central face, nipples, and ulnar forearms.

Tabes dorsalis is often (>90%) accompanied by a pupillary abnormality known as Argyll Robertson pupil. The pupils are irregular and small. They react poorly to light, but do react well to the near reflex. Optic atrophy with resultant visual loss may also be present. Aortitis may also accompany tabes dorsalis.

Diagnosis. As described earlier, serum MHA-TP is positive; serum VDRL may be negative. The CSF VDRL may be positive or negative. CSF examination may be normal or demonstrate a mononuclear pleocytosis, with elevated protein, normal glucose, elevated immunoglobulin G (IgG), and oligoclonal bands.

Treatment. Tertiary syphilis is treated with intravenous penicillin as described in the section on CNS disorders.

Tuberculosis

Presentation and Progression. Tuberculosis can produce vertebral osteomyelitis and associated radiculopathy via epidural space extension and compression of the involved nerve root(s) by either a pathologic fracture or a tubercular abscess. Back pain usually precedes the development of radicular pain, along with loss of sensory, motor, and autonomic function consistent with the site of involvement. Injury to multiple lumbosacral roots, the cauda equina syndrome, can result from a lumbar or vertebral tubercular process.

Diagnosis. Neuroimaging of the involved spinal segment(s) will reveal the extent and the location of the vertebral and epidural processes.

Treatment. Treatment includes possible neurosurgical decompression and stabilization along with antituberculous medication (see above).

Myopathy: Pyomyositis/Lymphomatous Infiltration of Muscle

Presentation and Progression. *Cryptococcus*, CMV, MAI, and *Toxoplasma* can infect muscle (pyomyositis) and produce painful muscular swelling along with weakness. Lymphoma (discussed below) can also infiltrate muscle.

Diagnosis. Imaging of the involved muscle(s) with MRI or CT scanning may reveal the location and distribution of the abnormality. Similarly, electromyography may demonstrate the presence of a destructive focal or multifocal myopathic process. Muscle biopsy is necessary to make a specific etiologic diagnosis and direct treatment.

Treatment. Antibiotic treatment is guided by the specific infectious agent. Lymphoma is treated with systemic chemotherapy. Adjunctive radiation therapy directed at involved muscle(s) can be added if necessary.

Neoplastic Disorders
Lymphoma
Presentation and Progression. A subacute motor neuronopathy can develop as a paraneoplastic manifestation in patients with lymphoma. A symmetric, painless, and often mild lower motor neuron weakness of the arms greater than legs develops progressively and then stabilizes. Bulbar muscles are usually spared. No upper motor neuron manifestations are noted.

Diagnosis. CSF examination demonstrates no cells and a mild elevation of protein with normal glucose. MRI scanning of the spinal cord and roots is normal. Electromyography demonstrates an active, multisegmental lower motor neuron process. Motor nerve conduction may reveal lower motor amplitudes but preservation of motor conduction velocity. Sensory conduction is normal or relatively spared.

Treatment. The syndrome may respond to treatment of the underlying lymphoma with chemotherapeutic agents.

Lymphomatous Meningitis
Presentation and Progression. Lymphomatous meningitis is common, presenting with headache, cranial neuropathies, confusion, or seizure; however, it may be asymptomatic. Lymphomatous infiltration of nerve roots is usually associated with simultaneous infiltration of the leptomeninges. This process results in injury to axons within the motor and sensory roots of the lumbar and sacral regions along with cranial nerves, which are present within the subarachnoid space. Roots at the cervical and thoracic levels are less often affected. Progressive, usually painless, and asymmetric weakness in the lower extremities develops. This may be accompanied by multiple cranial neuropathies, typically involving nerves III, V, VI, and VII. Sphincter dysfunction and a predominance of pain or sensory loss are atypical.

Diagnosis. CSF usually demonstrates a mononuclear pleocytosis with elevated protein and normal glucose. CSF cytology may demonstrate atypical or frankly malignant lymphocytes. Flow cytometry can demonstrate a clonal population of malignant lymphoid cells. The diagnosis of paraspinal lesions depends on imaging studies.

Treatment. Treatment of lymphomatous meningitis consists of craniospinal irradiation along with intrathecal chemotherapy, usually administered through an Ommaya reservoir into the lateral ventricle.

Neurologic Complications of Treatment: Medication-Induced Neuropathy
Presentation and Progression. HIV-infected patients may develop neuropathy as a complication of one or more medications. HIV-infected patients using nucleoside analogues can develop a distal, symmetric, painful, and purely sensory neuropathy in the legs greater than the arms. This complication occurs in a dose-related fashion and is more common in the setting of preexisting neuropathy or with later-stage HIV disease. It occurs most commonly with zalcitabine (ddC) (25% to 65%) and stavudine (d4T) (15% to 55%), but can occur with didanosine (ddI) (12% to 34%).

Vincristine, used for treatment of HIV-related Kaposi's sarcoma or lymphoma, produces a sensory-motor neuropathy. Paresthesias begin in the hands and the feet. This is followed by distal weakness, including wrist and foot drop. Neuropathic pain can develop. It can be accompanied by cranial neuropathies (especially involving nerves VII and IX). Autonomic dysfunction including postural hypotension, bowel dysmotility, and bladder atony can occur. Recovery is slow and often incomplete. INH, used for the treatment of tuberculosis, can produce a sensory-predominant neuropathy, particularly in patients not receiving prophylaxis with pyridoxine (vitamin B_6).

Dapsone, used for prophylaxis against *Pneumocystis carinii*, produces a dose-related (usually >300 mg/day) motor-predominant polyneuropathy, which involves the arms greater than the legs. The neuropathy can progress even after the drug is stopped. Improvement occurs late following discontinuation of the drug.

Diagnosis. When nucleoside analogues are the cause of neuropathy, electromyography and nerve conduction studies demonstrate a disturbance of sensory conduction consistent with a sensory axonal neuropathy. Electromyography and nerve conduction studies in vincristine-induced neuropathy demonstrate evidence of an axonal sensory motor polyneuropathy. In INH-related neuropathy, electromyography and nerve conduction studies demonstrate evidence of a sensory axonal polyneuropathy, and in the case of dapsone, the findings indicate a motor-predominant axon loss polyneuropathy.

Treatment. If appropriate, the offending agent can be stopped or the dose reduced.

Myopathy: Zidovudine Myopathy
Presentation and Progression. Patients receiving AZT may develop proximal lower extremity greater than upper extremity weakness, muscle wasting, and myalgias.

Diagnosis. There is an elevated CK. Electromyography demonstrates evidence of a mildly irritative myopathy. Biopsy demonstrates mild inflammation, with muscle cell necrosis. Many cells may contain a proliferation of abnormal mitochondria, which on specific staining produce "ragged red" fibers.

Treatment. When AZT is discontinued, the symptoms usually resolve within 3 to 4 months.

Drug Interactions
Protease inhibitors interfere with the P450 enzyme system. As a result, the dosage of some medications may need to be adjusted. This is particularly true of anticonvulsant medications. Carbamazepine, ergotamine, and dihydroergotamine should not be coadministered with saquinavir. Triazolam, midazolam, and flurazepam should be avoided. Lorazepam, however, is considered safe.

When to Refer
Neurologic consultation should be considered for any HIV-infected patient who presents with complaints of motor, sensory, or cognitive dysfunction in association with focal neurologic findings on examination. Infectious disease specialists

should be involved in the management of patients with meningitis or abscess within the CNS, and oncologists should be consulted when a neoplasm is suspected on the basis of brain or spinal cord imaging.

SUGGESTED READINGS

Belman AL, Preston T, Milazzo M: Human immunodeficiency virus and acquired immunodeficiency syndrome. In Goetz CG, Pappert EJ, editors: *Textbook of clinical neurology,* Philadelphia, 1999, WB Saunders, pp 876-905.

Berger JR, Levy RM: The neurologic complications of human immunodeficiency virus infection, *Med Clin North Am* 77(1):1-23, 1993.

Berger JR: AIDS and the nervous system. In Aminoff M, editor: *Neurology and general medicine,* ed 2, New York, 1995, Churchill Livingstone, pp 757-778.

Gabuzda DH, Hirsch MS: Neurologic manifestations of infection with human immunodeficiency virus, *Ann Intern Med* 107: 383-391, 1987.

Quality Standards Subcommittee of the American Academy of Neurology: Evaluation and management of intracranial mass lesions in AIDS, *Neurology* 50:21-26, 1998.

Wulff EA, Simpson DM: Neuromuscular complications of the human immunodeficiency virus type 1 infection, *Semin Neurol* 19(2):157-164, 1999.

18 Neuropsychiatric Complications of HIV Infection

ROGER E. WEISS

Introduction

The case report in Box 18-1, unique in some ways, commonplace in others, is presented because it contains within it many of the problems that patients with the acquired immunodeficiency syndrome (AIDS) and the physicians who care for them often face. The various psychiatric symptoms that are encountered run the gamut from depression, anxiety, and confusion to dementia. Psychotic reactions and personality alterations are also seen. At times patients experience reactions to being ill in ways that are usual for them, and at other times they develop new psychiatric illnesses. Sometimes it is a purely psychological phenomenon, and sometimes it is a reaction to organic physical or central nervous system (CNS) disease. Additionally there are philosophical and social complications of being ill with AIDS. Sometimes a lack of a support system or intense shame about how the disease was contracted promotes an isolation that contributes to the problems of overall care.

Psychiatric complications of AIDS and human immunodeficiency virus (HIV) infection can be divided into three basic categories: psychiatric illness and psychological reactions, organic reactions, and mixed organic/psychological responses. These three categories will be discussed from the standpoint of their clinical presentations, differential diagnosis, and treatment approaches. Additionally, there will be separate discussions of the problems of suicidal ideation, pain syndromes, and sleep disturbance in patients with HIV infection and AIDS.

Psychiatric Illness
Mood Disorders
Reactive Depression

Presentation and Progression. Patients often experience symptoms of a mild depression or dysphoria when they find out they are HIV-positive. This is a feeling of mild sadness, and at times mild anxiety, and may come and go over the duration of the illness. It may be most intense when the patient is first diagnosed or when any actual symptoms appear. Its hallmarks are usually feelings of sadness and/or despair, helplessness, hopelessness, and a feeling of being out of control. These symptoms are often accompanied by feelings of guilt, shame, or embarrassment. Patients suffering from this form of reactive depression often experience a concurrent anxiety that may manifest itself with mild to moderate sleep disturbance, such as frequent awakenings and early morning awakening. Patients describe having a thought about being ill the moment they wake up and immediately becoming anxious. Getting back to sleep quickly will depend on the depth and intensity of the anxiety.

Another hallmark of reactive depression is shame and guilt. Even in diseases in which the patient played no role in contracting the illness there is often a feeling of guilt expressed as the thought, "what could I have done differently to prevent this from happening." Patients with various forms of cancer or patients recovering from an acute myocardial infarction often express these same sentiments. Their illness is experienced as a punishment for something that they did wrong. Patients with HIV-related illness have a particularly strong sense of guilt and shame as it applies to their illness. Some of these feelings are purely personal and stem from the general feeling described above of feeling that they are being punished in some way. Some of their feelings of guilt may arise from the way that they believe they contracted the disease and what they might have done to prevent it. In general, with all illnesses, patients often feel that they did something to bring about the illness as a means of subconsciously attempting to control the uncontrollable. If they caused it, then they can rid themselves of it. The general sense of guilt, however, contributes a great deal to the symptoms of reactive depression.

Shame is another element in the reaction to HIV illness. This psychological response is related more to a sense of society's view and the view of friends and family as perceived by the patient. It is a sense of being an outcast by virtue of having a dreaded disease. Patients feel more vulnerable and exposed by having to reveal that they have contracted the infection and, in their minds, what it implies. The potential for social isolation is heightened by these feelings. Reactive depression and adjustment disorders are terms applied to one's reaction to a traumatic event or the discovery of a major negative life change or medical illness.

Diagnosis. There are a number of patients for whom mild reactive symptoms are the prodrome to a severe major depressive or psychotic depressive episode. These patients must be watched for in the general population of patients with mild depressions and dysphorias. It is also most important to carefully note any change in mental status or mood in someone who has been diagnosed with HIV infection to rule out underlying changes in overall health and metabolic status, possible drug effects, or direct effect of CNS infection or secondary CNS infection.

Treatment. Patients with newly diagnosed HIV disease often report depressive symptomatology that is generally at a mild level of disturbance. The treatment of this reaction to an illness is best approached with either short-term supportive psychotherapy, education, or psychopharmacologic intervention. Medications often used under these circumstances range from minor tranquilizers (a short- or long-acting variety in the benzodiazepine family) to sleep medications and antidepressants. Generally, in an uncomplicated reactive depression that extends in duration no more than 3 months, short-acting benzodiazepines prescribed on a prn basis will be adequate treatment in conjunction with supportive psychotherapy and greater education about the illness.

Psychotherapy. In addition to the direct benefits of psychotherapy in providing an outlet for emerging feelings during the course of a newly diagnosed illness, it is extremely important in preventing isolation and alienation. Feeling understood is a very potent experience for reducing isolation. Patients diagnosed as HIV-positive or with AIDS run the additional risk of emotional withdrawal and isolation, even from close family and friends. The release of feelings such as anger, shame, guilt, grief, sadness, and embarrassment can help reduce overall feelings of depression and anxiety in patients. In patients with reactive depressions or adjustment disorders, there is a range in terms of the degree of anxiety that is associated with the depressive feelings. For some patients the release of their suppressed and hidden feelings in a safe confidential setting, where they are supported, will contribute greatly to a sense of well being and reduce the need for medication. For some patients a well-organized educational approach will help significantly in developing a greater sense of control, by strengthening intellectual defenses and by providing a sense of security that they will be effectively cared for.

Pharmacologic Treatment. It is important to note that patients with reactive depressions experience a varying amount of anxiety as a component of their depressive feelings, and patients with primarily anxiety-based reactions often experience some depressive symptoms as well. It is up to the clinician to determine by listening to the patient where the emphasis of the illness is. As a general rule, uncomplicated grief, reactive depression, and bereavement can be treated with psychotherapy alone. Medication is added as the symptomatology worsens in severity. If greater anxiety appears with sleep disturbance and difficulty with concentration, then minor tranquilizers are added. If necessary, small-dose hypnotics may be necessary in the short term to treat sleep disturbance.

KEY POINTS

REACTIVE DEPRESSION
- Symptoms: Mild feelings of sadness, (+/−) mild anxiety, (+/−) sleep disturbance, feelings of shame and guilt, often self-limiting
- Differential diagnosis: Grief reactions (bereavement), anxiety disorders, prodrome to major depressive disorder, prodrome to medical illness
- Treatment:
  Supportive psychotherapy
  Low-dose benzodiazepines (side effects include sedation and abuse potential)
   Lorazepam (Ativan)
   Oxazepam (Serax)
   Clonazepam (Klonopin)

BOX 18-1
Case Report

"After I was told that I was HIV-positive, everything in my life changed."

D.B.

D.B. was a 45-year-old gay white male who died of complications of AIDS after a 4-year period of having knowledge that he had been infected with the virus. He succumbed to the illness in the early 1990s after having been found in his apartment by a friend who had been unable to reach him for several days. He had lived alone, ever since his lover of 20 years had died the previous year, also from the consequences of AIDS.

Both of these men were extremely intelligent and worked in high-level technical capacities. D.B. was a mechanical engineer, who had traveled worldwide as a consultant working for large corporations. He had said that his I.Q. was 160, which actually seemed low when he revealed the encyclopedic amount of information and sophisticated understanding that he had possessed. He had a long history of chronic unipolar depression and described these episodes as being among the most painful and devastating experiences of his life. He was intermittently treated with combinations of antidepressant medication over a 20-year period. He loved to read, write poetry, listen to opera, and pursue scholarly undertakings of various kinds. He was an inherently kind and sensitive man. He was devastated by the knowledge that he was ill with AIDS. He had been sexually active in the late 1970s and early 1980s at a time when the virus was not as prevalent, and he thought that he had escaped the possibility of contracting it because he and his partner had a committed monogamous relationship for years. He was extremely upset by the news that he was HIV-positive because he had been reading about the devastation that AIDS was causing and knew immediately that his life had been shortened. He became obsessed with any bits of information that he could get his hands on to better understand the disease. Information helped with the intellectual defense that he tried to set up. Just knowing about the realities made him feel better and helped provide a feeling of psychological control. But the overall sense of his state of being was one of despair. After it became known that his lover was also HIV-positive, his depressive symptoms became much worse for a period of time. He was intermittently suicidal and needed several emergency interventions to bring him back under control. His lover was a nuclear physicist. He developed a more rapid course of the disease including AIDS dementia complex (ADC). Of all their physical and psychological capabilities, they both admitted that their intellect was their most prized attribute. His partner became disoriented, forgetful, and extremely anxious, and needed to be treated with anxiolytic medication and small-dose neuroleptics to reduce his extreme anxiety. He died several years after developing the illness. After his death, D.B. organized a memorial service for him, which was attended by several hundred people, including many friends, some family, and many professional associates from around the country. The loss was devastating to D.B. He felt totally isolated and extremely frightened about facing a fate similar to his lover. Losing his intellect and being aware that it was happening was his greatest fear. After his death it became known that he had bequeathed a large portion of his estate for research in affective disorders.

Only rarely should antidepressants be necessary in reactive depression and grief reactions, which should be self-limiting in nature. There are a group of patients, however, who will not recover fully from these symptoms without more aggressive pharmacologic intervention and who may even progress to more severe depressive illness unless treated. If depressive symptoms seem to be getting worse over time rather than improving, it is wise to consider an antidepressant, particularly a selective serotonin reuptake inhibitor (SSRI), to aid in the treatment.

Bereavement

Presentation and Progression. Over the course of a patient's life history with HIV/AIDS-related illness, the concept of loss may need to be addressed from time to time. Losses may be those of others with whom the patient had been closely involved or personal loss involving changes in levels of functioning or self-esteem. Diminished status due to an inability to function or having to change professional activity due to being HIV-positive can result in a loss of esteem. In certain vulnerable individuals even severe depressive symptomatology can occur. For some individuals, their professional lives are attached tightly to their overall sense of themselves, and they feel a huge loss of status along with intense feelings of worthlessness and humiliation. Loss of physical health and integrity of one's body is another area of significant loss with HIV disease. This can produce an increased sense of vulnerability and anxiety about the future. The adjustment from a state of well being to one that has with it constant reminders of being ill is another shift representative of loss. For some patients, the multiple medications required and their dosing schedules, the medication side effects, and the frequent doctor's visits act as constant reminders of the disease and of a shift from life prior to being ill.

Treatment. The best method for handling these feelings is by treating the patient with understanding and dignity. Recognition by the physician that the patient is faced with overwhelming circumstances will be of great help in addressing some of these losses. For an HIV-infected patient, to be respected and appreciated by those caring for him or her may at times be the best defense against loss of esteem. Of course, the emergence of more severe symptomatology must be addressed, since there are many adjustments to loss that these patients often experience over time that may progress to a more severe depressive disorder.

Major Depressive Disorder

Presentation and Progression. The hallmark of major depressive disorder is pervasive sadness and a depressed mood throughout the day. This feeling of sadness is often accompanied by feelings of emptiness. There is an increased amount of tearfulness, guilt, and self-recriminatory thoughts. Patients experience a generalized slowing down, with loss of interest in activities of everyday life, extreme loss of energy, psychomotor retardation, loss of appetite, and a lack of concentration. In treating patients with HIV who are already susceptible to self-recriminatory thoughts, one must be particularly vigilant to look for suicidal ideation when severe depressions occur. When patients view their illness as punishment, the concurrence of a severe depression can exacerbate these feelings, which are often a component of major depressions. Patients with major depressions can have feelings of worthlessness and loss of self-esteem that approaches delusional proportions. In its most severe form it can have psychotic manifestations including hallucinations and frank delusions, with recurrent thoughts of death. Patients with this disorder can present with either psychomotor retarded or agitated states. They often have an ambivalence related to decision making that is totally paralyzing. No decision seems right. Biologic manifestations also include severe sleep disturbance, either difficulty falling asleep or early morning awakenings, hypersomnia, severe anorexia with weight loss, restlessness, and loss of energy. It is often helpful to get a family and personal history of previous episodes of depression.

Diagnosis

Psychiatric Disorders. Depression is a spectrum, ranging from the mild forms of self-limiting depressions and dysphorias to severe incapacitating biologic depressions. In diagnosing major depressions, one must be aware that minor depressions and dysphorias can sometimes progress to major depressive proportions, particularly if they persist longer than 3 to 6 months. Patients with HIV who present with dysphoria (symptoms of sadness over long periods of time), mood swings (which may be indicative of cyclothymia or bipolar disorder), chronic bereavement, psychotic symptoms (which may indicate underlying schizoaffective disorder), severe adjustment disorders, underlying personality disorders, reactions precipitated by drug abuse, or mood disorder due to underlying medical condition must be distinguished from patients with a major depression. Symptoms that help distinguish major depression are severely depressed mood, loss of interest or pleasure in everyday events, sleep disturbance, and loss of energy. Without major changes in cognition, levels of consciousness, psychotic symptoms, agitation, or physical symptoms, one should think of major depression.

Medical Conditions. There are many organic illnesses that can cause symptoms that mimic severe depressive illness in patients with HIV/AIDS, including metabolic or endocrine disorders, systemic illness of any kind, secondary opportunistic infections, anemias, and HIV neurocognitive disorder—

▶ KEY POINTS

BEREAVEMENT

⊃ Symptoms: Depressive focus is loss, survivor guilt, intense anxiety if denial is utilized, sleep disturbance, appetite loss
⊃ Differential diagnosis: Primary anxiety disorders, major mood disorders, underlying medical illness
⊃ Treatment:
Supportive or uncovering
Psychotherapy
Benzodiazepines for anxiety (side effect of sedation)
  If progresses use low-dose tricyclic antidepressants (side effects include sedation, anxiety, constipation, and confusion)
    Desipramine (Norpramin)
    Nortriptyline (Pamelor)
Selective serotonin reuptake inhibitors (side effects include nausea, headache, and anxiety)
    Fluoxetine (Prozac)
    Paroxetine (Paxil)
    Sertraline (Zoloft)

> **BOX 18-2**
> **Antiretroviral Medications**
>
> **NUCLEOSIDE REVERSE TRANSCRIPTASE INHIBITORS (NRTIs)**
> Abacavir
> Didanosine
> Lamivudine
> Stavudine
> Zalcitabine
> Zidovudine
>
> **NON-NUCLEOSIDE REVERSE TRANSCRIPTASE INHIBITORS (NNRTIs)**
> Delavirdine
> Efavirenz
> Nevirapine
>
> **PROTEASE INHIBITORS (PIs)**
> Amprenavir
> Indinavir
> Nelfinavir
> Ritonavir
> Saquinavir

From Feucht CL, Weissman SB: *TEN* 2(11), 2000.

minor or progressing to dementia (AIDS dementia complex [ADC])—which can mimic depression, with symptoms of anergy, withdrawal, apathy, and depressed mood. Careful neurologic examination and mental status examination should be utilized to help make this distinction, since the depressive symptoms may be a manifestation of centrally active virus on the CNS. Treatment in this case would involve antiviral therapy alone or in addition to antidepressants.

Medication Side Effects. There are many drugs utilized in the treatment of AIDS patients that can precipitate depressive symptoms. These include steroids, interferon, zidovudine (ZDV), isoniazid, and others. The possibility of drug effects or drug-drug interactions must always be considered when attempting to distinguish depressions in medically ill individuals (Box 18-2 and Tables 18-1 and 18-2).

Treatment

Psychotherapy. There are a number of psychotherapeutic treatment modalities that are useful in approaching a patient with major depressive disorder. In some cases a combination of treatments is appropriate, depending on the clinical situation. Many patients suffering from this disorder experience a great deal of despair and hopelessness that is best addressed with a supportive approach. Patients need to know that they will improve and that their symptoms are treatable. There may be many social, familial, and work-related problems that may require family intervention. The depressive episode may be an entirely new experience for the patient, stemming from the overwhelming stress of being ill with HIV disease or a recurrence of a premorbid condition. It may be a manifestation of direct CNS involvement of the virus. It is important to distinguish the differences so that patients can be more effectively treated and communicated with. Reducing patients' isolation, alienation, and loss of control and guilt is an important element of supportive psychotherapy. There are times when a deeper orientation is warranted, for example, when longer standing or more deeply held negative self-concepts are noted. In these cases, cognitive therapy or insight-oriented psychotherapy can be useful. Patients may be struggling with chronic conflicts over dependency, trust, rejection, fears of loss of cognitive ability, and guilt, which require a deeper form of intervention. Issues relating to death and dying can emerge at any time during the course of illness with HIV disease. Medical or psychiatric hospitalization must always be considered as an option. Suicidal ideation must be determined and asked about in any patient suffering from a major depression. It must be asked directly because patients with this illness are often reticent to volunteer suicidal feelings, although they are very common in depressed individuals. A determination of the seriousness of these thoughts helps in determining whether hospitalization is warranted. It must be remembered that in addition to the depressive illness, these patients are experiencing the physical and emotional stresses of having HIV disease.

Pharmacotherapy. Medications used to treat major depression in patients with AIDS must be carefully selected so as to not interfere with other medications being utilized for treatment of coexisting medical conditions or antiviral therapy. Since protease inhibitors and antidepressant medications are both metabolized by the cytochrome P450 system, drug-drug interactions must be carefully monitored. The degree of protein binding is another area for close consideration. In general, it is best to start drug treatment at lower than therapeutic levels in patients who are medically compromised and to increase doses slowly. Patients with major depression in conjunction with HIV and AIDS have about the same rate of response to antidepressant medication as the general population of severely depressed individuals. Response rates of approximately 75% have been reported in both populations. Even patients with significant physical illness secondary to AIDS respond well to antidepressant medication for the treatment of their depressions. Depression and mood disorders in general have a very high prevalence rate among HIV-infected and AIDS patients (20% and 50%, respectively). Of the antidepressant groups available, the SSRIs are probably the safest and easiest to use in medically compromised individuals. The side effects include decreased libido and sexual dysfunction, nausea, increased anxiety, and decreased appetite. Although these side effects are usually not troublesome and sometimes transitory, they must be monitored to achieve good compliance. In general, lower than recommended doses can be initiated and titrated upward. It is possible that a

KEY POINTS

MAJOR DEPRESSIVE DISORDER

⊃ Symptoms: Severe feelings of sadness, anergy, loss of interest in daily living, loss of appetite, severe sleep disturbance and restless sleep, many awakenings, psychomotor retardation, (+/−) psychotic symptoms, (+/−) irritability
⊃ Differential diagnosis: Dysthymia, reactive depression, bipolar disorder, pathologic grief, schizoaffective disorder, organic medical or CNS disease, drug toxicity
⊃ Treatment:
Tricyclic antidepressants in higher doses (side effects include sedation, anxiety, constipation, and confusion)
Selective serotonin reuptake inhibitors:
  Fluoxetine (Prozac)
  Paroxetine (Paxil)
  Sertraline (Zoloft)
Also:
  Venlafaxine (Effexor)
  Citalopram (Celexa)

TABLE 18-1
Neuropsychiatric Side Effects of Selected Medications Used in HIV Disease

Drug	Target illness	Side effects
Acyclovir	Herpes encephalitis	Visual hallucinations, depersonalization, tearfulness, confusion, hyperesthesia, hyperacusis, thought insertion, insomnia
Amphotericin B	Cryptococcosis	Delirium, peripheral neuropathy, diplopia
β-Lactam antibiotics	Infections	Confusion, paranoia, hallucinations, mania, coma
Co-trimoxazole	*Pneumocystis carinii* pneumonia	Depression, loss of appetite, insomnia, apathy
Cycloserine	Tuberculosis	Psychosis, somnolence, depression, confusion, tremor, vertigo, paresis, seizure, dysarthria
Didanosine	HIV	Nervousness, anxiety, confusion, seizures, insomnia, peripheral neuropathy
Efavirenz	HIV	Nightmares, depression, confusion
Foscarnet	Cytomegalovirus	Paresthesias, seizures, headache, irritability, hallucinations, confusion
Interferon-α	Kaposi's sarcoma	Depression, weakness, headache, myalgias, confusion
Isoniazid	Tuberculosis	Depression, agitation, hallucinations, paranoia, impaired memory, anxiety
Lamivudine	HIV	Insomnia, mania
Methotrexate	Lymphoma	Encephalopathy (at high dose)
Pentamidine	*P. carinii* pneumonia	Confusion, anxiety, lability, hallucinations
Procarbazine	Lymphoma	Mania, loss of appetite, insomnia, nightmares, confusion, malaise
Quinolones	Infection	Psychosis, delirium, seizures, anxiety, insomnia, depression
Stavudine	HIV	Headache, asthenia, malaise, confusion, depression, seizures, excitability, anxiety, mania, early morning awakening, insomnia
Sulfonamides	Infection	Psychosis, delirium, confusion, depression, hallucinations
Thiabendazole	Strongyloidiasis	Hallucinations, olfactory disturbance
Vinblastine	Kaposi's sarcoma	Depression, loss of appetite, headache
Vincristine	Kaposi's sarcoma	Hallucinations, headache, ataxia, sensory loss
Zalcitabine	HIV	Headache, confusion, impaired concentration, somnolence, asthenia, depression, seizures, peripheral neuropathy
Zidovudine	HIV	Headache, malaise, asthenia, insomnia, unusually vivid dreams, restlessness, severe agitation, mania, auditory hallucinations, confusion

From Grant I, Atkinson JH Jr: Neuropsychiatric aspects of HIV infection and AIDS. In Sadock BJ, Sadock VA, editors: *Kaplan and Sadock's comprehensive textbook of psychiatry*, Philadelphia, 1999, Lippincott Williams & Wilkins, pp 308-336.

particular patient will be intolerant to one drug in this class but will do fine on another. The tricyclic antidepressants are the other major class of antidepressant medication. Many are highly anticholinergic and antihistaminic. Their side effects can therefore be quite intolerable to those patients who are already fatigued, somnolent, confused, or constipated. They can be useful at times, however, in smaller than usual doses to reduce anxiety, induce sleep, and encourage weight gain. Psychostimulants can be used at times as a third line of treatment for decreased energy. They can at times augment the efficacy of tricyclic antidepressants if used in very small doses. In rare circumstances electroconvulsive therapy can be utilized if medication is not tolerated and the seriousness of the patient's depression justifies its use.

TABLE 18-2
Potential Drug Interaction Effect with Antiretrovirals on Antidepressants

Antidepressant	Mild to moderate 3A4 inhibitors (indinavir, nelfinavir, saquinavir, amprenavir, delavirdine, efavirenz*)	Potent CYP inhibitor (ritonavir)	CYP 3A4 inducers (nevirapine, efavirenz*)
Amitriptyline	Potential ↑ TCA	Potential ↑↑ TCA	Potential ↓ TCA
Clomipramine	Possible ↑ TCA	Potential ↑↑ TCA	Potential ↓ TCA
Desipramine	No anticipated effect	Potential ↑↑ TCA	No anticipated effect
Imipramine	Potential ↑ TCA	Potential ↑↑ TCA	Potential ↓ TCA
Nortriptyline	No anticipated effect	Potential ↑↑ TCA	No anticipated effect
Fluoxetine	No anticipated effect	Potential ↑↑ SSRI	No anticipated effect
Paroxetine	No anticipated effect	Potential ↑↑ SSRI	No anticipated effect
Sertraline	Potential ↑ SSRI	Potential ↑↑↑ SSRI	Potential ↓ SSRI
Fluvoxamine	No anticipated effect	Potential ↑ SSRI	No anticipated effect
Venlafaxine	Potential ↑ venlafaxine	Potential ↑↑ venlafaxine	Potential ↓ venlafaxine
Bupropion	Potential ↑ bupropion	Potential ↑↑ bupropion	Potential ↓ bupropion
Trazodone	Potential ↑ trazodone	Potential ↑↑ trazodone	Potential ↓ trazodone
Nefazodone	Potential ↑ nefazodone	Potential ↑↑↑ nefazodone	Potential ↓ nefazodone
Mirtazapine	Potential ↑ mirtazapine	Potential ↑↑ mirtazapine	Potential ↓ mirtazapine

*Efavirenz is both an inhibitor and an inducer of CYP 3A4 isoenzyme. Drug interactions are difficult to predict.
TCA, Tricyclic antidepressant; SSRI, selective serotonin reuptake inhibitors; CYP, cytochrome P450 system.
From Feucht CL, Weissman SB: TEN 2(11), 2000.

Bipolar Disorder: Mania

Presentation and Progression. The hallmarks of mania are a generalized increase in the level of activity and rapidity of thought, flight of ideas, grandiosity, diminished sleep, and distractibility. One of the most helpful diagnostic characteristics of this disorder is the patient reporting racing thoughts that generate anxiety and that are described by the patient as being very uncomfortable. They will often report a difficulty in choosing which of the thoughts that they are being inundated with they should say. This symptom contributes to their anxiety. They can appear extremely talkative or withdrawn depending on how much difficulty they are having with thought selection. They can present with or without an agitated component to their disorder. Manic patients can be highly activated toward unrestrained sexual activity or buying sprees, both of which can have devastating consequences. Mania in the HIV/AIDS population must be evaluated from both an organic and a psychiatric basis. It can represent a primary illness in response to a traumatic life event or without evidence of a precipitating event. Patients can present with mania secondary to a primary CNS disease, infection, or metabolic abnormality, or in response to drug use or prescribed medication (i.e., steroids). It can represent a recurrence of a preexisting condition or a new illness. Symptoms generally include flight of ideas, grandiosity, pressured speech, restlessness, and impaired judgment. Psychotic features (hallucinations, delusions) may or may not be present. Hypomanic symptoms represent an attenuated, less severe form of full manic symptoms. The patient often presents with simply an elevated level of energy, with mild grandiose ideation and expansiveness. There is usually a diminished need for sleep. Patients in this state may manifest an inflated sense of self-esteem and an increased activity level, but in a relatively organized, if exaggerated, manner.

Diagnosis
1. Bipolar type 1 disorder versus type 2. The primary distinguishing characteristic is the severity of the manic symptom. The depressive aspect of both disorders is indistinguishable. In type 1, manic symptoms are florid, as opposed to hypomanic symptoms in type 2.
2. Cyclothymia
3. Schizoaffective schizophrenia
4. Substance abuse
5. Secondary to a medical condition: HIV-1–associated dementia (HAD) presenting as mania; mania secondary to

TABLE 18-3
Potential Drug Interaction Effect with Antiretrovirals on Antipsychotics

Antipsychotic	Mild to moderate 3A4 inhibitors (indinavir, nelfinavir, saquinavir, amprenavir, delavirdine, efavirenz*)	Potent CYP inhibitor (ritonavir)	CYP 3A4 inducers (nevirapine, efavirenz*)
Chlorpromazine	No anticipated effect	Potential ↑↑ chlorpromazine	No anticipated effect
Perphenazine	No anticipated effect	Potential ↑↑ perphenazine	No anticipated effect
Thioridazine	No anticipated effect	Potential ↑↑ thioridazine	No anticipated effect
Haloperidol	Potential ↑ haloperidol	Potential ↑↑ haloperidol	Potential ↓ haloperidol
Pimozide	Potential ↑ pimozide	Potential ↑↑ pimozide (contraindicated)	Potential ↓ pimozide
Clozapine	No anticipated effect	Potential ↑↑ clozapine	No anticipated effect
Olanzapine	No anticipated effect	Potential ↑ olanzapine	No anticipated effect
Risperidone	No anticipated effect	Potential ↑↑ risperidone	No anticipated effect

*Efavirenz is both an inhibitor and an inducer of CYP 3A4 isoenzyme. Drug interactions are difficult to predict.
CYP, Cytochrome P450 system.
From Feucht CL, Weissman SB: *TEN* 2(11), 2000.

medication neurotoxicity (e.g., steroids, antiretroviral medications, isoniazid, sympathomimetics, antidepressants); opportunistic infections and malignancies of the CNS that can present as mania (e.g., toxoplasmosis, cryptococcal meningitis, neurosyphilis, herpes); B_{12} deficiency; and drug abuse—particularly cocaine and amphetamines.

Treatment. For decades the mainstay of the treatment of patients with manic symptoms has been lithium carbonate. This drug is also useful in patients with HIV infection, but must be more carefully monitored for neurologic and gastrointestinal side effects. Particularly in the extremely ill patient, lithium may be difficult to use because of poor hydration, diarrhea, and diminished appetite, which may lead to elevated lithium levels and even toxicity. Valproic acid (Depakote) can be a very effective medication in the treatment of manic symptoms. Liver function must be monitored and care must be given to zidovudine levels, since they can be elevated by Depakote. Clonazepam (Klonopin) is useful in many varieties of anxiety states including mania. It is a relatively safe drug and can be used to reduce manic symptoms and control anxiety. Antipsychotic medication is extremely useful in controlling manic symptoms in patients. In HIV-infected individuals, one must be careful in the use of the high-potency antipsychotic medications haloperidol (Haldol) and thiothixene (Navane) to not worsen neurologic symptoms, such as parkinsonian and extrapyramidal symptoms. These drugs, however, are extremely effective, even in low doses, in lessening manic symptoms. Newer atypical antipsychotics such as olanzapine (Zyprexa) and risperidone (Risperdal) can also be useful. Low-potency antipsychotics are problematic, in general, in the medically ill because of their tendency to produce blood pressure abnormalities and sedation (Tables 18-3 and 18-4).

KEY POINTS

BIPOLAR DISORDER
- Symptoms: Type 1: Hypomanic episodes, mild euphoric states, anxiety, flight of ideas, sleep disturbance. Type 2: Full manic states, agitation, pressured speech, impaired judgment, (+/−) psychosis. Cyclical severe depressions (Type 1&2), highest suicide rate
- Differential diagnosis: Cyclothymia, hypomania vs. manic state, schizoaffective disorder, organic medical illness, medication toxicity, opportunistic infections, HIV dementia, drug abuse
- Treatment:
    Antipsychotic (neuroleptic) medications, high potency better than low potency (side effects include extrapyramidal and parkinsonian symptoms)
    Anxiolytics (Klonopin) (side effects include sedation)
    Lithium carbonate (side effects include GI [nausea, diarrhea, dehydration] and neurologic [tremor, toxicity])
    Valproic acid (Depakote) (side effects include liver toxicity)
    Tricyclic antidepressants (side effects include sedation, anxiety, constipation, and confusion)
    SSRIs (side effects include sedation, anxiety, constipation, and confusion)

Anxiety Disorders

Presentation and Progression. Anxiety is a common symptom in patients who are medically ill. Its hallmarks are feelings of intense fearfulness and worry, apprehension, and impending doom, which generally include an exaggeration of one's circumstances to catastrophic proportions. Patients with

TABLE 18-4
Potential Drug Interaction Effect with Anticonvulsants on Antiretrovirals

Antipsychotic	Mild to moderate 3A4 inhibitors (indinavir, nelfinavir, saquinavir, amprenavir, delavirdine, efavirenz*)	Potent CYP inhibitor (ritonavir)	CYP 3A4 inducers (nevirapine, efavirenz*)
Carbamazepine	Potential ↓ PI/NNRTI (avoid combination)	Potential ↓ PI/NNRTI (avoid combination)	Potential ↓ PI/NNRTI (avoid combination)
Phenytoin	Potential ↓ PI/NNRTI (avoid combination)	Potential ↓ PI/NNRTI (avoid combination)	Potential ↓ PI/NNRTI (avoid combination)
Phenobarbital	Potential ↓ PI/NNRTI (avoid combination)	Potential ↓ PI/NNRTI (avoid combination)	Potential ↓ PI/NNRTI (avoid combination)
Valproic acid	No anticipated effect (possible ↓ valproic acid)	No anticipated effect (possible ↓ valproic acid)	No anticipated effect
Lamotrigine	No anticipated effect (possible ↓ lamotrigine)	No anticipated effect (possible ↓ lamotrigine)	No anticipated effect
Gabapentin	No anticipated effect	No anticipated effect	No anticipated effect

*Efavirenz is both an inhibitor and an inducer of CYP 3A4 isoenzyme. Drug interactions are difficult to predict.
PI/NNRTI, Protease inhibitors/non-nucleoside reverse transcriptase inhibitors.
From Feucht CL, Weissman SB: *TEN* 2(11), 2000.

HIV infection experience a high level of anxiety, which increases as the severity of the illness worsens. As the realization of physical symptoms occurs and the interface with the medical establishment becomes more frequent, the general sense of helplessness and loss of control increases and, with it, anxiety. Uncertainty about the future, isolation, and shame can all contribute to increased anxiety. Anxiety can sometimes be a secondary symptom of depression, particularly in patients experiencing delayed or suppressed grief reactions. Depressive symptoms can also appear in situations of unremitting anxiety states as the patient becomes more despondent over being in a state of continuous anxiety. It must be remembered that all patients experience some level of anxiety and apprehension when encountering the medical community. This is a normal response to a loss of control and increased dependency. Patients who are predisposed to anxiety and fearfulness, in general, will react more negatively to finding out that they are HIV-positive and will become more anxious and terrified as they become ill. Any recognition of loss of function, physically or cognitively, can cause severe anxiety in susceptible individuals. Patients who have known anxiety disorders prior to being ill will worsen after the discovery of their illness. It is extremely important to attempt to elicit symptoms of anxiety from patients, even where there is no prior history, since chronic anxiety carries with it considerable morbidity. It can affect one's overall performance in life and at work and can make every task painful. It can affect sleep, appetite, sexual function, and social interaction. It can encourage noncompliance from fear of discovering negative news about the disease and encourage self-medication and drug abuse to treat symptoms. It is the physician's role to try to reduce stigmatization, isolation, and confusion about treatment and diagnostic approaches. Treating patients in an empathic and respectful manner can help reduce anxiety and develop trust, so that symptoms of anxiety and apprehension will be more easily revealed by the patient.

Diagnosis. Anxiety in medically ill HIV patients can manifest itself in the form of many somatic and autonomic symptoms. Chest pain, hyperventilation, palpitations, tachycardia, flushing, tension, fatigue, diarrhea, and headache can all be somatic manifestations of anxiety. Anxiety can manifest itself directly as an expression by the patient of feeling tense and frightened, through somatic expressions or through a variety of phobic responses. It can result from drug withdrawal syndromes (i.e., opiate, benzodiazepine, alcohol withdrawal). It can sometimes result as a side effect from steroids, antidepressants, thyroid preparations, and other medications used in the treatment of HIV. Anxiety can also appear as a manifestation of CNS disease of a primary or secondary (i.e., metabolic, infectious) variety.

Treatment

Pharmacologic. The mainstay of the treatment of anxiety are the benzodiazepines. In general they are a very effective and safe group of drugs that can significantly reduce the morbidity of anxiety in patients. They fall into two basic groups: long acting, such as diazepam (Valium), chlordiazepoxide (Librium), and clonazepam, and short and intermediate acting, such as lorazepam (Ativan) and alprazolam (Xanax). When prn intermittent dosing is preferred, the short-acting variety can be useful. When it is preferable to place a patient on a standing dose, the long-acting variety has an advantage in needing fewer doses per day, with less breakthrough of anxiety between doses. However, the longer acting benzodiazepines must be used with caution and in small doses in patients who are medically compromised, since they have active metabolites that can accumulate and produce side effects. Oxazepam and lorazepam have no active metabolites and are particularly well suited for use in medically ill patients. The smallest dose that satisfactorily reduces anxiety, without producing undue sedation, is the easiest way to establish treatment regimens with patients. Since there are no clinically significant drug interactions with this group of medications, they can be used judiciously to help patients reduce their anxiety. Other classes of drugs that can be useful in treating anxiety are buspirone, β-adrenergic blocking agents, and antidepressants such as SSRIs and tricyclics. Neuroleptics can also be useful in certain instances when benzodiazepines are either ineffective or not well tolerated. In these situations small-dose neuroleptics of either the low- or high-potency variety can be useful.

Psychotherapy. Various forms of psychotherapy can also be helpful in treating the anxiety that stems from being physically ill. Supportive, cognitive, and educational approaches can add a great deal in helping to abate a patient's anxiety. At times, insight-oriented psychotherapy can also be helpful, as can relaxation techniques. In many ways, the selection of a particular course of psychotherapy is determined by the cognitive, intellectual, and personality style of the particular patient.

KEY POINTS

ANXIETY DISORDER

- Symptoms: Feelings of impending doom; fear of losing control, hypervigilance, dizziness, tremors; palpitations, hyperventilation; paresthesias, choking sensations; GI symptoms
- Differential diagnosis: Panic disorder; general anxiety disorder; bereavement, delirium, depressive disease; drug abuse and withdrawal, drug toxicity; dementia, medical illness (metabolic abnormality)
- Treatment:
  Psychotherapy
  Benzodiazepines: short, intermediate acting preferred
    Oxazepam (Serax)
    Lorazepam (Ativan)
  Long acting, use in small doses
    Clonazepam (Klonopin)
  High-potency antipsychotics, in small doses
    Haloperidol (Haldol)
    Thiothixene (Navane)

Organic Manifestations
Delirium

Delirium is an acute confusional state representing a disturbance in cognition. It is generally of acute onset, with a duration lasting hours to weeks. The clinical symptoms of delirium are similar in many ways to dementia and certain types of psychosis, and it is therefore frequently misdiagnosed. Hallmarks of delirium include disturbance of consciousness, with reduced clarity of awareness of the environment; memory loss; disorientation to time, place, or person; and changes in cognition, including language and perceptual disturbances. There is a loss of ability to maintain focus and attention. Patients appear easily distractible. Levels of consciousness and orientation are extremely labile and may change within a period of hours or days. Patients can at times appear extremely incoherent, making an interview very difficult. They can experience perceptual disturbances, which include illusions, hallucinations, and misperceptions of events going on around them. Behavioral changes can vary from extreme agitation to lethargy. Emotional reactions such as anxiety, fear, depression, irritability, anger, and paranoia are common during episodes of delirium. Delirium has been noted in over 50% of patients with late-stage AIDS. It is a symptom complex that implies a direct or indirect (endogenous or exogenous) disturbance of CNS functioning.

TABLE 18-5
Central Nervous System Manifestations of HIV-1 Infection

Type of manifestation	Condition
Acute HIV-1 infection	Viral meningitis Encephalitis Ascending polyneuropathy
Opportunistic infections (late HIV-1 infection)	Toxoplasma cerebritis Cryptococcal meningitis Progressive multifocal leukoencephalopathy Neurosyphilis *Mycobacterium tuberculosis* meningitis Cytomegalovirus encephalitis Herpes simplex encephalitis
Neoplastic disease (late HIV-1 infection)	CNS lymphoma Kaposi's sarcoma
Other manifestations	HIV-associated dementia HIV-associated minor cognitive motor disorder

From McDaniel JS, Purcell DW, Farber EW: Severe mental illness and HIV-related medical and neuropsychiatric sequelae, *Clin Psychol Rev* 17:311-325, 1997.

Diagnosis. The most common diagnosis that delirium is confused with is dementia or a combination of delirium superimposed on a preexisting dementia. The distinguishing characteristic of delirium is the always-present changes in levels of consciousness and clouding of sensorium. The list of possible medical causes of delirium is long and even includes some of the medications used in the treatment of HIV disease. Diagnostic work-up includes laboratory blood work, cerebrospinal fluid (CSF) examination, electroencephalography, and brain imaging. Additionally, delirious patients who present with symptoms of a thought disorder, hallucinations, and delusions must be distinguished from schizophrenic patients and patients with other primary psychiatric disorders with psychotic symptoms (Tables 18-1 and 18-5 and Box 18-3).

Treatment. The essence of treating delirium is first diagnosing and then treating whatever underlying medical condition is causing the delirium. Treatment may range from antiviral therapy for direct viral infection of the CNS to treatment for secondary infection or metabolic derangements of various kinds. Treatment of the psychiatric symptoms of delirium includes the use of small dose antipsychotic medication to help reduce anxiety and cognitive disturbances such as hallucinations and delusions. Haloperidol in doses of 0.5 to 2 mg is often useful in treating these symptoms, as well as in helping to control agitation and irritability. Support and reassurance are extremely important in treating delirious patients, since they experience a high level of fear and anxiety. Additionally, they must be carefully monitored and are often best cared for in intensive care units or special care units where direct visualization of the patient is possible.

KEY POINTS

DELIRIUM

- Symptoms: Disturbance of level of consciousness, clouded sensorium, acute onset, disorientation, cognitive deficits, rapid fluctuations, reduced attention, (+/−) hallucinations
- Differential diagnosis: Primary or secondary infections, CNS disease, metabolic abnormalities, vitamin deficiencies, other medical conditions; primary psychotic disorders, severe depression, HIV-associated dementia
- Treatment:
  Diagnosis and treatment of underlying medical condition
  Use of low-dose antipsychotic medications to help control agitation, anxiety, and disorientation
  Antiviral therapy

Dementia

Dementia is defined as a CNS disorder characterized by the development of multiple cognitive deficits that include memory impairment and disturbances in cognition. Patients with dementia show impairment in their ability to learn new material and a loss of recall of previously learned information. Cognitive symptoms may involve the naming and recall of common objects, deterioration of language function, and impaired ability to carry out motor activities. The dementia associated with HIV disease is judged to be the direct effect of HIV on the CNS. Neuropathologic findings most commonly involve diffuse, multifocal destruction of the white matter and subcortical structures. HIV is known to enter the CNS soon after infection. Symptoms of the dementia in HIV-infected individuals include psychomotor retardation, poor concentration, and forgetfulness. Behavioral manifestations include apathy and social withdrawal. Hallucinations, delusions, and delirium may be present on occasion. Neurologic symptoms include hypertonia, frontal release signs, tremors, and impaired ability to complete repetitive movements. Dementia associated with HIV/AIDS can be divided into two diagnostic categories, depending on the severity of the dementia: (1) HAD complex and (2) HIV-1-associated minor cognitive/motor disorder (MCMD).

Categories

HIV-1-Associated Dementia Complex. Early symptoms of HAD include apathy, lethargy, and social withdrawal. Depressive symptoms may be apparent, but less severe than in major depressive disorder. Patients may self-report slowness in thinking and forgetfulness, loss of concentration, and poor retention of new material. Major neurologic symptoms include unsteady gait, leg weakness, and mild tremors. Later symptoms can extend to psychotic-like features, severe mem-

---

BOX 18-3
Etiologies of Delirium in HIV/AIDS Patients

INTRACRANIAL
Seizures
Infections
Cryptococcal meningitis
Encephalitis due to HIV, herpes, cytomegalovirus
Progressive multifocal leukoencephalopathy
Mass lesions
Lymphoma
Toxoplasmosis

EXTRACRANIAL
Medications and other drugs (not exhaustive)
  Amphotericin B
  Acyclovir
  Ganciclovir
  Ethambutol
  Trimethoprim-sulfamethoxazole
  Pentamidine
  Foscarnet
  Ketoconazole
  Sedative/hypnotics
  Cycloserine
  Opiate analgesics
  Isoniazid
  Rifampin
  Zidovudine or didanosine
  Vincristine
  Dapsone
Drug or alcohol withdrawal
Infection/sepsis
Endocrine dysfunction/metabolic abnormality
  Hypoglycemia due to pentamidine, protease inhibitors
  Hypoxia due to pneumonia
Nonendocrine organ dysfunction
  Renal failure due to HIV nephropathy or medication toxicity
  Liver failure due to comorbid hepatitis and medication toxicity
Nutritional deficiencies
  Wasting syndrome
  Failure to replace trace elements or vitamins in total parenteral nutrition

From Bialer PA, Wallack JJ, McDaniel JS: Human immunodeficiency virus and AIDS. In Stoudemire A, Fogel BS, Greenberg DB, editors: *Psychiatric care of the medical patient*, New York, 2000, Oxford University, pp 871-888.

---

ory loss, attention deficit, and overall loss of vitality. Personality changes can appear, along with severe irritability and severe depressions. Ataxia and prominent tremors can be present. Mutism, delusions, and hallucinations can appear in later stages.

HIV-1-Associated Minor Cognitive/Motor Disorder. MCMD is a change in mental functioning characterized by symptoms less severe than required for a diagnosis of dementia. The primary cognitive complaint is that of memory disturbance. There is an absence of sufficient intellectual impairment for a diagnosis of dementia, but there is an abnormally delayed recall. There can be a mental slowing and some evidence of impaired coordination. Diminished concentration and attention with some irritability can be present but to a lesser degree than in HAD. Overall, neuropsychologic impairments and limitations of activities of daily living are

BOX 18-4
American Academy of Neurology AIDS Task Force Nomenclature and Research Case Definitions for Neurologic Manifestations of Human Immunodeficiency Virus-Type 1 (HIV-1) Infection

A. Criteria for clinical diagnosis of HIV-1–associated minor cognitive/motor disorder
  1. Cognitive/motor/behavioral abnormalities (each of the following)
     a. At least two of the following present for at least 1 month:
        1. Impaired attention or concentration
        2. Mental slowing
        3. Impaired memory
        4. Slowed movements
        5. Incoordination
        6. Personality change, irritability, or emotional lability
     b. Acquired cognitive/motor abnormality verified by clinical neurologic examination or neuropsychological testing (e.g., fine motor speed, manual dexterity, perceptual motor skills, attention/concentration, speed of processing information, abstraction/reasoning, visuospatial skills, memory/learning, or speech/language)
  2. Disturbance from #1 causes mild impairment of work or activities of daily living.
  3. Does not meet criteria for HIV-1–associated dementia complex or HIV-1–associated myelopathy (see below)
  4. No evidence of another etiology, including active CNS opportunistic infection or malignancy, severe systemic illness, active alcohol or substance use, acute or chronic substance withdrawal, adjustment disorder, or other psychiatric disorders
  5. HIV seropositivity (ELISA test confirmed by Western blot, polymerase chain reaction, or culture)
B. Criteria for clinical diagnosis of HIV-1–associated cognitive/motor complex
  1. HIV-1–associated dementia complex
     Each of the following:
     a. Acquired abnormality in at least two of the following cognitive abilities for at least 1 month: attention/concentration, speed of processing information, abstraction/reasoning, visuospatial skills, memory, and speech/language. Cognitive dysfunction causes impairment of work or activities of daily living; should not be attributable solely to severe systemic illness.
     b. At least one of the following:
        i. Acquired abnormality in motor function or performance verified by clinical examination, neuropsychological testing, or both
        ii. Decline in motivation or emotional control or change in social behavior
     c. Absence of clouding of consciousness during a period long enough to establish the presence of #1
     d. No evidence of another etiology, including active CNS opportunistic infection or malignancy, other psychiatric disorders (e.g., depression), active alcohol or substance use, or acute or chronic substance withdrawal
     e. HIV seropositivity (ELISA test confirmed by Western blot, polymerase chain reaction, or culture)
  2. HIV-1–associated myelopathy
     Each of the following:
     a. Acquired abnormality in lower-extremity neurologic function disproportionate to upper-extremity abnormality verified by reliable history and neurologic examination
     b. Myelopathic disturbance is severe enough to require constant unilateral support for walking
     c. Criteria for HIV-1–associated dementia complex not fulfilled
     d. No evidence of another etiology, including neoplasm, compressive lesion, or multiple sclerosis
     e. HIV seropositivity (ELISA test confirmed by Western blot, polymerase chain reaction, or culture)

Modified from Jansen RS et al: American Academy of Neurology AIDS Task Force. Nomenclature and research case definitions for neurologic manifestations of human immunodeficiency virus-type-1 (HIV-1) infection, *Neurology* 41:778-785, 1991.

mild to moderate compared with those found in patients with HAD.

Diagnosis. Diagnosis of these disorders is made by a combination of history and neurologic and psychiatric examinations. Brain imaging, neuropsychologic testing, CSF examination, and blood tests can all be useful in establishing a diagnosis. It is important to look for treatable causes of dementia such as folate and B_{12} deficiency, anemia, thyroid dysfunction, and electrolyte abnormalities. Particularly in the early stages of HIV-related dementias, cognitive findings may be subtle and difficult to tease out. If suspected, or subjective complaints about cognition are reported by patients, neuropsychologic testing and medical work-up for dementia are indicated (Boxes 18-4 and 18-5 and Fig. 18-1).

Treatment
Antiviral. Antiviral drug therapy is the primary treatment for dementias related to AIDS. Initiation of treatment of this kind can significantly improve cognitive function of patients with AIDS-related dementias over the short term and may have a protective effect in helping to delay progression. The drug of choice for the treatment and prevention of dementias in AIDS patients is zidovudine. Other drugs are being consid-

BOX 18-5
HIV-1–Associated Cognitive/Motor Complex

- HIV-1–associated dementia complex (HIV-1–associated dementia, AIDS dementia complex, HIV encephalopathy, subacute encephalitis, AIDS-related dementia)
- HIV-1–associated minor cognitive/motor disorder (HIV-1–associated mild neurocognitive disorder, HIV-1–associated neurocognitive disorder, HIV-associated neurobehavioral abnormalities)
- Asymptomatic neuropsychologic impairment

From Halman M: *Complications and disorders: HIV and the brain. Part I: Clinical and neuropsychiatric dimensions of HIV disease: AIDS training,* American Psychiatric Association Annual Meeting, May 18, 1999, Washington, DC.

ered to treat and prevent this condition but are limited in value, depending on their ability to cross the blood-brain barrier. Zidovudine is particularly effective because its penetration of the blood-brain barrier is particularly good. There is a growing concern, however, of viral resistance developing in patients who have been treated with zidovudine for long periods of time. Newer agents are being studied for use in the event that this occurs.

Psychopharmacologic. The treatment of symptoms related to HAD such as decreased concentration, dysphoria, apathy, psychomotor retardation, and lethargy is best handled with small dose psychostimulants such as methylphenidate (Ritalin) or dextroamphetamine (Dexedrine). Side effects seem to be fewer with Ritalin than Dexedrine. Dose scheduling for Ritalin should be on a tid basis since the drug is short acting. Treatment should begin with doses of 5 mg bid-tid and titrated upward, as necessary, on a very gradual schedule. Side effects to be particularly vigilant for are appetite suppression and increased anxiety, irritability, and the development of new-onset psychotic symptoms. Patients suffering from HAD with preexisting psychiatric illness or new-onset illness must be treated in a manner similar to patients without dementia. Patients who develop psychotic symptoms or severe anxiety or agitation will benefit from small doses of antipsychotic medication. It is important to weigh the advantages of high-potency antipsychotic medications, which produce less sedation and less cardiovascular problems, but more neurologic side effects, against the low-potency drugs of this class that produce greater problems with sedation and cardiovascular instability. Small doses (0.5 to 5 mg) of haloperidol, a high-potency antipsychotic, are generally well tolerated by patients with organic brain syndromes of various kinds. Some of the newer agents such as olanzapine and risperidone hold out promise for use with patients with HAD, since they are low in extrapyramidal- and orthostatic-producing side effects. Patients with manic symptoms and HAD can be treated with lithium carbonate. Care must be taken, however, to carefully monitor renal function, neurologic side effects, and hydration. If lithium is not tolerated, clonazepam in small doses (2 mg/day) can be used to treat manic symptoms. Small doses of antipsychotics as described above are also useful for this condition. Antidepressant medications used in patients with dementias are best reserved for those patients demonstrating clear evidence of depressive symptoms. Avoid using them for symptoms of lethargy, since they do not work well in stimulating diminished activity levels. Depressions, however, occur very frequently with mild to moderate dementias. Of the tricyclic antidepressants, desipramine (Norpramin) in small doses is well tolerated by patients, particularly if there is a component of anxiety with the depressive symptoms. Doses as small as 10 mg bid-tid can be effective, ranging up to divided doses of 100 mg per day. Another tricyclic, nortriptyline (Pamelor), can be useful in doses ranging from 30 to 60 mg per day. This drug offers the additional advantage of reliable blood levels, with a therapeutic window of 50 to 100 ng/ml. One must be careful of drug-drug interactions, particularly with protease inhibitors (inhibitor of cytochrome P450 isoenzyme in the liver). SSRIs can be very useful, since their tendency to alter blood pressure or produce sedation is minimal. Sertraline (Zoloft) is beneficial, since its inhibition of the CYP2D6 isoenzyme in the liver is less than with other drugs in the class. Other SSRIs such as paroxetine (Paxil), fluoxetine (Prozac), venlafaxine (Effexor) (inhibitor of serotonin and norepinephrine), and celexa can be useful, depending on the situation.

Psychotherapy. Patients suffering from various degrees of dementia and cognitive disturbance often need a great deal of emotional support, and at times social support. Family and friends must be mobilized to help if significant changes in activities of daily living have occurred. All patients feel better if they feel understood, and even patients suffering the anxiety of intellectual deterioration respond positively knowing that they are understood. This process reduces a feeling of isolation and therefore reduces anxiety.

KEY POINTS

DEMENTIA

- Symptoms: Slow, insidious, onset; cognitive deficits; poor concentration and attention; recent memory disturbance; apathy, slowness, frontal release signs; secondary depression; (+/−) hallucinations
- Differential diagnosis: Metabolic abnormality, primary or secondary CNS disease, depression, schizophrenia, drug side effects
- Treatment:
  Low-dose antipsychotic medication for control of anxiety and increased irritability (side effects include extrapyramidal and parkinsonian symptoms)
  Stimulants for apathy and depression
  Tricyclics: low dose (side effects include sedation, blood pressure instability)
  SSRIs (side effects include loss of appetite)
  Antiviral therapy

Mixed-Psychotic Disorders: Delirium
Diagnosis

There are many possible etiologies of psychotic disorders in patients with HIV and AIDS. They range from preexisting disorders such as schizophrenia, schizoaffective, and bipolar disorders to delirium that results from direct CNS viral involvement, secondary infections, or metabolic abnormalities. Any patient with a diagnosis of HIV/AIDS must be carefully evaluated medically if a change in mental status occurs. Patients with pre-

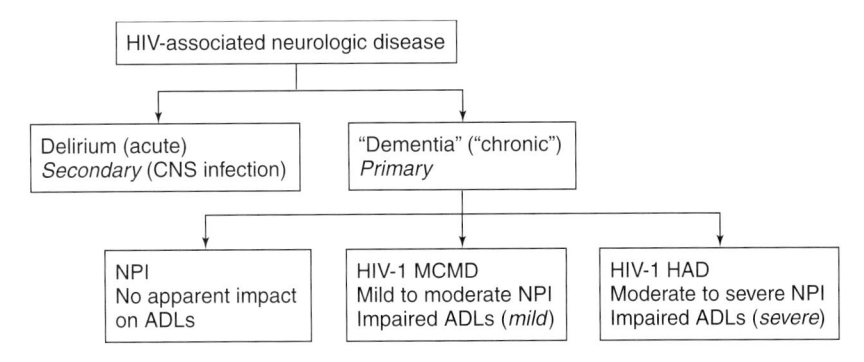

FIG. 18-1 Classification of HIV-related brain impairments. *NPI,* Neuropsychologic impairment; *ADL,* activities of daily living; *HIV-1 MCMD,* HIV-1–associated minor cognitive/motor disorder; *HIV-1 HAD,* HIV-1–associated dementia complex. (From Halman M: *Complications and disorders: HIV and the brain. Part I: Clinical and neuropsychiatric dimensions of HIV disease: AIDS training,* American Psychiatric Association Annual Meeting, May 18, 1999, Washington, DC.)

existing histories of psychosis and chronic psychotic disorders have higher rates of acquiring HIV infection due to dangerous behaviors (i.e., unprotected sexual behavior and dangerous drug abuse activity). Drug abuse in general is another etiology of acute psychosis that must always be ruled out in the differential diagnosis of psychosis in patients with or without a premorbid history. Distinguishing between psychotic reactions that are organically based and those that are primarily psychiatric in origin is of utmost importance from a diagnostic and treatment perspective. In general, the hallmark of organic major mental status changes (delirium) is a disturbance in orientation to time, place, and person. Symptoms of anxiety, bizarre behavior, and hallucinations, generally visual rather than auditory, can occur, but confusion and disorientation are always present if the patient is carefully interviewed. Complicating the clinical picture may be preexisting psychotic disorders. The features of disorientation and confusion superimposed on the previous conditions should point the clinician toward a diagnosis of delirium. There are times, however, when it is difficult to distinguish a reactive psychotic reaction from an organic etiology in change in mental status. Of particular note are patients who develop psychotic reactions from direct viral CNS infection. Symptoms of delusions, hallucinations, mood disturbance, and thought disorders can occur under these circumstances. Generally some cognitive disturbance will be noted in these patients, pointing the evaluation in an organic direction. Patients with delirium in general are less stable and more labile than patients with primary psychiatric disorders. Their symptoms tend to worsen secondary to fluctuations in the underlying medical condition causing the derangement. Waxing and waning symptoms are another characteristic distinguishing delirium. The list of possible causes of delirium is long and includes direct and indirect organic possibilities. Patients with HIV/AIDS syndromes who develop psychotic disorders, either exacerbations of preexisting conditions or new-onset psychosis, will have the hallmarks of whatever diagnostic category is being manifest. Symptoms can range from paranoia, thought insertions, persecutory fantasies, somatic delusions, bizarre behavior, hallucinations of various kinds, and disorganized speech to a mixture of these symptoms with mood disturbances. Distinguishing symptoms becomes important in differentiating between schizophrenic episodes and bipolar psychotic reactions. It is always important to try to assess patients for cognitive disturbances as an indicator of possible direct effects of HIV on the CNS as cause of the psychotic reaction. Computed tomography (CT) scans, magnetic resonance imaging (MRI) scans, and electroencephalograms may be useful at times in making this distinction. At times, neuropsychiatric psychological testing can be useful in teasing out subtle symptoms of cognitive dysfunction. At the far end of the psychotic spectrum in patients with HIV/AIDS are patients with cognitive dysfunction, ranging from mild cognitive disturbance to severe ADC. These patients may present a psychotic picture as a direct effect of CNS dysfunction or a reactive psychosis stemming from the knowledge of a loss of intellectual function. Reactive psychotic episodes in HIV-infected patients can also be related to bereavement and loss, the trauma of being ill, and the change in life that it all represents. These episodes may be discrete, short lived, responsive to treatment, and nonrecurrent. Any major change in mental status in patients with HIV/AIDS must be followed up with complete medical and neurologic work-ups before an assumption is made that the diagnosis is purely psychiatric in origin.

Treatment

It may be necessary to begin treatment of an acute psychotic state before complete diagnostic work-up is complete. This will depend on the degree of morbidity, level of agitation and disruption, level of dangerousness to self or others, or ability to comply with the work-up. Ideally, since this is a complex illness with many overlaps between the organic and psychiatric, it would be beneficial to complete the work-up first. It is particularly important to determine whether the psychosis is secondary to self-medication or drug abuse or is a side effect of prescribed drug regimens. In general, antipsychotic agents (neuroleptics) are used to treat acute and chronic psychotic states. In patients who are medically ill, smaller than usual doses are recommended since they seem to cross the blood-brain barrier more readily and produce greater effect and greater side effects at smaller doses. High-potency neuroleptics run the risk of greater extrapyramidal side effects, and low-potency neuroleptics cause greater anticholinergic effects and sedation. In general, the high-potency and atypical newer antipsychotics are safer and of greater benefit in this population. In addition, they will be better tolerated, producing greater compliance.

> **KEY POINTS**

PSYCHOTIC DISORDERS
- Symptoms: Paranoia, grandiosity, religiosity, thought disorder, delusions, hallucinations, catatonia
- Differential diagnosis: CNS infection, CNS malignancy, severe depression, schizoaffective disorder, bipolar disorder, drug toxicity, drug abuse, metabolic abnormality, HIV-associated dementia
- Treatment:
  High-potency antipsychotic medications (side effects include extrapyramidal and parkinsonian symptoms), preferably
  Haloperidol (Haldol)
  Thiothixene (Navane)
  Atypical antipsychotic medications (side effects include weight gain)
  Olanzapine (Zyprexa)
  Risperidone (Risperdal)

Suicide

The psychiatric evaluation of every patient must include an assessment for suicidal ideation. This evaluation can sometimes be by assessment of the overall severity of the symptomatology, without directly addressing the issue with patients. However, the greatest mistakes in this assessment are made by not directly asking patients about suicidal feelings, ideation, or plans. It is imperative that with any depressed individual or any patients with psychotic symptomatology questions about suicidal feelings be addressed. This is particularly true with patients with HIV/AIDS, since the overall rate of suicide is higher than in the general population. Fears and anxiety over impending illness, fears of dependency, and concerns about experiencing pain, isolation, and shame are all issues that must be assessed when working with this population of patients. Maintaining a nonjudgmental supportive relationship can help develop greater trust and openness from the patient. This becomes particularly important in assessing areas that patients tend to be ashamed of or frightened by. As with drug abuse and sexual practices, suicidal feelings are subjects that are particularly difficult for patients and physicians to deal with. They are areas that are often neglected in assessing patients but are of utmost importance with this population. It is always better to err on the side of extra caution and be overly vigilant in asking about suicidal feelings with this group of patients. Any major change in mood, cognition, life circumstance, behavior, or progression of the illness should cause one to be concerned about this issue. Proper psychiatric intervention must be sought if the physician's concerns are heightened after exploring these issues with a patient.

Pain Syndromes
Presentation and Progression

Some of the most disturbing symptoms experienced by patients with HIV/AIDS are various kinds of pain syndromes and the anticipation of recurrent pain. The experience of pain is intensified by feelings of anxiety and depression. The most common pain experienced by patients with HIV is peripheral neuropathy, affecting up to 35% of patients with HIV/AIDS. It generally presents as a distal symmetrical polyneuropathy that can be caused or triggered by antiviral agents. The diagnosis is made with neurologic examination and electromyelogram, but is often difficult to make. Overall, estimates of pain of various kinds in patients with HIV/AIDS vary, depending on the study, with a range of between 30% and 80%. Even asymptomatic patients who are HIV-positive can report pain experiences to varying degrees. Overall, patients with AIDS report increasingly higher levels of pain as the illness progresses and eventually reach levels comparable with patients with advanced cancer. As a group, patients with AIDS are undertreated for their symptoms of pain. Undertreatment seems to relate to a tendency to underutilize opioid analgesics in the treatment of pain syndromes in this population. This is particularly true if patients have previous drug histories or communicate poorly about their internal experiences. They may have a tendency to want to be good patients, without complaints, or physicians may view pain as being subjective and controllable by patients. Adjuvant analgesic drugs, such as antidepressants and tranquilizers, also tend to be underutilized in AIDS patients. In general, women tend to be undertreated more than men, even though they tend to experience greater levels of pain.

The impact of chronic severe pain on the lives of patients who have AIDS is enormous. Depression and disability are highly correlated with increasing levels of pain. For some patients, the experience of pain is a reminder of their underlying illness, making them feel sicker than they may actually be. It is the harbinger of future negative events, causing greater distress than for those who do not have these associations. For some patients, pain that is unremitting equals hopelessness and loss of control. The most common pain syndromes in patients with AIDS are sensory peripheral neuropathy, pain due to Kaposi's sarcoma, headache, oral and pharyngeal pain, abdominal pain, chest pain, arthralgias, myalgias, and painful dermatologic conditions. Most pain syndromes in patients with AIDS are related to either (1) direct consequences of infection or the immunosuppression effects of treatment (e.g., HIV peripheral neuropathies, myelopathy, secondary infections, arthritis, vasculitis) or (2) toxic neuropathies due to antiviral agents and chemotherapy. Pain of the gastrointestinal tract secondary to infections and neoplasms is the most common chronic pain in AIDS patients. Painful neurologic complications of HIV disease include headaches, the most common neurologic complaint, and neuropathies. Rheumatologic pain syndromes include arthritis and arthropathies, psoriasis and psoriatic arthritis, HIV-associated arthritis, myopathies, and myositis.

Diagnosis

In all cases in which the patient is experiencing extreme pain, there should be an attempt to diagnose and treat the underlying cause of the pain. However, treatment of underlying disease processes or diagnostic work-ups may be lengthy, and treatment of pain should not be delayed until after they are completed. One always wants to avoid allowing patients to remain in pain too long both from a humanitarian standpoint and because pain is best and most effectively treated early. In the case of severe pain, pain cycles are best broken by aggressive around-the-clock use of analgesics rather than treating pain on an as-needed basis. Mild to moderate pain may be treated less aggressively. This approach helps reduce the anticipation and anxiety that come from the return of acute unremitting pain, which intensifies the response and makes treatment more difficult. Pain can be characterized to help determine a proper course of therapy. One should assess pain from the perspective of its onset, location, quality, duration, intensity, modifiers, effects on daily living, associated physical signs and symptoms, and emotional consequences. It is also important to take a history of previous drug use and tolerance to analgesic medication.

Treatment
Pharmacologic. The treatment of pain in AIDS patients is similar to the treatment of cancer patients. For mild to moderate pain syndromes the nonopioid analgesics should be used, such as nonsteroidal antiinflammatory drugs. For persistent and moderate to severe pain the opioid analgesics should be employed in increasing potency and dosage as needed to eliminate pain. Adjunctive therapy includes anxiolytics, neuroleptics, corticosteroids, anticonvulsants, stimulants, and antidepressants. It is often useful to combine a primary and adjunctive medication to help reduce the dosage needed with analgesics. In this way, unwanted side effects such as gastrointestinal disturbance and oversedation can be avoided. Analgesic medication should always be titrated from weakest to strongest and from lower to higher dosages. Choices have to be made concerning dosage schedule, shorter versus longer acting preparations, and routes of administration. In the case of chronic pain, it is preferable to establish a standing dosage schedule rather than prn dosing. Side effects that can be troublesome in the utilization of opioid analgesics include sedation, gastrointestinal disturbance, respiratory depression, and delirium, and necessitate careful monitoring of patients, particularly in higher dosage ranges. Adjunctive therapies to help reduce opioid doses can often be helpful in reducing side effects.

Nonpharmacologic. Nonpharmacologic treatments can also be helpful in reducing anxiety, enhancing well being, and reducing pain experience. Supportive psychotherapy, biofeedback, relaxation therapy, and behavioral therapy all have their place in the treatment of pain syndromes. Patients with AIDS who are chronic drug abusers require special attention. These patients also deserve pain control treatment but are easily discredited because of their histories. They may present special problems in terms of dosing and tolerance and present a special challenge from the standpoint of trust with the treating physician. It is particularly important with this group of patients to utilize a multidisciplinary team approach.

Sleep Disturbance
Presentation and Progression
There are various causes of insomnia in patients with AIDS including the degree of CNS disease, medical illness in general, HIV infection, depression, and chronic pain. Negative consequences of insomnia include fatigue, cognitive deficits, memory loss, depression, and anxiety. Patients with HIV infection have characteristic sleep patterns including shorter total sleep time, longer sleep latency, more frequent awakenings, increase in stage-1 sleep, and decrease in stage-2 sleep. Hypersomnia is usually associated with advanced disease and can contribute significantly to morbidity and disability.

Diagnosis
The diagnosis of sleep disturbances in patients with AIDS includes primary and secondary insomnias. Secondary insomnias include sleep disturbances caused by psychiatric disorders such as major depressions, anxiety disorders, and mania; medical conditions such as pain syndromes and physical symptoms that cause altered sleep patterns; psychoactive drug and alcohol effects; and disturbed sleep secondary to side effects of prescribed medication utilized in the treatment of HIV. Treatment for insomnia varies from behavior therapy and relaxation techniques to medication. General sleep hygiene approaches include learning to not create pressure about sleep; developing a proper exercise regimen; avoiding liquids, alcohol, and caffeine drinks in the evening; and learning to regularize bedtime.

Treatment
1. *Sedative hypnotics:* Benzodiazepines with short to intermediate half-lives are generally preferable in AIDS patients, since their tendency for accumulation, daytime drowsiness, ataxia, and amnesia is less than with longer acting varieties. Lorazepam, temazepam, and oxazepam are frequently used. Since they bypass the hepatic oxidative pathways, they are theoretically safer to use with patients receiving protease inhibitor therapy. Although longer acting agents such as clonazepam and flurazepam may be useful when the difficulty is sleeping throughout the night rather than falling asleep, they must be monitored carefully for side effects.
2. *Antidepressants:* Tricyclic antidepressants in low dose can be helpful at times to treat insomnia when anxiety and depression also play a role in the disorder.
3. *Trazodone:* Trazodone in doses ranging from 25 to 100 mg can at times provide a mild hypnotic effect that can be useful.

> ### KEY POINTS
>
> ***PAIN***
> - Symptoms: GI tract most common pain site, neuropathies, rheumatologic, migraine myopathies
> - Differential diagnosis: Medical diagnosis of pain source; description, nature, quality, and frequency of pain
> - Treatment:
>   Assess nature of pain
>   Graduate treatment:
>   Nonopioid (NSAID)—mild (side effects include GI disturbance, peptic ulcer, and renal/hepatic failure)
>   Weak opioid—moderate (side effects include sedation, nausea, constipation, delirium, and respiratory depression)
>   Strong opioid—severe (side effects include sedation, nausea, constipation, delirium, and respiratory depression)
>   Add adjuvant rx to each of above as necessary:
>   Tricyclics
>   SSRIs
>   Antipsychotics
>   Benzodiazepines

4. *Remeron:* A new antidepressant, Remeron is very sedating, and also in low doses (7.5 to 15 mg) it can be a useful sleep aid while promoting an antidepressant effect.
5. *Antihistamines:* Antihistamines such as Atarax and Benadryl can contribute something to the overall treatment of insomnia in cases in which a very mild medication is needed.

KEY POINTS

SLEEP DISTURBANCE

- Symptoms: Frequent awakenings, long sleep latency, less time asleep, decrease in stage 2 sleep, increase in stage 1 restless sleep
- Differential diagnosis: Primary insomnia, secondary insomnia due to medical conditions, pain, major depression, delirium, mania, anxiety disorders, medication side effects, stimulants
- Treatment:
  Avoid stimulants
  Increase level of exercise
  Avoid barbiturates
  Benzodiazepines (short/intermediate half-life) (side effects include drowsiness, ataxia, amnesia, and confusion)
      Lorazepam (Ativan)
      Temazepam (Restoril)
      Oxazepam (Serax)
  Avoid long-acting benzodiazepines
  Nonbenzodiazepine hypnotic
      Zolpidem (Ambien) (well-tolerated short half-life)
  Also useful are small-dose tricyclics

When to Refer

A referral should be made:
1. If, in the opinion of the primary physician, psychotherapy would be valuable in the overall treatment plan.
2. If there are diagnostic questions from a psychiatric perspective.
3. If there is a sudden or chronic change in mental status or cognitive function.
4. If a patient being treated for psychiatric symptoms demonstrates a deepening or worsening of symptoms over time.
5. If there are concerns about the interaction between psychotropic medications and drugs being used in the treatment of AIDS.
6. If side effects from psychotropic medications appear.
7. If there is suicidal ideation.

Summary

Attention to the psychiatric complications of HIV/AIDS involves the complex interaction between psyche and soma. From a purely psychiatric standpoint the effects of the illness can promote the reemergence of preexisting psychiatric disorders, either from the direct effect of viral infection or from the simple stress of being ill. It can precipitate the emergence of new, never-before-experienced psychiatric disturbance, either from primary or secondary effects of HIV, or from an intense reaction to being ill. There are cognitive impacts of the disease and psychological reactions to these changes. Literally, the whole spectrum of psychiatric diagnosis can be drawn on, since the illness affects patients with many different personality types and reactions to physical illness. Major issues encountered with this disease also involve bereavement, loss, guilt, shame, and isolation, which must be dealt with to effectively reduce the morbidity of the disorder. In recent years, major breakthroughs in the treatment of HIV infection have occurred, most notably the treatment of opportunistic infections and highly active antiretroviral therapy (HAART). The consequences of these therapies have significantly reduced the psychological morbidity of the disorder. It is hoped that as time progresses and the treatments continue to improve, the traumatic impact of this infection will diminish.

SUGGESTED READINGS

American Psychiatric Association: *Diagnostic and statistical manual of mental disorders,* ed 4, Washington, DC, 1994, American Psychiatric Press.

American Psychiatric Association: *HIV-related neuropsychiatric complications and treatments,* Washington, DC, 1998, American Psychiatric Press.

Gelenberg AJ, Bassuk EL, editors: *The practitioner's guide to psychoactive drugs,* ed 4, New York, 1997, Plenum Publishing.

Practice Guideline for the treatment of patients with HIV/AIDS, *Am J Psychiatry* 157(11):1-49, 2000.

Rundell JR, Wize MG, editors: *The textbook of consultation and liaison psychiatry,* Washington, DC, 1996, American Psychiatric Press, pp 832-877.

The psychiatric manifestations of HIV/AIDS," *Prim Psych* 6(5):34-90, 1999.

19 Gastrointestinal Disease

ROBERT GROSS

Introduction

Gastrointestinal (GI) disorders constitute the most common manifestations of progressive human immunodeficiency virus (HIV) infection. Opportunistic pathogens are almost invariably the cause of these disorders, rather than HIV itself. Anatomically, any region of the GI tract can be involved, although it is uncommon for the entire GI tract to be involved in any one process. Identifying the anatomic site of the disorder is the first step in determining the etiology of the problem. This chapter is divided into sections based on disease entity, and the most common causes of each disease are discussed in turn.

Esophagitis
Presentation and Progression

Cause. Esophageal disorders are extremely common in HIV, with more than one third of all acquired immunodeficiency syndrome (AIDS) patients having esophageal disease at some time. These diseases almost exclusively occur in the setting of profound immunosuppression and therefore are almost always indicative of advancing disease. The most common cause of odynophagia (pain on swallowing) in HIV is esophageal candidiasis. Several other diseases, especially viral infections such as cytomegalovirus (CMV), also cause esophageal disease. Interestingly, one of the most common opportunistic pathogens in HIV, herpes simplex virus (HSV), only rarely causes esophagitis.

Candidal infections, including oropharyngeal candidiasis (thrush) and recurrent vaginal candidiasis, are the most common clinical indications of progressive HIV infection. Esophageal candidiasis is less common than infection at these other sites, but represents the cause of approximately three fourths of esophageal disease in HIV. Although esophageal candidiasis is generally an extension of the more common oropharyngeal candidiasis, esophageal candidiasis must be thought of as a more invasive infection and generally occurs in individuals with more advanced disease. Thus, unlike these other candidal infections, the Centers for Disease Control and Prevention (CDC) criteria classify esophageal candidiasis as an AIDS-defining illness.

Esophageal candidiasis is most commonly seen in individuals with concurrent thrush. However, esophageal candidiasis can occur in the absence of oropharyngeal infection. In addition, since thrush is so common, only a small percentage of individuals with thrush will have esophageal candidiasis, and the presence of thrush does not necessarily guarantee that the esophageal symptoms are due to *Candida*. *Candida albicans* is the most common species to cause this infection, although other species of *Candida* can be involved.

The second most common cause of odynophagia in HIV is the idiopathic esophageal ulcer. These lesions, also referred to as HIV-associated esophageal ulcers or aphthous ulcers of the esophagus, constitute somewhat less than one third of causes of odynophagia. They occur typically in severely immunocompromised individuals. As their name suggests, their etiology remains unknown, and neither risk factors nor causative agents have been identified.

CMV is the most common viral cause of esophagitis in HIV patients. However, it is less common than *Candida* and idiopathic ulcers. Since CMV maintains latent infection in all individuals exposed, and 90% of HIV-infected patients have past exposure (as evidenced by antibodies), a substantial number of patients are at risk for disease. However, the probability of end organ disease is directly related to degree of immunosuppression and is quite uncommon in subjects with CD4+ counts above 100 cells/mm^3.

Presentation. It is not possible to reliably distinguish among the causes of esophagitis by clinical presentation alone. Esophageal diseases typically present with odynophagia. Esophagitis tends to be quite symptomatic and therefore usually comes to medical attention quickly. Other modes of presentation include dysphagia (the feeling of food "sticking" retrosternally) and much less commonly singultus ("hiccups"). As mentioned above, esophageal candidiasis is overwhelmingly the most common cause, and symptomatic patients are generally treated empirically for this. Individuals who do not respond to such treatment undergo endoscopy to help distinguish among the other causes. If ulcers are found on endoscopy, the differential diagnosis broadens to include pill esophagitis from zidovudine (AZT), zalcitabine (ddC), or doxycycline.

Diagnosis

Since esophageal candidiasis is so common and the treatment generally very effective, the approach most often used to diagnose esophagitis is "test of cure." Fig. 19-1 is an algorithm for the evaluation of odynophagia/dysphagia in HIV. This empiric approach is the most cost-effective approach to odynophagia in HIV. Treatment with any of the anti-*Candida* regimens is usually effective. If symptoms are debilitating and prevent oral alimentation, then hospital admission and a diagnostic procedure are warranted. If a patient is able to swallow, a barium swallow typically demonstrates a "moth-

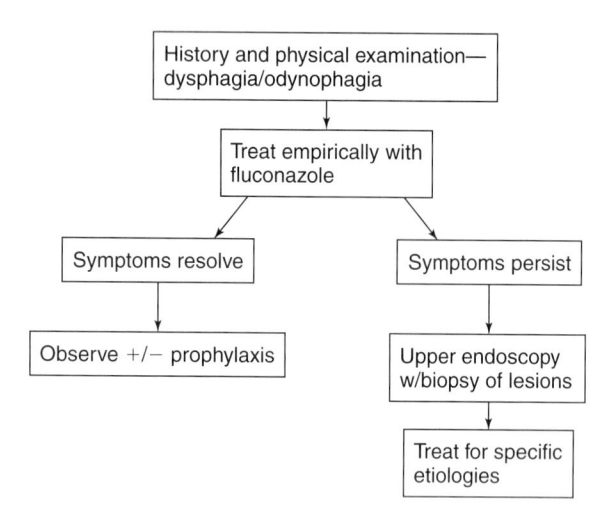

FIG. 19-1 Algorithm of evaluation and treatment of esophagitis. (Modified from Dieterich DT et al. In Merigan TC Jr, Bartlett JC, Bolognesi D, editors: *Textbook of AIDS medicine*, ed 2, Baltimore, 1999, Williams & Wilkins.)

eaten" appearance in esophageal candidiasis. However, this test is not definitive, since the mucosa is not directly visualized and specimens cannot be obtained for culture and histopathology. Therefore upper endoscopy is the preferred approach if symptoms do not resolve with a course of antifungal therapy.

Idiopathic esophageal ulcers are diagnosed by gross and histologic appearance on upper endoscopy. They are either solitary or multiple ulcers with a discrete border and are frequently quite large. Biopsy generally reveals granulation tissue without identifiable pathogens.

As with idiopathic esophageal ulcers, the diagnosis of CMV esophagitis is made on endoscopy. Large shallow ulcers or diffuse mucosal inflammation may be present. Histology of the ulcers on biopsy reveals characteristic "owl's eye" virologic inclusions in the mucosal cells. Culture for CMV is of limited value because false-positive results often occur. Patients at risk for this disease often have reactivated CMV in their blood, but it is not causing end organ disease, and the biopsy specimen is often contaminated with blood. Thus culture of this material will grow CMV even in the absence of end organ disease. Therefore only if pathologic changes are seen on histology in the biopsy specimen should the diagnosis of CMV disease be considered definitive.

Natural History and Treatment

Treatment of esophageal candidiasis consists of a combination of supportive care and antifungal agents. If oral alimentation is precluded by pain, intravenous hydration should be instituted. Response to therapy is typically rapid, and therefore parenteral alimentation is not usually needed. Pain should be managed with narcotics, as needed. Non-oral routes of narcotic administration (e.g., parenteral, transcutaneous) should be considered if the patient is unable to swallow pills.

Several antifungal agents are effective. Fluconazole is the first-line agent to be used, unless the individual has had thrush that has been refractory to high doses of fluconazole in the past and resistant *Candida* is suspected. Treatment is generally started with 200 mg (IV/po) followed by 100 mg daily for approximately 2 to 3 weeks. If the individual has been on increasing prophylactic doses of fluconazole, the daily dose should be increased concomitantly. If the prophylactic dose is maximized (i.e., 400 mg), the individual does not tolerate fluconazole, or the regimen fails, other effective agents include itraconazole (tablets or liquid suspension) and amphotericin B. Itraconazole oral solution is dosed 100 mg daily for 3 weeks. If parenteral therapy is required, low-dose amphotericin B is quite effective at 0.3 mg/kg/day IV. Symptoms typically remit within a week in most responders. Lack of remission of symptoms in an individual with odynophagia treated empirically with antifungals is an indication for endoscopy. As is common in HIV, more than one pathogen may be causing the symptoms. When this is the case, patients tend to improve only partially when the *Candida* is treated. Endoscopy will identify the majority of other diagnoses that may be causing the dysphagia.

Treatment of idiopathic esophageal ulcers includes supportive care regarding alimentation. Controlled trials have not been performed, but observational studies have demonstrated benefit of therapy with prednisone and thalidomide. Therapy with prednisone is generally initiated at a dose of 40 mg per day and tapered by 10 mg per week for a 4-week course. Thalidomide is an inhibitor of tumor necrosis factor (TNF)-α production, suggesting a cytokine-mediated etiology to these lesions. It is utilized in patients who do not respond to prednisone or require multiple courses for recurrent ulcers. Of course, with the known teratogenic potential of thalidomide, this agent should be avoided in pregnant women at all costs.

The treatment of CMV esophagitis is limited to the three available agents active against CMV, ganciclovir, foscarnet, and cidofovir. Cidofovir is the newest agent with anti-CMV activity and has an extremely long half-life, allowing it to be dosed infrequently. All have important potential toxicities. Ganciclovir can cause bone marrow suppression. Foscarnet and cidofovir are both nephrotoxic.

Therapy is generally initiated with ganciclovir at 5 to 10 mg/kg IV daily for 2 to 4 weeks. Once the acute episode is resolved, options include switching the ganciclovir to oral maintenance therapy with valganciclovir or observing for other evidence of end organ disease.

If induction with ganciclovir fails, switching to or adding foscarnet or cidofovir is a viable option. Foscarnet is dosed 60 mg/kg IV tid or 90 mg/kg IV bid. Cidofovir is dosed at 5 mg/kg IV once a week for the first 2 weeks and then every other week thereafter. On the day of administration, probenecid is administered at a dose of 500 mg po qid. Unfortunately, neither foscarnet nor cidofovir is orally bioavailable and so the maintenance options are oral valganciclovir or watchful waiting. Continued IV therapy as is frequently used in CMV retinitis is probably not warranted in most situations.

When to Refer

As long as the patient is able to maintain adequate nutrition and hydration, esophageal disease in patients with HIV can be managed as an outpatient. Referral to a gastroenterologist is warranted in the patient who does not respond to antifungal agents because endoscopy is the next step in the diagnostic algorithm.

KEY POINTS

- *Candida* is the most common cause of esophagitis in HIV disease
- Failure of empiric antifungal therapy requires endoscopy
- Biopsy is required for the diagnosis of CMV esophageal ulcer

Diarrhea

Diarrhea is arguably the most common complaint of individuals infected with HIV. Over half of individuals with HIV in the developed world will have diarrhea at some point in their illness. This percentage is substantially higher in the developing world, where food and water supplies are more likely to be contaminated with pathogens to which these individuals are particularly susceptible.

The causes of diarrhea include protozoal, viral, mycobacterial, and routine bacterial pathogens. Since infections with protozoal and bacterial pathogens are common in nonimmunocompromised hosts, they are not always indicative of progression of HIV. However, diarrhea caused by CMV or *Mycobacterium avium* complex (MAC) occurs exclusively in the setting of profound immunosuppression and is invariably associated with advancing disease. Unfortunately, law of parsimony ("Ockham's razor") often does not hold in the setting of AIDS. That is, several pathogens may in fact be causing a particular GI syndrome in this setting simultaneously. Therefore identification of one pathogen should not eliminate one's suspicion of another organism causing the same effect. The topic of diarrhea in patients with HIV infection is covered extensively in Chapter 21.

Hepatitis

Presentation and Progression

Cause. Abnormalities of liver tests are extremely common in HIV. The list of causes of abnormal liver tests is extensive. The potential causes range from drug-induced abnormalities to infections with numerous viruses, mycobacteria, fungi, and parasites. The viruses in particular, such as hepatitis B (HBV) and hepatitis C (HCV), tend to be much more common in HIV-infected individuals than in the general population because of shared risk factors for transmission with HIV (i.e., exposure to blood and body fluids of infected individuals). Furthermore, the natural history of disease is generally altered by HIV coinfection. Other causes of abnormal liver tests are opportunistic pathogens that almost never cause disease outside of the setting of HIV. Of course, HIV-infected individuals may have substance abuse problems (i.e., alcoholism) that cannot be overlooked as the cause of abnormal liver tests and liver function.

Abnormal liver tests are so prevalent in HIV that they are often ignored unless they are markedly abnormal, are progressively worsening, or are accompanied by other symptoms indicative of an important and potentially treatable underlying process.

The most common cause of abnormal liver tests depends on the individual's risk factor for acquiring HIV. Among in-

---

BOX 19-1
Potentially Hepatotoxic Drugs Used in HIV

HEPATOCELLULAR	CHOLESTATIC
Zidovudine	Macrolide antibiotics
Didanosine	Indinavir
Azole antifungals	Albendazole
Isoniazid	
Rifamycins	
Pentamidine	
Pyrazinamide	
Metronidazole	
Tetracyclines	
Ganciclovir	
Ritonavir	
Saquinavir	
Nelfinavir	
Trimethoprim-sulfamethoxazole	

Modified from Dieterich DT et al: Gastrointestinal manifestations of HIV disease, including the peritoneum and mesentery. In Merigan TC Jr, Bartlett JC, Bolognesi D, editors: *Textbook of AIDS medicine,* ed 2, Baltimore, 1999, Williams & Wilkins.

---

jecting drug users (active or former), the most common liver infection is HCV. The prevalence of HCV in injecting drug users is on the order of 80%. Despite this overwhelming number, several other causes of abnormal liver tests may be present in these individuals, and therefore further evaluation is often warranted despite positive HCV serology.

The rate of sexual transmission of HCV is low. In fact, other than injection with contaminated blood products, the principal risk factors for HCV transmission are currently poorly understood. Thus HIV-infected individuals who are not injecting drug users are at much lower risk for HCV.

Among non–HCV-infected subjects, the most common cause of abnormal liver tests is drug toxicity. The list of medications that have been reported to cause abnormal liver tests is too extensive to be practically useful. The most commonly implicated medications are listed in Box 19-1. Of all the potential causes, the most ubiquitous medication is trimethoprim-sulfamethoxazole. Since this medication is a mainstay in the prevention of opportunistic infections, including *Pneumocystis carinii* pneumonia and *Toxoplasma gondii* encephalitis, this drug is the one that clinicians are most hesitant to stop. Other causes include the azole antifungals, commonly used to treat and prevent thrush and cryptococcosis, as well as antiretroviral agents themselves, including protease inhibitors. Many patients take one drug from each of these classes simultaneously, making it difficult to sort out the offending agent.

MAC is a common cause of liver test abnormality in individuals with low CD4+. MAC is uncommon in individuals with CD4+ counts greater than 100 cells/mm^3 and much more common in individuals with CD4+ counts below 50 cells/mm^3. MAC is a systemic illness, and therefore other abnormalities or symptoms are often present when a patient has liver test abnormalities due to MAC. These may include fever, sweats, diarrhea, weight loss, and hepatosplenomegaly.

Past or ongoing infection with HBV is evident in a very high proportion of HIV-infected subjects, since this virus shares transmission patterns with HIV, yet is substantially more transmissible. Like HCV, primary infection with HBV is often asymptomatic and therefore often only detected on serology. However, HBV goes on to chronic hepatitis much less commonly than does HCV, especially if infection occurs in adulthood. However, in HIV-infected subjects, rates of chronic infection after newly acquiring HBV may be as high as 20%, compared with less than 10% in the general population. Resolution of new infection is probably related to the degree of immunosuppression at the time of infection. Of note, reactivation after apparent resolution is not uncommon in HIV, in contrast to the non-HIV setting. Reactivation is recognized by the return of hepatitis B surface antigen and loss of antibodies to hepatitis B surface antigen. The absence of hepatitis B e antigen cannot be used to rule out reactivation.

As discussed previously, reactivation of CMV infection is one of the most problematic issues in advanced HIV. CMV often causes hepatitis when initial infection is established and is one of the causes of mononucleosis-like syndromes. However, hepatitis is one of the less common and generally less severe manifestations of CMV disease in HIV. Another herpesvirus, HSV, can also cause hepatitis in HIV.

Fungal pathogens that cause systemic disease can also infect the liver, although rarely as an isolated site. These include histoplasmosis, coccidioidomycosis, and cryptococcosis. A history of potential exposure (i.e., travel or other activity) is useful in raising suspicions regarding these organisms. Unfortunately, there are no characteristic findings to suggest any of these etiologies over the others.

Bacillary angiomatosis involving the liver can result in "peliosis hepatis." The syndrome is caused by one of the *Bartonella* species, either *B. henselae* or *B. quintana*. It is characterized by findings of blood lakes in the liver seen on either ultrasonography or CT scan. Peliosis hepatis due to *Bartonella* species can be seen in patients with and without the violaceous, raised skin lesions of bacillary angiomatosis.

Common neoplasms in HIV such as Kaposi's sarcoma and lymphoma can also involve the liver. However, at the point the liver is involved, the disease is typically advanced. The liver abnormalities are not the clinically most important aspect of these diseases.

Presentation. The presentation of hepatitis is as varied in HIV-infected patients as it is in non–HIV-infected patients, ranging from asymptomatically elevated liver tests and mild jaundice to severe right upper quadrant pain and fulminant hepatic insufficiency.

Diagnosis

As with all clinical problems in HIV-infected patients, the approach begins with consideration of the CD+ cell count of the patient, since this is a useful predictor of which opportunistic infections the patient is at risk for. In addition, a review of prior liver tests and prior serologies is critical. If the increased liver tests are found to be new, suspicion about medications and acute infectious processes should be heightened. If the increased liver tests are chronic, then chronic processes (e.g., HCV, alcohol ingestion) are more likely to be the etiology. The timing of the onset of the abnormalities and the institution of new medications can be useful for determining etiology. However, one must be aware that longstanding medications may be responsible for newly elevated liver tests. Thus there is no hard and fast rule regarding the acuity of the liver test abnormality and the etiology.

The only way to prove that an individual medication is the cause of the abnormal liver test is to stop the potentially offending drug ("dechallenge"), wait for the liver tests to normalize, resume only that drug, and watch for the abnormality to recur ("rechallenge"). In reality, this approach may be impractical and potentially dangerous in the majority of cases, particularly when drugs are required to be given together (i.e., not to be used alone). Thus isolating one drug at a time can be difficult.

A common approach is to stop all medications that can be safely stopped and to follow the liver tests. If and when they return to normal, all unnecessary or marginal drugs are withheld, as is the most likely offender of the remaining vital drugs. Often another drug is substituted for a potentially offending but vital drug. If the abnormality recurs, the process is repeated and the most likely offender of the remaining medications is withheld. Although this approach is entirely empirical, it tends to isolate the offending medication after one or two attempts. In the event that the liver test abnormality does not resolve, drugs are unlikely to be the cause and a more extensive evaluation is warranted.

Patients at high risk (i.e., low CD4+ counts) and/or with a clinical syndrome consistent with MAC should be evaluated with lysis-centrifugation blood cultures looking for mycobacteremia. Whether or not hematologic abnormalities are prominent, some clinicians also choose to perform a bone marrow biopsy with stain and culture for mycobacteria. Liver biopsy is rarely required to make the diagnosis, and the yield is somewhat low due to the small numbers of organisms. Culture of biopsy specimens should be sent to increase the diagnostic yield.

Other pathogens can be identified by histopathology of liver biopsy specimens. Stains for fungi and *Bartonella* species should be performed. Lymphoma and Kaposi's sarcoma are usually detected by light microscopy. Fig. 19-2 is an algorithm for the evaluation of hepatic disease. Although the list of organisms that cause liver disease in HIV is extensive, the yield of liver biopsy is poor. Thus, especially in the absence of a focal lesion, most clinicians forgo this procedure.

Natural History

Some controversy exists at present on the natural history of HCV disease in HIV. Although little doubt exists about the fact that HCV viral loads are higher in HIV-infected individuals than in non–HIV-infected individuals, whether this translates to worse clinical outcomes is still being debated and researched.

Although rates of chronic infection with HBV are higher in HIV, as are levels of hepatitis B e antigen (a measure of the activity of hepatitis B), ample data demonstrate that the severity of the liver disease caused by HBV is *less* than in non–HIV-infected patients. Although this phenomenon may seem counterintuitive, the mechanism is probably explained by the fact that the liver disease caused by HBV is due to immunologic response to the infection. Since these patients have impaired T cell immunity, their ability to destroy hepatocytes,

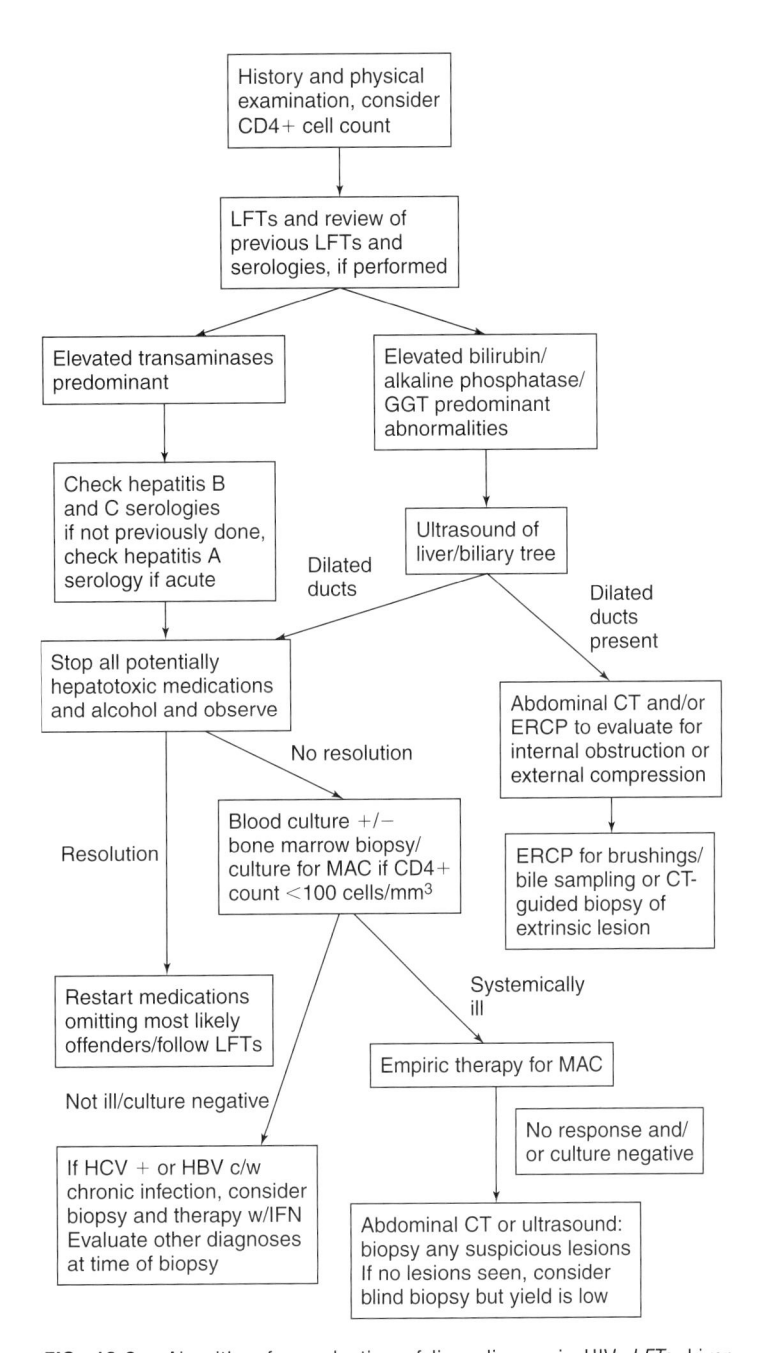

FIG. 19-2 Algorithm for evaluation of liver disease in HIV. *LFTs,* Liver function tests; *GGT,* γ-glutamyltranspeptidase; *MAC, Mycobacterium avium* complex; *HCV,* hepatitis C virus; *HBV,* hepatitis B virus; *ERCP,* endoscopic retrograde cholangiopancreatography; *IFN,* interferon. (Modified from Dieterich DT et al. In Merigan TC Jr, Bartlett JC, Bolognesi D, editors: *Textbook of AIDS medicine,* ed 2, Baltimore, 1999, Williams & Wilkins.)

and in turn, the severity of the disease, is decreased. However, in contrast, *reactivation* of HBV can be very severe and at times fatal.

Treatment

The standard of care for the treatment of HCV is the combination of oral ribavirin and parenteral pegylated interferon. Unfortunately, side effects limit the tolerability of the regimen. The most common side effects of the interferon include flu-like symptoms including malaise and myalgias. These symptoms can persist for long periods of time and can even include depression and a concomitant increase in suicide risk. Another important and inevitable side effect of this regimen is hemolysis. The median amount of hemolysis has been reported to result in a decrease in hemoglobin on the order of 3 g/dl. Particularly in HIV-infected patients, this side effect is often intolerable because they often already have underlying anemia.

In non–HIV-infected patients, the rate of eradication of HCV is on the order of 40%. However, mounting data suggest that the regimen is less effective in HIV. In addition, for patients with poorly compensated liver disease, debate exists as to whether or not treatment is indicated. The argument for treatment is that treatment may decrease the rate of hepatocellular carcinoma. The argument against treatment is that the treatment is arduous in patients with a poor prognosis. Thus the decision to treat an HIV-infected patient for HCV is a difficult one. With the increasing numbers of HIV-infected patients who have had a nice response to highly active antiretroviral therapy (HAART), control of HCV is particularly important. Therefore, for highly motivated patients without significant underlying anemia and well-controlled viral load, treatment is often a reasonable approach. However, further research on clinical outcomes from current therapies and drug development for future therapies are needed.

Hepatic drug toxicity can occur after the individual has been on the agent for a long period of time, even up to years in some cases (e.g., trimethoprim-sulfamethoxazole). Drug-induced liver disease resolves without sequelae in the vast majority of cases. Although case reports of death have been associated with the use of protease inhibitors and other HIV medications, these events are rare. Thus, as demonstrated in the algorithm in Fig. 19-2, since the course tends to be benign in most cases and an invasive work-up unwarranted, stopping medications whenever one notes important elevations in liver tests is the recommended course of action.

The course of MAC infection has been altered by the advent of antiretroviral therapy. Individuals with MAC who receive effective antiretroviral therapy in addition to their anti-MAC therapy often respond very well, with a decrease in symptoms, weight gain, and improvement in liver tests. Many clinicians who suspect MAC, especially in cases in which the patient appears ill, start therapy empirically while awaiting the blood culture results. First-line therapy for MAC includes a newer macrolide (azithromycin or clarithromycin) plus ethambutol. As outlined in the section on MAC-associated diarrhea, the dose of clarithromycin is 500 mg twice daily, the dose of azithromycin is 500 mg once daily, and the dose of ethambutol is 15 to 25 mg/kg daily. Therapy can usually be stopped in patients whose immune system has responded to HAART with a rise in CD4+ cell count to over 100 to 150 cells/mm^3 for more than 3 months.

Although their disease may be less severe, HIV-infected patients with HBV infection are *less* likely to respond to therapy with interferon. Fortunately, one of the nucleoside reverse transcriptase inhibitors used to treat HIV, lamivudine (3TC, Epivir), has activity against HBV. Although the long-term effects are still being determined, it is a reasonable approach to include lamivudine whenever possible in antiretroviral regimens for patients with chronic HBV infection.

When to Refer

A liver biopsy is often avoided in the work-up of hepatitis in HIV-infected patients. If required, however, most liver biopsies are performed by experienced gastroenterologists. The treatment of HBV and HCV is complicated even without the concomitant HIV infection. Referral to a specialist skilled in the treatment of HBV and HCV is strongly recommended.

KEY POINTS

- About 80% of injecting drug users are infected with hepatitis C
- Medication-induced hepatitis can occur at any time in the course of therapy
- Chronic hepatitis B tends to be less severe in HIV-infected patients than in non–HIV-infected patients
- Current pharmacotherapy for hepatitis B and hepatitis C may be less effective in HIV-infected patients than in the general population

Biliary Tract Disease

Presentation and Progression

Cause. Biliary tract disease is a much less common cause of jaundice in HIV than is hepatocellular dysfunction. The most common causes of cholestasis in HIV are medications. Of particular note, indinavir (Crixivan) commonly causes a benign, Gilbert syndrome–like elevation of indirect bilirubin. Other processes that can cause biliary tract disease in HIV present as an acalculous cholecystitis and have been called "HIV-associated cholangiopathy." Several pathogens other than HIV have been implicated as potential causes of cholangiopathy in HIV-infected patients, including cryptosporidia, microsporidia, and CMV. In addition, although uncommon, HIV-associated lymphomas can also cause obstruction at the porta hepatis and result in jaundice.

Presentation. Each of the causes of biliary tract disease presents similarly. They are generally associated with jaundice, malaise, and loss of appetite. It can be painless or a more acute presentation of cholangitis, with the attendant fever, right upper quadrant pain, and increased white blood cell count.

Diagnosis

The evaluation of jaundice begins with a history, physical examination, and liver test panel. Elevated total and direct bilirubin accompanied by an alkaline phosphatase elevated out of proportion to the other liver tests suggests cholangiopathy. The next step is to obtain an ultrasound of the liver and gallbladder to evaluate the size of the common bile duct. A dilated duct suggests intrinsic obstruction (e.g., gallstone) or extrinsic compression (e.g., tumor). A normal appearing duct favors drug-induced or HIV-associated cholangiopathy.

Most clinicians initially choose to discontinue all potentially offending medications and follow bilirubin and alkaline phosphatase levels. If the jaundice does not resolve, endoscopic retrograde cholangiopancreatography (ERCP) is a useful tool in looking for a specific biliary opportunistic pathogen. Brushings as well as aspirated bile can be taken from the biliary tree and examined for the presence of organisms.

If extrinsic compression is identified by ultrasound, computed tomography (CT) scan of the abdomen is indicated to better define the anatomy. CT-guided or endoscopic-guided biopsy can often yield a diagnosis. Tissue should be sent for histopathology, including special stains to look for fungi, mycobacteria, and protozoa. Culture for fungi and mycobacteria should be performed, although these etiologies are very rarely the cause of obstructive masses in this area.

Natural History and Treatment

In general, unless the cause of the jaundice is drug-induced cholestasis, the outcome tends to be variable. Treatments for cryptosporidia and microsporidia are poor, as outlined in Chapter 21. Treatment for CMV is, of course, available. However, response rates are not known due to the rarity of the syndrome.

When to Refer

If a patient has suspected biliary tract disease without dilated ducts and has failed to respond to changes in medications, referral for ERCP may be indicated. If dilated ducts are present on ultrasound, referral for further imaging and possible biopsy and/or ERCP is warranted.

KEY POINTS

- Medications are the leading cause of cholestasis in HIV disease
- Several microorganisms that cause enteric infections in HIV-infected patients may cause HIV-associated cholangiopathy
- Response to therapy for infectious causes of biliary tract disease is poor

Anorectal Lesions

Presentation and Progression

Cause. HSV is one of the most common sexually transmitted diseases in the world. Of the two types of HSV, HSV-1 and HSV-2, HSV-2 is much more commonly associated with anogenital disease. It is estimated that approximately one in five individuals in developed countries has been infected with HSV-2 at some point. These rates are substantially higher in developing countries and, because of shared risk factors, in individuals with HIV. Furthermore, as a major cause of genital ulcer disease, HSV plays an important role in the sexual transmission of HIV.

Herpesvirus infections are lifelong, yet they generally remain latent due to the suppressive effect of an intact immune system. The immunodeficiency associated with HIV infection can profoundly affect the host's capacity to suppress herpesvirus infections including HSV, CMV, and varicella-zoster virus. As a result, herpes simplex outbreaks in HIV tend to be both more common and more severe than in non–HIV-infected individuals. These outbreaks are usually due to reactivation of latent infection.. Recurrent and/or severe herpes outbreaks may be a tip-off to coinfection with HIV. Human papillomavirus (HPV) causes both benign and malignant diseases. It is the cause of non–sexually transmitted warts, sexually transmitted genital warts (anogenital condyloma acuminatum), and cervical neoplasia and cervical cancer in women. In addition, it is the cause of squamous cell carcinoma of the anus. Different viral types are associated with different diseases. Two types in particular, HPV 16 and 18, are associated with cervical cancer and anorectal malignancy. The virus transforms epithelial cells via a unique mechanism involving prevention of normal mechanisms of programmed cell death (apoptosis).

Perianal condylomata make up the majority of the disease caused by HPV in HIV. However, in subjects with advanced immunosuppression, serious anorectal disease can be seen. Since this virus is sexually transmitted, it is particularly prevalent in subjects whose risk factor for acquisition of HIV was sexual contact. The prevalence of HPV is probably between one fourth and one half of the HIV-infected population.

Presentation. Although HSV does cause esophagitis, its principal role in GI disease is as the cause of anorectal ulcers. Anorectal disease due to HSV is more common in individuals who have engaged in anal receptive intercourse. It generally presents with painful vesicles that appear after a prodrome of hyperesthesia or paresthesia in the area of the outbreak. The vesicles are generally filled with clear fluid on a base of erythematous skin ("dewdrop on a rose petal"). They then coalesce, break down, and ultimately result in a painful, tender ulcer with an irregular border. Due to the difficulty of visualization for the patient, the preceding phases are often missed and the patient often presents with a painful perianal ulcer. HSV can also cause rectal disease, which presents with painful defecation, tenesmus, rectal discharge, and constipation. In severe cases, neurologic involvement can occur, and the patient can present with a cauda equina syndrome.

The differential diagnosis of anorectal HSV depends on the stage and location of the lesions at the time of presentation. If the classical vesicular lesions are seen, while varicella-zoster virus (i.e., shingles) may be the cause, the diagnosis in most cases will be HSV. However, if the patient presents after the lesions have ulcerated, the differential diagnosis includes other genital ulcer diseases, such as chancroid and syphilis. Finally, the differential diagnosis of rectal HSV includes other diseases presenting with rectal discharge and/or pain, such as gonorrhea and CMV.

Condylomata caused by HPV are soft, sessile lesions whose surface can vary from rough to smooth. They can occasionally achieve large size, often described as "cauliflower-like." When the lesions become large and are located either in the perianal area or within the anal canal, they can obstruct fecal flow and lead to constipation. The differential diagnosis in this setting is rarely in doubt. However, large condylomata in the anal canal can be mistaken for colonic mucosal polyps on digital rectal examination. The next step in the evaluation generally includes flexible sigmoidoscopy, which is able to rule out the diagnosis of colonic polyps.

HPV is also the cause of squamous cell carcinoma of the anus. This disease is much more common in men and women who engage in anal receptive intercourse. HPV infection of the anus is usually asymptomatic and generally cannot be seen on examination. Squamous cell carcinoma of the anus, when symptomatic, often presents simply as pruritus ani or blood on toilet paper. Furthermore, condylomata themselves can undergo malignant transformation and result in verrucous anal carcinoma. The differential diagnosis for squamous cell carcinoma depends on the presenting symptoms. The differential diagnosis includes benign condylomata; other causes of pruritus ani, such as pinworm infection; and other causes of perianal bleeding, such as hemorrhoids.

Diagnosis

The diagnosis of anorectal HSV infection depends on whether the perianal area or the rectum is the site affected. On the skin, a Tzanck smear of a vesicle base will often reveal characteristic multinucleated giant cells. This test is unable to distinguish between HSV and varicella-zoster virus infections. However, the anogenital location is strongly suggestive of HSV. Culture of vesicle fluid does distinguish between the two herpesviruses. Viral culture requires special transport medium; it has a turnaround time on the order of days and is quite sensitive if the material is obtained from vesicles less than 2 days old.

Rectal symptoms usually prompt sigmoidoscopy, which typically reveals vesicles or ulcerated, friable mucosa. This material should be sent for viral culture and pathology. As noted previously, caution should be exercised if the culture results yield CMV, since culture of CMV is generally considered nondiagnostic. This diagnosis is made by finding the characteristic "owl's eye" cellular inclusions.

The diagnosis of condyloma acuminatum is usually made on visual inspection of the lesion and the location. Occasionally, histopathology is needed on a biopsy specimen to confirm the diagnosis. The diagnosis of condyloma acuminatum in the anal canal is generally made on surgical examination under anesthesia after a flexible sigmoidoscopy rules out a colonic neoplasm. The diagnosis of squamous cell carcinoma of the anus or of verrucous carcinoma can only be made by biopsy of suspicious lesions.

Natural History and Treatment

Several agents, both parenteral and oral, are available for the treatment of HSV infections. Acyclovir had been the mainstay of treatment for many years. However, with the advent of newer, better orally bioavailable agents such as valacyclovir and famciclovir, acyclovir may be preferred for parenteral use only. All of these agents are generally effective in reducing the time to healing of HSV lesions. However, the treatment of proctitis may not decrease the duration of symptoms. Valacyclovir is dosed at 500 mg po bid, famciclovir is dosed at 125 mg po bid, and acyclovir is dosed at 200 mg po 5×/day. If oral therapy is not possible, acyclovir at 5 mg/kg IV q8h can be used. Treatment generally lasts for 5 to 10 days, depending on the rapidity of healing.

Some HSV ulcers in patients with advanced HIV disease do not respond to treatment with one of the above agents. Although resistance had been demonstrated in HSV specimens in the laboratory, clinical resistance has only been seen in AIDS patients. Although resistance testing can be performed, the diagnosis of resistant HSV is usually made on clinical grounds. Risk factors, other than advanced HIV, have yet to be determined. In patients whose HSV demonstrates clinical resistance to first-line agents, foscarnet or cidofovir can be tried. The mutations that confer resistance to acyclovir also confer resistance to ganciclovir, and therefore this drug is not a viable option in this setting. The dose of foscarnet is 40 mg/kg IV q8h until substantial healing has occurred. The nephrotoxicity of foscarnet can be decreased by volume repletion prior to infusion. The appropriate dose of cidofovir is not currently known and consultation is recommended if its use is planned.

As opposed to a lack of response to treatment, if HSV lesions recur in these subjects, the virus is generally still sensitive to first-line agents. Therefore, in most cases, retreatment with a first-line agent is indicated, and treatment with a second-line agent (i.e., foscarnet) is instituted only if they fail to respond to the therapy.

Prophylactic use of one of the first-line agents is an effective strategy for decreasing the frequency and severity of recurrent HSV. Prophylaxis is recommended if the patient has four or more outbreaks of anogenital herpes simplex per year. The dose of acyclovir is 400 mg po bid, valacyclovir 500 mg po once daily, and famciclovir 250 mg po bid.

The goals of treatment of condylomata acuminata can be to improve cosmetics, to prevent or remove an uncomfortable or obstructing lesion, or to prevent or treat a carcinoma. Eradication of the virus is not currently possible, and therefore host immunity is the only mechanism for suppression of viral replication.

Topical treatments used to destroy the lesions include podophyllin resin or podophyllotoxin, liquid nitrogen, interferon-α, or imiquimod. Podophyllin resin in tincture of benzoin is applied directly onto the lesion and allowed to remain for 4 to 6 hours, after which it is washed off. This procedure is repeated weekly until resolution. Podophyllotoxin can be self-applied twice daily, three times per week for up to a month. Imiquimod, an agent with unclear mechanism of action but demonstrated efficacy, is applied two to three times per week. Interferon-α is injected directly into the lesions three times a week. Cryotherapy with liquid nitrogen is also effective. For large lesions, lesions in the anal canal, or lesions suspicious for malignancy, excisional biopsy is indicated.

When to Refer

For large condylomata that are not amenable to topical therapy, referral to a surgeon for excision may be required. Malignant lesions should be evaluated by both a surgical and a medical oncologist to determine optimal management.

KEY POINTS

- Anorectal ulcers are the most important GI disease caused by HSV
- HPV is a cause of condyloma and squamous cell carcinoma of the anus
- Drug-resistant HSV can be a significant problem in HIV-infected patients

Gastrointestinal Bleeding

Presentation and Progression

Cause. The common causes of GI bleeding in the non-HIV setting are the most common causes in HIV as well. These include gastroduodenal ulcer disease and variceal bleeding due to portal hypertension. However, there are causes of GI bleeding that are somewhat unique to HIV, including Kaposi's sarcoma and lymphoma.

Kaposi's sarcoma is a tumor of vascular epithelial origin that was very uncommon before the HIV pandemic. However, in the pre–protease inhibitor era, it became very common, particularly among men who have sex with men. Since the advent of HAART, the incidence of Kaposi's sarcoma has decreased substantially. Kaposi's sarcoma can cause bleeding when it involves the mucosa of the GI tract. Within the last several years, an etiologic agent has been discovered and termed "Kaposi's sarcoma herpesvirus" or "human herpesvirus 8."

Both non-Hodgkin's lymphoma and Hodgkin's disease have been recognized to be more common in HIV, with non-Hodgkin's lymphoma being the more common. Although all HIV-infected patients are at increased risk of lymphoma, lower CD4+ counts are associated with a greater risk.

Presentation. The typical manifestation of Kaposi's sarcoma is a violaceous raised, nonblanching lesion, often first noted on the skin or mucous membranes. Occasionally, the disease presents in other organs, particularly in the respiratory or GI tract without apparent cutaneous involvement. Lymphomas generally present in the same manner as they do in non–HIV-infected patients. However, they present in unusual sites more commonly than in non–HIV-infected patients. The presentation generally includes one or more enlarged lymph nodes, and may include weight loss, fever, other constitutional symptoms, and splenomegaly. If only intraabdominal lymph nodes are enlarged, the symptoms may closely resemble MAC infection. The symptomatology of lymphoma in the GI tract depends on the site of involvement. For example, gastric lymphoma may present with early satiety. However, lymphoma in any of the GI sites can present with bleeding.

Diagnosis

Kaposi's sarcoma is diagnosed by biopsy of a suspicious lesion. Microscopic examination reveals swirls of poorly formed blood vessels with spindle cells and extruded erythrocytes. On colonoscopy, the characteristic lesions are readily seen. Biopsy is often nonspecific, but the clinical scenario of cutaneous Kaposi's sarcoma with bleeding lesions in the GI tract strongly suggests the diagnosis.

The diagnosis of lymphoma is made definitively by biopsy, although physical examination and radiographic findings can be highly suggestive. On CT scan, hypodense intraabdominal lymph nodes can be seen. This appearance is similar to that of disseminated MAC or Whipple's disease. Thus the diagnosis can be delayed while awaiting the results of MAC cultures and empiric treatment. Lymph node biopsy, when possible, is the preferred means of making the diagnosis of lymphoma. However, infiltrating lymphocytes detected on histopathology of a mucosal biopsy obtained during colonoscopy may make the diagnosis as well.

Treatment

The treatment of Kaposi's sarcoma after it has disseminated consists of systemic chemotherapy. The first-line choice should be one of the liposomal anthracyclines (liposomal doxorubicin or liposomal daunorubicin). The majority of patients have at least a partial response and a large proportion have a complete response. Response is probably even better when HAART is given concomitantly. Paclitaxel is potentially more active against Kaposi's sarcoma, but has substantially more toxicity. Therefore it is generally reserved for refractory cases, where it has been shown to have benefit in a large percentage of patients.

Lymphoma not involving the central nervous system is treated with systemic chemotherapy. Chemotherapy regimens can result in clinical remission in upward of half the patients treated. Response rates depend on the extent of disease and degree of immunosuppression. New approaches are under development.

When to Refer

GI bleeding in HIV-infected patients can be a medical emergency, as it can in non–HIV-infected patients. Urgent diagnostic and therapeutic interventions by a gastroenterologist may be required. Even in less acute cases, endoscopy is usually required. Treatment of Kaposi's sarcoma or lymphoma should be managed by physicians skilled in the use of chemotherapeutic agents.

KEY POINTS

- The most common causes of GI bleeding in HIV-infected patients are the same as in the general population
- HIV-associated malignancies, Kaposi's sarcoma, and non-Hodgkin's lymphoma are additional important causes of GI bleeding

SUGGESTED READINGS

Dieterich DT et al: Gastrointestinal manifestations of HIV disease, including the peritoneum and mesentery. In Merigan TC Jr, Bartlett JC, Bolognesi D, editors: *Textbook of AIDS medicine,* ed 2, Baltimore, 1999, Williams & Wilkins.

Forsmark CE: AIDS and the gastrointestinal tract, *Postgrad Med* 93(2):143-148, 151-152, 1993.

Main J et al: Liver disease and AIDS. In Merigan TC Jr, Bartlett JC, Bolognesi D, editors: *Textbook of AIDS medicine,* ed 2, Baltimore, 1999, Williams & Wilkins.

Redvanly RD, Silverstein JE: Intra-abdominal manifestations of AIDS, *Radiol Clin North Am* 35(5):1083-1125, 1997.

Smith PD et al: NIH conference: gastrointestinal infections in AIDS [see comments], *Ann Intern Med* 116(1):63-77, 1992.

Tanowitz HB et al: Gastrointestinal manifestations, *Med Clin North Am* 80(6):1395-1414, 1996.

Tanowitz HB, Simon D, Wittner M: Medical management of AIDS patients: gastrointestinal manifestations, *Med Clin North Am* 76(1):45-62, 1992.

Part III

LATE INFECTION

Section 1 Differential Diagnosis of Common Syndromes

20 Pneumonia

MICHAEL N. BRAFFMAN

Introduction

Despite the rapid advances in the treatment of patients infected with the human immunodeficiency virus (HIV) over the past several years, pulmonary infections continue to be a major cause of morbidity and mortality among this patient population. From 1987 to 1992 the incidence of *Pneumocystis carinii* pneumonia (PCP) as a cause of death fell from 35% to less than 15% as prophylaxis became commonplace, even though the number of acquired immunodeficiency syndrome (AIDS)-related deaths steadily rose. However, mortality from pneumonia remained constant at 15% to 20%, as bacterial pneumonia became the leading cause of death due to pulmonary infection. With the advent of highly active antiretroviral therapy (HAART) in 1996, mortality due to PCP has continued to decline, and early data suggest that the incidence of bacterial pneumonia in HIV-infected patients is dropping as well. Despite these promising signs, there is still a disconcerting number of patients to whom HAART is not available, who have developed resistance to the available agents, or who remain poorly compliant with the complex medication regimens. The lung continues to be the most common site of infectious and noninfectious complications in HIV-infected patients.

In this chapter, the spectrum of pulmonary disease in patients with HIV infection will be reviewed, and then diagnostic and therapeutic approaches as well as the clinical management of these patients will be discussed.

Spectrum of Pulmonary Disease

The differential diagnosis of pneumonia in patients with HIV infection is vast. The list spans a wide spectrum of organisms, including bacteria, viruses, protozoa, fungi, and mycobacteria (Box 20-1). A host of noninfectious diseases, both inflammatory (e.g., interstitial pneumonitis) and neoplastic (e.g., lymphoma, Kaposi's sarcoma [KS], carcinoma), can present indistinguishably from infectious etiologies. Furthermore, the likelihood of any disease varies depending on host factors, geography, and demographics. For example, *Mycobacterium tuberculosis* is more likely to be found in an HIV-infected person who is an intravenous drug abuser in a large northeastern U.S. city, whereas histoplasmosis is much more common in a homosexual non–intravenous drug abusing patient residing in Indiana.

The most critical risk factor for developing an opportunistic pneumonia such as PCP, cytomegalovirus (CMV), *Cryptococcus*, or a more severe lower respiratory infection with a bacterial or mycobacterial infection is the degree of immunosuppression, as measured by a CD4+ lymphocyte count (T cell count) of less than 200 cells/mm^3. This has been well documented since the onset of AIDS and elegantly confirmed in the multicenter "Pulmonary Complications Study."

Furthermore, the CD4+ count can influence disease presentation. For example, with a CD4+ count above 200 to 250 cells/mm^3, *M. tuberculosis* presents much as it does in other patients, with upper lobe cavitary findings. At low CD4+ counts, atypical findings such as diffuse bilateral infiltrates (mimicking PCP) or nodular disease (mimicking fungal infection) are much more common.

Specific Pulmonary Infections and Processes
Pneumocystis carinii Pneumonia (see Chapter 7)

Although the incidence of and mortality due to PCP are declining, it is still the most common AIDS-defining illness in the United States. Despite the availability of widespread prophylaxis, PCP continues to occur in individuals unaware of their HIV seropositive status and in those who cannot tolerate or are poorly compliant with effective prophylaxis.

Presentation and Progression. The vast majority of patients with PCP have CD4+ counts below 200 cells/mm^3. An insidious onset of symptoms is the rule. Constitutional symptoms, including fever, fatigue, weight loss, and a nonproductive cough, are often present for weeks. Exertional dyspnea then develops, and progresses to more severe shortness of breath as gas exchange worsens, culminating in dyspnea at rest. Retrosternal discomfort or tightness with inspiration is a common feature.

Physical examination is often nonspecific. The lungs are generally clear, although in severe disease fine crackles may be present. Tachypnea is present in the setting of significantly advanced disease. Along with other manifestations of advanced HIV infection, oral thrush and seborrheic dermatitis may be present. Up to 10% of patients present with spontaneous pneumothorax, especially if there is a smoking history, with characteristic sharp chest pain.

Hypoxemia is usually present, and its degree is associated with increasing mortality. Serum lactate dehydrogenase (LDH) levels are characteristically elevated, but not always. The classic chest radiograph finding is a bilateral diffuse interstitial ground-glass infiltrate, seen in about 80% of patients. However, almost every pattern of abnormality has been described, including nodules, cysts, focal infiltrates, alveolar infiltrates, cavities, bullae, blebs, and pleural effusions. In earlier disease, the chest radiograph may appear entirely normal.

BOX 20-1
Spectrum of Pulmonary Disease

INFECTIOUS
Pneumocystis carinii

Mycobacteria
Mycobacterium tuberculosis

Nontuberculous Mycobacteria
M. kansasii

Other Bacteria
Streptococcus pneumoniae
Haemophilus influenzae
Pseudomonas aeruginosa
Staphylococcus aureus

Gram-negative Aerobic Bacilli
Nocardia asteroides
Rhodococcus equi
Legionella
Mycoplasma pneumoniae

Fungi
Cryptococcus neoformans
Histoplasma capsulatum
Coccidioides immitis
Blastomyces dermatitidis
Aspergillus species
Penicillium marneffei
Candida species

Viral
Cytomegalovirus
Herpes simplex virus
Varicella-zoster virus

Other
Toxoplasma gondii
Strongyloides stercoralis

NONINFECTIOUS
Neoplastic
Lymphoma
Kaposi's sarcoma
Bronchogenic carcinoma

Inflammatory
Nonspecific interstitial pneumonitis
Lymphoid interstitial pneumonitis

Other
Bronchiectasis
Bronchiolitis obliterans with organizing pneumonia

Diagnosis. The diagnosis of PCP is made by visualization of the organism in induced sputum or from bronchoalveolar lavage (BAL) fluid. Infrequently, transbronchial lung biopsy is necessary to establish the diagnosis. The organism can persist in specimens for weeks after completion of successful therapy.

Treatment. Multiple studies have established the supremacy of trimethoprim-sulfamethoxazole (TMP-SMX [Bactrim, Septra]) as first-line treatment for PCP. Although highly effective, the drug has a significant risk of rash and can also cause nausea, vomiting, leukopenia, and hepatitis. Second-line therapy for treatment failure or for unacceptable toxicity to TMP-SMX includes pentamidine, atovaquone, TMP-dapsone, trimetrexate, and clindamycin-primaquine. Clinical improvement on any drug treatment for PCP usually requires 5 to 7 days, and it is recommended that therapy should not be changed before this period of time. Adjunctive high-dose systemic corticosteroids are indicated for all patients with an alveolar-arterial gradient (A-a gradient) of greater than 30 mm Hg or Po_2 of less than 70 mm Hg. In these situations, corticosteroids have been shown to prevent clinical deterioration and reduce mortality. Pneumothorax complicating PCP can be effectively treated by chest tube and by surgical repair. Despite these interventions, the development of pneumothorax carries a higher mortality.

PCP Prophylaxis. For patients with a CD4+ count of less than 200 cells/mm³ and for patients who have already experienced PCP, prophylaxis with TMP-SMX is highly effective (95% to 100%) at preventing the disease or a relapse of the disease and is a standard of care. Alternative therapies (aerosolized pentamidine, atovaquone, dapsone) are also effective prophylactic agents but have a higher failure rate of approximately 15% to 20%.

When to Refer. Recognition of risk factors for HIV, signs of significant immunodeficiency, and features suggestive of PCP remains the obligation of the primary care provider. Since the diagnosis of PCP frequently requires bronchoscopy, a pulmonologist should be consulted when the diagnosis of PCP is suspected. Consultation with the infectious diseases service may be necessary to assist in the treatment of PCP and concomitant infection, as well as to address the overall management of the patient with advanced HIV disease.

▶ KEY POINTS

- PCP is almost always limited to patients with significant immune depletion, specifically with a CD4+ below 200 cells/mm³
- Most patients present with indolent symptoms, progressing from cough to fever and dyspnea, over several weeks
- Diagnosis of PCP requires special stains of induced sputum or of pulmonary secretions obtained by bronchoscopy
- TMP-SMX remains the drug of choice for treatment and prophylaxis but has a high incidence of rash
- Corticosteroids are an important adjunct to treatment

Bacterial Infections

Bacterial infection of the lower respiratory tract is currently the most common serious complication of HIV infection. Its incidence is higher in HIV-infected individuals than in uninfected individuals and higher still in those patients with lower CD4+ counts, especially in intravenous drug abusers and cigarette smokers.

Presentation and Progression of Common Bacteria

Cause. *Streptococcus pneumoniae* is the leading cause of community-acquired pneumonia in adults with HIV infection, often at a rate greater than 100 times more common than in the general population. Pneumococcal pneumonia presents as it typically does in other hosts, with fever, cough, pleuritic chest pain, dyspnea, and chills. The sputum is often rust colored, and the chest radiograph reveals segmental lobar or multilobar consolidation. Diagnosis is usually made by identification of *S. pneumoniae* in sputum by Gram's stain and culture, and frequently by positive blood cultures. The rate of pneumococcal bacteremia is higher in the HIV-infected patient population. In addition, the rate of drug resistance to penicillin, tetracycline, and TMP-SMX is higher in these patients, requiring empirical therapy with vancomycin or ceftriaxone pending susceptibility testing. Pneumococcal vaccine should routinely be administered to all HIV-infected patients, preferably as soon as the seropositive status is established.

Haemophilus influenzae is another common pathogen, and is frequently isolated from BAL specimens. It often produces an interstitial pattern on chest radiograph and can mimic PCP. *Pseudomonas aeruginosa* is an important cause of both nosocomial and community-acquired pneumonia, especially in advanced HIV infection. Tendency to necrosis, cavitation, relapse, and extrapulmonary sites of infection are hallmarks of *P. aeruginosa* in this population. Awareness of this pathogen should prompt the use of broad-spectrum, antipseudomonal β-lactam antibiotics, perhaps with an aminoglycoside, especially if gram-negative rods are seen on Gram's stain. Other gram-negative aerobic bacilli (*Klebsiella, Escherichia coli*) and *Staphylococcus aureus* are recognized frequently as pathogens, the latter particularly in intravenous drug abusers.

Presentation of Unusual Pathogens. Among more unusually seen organisms, *Rhodococcus equi* can be an important pathogen in HIV-infected patients. Before AIDS, this organism was seen by veterinarians as a pulmonary pathogen of horses. It can cause a subacute or chronic pneumonia in patients with advanced HIV infection. Presentation is typically with the insidious onset of fever, cough, fatigue, chest pain, and weight loss. The characteristic radiographic appearance is cavitation, although focal infiltrate, masslike lesion, and pleural effusion can be seen. The diagnosis can be difficult unless a high index of clinical suspicion is maintained. The organism, which can be overlooked as normal flora or as a contaminant, is a pleomorphic, gram-positive coccobacillus that can be seen on smear or on aerobic culture. Combination antibiotic treatment with vancomycin or imipenem plus ciprofloxacin, erythromycin, or rifampin for several months is necessary. The high frequency of relapse necessitates long-term antibiotic suppression or surgical resection and drainage of persistent abscesses.

Nocardia asteroides, in general a seldom seen pathogen, occurs with some frequency in HIV-infected patients. Clinical presentation with pulmonary nocardiosis can be acute, subacute, or chronic, and like other illnesses is associated with fever, cough, dyspnea, pleuritic pain, weight loss, and on occasion hemoptysis. Chest radiograph usually shows an alveolar infiltrate, but cavitation and a wide variety of presentations are described. As with *R. equi,* a high clinical index of suspicion is necessary to make the diagnosis. The organism grows very slowly on culture (over several weeks). Diagnosis is best made by the appearance of gram-positive, filamentous, beaded, branching, modified acid-fast rods in sputum or BAL samples. The treatment of choice is TMP-SMX, usually for extended courses.

Legionella pneumophila is uncommonly seen in HIV-infected patients but should remain in the differential diagnosis.

Diagnosis. In general, as in non–HIV-associated bacterial pneumonias, Gram's stain evaluation of sputum or BAL samples can provide an invaluable clue to the etiology of pneumonia in HIV-infected patients and can greatly hasten the choice of appropriate antibiotic therapy. Cultures of respiratory samples remain the mainstay of diagnosis.

When to Refer. The primary care provider should readily be able to establish the diagnosis of bacterial pulmonary infections in the setting of HIV disease. As with PCP, when a diagnosis has not yet been made, the assistance of a pulmonologist for bronchoscopy will be necessary. Infectious diseases consultation will be helpful in the choice of specific antibiotic therapy, especially if more unusual pathogens are present.

KEY POINTS

- Common bacterial pathogens, especially pneumococcus, are more frequently seen in HIV-infected patients
- There is a higher incidence of severe, community-acquired pneumonia with pathogens not typically seen in the outpatient setting, especially *P. aeruginosa*
- Unusual bacterial pathogens have a higher frequency in this population (*Nocardia, Legionella, Rhodococcus*)
- The chest radiograph is not specific for any one pathogen

Mycobacterial Infections

Mycobacterium tuberculosis. Since the onset of the AIDS epidemic, HIV infection has been recognized as a significant risk factor for the development of tuberculosis, regardless of the degree of immunosuppression. The risk of developing clinical disease after *M. tuberculosis* infection is estimated as high as 10% per year, as opposed to 5% to 10% over the lifetime of uninfected individuals. Furthermore, there is increased risk of reactivation of latent disease. The risk of developing active tuberculosis is highest in patients residing in the eastern United States, in recent tuberculin skin test converters, in intravenous drug abusers, and in patients with CD4+ counts of less than 200 cells/mm^3. Currently, it is recommended that all patients with tuberculosis be tested for HIV; conversely, all HIV-infected patients should be regularly screened for tuberculosis.

Presentation and Progression. The clinical presentation of tuberculosis is characterized by fever, weight loss, cough, and other nonspecific constitutional symptoms. The radiographic appearance varies dependent on the degree of immunosuppression. In patients with minimal to mild immunosuppression, characteristic upper lobe infiltrates and cavitation are the rule. With progressively lower CD4+ counts, especially below 200 cells/mm^3, the findings are more often characterized by lower lobe or diffuse infiltrates, pleural effusion, hilar and/or mediastinal adenopathy, and a miliary pattern. The infiltrates can be confused with bacterial pneumonia or PCP. Patients with advanced HIV disease are also more likely to develop disseminated disease and have mycobacteremia.

Diagnosis. The diagnosis is usually made by the presence of acid-fast bacilli (AFB) in expectorated and induced sputa and on BAL specimens. On occasion, transbronchial biopsy is necessary to make the diagnosis. Patients with extremely low CD4+ counts may have a lower rate of acid-fast smear positivity. Conversely, the presence of AFB in respiratory secretions has a high predictive value for pulmonary tuberculosis, and such patients should be treated accordingly.

Treatment. Treatment of pulmonary tuberculosis with a standard first-line four-drug regimen of isoniazid (INH), rifampin, pyrazinamide, and ethambutol is indicated for HIV-infected patients as well. It is often necessary to substitute rifabutin for rifampin due to the latter drug's interaction with antiretroviral medications. Culture and sensitivity are still mandatory to help refine therapy, especially because many HIV-infected patients who develop tuberculosis are also at risk for multidrug resistant (i.e., INH- and rifampin-resistant) tuberculosis. Newer diagnostic techniques are significantly shortening the time to culture positivity. Therapy should be continued for 9 to 12 months (compared with the 6 months in HIV-negative patients) and for even longer in miliary, meningeal, and bone disease. It is highly preferable to treat patients using directly observed therapy (DOT) semiweekly to ensure compliance and to prevent the development of resistant disease.

When to Refer. Proper index of suspicion for the possible diagnosis of pulmonary tuberculosis is essential on the part of the primary care physician. If bronchoscopy will be necessary to establish (or exclude) the diagnosis, consultation with a pulmonologist will be necessary. Subspecialty consultation may be necessary in deciding the choice and duration of antituberculous therapy, as well as in assessing infectious risk to others and infection control procedures.

KEY POINTS

- HIV-infected patients exposed to and infected with *M. tuberculosis* have a very high likelihood of developing clinical tuberculosis
- The presentation of pulmonary tuberculosis is dependent on the degree of immunosuppression; the higher the CD4+ count, the more "typical" the chest x-ray and clinical presentation, and the lower the CD4+ count, the more unusual the chest x-ray and clinical course
- All HIV-infected patients should be screened for tuberculosis, and all patients with tuberculosis should have HIV testing offered

Nontuberculous Mycobacteria

Presentation and Progression, Diagnosis, and Treatment. The most important of these organisms to cause pulmonary disease in HIV-infected patients is *M. kansasii*. This usually occurs in patients with advanced HIV disease, often with a CD4+ count of less than 50 cells/mm^3. Presentation is with fever, cough, weight loss, chest pain, dyspnea, hemoptysis, and constitutional symptoms. The chest radiograph is highly variable and nondiagnostic, including interstitial or lobar infiltrates, cavities, hilar adenopathy, and nodules. Disease tends to be confined to the lungs. The diagnosis can only be made by culture, and patients are often treated as having tuberculosis until cultures identify *M. kansasii*. Optimal treatment is poorly defined but usually includes isoniazid, rifampin, and ethambutol for well over 1 year.

M. avium complex (MAC) is commonly isolated from sputum and respiratory secretions, especially in advanced HIV infection with a CD4+ count of less than 50 cells/mm^3, but is a rare cause of pulmonary disease in AIDS. The presence of MAC in sputum is often a predictor for the development of disseminated symptomatic disease. A frequent pulmonary manifestation of disseminated MAC is mediastinal lymphadenopathy. The diagnosis of the rare case of MAC pneumonia in AIDS requires the presence of repeated growth of the organism, an infiltrate, the lack of any other pathogen, and the presence of acid-fast organisms in tissue. Treatment of MAC infection is detailed in Chapter 8.

Finally, other mycobacteria (hemophilum, scrofulaceum, xenopi, and simiae) are all reported as causing HIV-associated pulmonary disease but are all unusual.

When to Refer. The diagnosis of most of these infections will be made by bronchoscopy. Their treatment will usually require consultation with an infectious diseases physician.

KEY POINTS

- Numerous nontuberculous mycobacteria can cause pulmonary disease in the HIV-infected patient
- MAC is an extremely common cause of disseminated infection in AIDS but a rare cause of pulmonary infection

Fungal Disease

Invasive fungal disease and fungal pneumonias occur in the setting of advanced HIV disease with low CD4+ counts, usually less than 100 cells/mm^3. They usually occur as reactivation of prior infection but can be a result of primary infection as well. Obtaining a history of travel to or residence in endemic areas is critical when developing a differential diagnosis of AIDS-associated pneumonia.

Pulmonary Cryptococcosis

Presentation and Progression. After the central nervous system (CNS), the lung is the most common site of infection with *Cryptococcus neoformans*. Most patients present with subacute symptoms, characterized by cough, fever, dyspnea, and hypoxemia, not unlike PCP. Diffuse, bilateral interstitial infiltrates are the most common radiographic finding, although alveolar infiltrates, focal infiltrates, nodular disease, adenopathy, and pleural effusion are described.

Diagnosis. The diagnosis is made by demonstration of the organism in respiratory secretions, especially by BAL. With both meningitis and pulmonary disease, the serum cryptococcal antigen is frequently positive as well. Up to one third of patients with pulmonary cryptococcosis have a coexisting opportunistic pulmonary infection (e.g., PCP, CMV). As many as 60% to 70% of patients with pulmonary cryptococcosis have meningitis as well, and lumbar puncture should be performed on these patients.

Treatment. Treatment with amphotericin B and flucytosine, well delineated for meningitis, is effective for pulmonary cryptococcosis. Following clinical improvement, patients can be switched to oral fluconazole, and must remain on this for chronic suppression until the CD4+ count can be elevated by HAART, if possible. For patients with mild disease, fluconazole can successfully be used from the outset.

Histoplasmosis

Presentation and Progression. Although histoplasmosis is found worldwide, it is especially prevalent in the Ohio and Mississippi River valleys, southern Mexico, Central America, and the Caribbean, including Puerto Rico. The disease occurs predominantly in endemic areas but also is seen in patients who have moved to nonendemic areas. Histoplasmosis usually presents as disseminated disease in advanced HIV infection, with liver, spleen, lymph node, and bone marrow involvement. The majority of patients with disseminated disease have pulmonary involvement. Patients present with fever, weight loss, cough, and dyspnea, and the typical chest radiograph shows diffuse, bilateral interstitial, nodular or reticulonodular infiltrates. In disseminated disease, a sepsis syndrome can predominate, and patients are often pancytopenic, have significant hepatosplenomegaly, and have a characteristic diffuse papular rash.

Diagnosis. The diagnosis of histoplasmosis is made by isolation of the organism from respiratory secretions (mostly in BAL secretions) or blood or bone marrow, or by histopathologic examination of BAL or tissue revealing intracellular organisms. In more severe disease, the organism can be detected in blood by careful examination of a peripheral smear or buffy coat. Antigen detection in urine and serum can also provide a rapid diagnosis with a high degree of specificity.

Treatment. Treatment involves high-dose amphotericin B followed by chronic suppression with oral itraconazole.

Coccidioidomycosis

Presentation and Progression. *Coccidioides immitis* pulmonary disease is largely restricted to endemic areas, notably in the arid areas of the southwestern United States and northern Mexico, where it is one of the most common opportunistic infections in AIDS patients. The lung is the most common site of involvement, and nonspecific presentation with fever, cough, and weight loss is characteristic. Chest radiograph typically reveals diffuse reticulonodular disease, although focal infiltrates and even normal chest films are described.

Diagnosis. Diagnosis is made by culture of respiratory secretions and by the identification of pathognomonic spherules on cytologic evaluation of sputum, BAL secretions, and transbronchial biopsy tissue. Unlike histoplasmosis, blood cultures and serology are infrequently positive. Spherulin skin testing is not helpful in the diagnosis.

Treatment. Amphotericin B is the treatment of choice, although fluconazole and itraconazole have some efficacy. In the laboratory, *C. immitis* is highly contagious, and laboratory personnel should be appropriately warned if the disease is suspected.

Blastomycosis

Presentation and Progression. *Blastomyces dermatitidis* is endemic in the midwestern United States, but unlike the other endemic fungi, it is an uncommon cause of infection in patients with AIDS or advanced HIV infection. The lung is the prime site of infection and up to 80% of patients at initial presentation have pulmonary involvement. Fever, weight loss, and cough are typical. Chest radiograph frequently shows cavitary disease, but the spectrum of findings is broad, including lobar disease, diffuse interstitial markings, nodules, and pleural disease.

Diagnosis. Diagnosis is made by smear and culture of bronchoscopic secretions; serology is unhelpful and there is no skin testing available.

Treatment. Amphotericin B is the treatment of choice in disseminated and extensive pulmonary disease. Oral itraconazole is used for chronic suppression as well as for more mild disease.

Aspergillosis

Presentation and Progression. Aspergillosis is well recognized as an ominous but uncommon disease in patients with advanced HIV infection, especially (although not necessarily) in the setting of concomitant neutropenia, corticosteroid use, or hematologic malignancy. Invasive pulmonary aspergillosis is characterized by fever, cough, and pleuritic chest pain. With tracheobronchial involvement, dyspnea and wheezing are characteristic, and bronchoscopy can reveal bronchial plaques and ulceration. *Aspergillus* can disseminate widely, especially to the brain and other solid organs. Chest radiographs characteristically show diffuse or nodular infiltrates, with frequent progression to cavitation and necrosis.

Diagnosis. Diagnosis is established by the presence of the organism, usually *A. fumigatus,* on culture or the presence of invasive hyphal elements on transbronchial biopsy.

Treatment. Treatment is with high-dose amphotericin B, but the response to therapy is poor and the mortality with invasive disease is disappointingly high.

Other Mycoses. *Penicillium marneffei* is endemic to China and Southeast Asia and is a common opportunistic infection in HIV-infected patients from these regions. It typically presents with disseminated disease and skin lesions but frequently involves the lung. It can present with focal densities, cavitation, and abscess formation on chest radiograph. Diagnosis is made by isolation from blood, skin, and respiratory secretions. It can be confused microscopically with histoplasmosis, also an intracellular organism, and the laboratory should be alerted if the patient is known to come from an endemic area so that this distinction can be kept in mind.

Candida is a rare cause of pneumonia in advanced HIV infection and can be difficult to establish antemortem. It probably develops as an extension of severe upper airway disease in patients with advanced HIV infection. Diagnosis requires detection in lung tissue and growth of the organism.

When to Refer. As with other pulmonary infections in this setting, the assistance of an experienced bronchoscopist may be necessary to establish the diagnosis of fungal pneumonia. Infectious diseases consultation is strongly recommended, especially if the diagnosis is made in a patient residing in a nonendemic area for a specific fungus, to assist in selection and duration of antifungal management.

KEY POINTS

- A history of residence in endemic regions is crucial to more quickly making the diagnosis of fungal pneumonias
- The spectrum of radiographic findings is too diverse to be specific. However, fungal pneumonia should be considered if nodules or cavities are seen on the chest radiograph
- Amphotericin B and azoles each have roles in the treatment of fungal pneumonia

Viral Diseases

Cytomegalovirus

Presentation and Progression. CMV is by far the most important viral pulmonary pathogen in AIDS patients. It is only seen in advanced HIV infection, typically with a CD4+ count of less than 50 cells/mm^3. The presentation of CMV pneumonia is nonspecific, with fever, cough, dyspnea, and hypoxemia, not unlike PCP. The chest radiograph characteristically reveals diffuse, often fine interstitial infiltrates, although nodular disease and alveolar consolidation are reported less commonly. Pneumonia may be the only clinically involved end organ with CMV, but it can also occur with or after the diagnosis of CMV retinitis or gastrointestinal disease. The diagnosis of CMV pneumonitis should prompt a thorough funduscopic examination by an ophthalmologist.

Diagnosis. The diagnosis of CMV pneumonitis can be a difficult one. CMV is a frequent colonizer of the upper and lower respiratory tracts in patients with HIV disease, and the isolation of CMV from pulmonary secretions is extremely common. To further complicate matters, CMV pneumonia often presents with other concomitant opportunistic infections such as PCP. A definitive diagnosis of CMV pneumonia requires the isolation of CMV, absence of other pathogens, and most importantly confirmatory histopathology, with multiple CMV inclusions on cytology or in lung tissue. The isolation of CMV from BAL alone without clear histopathology should not be treated with anti-CMV agents but rather requires a continued search for another diagnosis.

Treatment. Treatment for CMV pneumonitis is with ganciclovir, foscarnet, or cidofovir, all administered intravenously. The duration of therapy for isolated CMV pneumonia, unlike CMV retinitis, need not be indefinite, and is usually several weeks to months, until clinical resolution occurs.

When to Refer. An experienced ophthalmologist should examine the fundi for evidence of mild or subclinical CMV retinitis in any patient with CMV pneumonitis. The diagnosis of CMV pneumonia almost always requires bronchoscopy. As with most opportunistic infections, the infectious diseases consultant can assist with the selection and duration of anti-CMV therapy.

KEY POINTS

- CMV pneumonia remains the most common viral pneumonia in the patient with advanced HIV infection
- Diagnosis can be difficult and requires the presence of specific viral pathology on cytologic or tissue examination along with positive cultures
- CMV shedding is common in advanced HIV. The isolation of CMV from respiratory secretions without concomitant specific cytopathology should not lead to reflexive treatment for CMV pneumonia

Other Viruses. Other viral infections of the lung are much less common as significant causes of opportunistic disease. Herpes simplex virus (HSV) can present much like CMV. Varicella-zoster virus, measles, and adenovirus have all been reported. Although influenza and respiratory syncytial virus occur in HIV-infected patients as well, their incidence and severity appear no greater than in the general population. Influenza vaccine is indicated for all HIV-infected patients, to help prevent postinfluenza pulmonary complications.

Other Pneumonias
Toxoplasmosis
Presentation and Progression. Other than PCP, the only significant protozoal infection of the lung is *Toxoplasma gondii*. Pulmonary disease, like CNS disease, is more prevalent in AIDS patients in Europe and Latin America, where *Toxoplasma* seroprevalence is much higher than in the United States. Most patients have advanced HIV infection, often with a CD4+ count of less than 50 cells/mm³. As with other opportunistic infections, disease presents with fever, cough, and dyspnea. Less commonly, patients present with a diffuse, fulminant pneumonia resembling adult respiratory distress syndrome (ARDS). The chest radiograph reveals diffuse bilateral interstitial infiltrates and can be difficult to distinguish from PCP; nodular disease and pleural effusions have also been described.

Diagnosis and Treatment. The diagnosis of *Toxoplasma* pneumonia first requires a sufficient index of suspicion and is best made by observation of tachyzoites on Giemsa stain or indirect immunofluorescence of BAL fluid. Most patients are seropositive for *T. gondii*, but serology is not helpful in establishing the diagnosis of pulmonary toxoplasmosis.

Treatment of *Toxoplasma* pneumonia is with pyrimethamine and either sulfadiazine, dapsone, or high-dose clindamycin.

Strongyloides stercoralis
Presentation and Progression. *Strongyloides stercoralis*, a nematode, is ubiquitous in the developing world and can lay dormant for many years, only to become active later in life when the host develops immunosuppression. It can cause a hyperinfection syndrome with pulmonary involvement as the larvae burrow from the portal circulation through the diaphragms and into the lung, causing diffuse patchy infiltrative disease.

Diagnosis and Treatment. The larvae can be visualized in respiratory secretions. Treatment with thiabendazole can be lifesaving. It should be considered in HIV-infected patients who hail from or have resided in the developing world.

KEY POINTS

- Unusual causes of pneumonia should always be considered in the patient with advanced HIV disease, especially in patients with exposure (e.g., cats) or travel histories

Noninfectious Pulmonary Disease
Kaposi's Sarcoma
Presentation and Progression. Respiratory tract involvement with KS can be variable and widespread, including the lung, pleura, and tracheobronchial tree. KS occurs predominantly in men who have had sex with men and is unusual in heterosexual intravenous drug abusers and women. Pulmonary KS occurs predominantly in patients with advanced HIV infection. Skin and mucocutaneous involvement is absent in 10% to 20% of patients with pulmonary disease, sometimes making the diagnosis more difficult to establish. Radiographs characteristically show nodular or dense infiltrates, often in the perihilar region, and occasionally pleural effusions. However, similar to the other entities reviewed above, the findings can be variable.

Diagnosis. Definitive diagnosis is made by observation of characteristic endobronchial violaceous papules or by histologic examination of lung tissue obtained by biopsy. A significant proportion of patients with pulmonary KS have concomitant opportunistic pulmonary infections, and this should be kept in mind when diagnostic studies are being performed.

Other Malignancies
HIV-associated pulmonary non-Hodgkin's lymphoma can occur, and presents with infiltrative, nodular, or masslike

disease on chest radiograph. Unlike many other opportunistic entities, lymphoma can occur at earlier stages of HIV disease. There is a suggestion in the literature that HIV-infected patients may be at increased risk for adenocarcinoma of the lung.

When to Refer. The diagnosis of KS or any pulmonary malignancy should prompt referral to an experienced oncologist.

KEY POINTS

- Pulmonary involvement with Kaposi's sarcoma is usually but not always associated with concomitant cutaneous involvement
- Pulmonary KS is usually a complication of advanced HIV disease
- Pulmonary and extrapulmonary lymphoma may be seen at any stage of HIV disease

Nonspecific Interstitial Pneumonitis

Presentation and Progression. Nonspecific interstitial pneumonitis (NSIP) is a poorly understood process that presents virtually indistinguishable from PCP, with dyspnea, cough, and fever, and interstitial infiltrates on chest radiography. Many patients are treated as if having PCP but bronchoscopy fails to show the typical organisms of *P. carinii*. Unlike PCP and many other opportunistic pathogens, the mean CD4+ count in patients with NSIP is much higher, often well above 200 cells/mm^3, and should be a clue to the diagnosis.

Diagnosis and Treatment. Transbronchial biopsy, when performed on these patients, reveals a mild to moderate mononuclear infiltrate with macrophages and lymphoid aggregates. Although this process appears to resolve spontaneously, in reality many patients are treated as if they have PCP and improve on corticosteroids and TMP-SMX. Whether the etiology of this process is infectious or inflammatory has not been determined.

Other Pulmonary Processes

Many other processes can involve the lung in patients with HIV infection or AIDS, some of which may mimic infectious processes, others not, any of which can be associated with concomitant opportunistic infections. This list includes bronchiectasis, bronchiolitis obliterans with organizing pneumonia (BOOP), pulmonary embolism, congestive heart failure, pulmonary hypertension, pulmonary hemorrhage, and pulmonary sequelae of intravenous drug use. Lymphoid interstitial pneumonitis is rare in adults with AIDS, but can occur in HIV-infected children.

KEY POINTS

- Nonspecific interstitial pneumonitis can mimic PCP but is usually seen in patients with higher CD4+ counts and frequently nondiagnostic bronchoscopic evaluations
- A large number of noninfectious and nonmalignant causes must always be considered in the patient with HIV infection

Diagnostic Tools, Clinical Assessment, and Approach

In order to wade through the extensive differential diagnosis of pulmonary disease in HIV-infected patients and to prioritize the diagnostic possibilities, it is necessary to review the diagnostic tools available to the clinician.

History

Before considering other tools, the accurate recording of a patient history remains a critical part of evaluating the patient. A thorough history is unlikely to lead to a specific diagnosis, but it will prove valuable in narrowing the focus of the differential diagnosis and will be helpful in guiding the diagnostic approach. Risk factors for HIV infection can affect the differential diagnosis. Intravenous drug abusers or homeless individuals are at greater risk for tuberculosis, for example, as well as for bacterial pneumonias. Homosexual men are at greater risk for the development of KS and concomitant pulmonary involvement. HIV disease status (history of opportunistic infections, CD4+ count, viral load) is critical in assessing likelihood of significant immunosuppression. For example, the patient's describing oral thrush helps to identify the patient as significantly immunocompromised; a prior history of PCP indicates a risk for recurrence. History of exposure to tuberculosis or prior purified protein derivative (PPD) testing helps assess the risk of tuberculosis. Specific medication use, especially the use of and compliance with prophylactic medications such as TMP-SMX, can be of great assistance in deciding whether specific opportunistic infections, such as PCP, are likely or not. Use of less effective prophylactic agents, such as aerosolized pentamidine, may make suspicion for PCP higher, for example. Use of recreational drugs such as smoking marijuana can increase risk for *Aspergillus*, as will the use of corticosteroids and broad-spectrum antibiotics. Knowledge of region or country of origin, places of residence, and both recent and remote travel history are critical in gauging the risk of endemic diseases, particularly the fungal infections histoplasmosis, coccidioidomycosis, and blastomycosis. Residence in the eastern United States increases the risk for developing tuberculosis, presumably due to a greater frequency of exposure. HIV-infected patients returning from or raised in Southeast Asia should prompt a consideration of *P. marneffei* or *Strongyloides*. A history of animal exposure should raise concerns for *R. equi*.

Certainly, the history of the present illness can give valuable clues as to the etiology of the process. The onset, type, and duration of symptoms are helpful in differentiating the cause of the symptoms. An abrupt onset of symptoms is more consistent with a bacterial pneumonia; a more indolent presentation, with progressive cough, fever, and increasing dyspnea over several weeks, makes PCP, fungal, and other diseases more likely. The presence of hemoptysis can further focus the differential diagnosis to entities such as tuberculosis, aspergillosis, or pulmonary KS.

Physical Examination

Along with a thorough history, a standard physical examination can assist greatly in developing an appropriate diagnostic list, although it too infrequently leads to a specific diagnosis. The presence of mucocutaneous candidiasis is consistent with

> **BOX 20-2**
> **Likelihood of Pulmonary Disease Based on CD4+ Count**
>
> **CD4+ ABOVE 200-250**
> Bacterial pneumonia
>   *Streptococcus pneumoniae,* community viral respiratory pathogens (influenza, respiratory syncytial virus, adenovirus)
>   *Mycoplasma pneumoniae/Chlamydia*
>   *Staphylococcus aureus* (intravenous drug abusers)
> *Mycobacterium tuberculosis*
>   Typical presentation
> Nonspecific interstitial pneumonitis
> Lymphoma
>
> **CD4+ BELOW 200**
> Bacterial pneumonia
>   *S. pneumoniae* with bacteremia
>   *Pseudomonas aeruginosa*
>   *Rhodococcus equi*
>   *Nocardia*
> *Mycobacterium tuberculosis*
>   Atypical presentation
> Nontuberculous mycobacteria
> Endemic fungi
>   Histoplasmosis, blastomycosis, coccidioidomycosis, *Penicillium marneffei*
> Other fungi
>   *Cryptococcus, Aspergillus*
> Cytomegalovirus
> Toxoplasmosis
> *Strongyloides*
> Neoplasms
>   Kaposi's sarcoma
> Lymphoma

a low CD4+ count and/or significant immunosuppression and includes an entire spectrum of pulmonary pathogens. The finding of cutaneous or mucous membrane KS increases the likelihood of pulmonary involvement. A skin lesion consistent with *Cryptococcus* likewise raises this possibility of pulmonary cryptococcosis. The presence of CMV retinitis can be associated with CMV pulmonary involvement. The lung examination may be extremely helpful (e.g., focal bronchial breath sounds suggesting lobar consolidation, diffuse crackles suggesting any one of the causes of a diffuse interstitial process). Frequently, the lung examination is normal, even in the setting of significant dyspnea or abnormal chest radiograph findings.

Laboratory Studies

By far the single most important laboratory value that helps define or focus the differential diagnosis of HIV-associated pneumonias is the CD4+ count. Above 200 to 250 cells/mm^3, the possibilities generally are limited to bacteria (particularly *S. pneumoniae,* but also other community-acquired bacteria, viral respiratory infections, and *Mycoplasma/Chlamydia*), *M. tuberculosis,* NSIP, lymphoma, and possibly *Nocardia.* PCP is unusual in this group, and endemic fungi, CMV, pulmonary toxoplasmosis, and *Rhodococcus,* for example, would be extremely unlikely and unrealistic considerations (Box 20-2). In one large series, 79% of patients with PCP had CD4+ counts below 100 cells/mm^3 and fully 95% had CD4+ counts below 200 cells/mm^3.

Other studies are useful as well. The tuberculin skin test as measured by reactivity to PPD can help aid in the diagnosis of pulmonary tuberculosis, despite the significant incidence of anergy in HIV-infected patients. A large multicenter Italian study showed that risk for developing subsequent tuberculosis in non-anergic patients directly correlates with the degree of tuberculin reactivity of 5 mm or greater, and is not affected by the degree of immunosuppression. Because there is a greater incidence of anergy, however, a negative reaction should not dissuade the clinician from pursuing a diagnosis of tuberculosis if other clinical factors suggest the diagnosis. A high serum LDH can tilt the diagnosis more toward PCP. A positive serum cryptococcal antigen increases the likelihood of pulmonary *Cryptococcus* in the setting of a characteristic radiograph. *Histoplasma capsulatum* antigen testing of urine and serum has a very high sensitivity for the diagnosis of disseminated histoplasmosis in the HIV-infected population. A negative urine antigen effectively excludes the diagnosis. A marked leukocytosis with bandemia is consistent with a bacterial pneumonia; marked neutropenia increases the risk for *Aspergillus.* Blood cultures remain valuable and can detect bacteremia (e.g., pneumococcus), fungemia *(Cryptococcus),* and mycobacteremia. Examination of the peripheral blood smear can reveal histoplasmosis.

Pulmonary function testing is often very helpful in establishing the presence of pulmonary disease in HIV-infected patients. Determination of the A-a gradient by blood gas and pulse oximetry can assess the severity of disease and can indicate significantly more impairment than is obvious from the patient's history, examination, or chest film findings. Pulmonary function testing is most useful in the diagnosis of PCP when the chest radiograph findings are normal or equivocal. In one study, an increase in the A-a gradient during exercise revealed 100% sensitivity and 65% positive predictive value for PCP in patients who were not receiving PCP prophylaxis. Since the negative predictive value of a normal study is 100%, a normal test effectively excludes PCP as a diagnosis. The diffusing capacity, as measured by the diffusing capacity for carbon monoxide (DLCO), can be used the same way but has less specificity.

Chest Radiograph

As reviewed in detail earlier, the radiographic findings of pulmonary processes in the HIV-infected population can be so variable and atypical that any specific pattern is of limited use in arriving at a single diagnosis. Findings range from diffuse interstitial/reticulonodular infiltrates to consolidation, cavitary disease, masslike lesions, nodules, effusions, adenopathy, and even a "normal" radiograph. Nevertheless, the chest radiograph is the most commonly obtained study in the initial evaluation of HIV-infected patients with pulmonary disease. The findings can help to focus the differential possibilities, to some extent, and to assist in deciding follow-up interventions such as bronchoscopy, thoracentesis, or biopsy (see below). The chest film must always be interpreted in the setting of other information as well. For example, identical diffuse infiltrates with fever and cough would suggest NSIP in a patient with a CD4+ count of 450 cells/mm^3 and undetectable viral load on HAART; it would suggest PCP, CMV, tuberculosis, or other opportunists in a patient with a CD4+ of 25 cells/mm^3 who is noncompliant with prophylactic TMP-SMX and HAART therapy. Pneumothorax on chest film should prompt a search for PCP, even if the parenchyma appears normal otherwise.

As a screening tool, chest radiography has no role in the asymptomatic HIV-infected patient. In the Pulmonary Complications Study, fewer than 2% of more than 5,000 asymptomatic patients were found to have an abnormality. Screening also failed to detect any abnormality in the vast majority of patients who developed a new pulmonary process within 2 months of the film. Chest radiography should only be employed for patients with pulmonary symptoms.

Chest Computed Tomography

Computed tomography (CT) of the chest can be helpful in delineating the nature and extent of disease and is often a useful adjunct to plain chest radiograph. CT scanning adds limited information in establishing a diagnosis if there are obvious chest radiograph abnormalities. However, CT is most useful in the setting of equivocal or normal chest films, where high-resolution and spiral CT scans can visualize abnormalities not well appreciated on chest radiograph. CT scan can also help direct diagnostic intervention by visualizing the location and extent of parenchymal lesions and allowing for more direct sampling by bronchoscopy or biopsy. In certain instances, CT scans can aid in the diagnosis of specific processes such as KS (the presence of multiple flame-shaped lesions originating from the hila) or lymphoma (large mediastinal, chest wall, or parenchymal mass lesions).

Gallium Scanning

Gallium-67 scans were used frequently for screening symptomatic patients for PCP at the outset of the AIDS epidemic in the early 1980s. Although useful then, current diagnostic techniques are much more sensitive. Their low specificity, cost, and time requirement have rendered them obsolete as a useful diagnostic tool.

Sputum Examination

Examination of expectorated and induced sputum remains a simple and very useful procedure. Although the yield of a diagnostic study may be somewhat reduced in patients with advanced HIV disease, Gram's stain and culture of expectorated sputum can readily reveal a bacterial pathogen, particularly pneumococcus, *H. influenzae,* or *P. aeruginosa.* Induced sputum (i.e., obtained by a respiratory therapist after inhalation of a saline mist) has been successful in diagnosing PCP. Induced sputum is stained by silver stain or a monoclonal antibody directed against PCP. It can help prevent the need for a more invasive procedure such as bronchoscopy, thereby reducing the cost of care and potential morbidity of a procedure. It is rapid and inexpensive, and generally has a high degree of sensitivity. The sensitivity of the test is greatest in patients not on chemoprophylaxis for PCP and lower in patients who are compliant with prophylaxis.

The yield of sputum induction in making a diagnosis of PCP will vary with how well the specimen was obtained and processed and is very institution- and personnel-dependent. Since tuberculosis is a common pathogen in this population and can present similar to PCP, appropriate precautions should be taken by medical personnel during sputum induction to prevent the airborne transmission of tuberculosis.

Sputum can also be obtained for acid-fast smear and culture in an attempt to diagnose tuberculosis or other mycobacteria. At least two induced sputa should be sent for AFB smear and culture to improve the diagnostic yield. Studies suggest that the majority (50% to 70%) of HIV-infected patients with active pulmonary tuberculosis are acid-fast smear–positive and that almost all (75% to 100%) are culture-positive. The vast majority (more than 80%) of all AFB smear–positive–induced sputa are due to tuberculosis and should be treated as such pending cultures.

Fiberoptic Bronchoscopy

Flexible fiberoptic bronchoscopy (FOB) remains the most valuable diagnostic intervention in the diagnosis of HIV-associated pneumonias and is performed when evaluation of induced sputum fails to make a specific diagnosis. FOB should be the initial diagnostic procedure when the patient is unable to perform an induced sputum, when the clinical presentation is atypical for PCP, or when the pulmonary process is progressing rapidly. FOB can assess all segments of the respiratory tree: airway, bronchi, lung parenchyma, and adjacent tissue. Pulmonary secretions are easily and generally safely obtained by BAL, and biopsies can be taken of bronchi, parenchyma, or specific lesions to obtain tissue for diagnosis. In general, the yield of the procedure is quite high, as numerous studies and much experience have demonstrated.

Currently, BAL without biopsy is the procedure of choice for diagnosing PCP and, initially, most other pathogens. It is highly sensitive and well tolerated by most patients. Some patients develop fever and small, localized infiltrates after the procedure. Lavage is usually obtained from the two lobes with the greatest degree of abnormality on chest radiograph. Diagnostic sensitivity for PCP by this technique of site-directed multilobe BAL approaches 100% in patients not on prophylaxis, and is almost as high in patients taking prophylaxis. For the diagnosis of *M. tuberculosis,* sputum induction is preferred when possible to reduce the risk of transmission to health care workers during bronchoscopy. FOB should be used for the diagnosis of tuberculosis when acid-fast smears and cultures are negative but where the diagnosis is still suspect. In addition, when FOB is being performed while another diagnosis is being considered, BAL fluid should be routinely sent for AFB smear and culture.

BAL fluid obtained by FOB can also be examined for a variety of specific fungal antigens, which can assist cytology and culture in diagnosis. Cryptococcal antigen titers of 1:8 or greater in BAL fluid are consistent with a diagnosis of pulmonary cryptococcosis. *Histoplasma* polysaccharide antigen detection in BAL fluid is a rapid method by which to diagnose pulmonary histoplasmosis, with sensitivity approaching 70%, similar to the sensitivity of silver or Giemsa staining.

Transbronchial biopsy is usually not necessary for the diagnosis of PCP and can carry with it a higher rate of pneumothorax and hemorrhage. The rate of pneumothorax is dependent on the bronchoscopist and the severity and extent of lung disease, and can be as high as 10% to 20% of all procedures. However, in instances in which the BAL is negative or nondiagnostic, repeat bronchoscopy with biopsy will be necessary. Biopsy is often necessary for the diagnosis of other processes, such as tuberculosis, CMV, fungal pneumonias, certain malignancies,

BOX 20-3
Assessment of Patient with HIV Disease and Pulmonary Processes

- History: risk factors, HIV disease status, exposures, medications, residence in endemic areas, travel, animals, history of present illness
- Physical examination
- Laboratory: CD4+ (essential); purified protein derivative, lactate dehydrogenase, serum cryptococcal antigen, *Histoplasma* antigens, blood cultures, peripheral smears
- Pulmonary function tests
- Chest radiograph: not specific for a diagnosis, but essential
- Chest CT scan
- Gallium scan: obsolete
- Sputum examination: Gram's stain; induced (for PCP); acid-fast bacilli smear/culture
- Fiberoptic bronchoscopy: bronchoalveolar lavage; transbronchial biopsy
- Lung biopsy: percutaneous fine needle aspirate; open lung; video-assisted thoracoscopic surgery

BOX 20-4
Issues to Consider

- Are the chest radiograph findings typical of PCP, with diffuse, bilateral interstitial infiltrates?
- Is the pulmonary disease mild (i.e., P_{O_2} above 70 mm Hg, A-a gradient below 30 mm Hg)?
- Is the CD4+ count low (below 200 cells/mm^3)?
- Has the patient not been on chemoprophylaxis for PCP with TMP-SMX?
- Are epidemiologic risk factors for tuberculosis or endemic fungi absent?
- Is the lactate dehydrogenase elevated?
- Is the patient likely to follow up with the clinician and remain compliant with medications?

BOX 20-5
Further Evaluation of PCP Diagnosis Not Confirmed

- The finding of a specific bacterial process by Gram's stain and culture should prompt the specific treatment with appropriate antibacterial antibiotics.
- Acid-fast smear and culture should be performed. If acid-fast bacilli are seen, then treatment for *M. tuberculosis* should commence.
- If the induced sputum is nondiagnostic, then bronchoscopy with bronchoalveolar lavage (BAL) should be performed. BAL will be either diagnostic or not.
- A specific diagnosis should be treated accordingly.
- If no diagnosis is made, bronchoscopy should be repeated and transbronchial biopsy for tissue should be performed.
- If a specific diagnosis is established, then appropriate therapy should begin.
- If transbronchial biopsy still has not revealed a diagnosis, then consideration should be given to needle aspirate of peripheral focal lesions or lung biopsy by open thoracotomy, minithoracotomy, or video-assisted thoracoscopic surgery.

and nonspecific or lymphoid interstitial pneumonitis. The combination of BAL and transbronchial biopsy increases the diagnostic yield to 98% to 99% for all diagnoses.

Close cooperation with an experienced bronchoscopist is invaluable in the care of HIV-infected patients with pulmonary disease.

Lung Biopsy

Lung tissue can be obtained by means other than bronchoscopy for diagnosis, although it is infrequently necessary for the diagnosis of HIV-associated pneumonias due to the overall high diagnostic yield of bronchoscopy.

Percutaneous transthoracic needle aspiration is extremely useful for sampling peripheral focal lesions of the lung in HIV-infected patients, such as masses, nodules, or localized infiltrates, with a fairly high yield. It can help to avoid more invasive or open procedures. The major complication is pneumothorax, occurring in as many as 20% of patients.

Open lung biopsy carries significant morbidity and in general has not been found to greatly enhance the ability to make a diagnosis in HIV-infected patients who have been extensively evaluated. However, in selected patients, the procedure can be safely performed and diagnostic. In several illnesses, larger amounts of tissue are on occasion necessary for diagnosis, including KS, lymphoma, NSIP, and BOOP. In addition, for patients who continue to deteriorate or fail to improve and still lack a diagnosis, it may be necessary to obtain tissue. In several studies of AIDS patients, the yield is greatest in those who had not undergone FOB (77%), lower in patients with nondiagnostic bronchoscopy (45%), and lowest in patients with continued progression of disease process despite appropriate treatment for a documented process (15%). The mortality of an open lung procedure is highest for patients who are ventilator-dependent.

An alternative to open lung biopsy is video-assisted thoracoscopic surgery (VATS), which significantly reduces morbidity associated with obtaining lung tissue. It is significantly less invasive and does not require a thoracotomy. Data are preliminary and limited for the use of this technique in the diagnosis of pulmonary processes in HIV-infected patients, but it is likely to be used much more frequently as the skill is refined.

Box 20-3 lists the key elements of assessing the patient with HIV disease and pulmonary processes.

Summary

Although there is no rigidly defined formula to follow, the approach to the HIV-infected patient with pulmonary symptoms outlined below is a reasonable consensus that synthesizes the information reviewed throughout this chapter. As in all clinical medicine, nothing replaces the judgment of the informed clinician who is presented with an ill patient. Each clinical situation must be individualized.

Establish the Degree of Immunocompromise: CD4+ Count

As emphasized repeatedly, the CD4+ count is the single most important piece of information that will help the clinician prioritize the focus of the differential diagnosis. Specifically, the spectrum of illnesses will be narrower when the count is greater than 200 to 250 cells/mm^3 and essentially wide open when the count is lower.

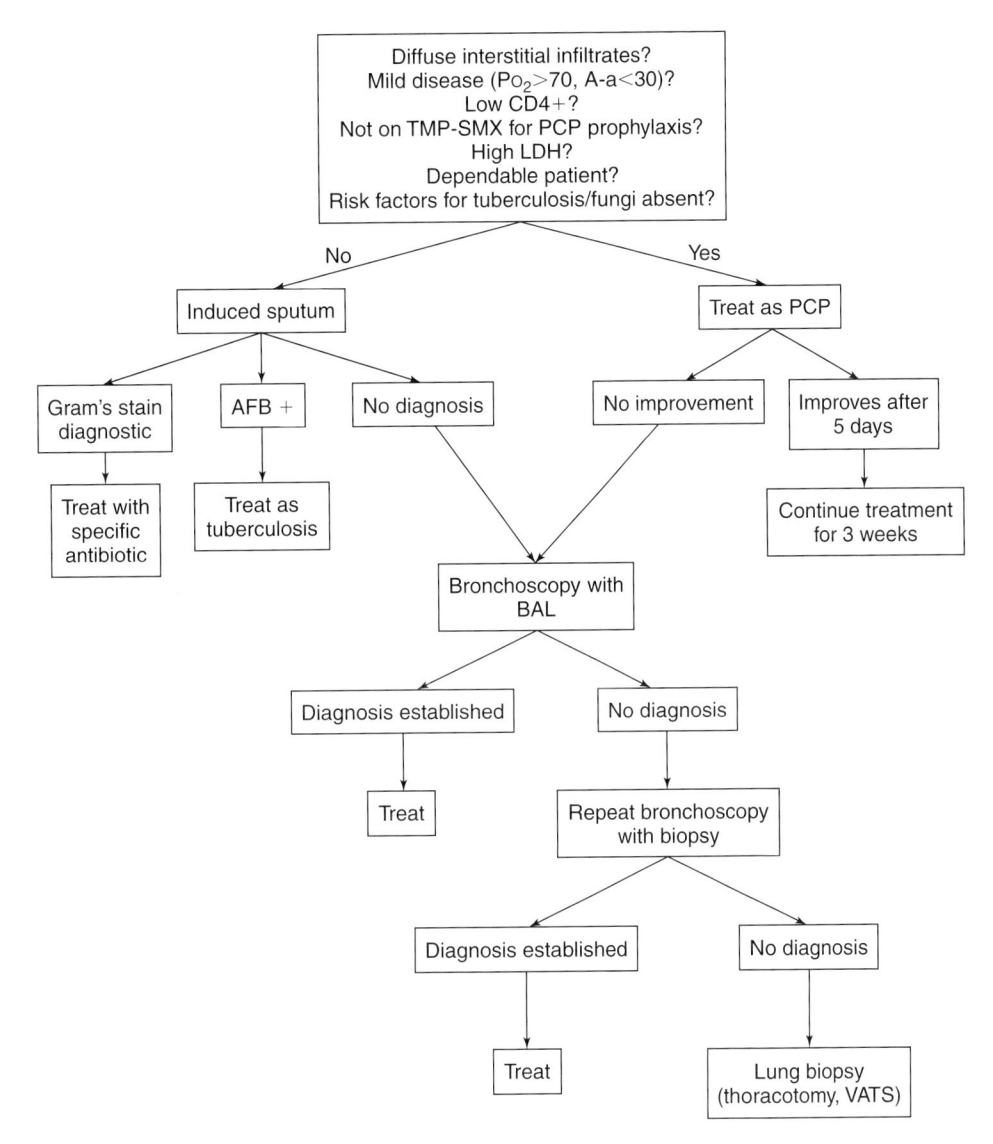

FIG. 20-1 Algorithm for the treatment and evaluation of the HIV-infected patient with pulmonary symptoms. *TMP-SMX*, Trimethoprim-sulfamethoxazole; *PCP*, *Pneumocystis carinii* pneumonia; *LDH*, lactate dehydrogenase; *BAL*, bronchoalveolar lavage; *VATS*, video-assisted thoracoscopic surgery.

Clinical Approach: Empirical Treatment for PCP Versus Continued Evaluation

Box 20-4 lists the questions that should be asked prior to initiating empirical treatment for PCP.

If the answer to all of these questions is affirmative, then PCP treatment should begin. If clinical improvement occurs within 5 days, then the patient should continue treatment, preferably with oral TMP-SMX for a full 21 days. However, if there is minimal to no improvement or worsening, then bronchoscopy with BAL should be performed for a specific diagnosis.

If, on the other hand, the answer to any or all of the questions above is no, then sputum induction should be performed. See Box 20-5 for the next steps to follow. This approach is summarized in Fig. 20-1. It should again be emphasized that there is no single approach to all patients. Careful review of the specifics of each case and thoughtful clinical judgment are necessary for establishing the diagnosis and formulating an appropriate treatment plan.

SUGGESTED READINGS

Bartlett J, Gallant J: *Medical management of AIDS,* Baltimore, 2000, Johns Hopkins University, pp 298-308.

Bartlett J: *Management of respiratory infections,* Philadelphia, 1999, Lippincott Williams & Wilkins, pp 89-109.

Falloon J: Pulmonary manifestations of human immunodeficiency virus infection. In Dolin R, Masur H, Saag M, editors: *AIDS therapy,* Philadelphia, 1999, Churchill Livingstone, pp 699-721.

Levine SJ: Diagnosing pulmonary infections in HIV-positive patients. Part I: Epidemiology, etiology, and evaluation, *Infect Med* 16(10):637, 1999.

Levine SJ: Diagnosing pulmonary infections in HIV-positive patients. Part II: Diagnostic approaches, *Infect Med* 16(12):814, 1999.

Mandell G, Bennett J, Dolin R, editors: *Principles and practice of infectious diseases,* ed 5, Philadelphia, 2000, Churchill Livingstone, pp 1415-1426.

Stover D: Approach to the HIV-infected Patient with Pulmonary Symptoms. In Rose B, editor: *Up-to-Date* CD Rom, vol 8, no 3, 2000.

21 HIV and Diarrhea

TODD D. BARTON, ANNE H. NORRIS

Introduction

Diarrhea is one of the most common complaints of HIV-infected individuals, occurring in 30% to 50% of American patients and 90% to 100% of the international population. Up to 15% of patients will complain of diarrhea at their first visit to an HIV practitioner. This problem was recognized early in the HIV epidemic as a quality of life issue, and has more recently been linked to mortality. Indeed, diarrhea lasting more than 1 month, associated with an unexplained weight loss of at least 10%, is an AIDS-defining condition. Like other clinical syndromes in HIV-infected patients, diarrhea is often an infectious problem. Causative agents span the spectrum of known microbes (Table 21-1). In the past, both detecting and treating HIV-associated diarrheal pathogens have been frustrating. The last 5 years, however, have brought improved detection methods for previously hard-to-find microbes, as well as a more well-defined approach to chronic diarrhea in HIV disease. Nevertheless, despite a thoughtful and complete work-up, up to 20% of cases of HIV-associated diarrhea will remain unexplained.

Patients, History, and Examination

Most studies of HIV-associated diarrhea are dominated by males (>90%), predominantly homosexual. Despite this, it is not clear that homosexual men are at an increased risk of developing diarrhea. One study actually found intravenous drug users to be at higher risk than homosexual men when matched for CD4+ count. Diarrhea occurs at all stages of HIV infection, but chronic diarrhea most often affects patients with CD4+ counts below 50 cells/mm^3. Certain pathogens (cytomegalovirus [CMV], *Mycobacterium avium* complex [MAC], microsporidia) occur almost exclusively in these severely immunocompromised patients.

Diarrhea may appear as an isolated symptom or may be accompanied by fever, abdominal pain, nausea, and/or vomiting. Unfortunately, the presence or absence of these symptoms does not correlate with any specific microbe. Furthermore, the character of the stool (bloody, watery) does not reliably point to a specific pathogen. Weight loss is common, on average 10 pounds at time of presentation. The likelihood of finding a new stool pathogen is highest in patients with a CD4+ count below 100 cells/mm^3. Weight loss in excess of 20 pounds and the presence of high stool volume also correlate with the successful identification of a stool pathogen.

Travel history is of less value in an HIV-infected host with diarrhea than in an immunocompetent host. However, a thorough review of the HIV-infected patient's medication list is imperative, particularly for those with advanced disease who may take dozens of pills daily.

Like the history, physical examination rarely points to a specific pathogen. Fever is common. Orthostatic changes in pulse and/or blood pressure may be present if vomiting or profuse diarrhea is prominent. Mild to moderate pain, often localizing to the lower quadrants, is typical and nonspecific. A careful examination of the perianal area should be undertaken, since local ulceration can indicate herpes simplex virus (HSV) or CMV. Rarely, some agents of diarrhea (particularly CMV) can be associated with abdominal catastrophe; a surgical abdomen must be immediately recognized and triaged accordingly.

Diagnosis

Routine laboratory tests may provide some insight into the severity of illness. Electrolytes such as sodium, potassium, and magnesium may be markedly abnormal and occasionally point toward an unusual cause of diarrhea such as adrenal insufficiency. An elevated creatinine may indicate gross clinical volume depletion. Serum albumin varies with the degree of malnutrition.

A critical diagnostic step in patients with HIV and diarrhea is the microscopic examination of stool. Although the sensitivity and positive predictive value vary widely according to pathogen, bacteria, parasites, and mycobacteria can all be detected by stool studies. Both upper and lower endoscopy have great value in the work-up of HIV-associated diarrhea because they allow the physician to obtain both duodenal and colonic tissue specimens. For most purposes, flexible sigmoidoscopy with biopsy is as useful as full colonoscopy, and at lower risk to the patient. Nonbiopsy specimens from the bowel, such as duodenal or jejunal aspirates, have proven to be of low yield. There is little role for noninvasive bowel imaging (i.e., barium enema) in the routine work-up of HIV-associated diarrhea.

Diagnosis and Treatment
Pathogens and Other Causes

Protozoa. The most common agents isolated from HIV-infected patients with diarrhea are species so unusual or new that they were rarely described as human pathogens before the AIDS epidemic. With the exception of microsporidia, these coccidian protozoa are now known to cause diarrheal illness associated with food-borne outbreaks in the immunocompetent, as well as the immunosuppressed, individual. Microsporidia and *Cryptosporidium parvum* are most prevalent.

Microsporidia. Microsporidia are obligate intracellular, spore-forming, protozoan parasites. There are hundreds of species, the most important among them being *Enterocytozoon bieneusi* and *Encephalitozoon intestinalis* (formerly *Septata intestinalis*). Thought to be food- and water-borne, these agents have been found in up to 25% to 50% of AIDS patients with chronic diarrhea. Affected patients are typically quite immunosuppressed, with less than 100 CD4+ cells/mm³. *E. bieneusi*, the more common of the two microsporidial agents, is associated with malabsorption, nonbloody diarrhea (three to 10 movements per day), and wasting without fever. *E. intestinalis* causes a similar enteric infection, but has also been linked rarely to sinusitis, conjunctivitis, bronchitis, peritonitis, and nephritis. Both species have been identified in up to 38% of AIDS patients with cholangitis and acalculous cholecystitis.

The diagnosis of microsporidiosis has been hampered by the organism's small size and poor staining qualities. Formerly electron microscopy of bowel biopsy specimens was the basis for diagnosis. However, recent advances in stool analysis have greatly improved detection of microsporidial spores. Modified trichrome stain and chemofluorescent stain have proven to have impressive sensitivity (88% to 100% and 73% to 98%, respectively) and specificity (88% and 100%). Polymerase chain reaction (PCR) is also under study.

Albendazole has been the most promising agent for treatment of microsporidiosis. Dramatic clinical responses and eradication of *E. intestinalis* have been achieved using albendazole. In contrast, there is no known effective therapy for *E. bieneusi* infection. Albendazole, metronidazole, atovaquone, pyrimethamine, trimethoprim-sulfamethoxazole (TMP-SMX), and octreotide have all offered symptomatic relief in selected patients, but none has successfully eliminated the parasite. Controlled clinical trials of albendazole, atovaquone, and thalidomide for treatment of *E. bieneusi* infection are all underway. Perhaps the most promising therapy for *E. bieneusi* infection is the initiation of highly active antiretroviral therapy (HAART). Several studies have demonstrated the elimination of the parasite from stool in patients successfully treated with antiretrovirals.

> **KEY POINTS**

- Single most common infectious cause of HIV-associated diarrhea
- Affects patient with marked immunosuppression (CD4+ less than 100 cells/mm³)
- Associated with gallbladder disease in up to one third of patients
- Diagnosed by trichrome or chemofluorescent staining of stool
- Optimizing HAART is best treatment; antimicrobials often fail

Cryptosporidium. In the last two decades, *C. parvum* has become recognized as a major cause of diarrhea in both immunocompetent and immunosuppressed hosts worldwide. Ten percent to 37% of AIDS patients with diarrhea in the United States and up to 50% of AIDS patients in the developing world are infected with *C. parvum*. A highly infectious intracellular protozoan, *C. parvum* is transmitted from infected

TABLE 21-1
Prevalence of Identified Pathogens in HIV-Associated Diarrhea

Pathogen	Prevalence (%)
PROTOZOA	
Microsporidia	25-40
Cryptosporidium parvum	10-37
Isospora belli	0.2-2
Cyclospora cayetanensis	?
Entamoeba histolytica	?
Giardia lamblia	?
BACTERIA	
Salmonella sp.	2-6
Campylobacter sp.	1-5
Shigella sp.	1-2
Yersinia sp., *Vibrio* sp., *Escherichia coli*	?
Clostridium difficile	10-25
Mycobacterium avium complex	25-40
VIRUSES	
Cytomegalovirus	13-19
Herpes simplex virus	?
NEOPLASM	2-3

food and water, from animal to person, and from person to person. In 1993 more than 400,000 people in Milwaukee developed cryptosporidiosis from contaminated drinking water. Typical of disease with this organism, immunocompetent patients did well. However, over 80 HIV-infected patients developed refractory diarrhea, many requiring hospitalization.

The spectrum of clinical illness with *C. parvum* varies from asymptomatic carriage to severe, life-threatening enteritis with biliary tract disease. Patients typically have voluminous, nonbloody diarrhea; abdominal pain; vomiting; and mild fever. The extent of illness correlates with the degree of immunosuppression. In patients with CD4+ counts above 150 cells/mm³, diarrhea generally resolves spontaneously within a month; advanced AIDS patients tend to have a protracted illness lasting months to years. The most common complication is biliary tract disease, seen in at least 15% of HIV-infected patients. Other complications include gastric outlet obstruction, toxic megacolon, and pneumatosis intestinalis. Interestingly, in one study 28% of AIDS patients with diarrhea were found to be coinfected with both microsporidia and *C. parvum*.

The diagnosis can be made by identification of the organism on modified acid-fast staining of stool. This test is less sensitive when applied to semiformed or solid stool. Several superior detection systems have recently been introduced. Direct immunofluorescence staining, for instance, has been reported to have a sensitivity of 93% to 100% and a specificity of 92% to 99%. A number of impressive enzyme immunoassays (EIA) are also available. PCR is under study as well. Because excretion of the oocyte is erratic and in small numbers, multiple specimens and concentrating techniques are necessary. Because of the patchy nature of intestinal cryptosporidiosis, biopsy is subject to significant sampling error and may be no more sensitive than stool studies.

Treatment of cryptosporidiosis has been disappointing. Literally over 100 drugs have been tried with no consistently reliable results. Paromomycin, a nonabsorbable, oral aminoglycoside, has been associated with symptomatic relief in small case series; however, an AIDS Clinical Trials Group (ACTG)-sponsored trial of paromomycin for AIDS patients with cryptosporidiosis found no benefit to the drug over placebo. Limited experiences with the newer macrolides, including clarithromycin, lactose-free azithromycin, and roxithromycin, have demonstrated some efficacy, but no large studies have been published yet. Numerous other approaches are under study, including the use of antimicrobials such as nitazoxanide, immunomodulators such as bovine colostrum, and antisecretory agents such as octreotide. The most effective treatment for cryptosporidiosis is reconstitution of the immune system with HAART. The symptoms of cryptosporidiosis, and indeed the presence of the organism in stool, resolve in most patients when their CD4+ count rises above 250 cells/mm³. However, in patients who fail HAART and experience a fall in their CD4+ count, diarrheal symptoms and the oocytes themselves recur, suggesting that the infection was never eliminated.

KEY POINTS

- A major cause of HIV-associated diarrhea, especially in the developing world
- Affects immunocompetent hosts, but disease is most severe in advanced AIDS patients
- Diagnosed by immunoassay or acid-fast staining of stool
- Immune reconstitution is the most effective treatment; no reliable antimicrobials have been found

Isospora belli. *Isospora belli* is another coccidian protozoan responsible for 0.2% to 2% of HIV-related diarrhea in the United States. In developing countries it causes up to 20% of diarrhea in AIDS patients. The clinical syndrome resembles mild cryptosporidiosis, with watery, nonbloody diarrhea and abdominal cramping. Biliary tract disease has also been reported. The organism is identified by modified acid-fast staining of stool, where the relatively large, oval oocytes are easily seen. The performance characteristics of stool acid-fast staining for isosporiasis are not known, but it is thought that intermittent shedding reduces the sensitivity of the test. Unlike *C. parvum* and *Microsporidium*, *I. belli* is quite susceptible to TMP-SMX. Response to therapy is excellent, but relapse rates exceed 50%, suggesting that chronic suppression is necessary in the absence of immune reconstitution.

The precise incidence of *Cyclospora cayetanensis* infection is unknown, but this coccidian protozoan occasionally causes HIV-related enteritis, with watery diarrhea, bloating, abdominal pain, extreme fatigue, and fever. The intensity of illness is related to the degree of immunosuppression, becoming severe and prolonged in patients with end-stage AIDS. *C. cayetanensis* is detected by acid-fast staining of stool. TMP-SMX is the treatment of choice; response rates are excellent, but relapse is common and long-term suppression is required. The routine use of TMP-SMX to prevent *Pneumocystis carinii* infection may explain the low incidence of both cyclosporiasis and isosporiasis in the developed world.

KEY POINTS

- Rare in the United States
- Diagnosed by stool acid-fast staining
- Responds well to TMP-SMX; relapse is common

***Entamoeba histolytica* and *Giardia lamblia*.** *Entamoeba histolytica* and *Giardia lamblia* are enteric protozoa that cause a minority of cases of diarrhea in the United States. The incidence of infection by these agents does not appear to be influenced by HIV status, but has been associated with homosexual sex. *E. histolytica* infection ranges in severity from asymptomatic carriage to severe, bloody dysentery, occasionally associated with liver abscess. Giardiasis also causes a range of symptoms, from occult infection to chronic malabsorption, with abdominal cramping, nausea, and watery stools. Both agents are detectable by examination of fresh stool for trophozoites or cysts. Concentrating techniques and serial studies enhance the yield. Newer stool studies have improved laboratories' ability to detect these protozoa. Immunofluorescent staining for *G. lamblia* is quite sensitive (96%) and specific (99%). *E. histolytica* monoclonal antibody detection and several EIA assays are also available. In some institutions, these superior tests have supplanted conventional ova and parasite light microscopy.

E. histolytica and *G. lamblia* are both successfully treated with metronidazole; amebiasis requires follow-up therapy with a nonabsorbable agent for eradication of intraluminal parasites. Iodoquinol and paromomycin are both effective.

KEY POINTS

- Rare causes of HIV-associated diarrhea in the United States
- Illness ranges from asymptomatic carriage to severe diarrhea
- Diagnosed by immunofluorescent staining, EIA, or traditional ova and parasite examination of stool
- Treatment with metronidazole is highly effective

Bacteria. Bacterial pathogens are found in 10% to 20% of HIV-infected patients with diarrhea. Although often the diarrheal symptoms are quite acute, they are not a reliable indicator of bacterial infection. The diagnosis is usually made by routine stool culture; however, bacteremia does occur in the absence of positive stool cultures (i.e., up to 30% of *Salmonella* cases). Treatment of bacterial diarrhea in immunocompetent hosts has been associated with a prolonged carrier state. Nevertheless, most authorities agree that HIV-associated bacterial diarrhea should be treated with antibiotics. Even with this intervention, 25% to 75% of cases will relapse and require retreatment.

Salmonella. Nontyphoidal *Salmonella* species are the most common bacteria to cause diarrhea in HIV-infected patients. The organism is usually acquired from infected foods or from person to person. The incidence of salmonellosis in AIDS patients is 100 times higher than in the immunocompetent population, and rates of bacteremia are extremely high, up to 80%. Bacteremia may be prolonged, despite antimicrobials. Treatment is based on susceptibility testing, generally using either ampicillin, TMP-SMX, or a quinolone. At least 2 weeks of treatment is usually advised and some authorities have recommended long-term suppression.

KEY POINTS

- One hundred times more common in HIV-infected individuals than in non–HIV-infected individuals
- Bacteremia occurs in 80% of cases of HIV-associated diarrhea, may be prolonged

Campylobacter. *Campylobacter* infection is also markedly (40 times) more common in HIV-infected patients than in the general population. The spectrum of clinical disease varies from asymptomatic shedding to severe dysentery. Ten percent of patients are bacteremic. Special selective media are required to isolate this slow-growing gram-negative rod. Treatment is generally with a quinolone or macrolide. Resistance to quinolones has been reported in numerous developing countries and in the United States. Guillain-Barré syndrome has been noted rarely following some cases of *Campylobacter* enteritis.

KEY POINTS

- Forty times more common in HIV-infected individuals than in non–HIV-infected individuals
- Requires selective media to grow
- May be resistant to quinolones

Shigella. *Shigella* infection in AIDS patients is similar in prevalence to that of the general population, but, like salmonellosis, is associated with a high rate of bacteremia (up to 50%). It is transmitted fecal-orally, and is easily spread in situations of crowding and poverty due to its low infective dose. Again, ampicillin, TMP-SMX, and a quinolone are the preferred treatment choices, depending on susceptibility data. The issue of long-term suppression is unresolved, but it appears that the rate of relapse is much lower than that of salmonellosis.

Less common bacterial pathogens. Several less common bacterial bowel pathogens are notable. *Yersinia* occasionally causes inflammatory HIV-related diarrhea associated with lymphadenitis, ulcerative mucosal lesions, and bacteremia. *Vibrio* species have an increased prevalence and severity in HIV-infected patients. Enteroadherent *Escherichia coli* may be a newly discovered cause of both acute and persistent diarrhea in AIDS patients.

Clostridium difficile. The rate of *Clostridium difficile* infection in HIV-infected patients parallels that of the general population: 10% to 25% of patients with diarrhea. Up to 75% of patients have a history of recent antibiotic therapy. The use of TMP-SMX for *P. carinii* prophylaxis does not appear to increase the risk of *C. difficile* colitis by much. The severity of disease ranges widely, from the asymptomatic carrier state to pseudomembranous colitis without abdominal symptoms to toxic megacolon with perforation and sepsis. There have been conflicting reports regarding the possible increased virulence of *C. difficile* in AIDS patients. There may be a delayed response to therapy as well. Most laboratories detect *C. difficile* using an EIA for toxin A or toxin B. The sensitivity of EIA approaches 100% with the examination of three stool specimens. Most *C. difficile* infections clear with oral metronidazole. The more expensive oral vancomycin is used for cases refractory to oral metronidazole. Relapse is common, but usually responds to retreatment.

KEY POINTS

- No more common, but perhaps more virulent and/or persistent in the setting of HIV infection
- About 25% of patients have no recent history of antibiotic use
- Treated with metronidazole or oral vancomycin; relapse is common

Mycobacterium. Disseminated MAC occurs in 25% to 40% of AIDS patients, usually when CD4+ counts have fallen below 50 cells/mm^3. About 50% of patients with disseminated MAC have diarrhea. MAC is the only identifiable cause of diarrhea in 5% to 25% of AIDS patients. The clinical scenario of disseminated MAC includes fever, weight loss, abdominal pain, lymphadenopathy, and hepatosplenomegaly. It is usually diagnosed by isolation of the organism from blood cultures, specially incubated to grow mycobacteria. Ubiquitous in the environment, food, and water, MAC may colonize the gastrointestinal tract. In the absence of positive blood cultures, isolation of MAC from stool does not confirm its role in causing diarrhea; bowel biopsy is required. Characteristic findings include atrophic villi, dilated lacteals, and infiltration of the lamina propria with PAS-positive macrophages. Treatment of MAC disease requires therapy with at least two agents. Typical choices include azithromycin or clarithromycin in combination with ethambutol, rifabutin, ciprofloxacin, or amikacin. Lifelong suppressive therapy has generally been recommended, although this recommendation is changing in the era of HAART.

> **KEY POINTS**
>
> - About 12% to 20% of advanced AIDS patients will develop MAC-associated diarrhea
> - Affects only severely immunosuppressed patients (CD4+ count usually below 50 cells/mm^3)
> - Diagnosed by culturing blood for mycobacteria; isolation from stool may reflect only colonization
> - Treatment requires at least two drugs, usually a macrolide plus ethambutol

Viruses. The precise incidence of virally induced HIV-associated diarrhea is not known, primarily because viral colitis is difficult to diagnose. Viruses may be more common causes of diarrhea than previously suspected. CMV is most prominent, but other agents, such as adenovirus, calicivirus, rotavirus, astrovirus, and picornavirus, have been implicated. Using careful detection methods, one study found enteric viruses in 35% of HIV-infected patients with diarrhea. Another study found adenovirus in 10% of AIDS patients with chronic diarrhea. However, other enteric agents were often found as well, clouding the role of viruses as pathogens. For most of these rarer agents, disease is probably self-limited, and no effective treatment is available.

Cytomegalovirus. The most serious and common virus to cause diarrhea in HIV infection is CMV. Disseminated infection from this ubiquitous herpesvirus has been found in up to 90% of AIDS patients at autopsy. Up to one third of AIDS patients will have gastrointestinal disease due to this agent, involving anywhere from mouth to anus (including the biliary tree). CMV has been identified in the gastrointestinal tract of 13% to 19% of AIDS patients with diarrhea, typically associated with fever, crampy lower abdominal pain, weight loss, and tenesmus. However, symptoms vary widely, from no gastrointestinal complaints to profuse diarrhea to toxic megacolon, gangrenous bowel, and massive gastrointestinal bleeding. In AIDS patients, CMV has also been associated with esophagitis, cholangitis, acalculous cholecystitis, gastritis, and pancreatitis. Endoscopic examination of the colon may reveal normal mucosa; diffuse erythema and friability; pseudomembranes; patchy, discrete ulcers; or diffuse, confluent colitis. Sigmoidoscopy will miss the 10% to 30% of cases that only involve the right side of the colon. Histologic diagnosis is based on the presence of CMV inclusions in the setting of inflammation.

Treatment is usually initiated with high-dose IV ganciclovir, followed by repeat endoscopy at 2 to 3 weeks to assess effectiveness. Ganciclovir is associated with neutropenia in 25% to 40% of patients and thrombocytopenia in 10% to 20% of subjects. Foscarnet is an alternative for patients with refractory disease or intolerable side effects. This agent is also highly toxic, causing renal insufficiency in up to 20% of patients. Cidofovir is also useful in the treatment of CMV infection, but its use is also limited by nephrotoxicity. Response to treatment for CMV colitis is not as good as that for CMV retinitis. The need for suppressive therapy has been uncertain. In the setting of immune reconstitution with HAART, it is certainly reasonable not to continue maintenance therapy, which is expensive, toxic, and difficult to administer intravenously, until a relapse occurs.

> **KEY POINTS**
>
> - Estimated prevalence of CMV infection in AIDS patients with chronic diarrhea is 13% to 19%
> - Causes a wide range of symptoms, from mild diarrhea to perforation
> - Definitive diagnosis requires intestinal biopsy; flexible sigmoidoscopy misses 10% to 30% of right-sided disease
> - Treated with ganciclovir, cidofovir, or foscarnet—may not require suppression if immune system reconstituted with HAART

Herpes Simplex. HSV commonly infects the anorectal area of homosexual men. Mild proctitis or distal colitis due to HSV can cause diarrhea or constipation, associated with pain, tenesmus, hematochezia, and perianal ulcers. The pain may be so severe that it leads to avoidance of defecation. Urinary dysfunction and sacral paresthesias occur as well. The endoscopic appearance can be similar to that of CMV colitis; characteristic Cowdry A inclusion bodies, viral culture, and immunohistochemical staining distinguish these two entities. HSV colitis responds well initially to acyclovir. Patients with advanced HIV disease may develop indolent, persistent HSV infection requiring long-term acyclovir suppression. Over time, resistance to acyclovir may evolve; foscarnet can be used in this setting, but resistance to both agents has been observed.

The role of HIV itself in enteropathy has yet to be clarified. It clearly infects enterocytes, but studies of its effect on mucosal cell functions are conflicting.

Noninfectious and Unexplained Causes. Protozoa, bacteria, viruses, and mycobacteria make up about 95% of identifiable causes of chronic diarrhea in HIV-infected patients in large case series reported to date. Neoplasms are detected in 2% to 3% of patients with chronic diarrhea, primarily small bowel lymphoma and Kaposi's sarcoma. Other rarely identified infectious agents include *Histoplasma* (and various other disseminated fungi), *Pneumocystis, Toxoplasma,* and *Leishmania.*

A critically important cause of diarrhea in HIV-infected patients is medications. Studies have found up to a 40% incidence of mild to moderate drug-induced diarrhea in patients on HAART. Drugs with a reported incidence of diarrhea exceeding 10% include didanosine (ddI), lamivudine (3TC), zidovudine (AZT), nelfinavir, ritonavir, and delavirdine. Predictably, the rate of enteric opportunistic infections has fallen precipitously with the widespread use of HAART. Recent studies have also noted the sustained resolution of enteric opportunistic infections in patients treated with effective antiretrovirals. With the widespread use of HAART, one can anticipate the ongoing rise in importance of medications rather than infectious agents as causes of chronic diarrhea in HIV.

Despite an extensive evaluation, 10% to 20% of diarrheal illness in HIV-infected patients will remain unexplained. This number has steadily declined from 30% to 35% over the last 10 years. Proposed mechanisms include unidentified pathogens, autonomic dysfunction, motility

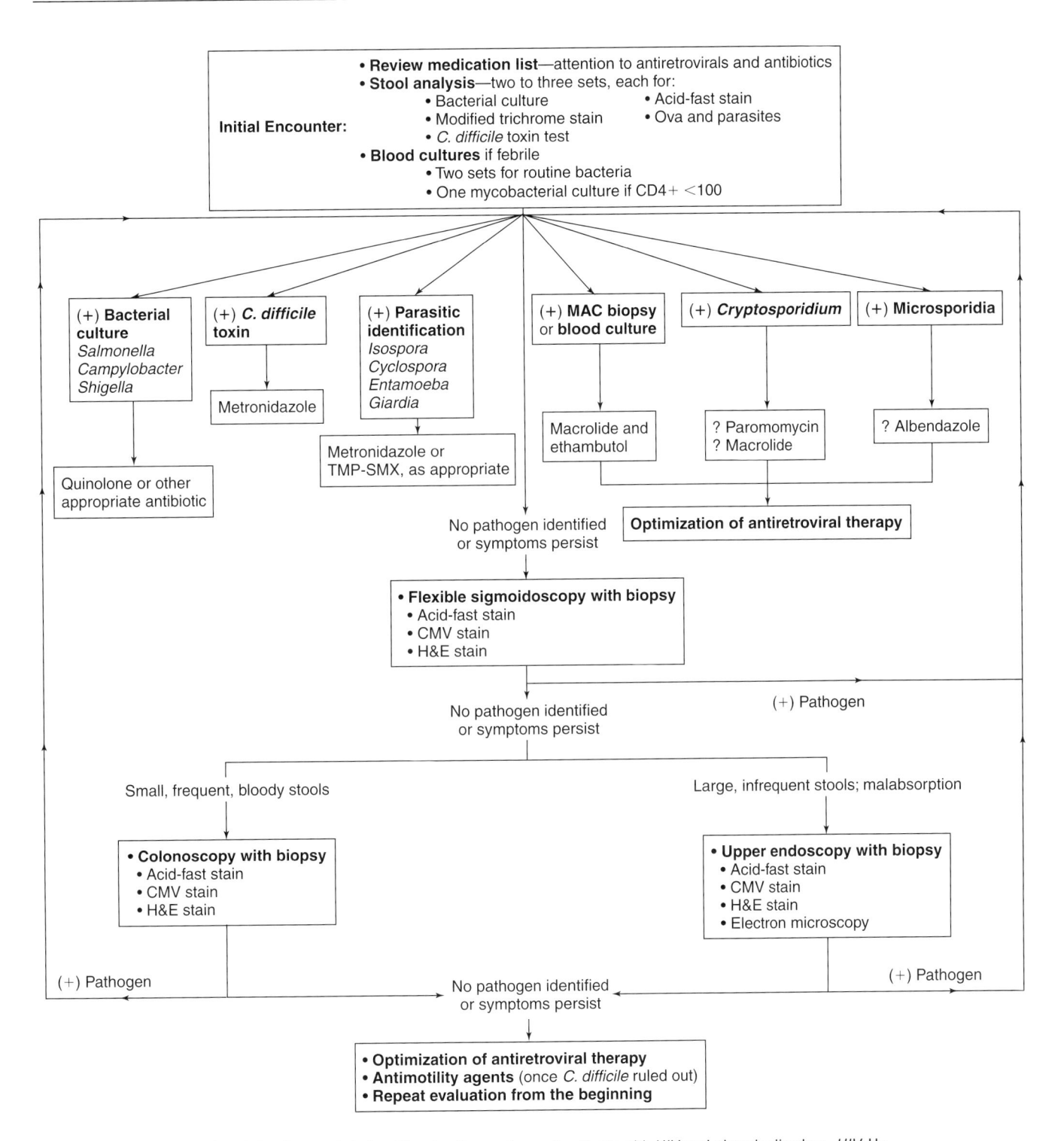

FIG. 21-1 Suggested algorithm for the work-up of patients with HIV and chronic diarrhea. *HIV*, Human immunodeficiency virus; *MAC*, *Mycobacterium avium* complex; *TMP-SMX*, trimethoprim-sulfamethoxazole; *CMV*, cytomegalovirus; *H&E*, hematoxylin and eosin.

disorders, dietary and alternative medicine habits, and bacterial overgrowth. The prognosis for patients with pathogen-negative diarrhea in HIV is good; in one study it was similar to HIV-infected patients without diarrhea, and much better than that of matched patients with an identified enteric pathogen.

Evaluation

The diagnostic work-up of HIV-associated chronic diarrhea is systematic (Fig. 21-1). Medication-induced diarrhea should be considered immediately. If the patient is febrile, blood should be cultured for bacteria, and if the CD4+ count is low, mycobacteria. Stool studies are the next step, including bacterial culture (e.g., for *Salmonella*), modified trichrome or fluorochrome stain (for microsporidia), modified acid-fast examination (for *Cryptosporidium, Isospora,* and *Cyclospora), C. difficile* assay, and ova and parasite examination (for *Giardia* and *Entamoeba.*) If available, immunofluorescent staining or EIA for *Cryptosporidium, Entamoeba,* and *Giardia* should be performed. Culture for viruses is not routinely performed. The growth of CMV from stool, in the absence of histologic evidence of invasion, is not adequate to prove CMV disease. It is not clear that other viruses (e.g., adenovirus, calicivirus) play a significant role in HIV-associated diarrhea, nor are there effective therapies to treat them if found.

To compensate for limited test sensitivity and erratic excretion of pathogens, multiple stool specimens should be evaluated. One recent large survey found that testing of two stool samples resulted in detection of 99% of bacterial agents. Two to three specimens for parasitology are recommended by most experts. Two to three samples may also be required to rule out *C. difficile,* although some institutions report up to 94% sensitivity with a single assay for *C. difficile* toxin. If time permits, samples should be submitted several days apart to allow for reporting of positive results before more studies are performed. Stool studies alone will identify the majority of pathogens in patients with CD4+ counts above 200 cells/mm^3.

When to Refer

If stool tests and blood cultures are unrevealing, endoscopy with biopsy should be performed. In most cases the test of choice is flexible sigmoidoscopy. If no focal lesions are present, multiple random biopsies should be obtained and stained for viral inclusions, acid-fast bacilli, and protozoa. A specimen may be reserved for later electron microscopy if initial studies are negative and microsporidiosis is suspected. If no enteric pathogen is identified by flexible sigmoidoscopy, the American Gastroenterological Association suggests proceeding to esophagogastroduodenoscopy (EGD) with duodenal biopsy, using the same diagnostic tests that were applied to colonic biopsies. This approach is certainly reasonable in patients with small bowel symptoms (malabsorption; infrequent, large-volume stools), once a good stool evaluation for microsporidia and *Giardia* is negative. Alternatively, full colonoscopy should be considered in patients with lower tract symptoms (frequent, small-volume, bloody, mucusy stools) and, in particular, in patients with a CD4+ count below 100 cells/mm^3. Several studies have found a significant incidence of lymphoma and CMV lesions beyond the reach of the flexible sigmoidoscope. Of note, recent prospective studies have not found the use of either upper endoscopy or colonoscopy to add much to flexible sigmoidoscopy, particularly if adequate stool studies have been performed. This may be due to enhanced awareness and detection of microsporidiosis, as well as the overall decreased incidence of CMV colitis that has come with the era of HAART.

Often, even after a pathogen has been identified and treated, many patients continue to have diarrhea. It is important to remember that AIDS patients very commonly have more than one enteric infection at a time. Repeat evaluation will often reveal additional occult, treatable agents. If thoughtful testing has failed to suggest an antiinfective, symptomatic relief with antidiarrheals is often successful. Luminal agents, such as fiber supplements, cholestyramine, and kaolin-pectin, reduce water and increase stool bulk. Antimotility agents, such as loperamide, diphenoxylate, and opiates, are often required. The use of these agents appears to be safe, once *C. difficile* colitis has been ruled out. A recent prospective evaluation of antimotility agents in the setting of HIV-associated diarrhea did not show increased risk of perforation or toxic megacolon. Octreotide, a synthetic somatostatin, showed tremendous initial promise; however, recent reports suggest that this agent is no more effective than placebo for chronic HIV-associated diarrhea. Although antimotility agents often fail to completely control diarrhea, it is important to remember that HIV-infected patients who have undergone a full but unrevealing diagnostic work-up have no increased mortality over matched controls without diarrhea.

SUGGESTED READINGS

American Gastroenterological Association medical position statement: guidelines for the management of malnutrition and cachexia, chronic diarrhea, and hepatobiliary disease in patients with human immunodeficiency virus infection. [Guideline. Journal Article. Practice Guideline] *Gastroenterology* 111(6):1722-1723, 1996.

Framm SR, Soave R: Agents of diarrhea: *Med Clin North Am* 81:427-447, 1997.

Hines J, Nachamkin I: Effective use of the clinical microbiology laboratory for diagnosing diarrheal diseases, *Clin Infect Dis* 23:1293-1301, 1996.

Kearney DJ et al: A prospective study of endoscopy in HIV-associated diarrhea, *Am J Gastroenterol* 94:596-602, 1999.

Lew EA, Poles MA, Dieterich DT: Diarrheal diseases associated with HIV infection, *Gastroenterol Clin North Am* 26:259-290, 1997.

Wilcox CM et al: Chronic unexplained diarrhea in HIV infection: determination of the best diagnostic approach, *Gastroenterology* 110:30-37, 1996.

Wilcox CM, Rabeneck L, Friedman S: AGA technical review: malnutrition and cachexia, chronic diarrhea, and hepatobiliary disease in patients with human immunodeficiency virus infection, *Gastroenterology* 111(6):1724-1752, 1996.

22 Wasting

JENNIFER L. ALDRICH, JOSEPH HASSEY

Introduction

Weight loss is a common problem in human immunodeficiency virus (HIV)-infected persons. The clinician needs to know how to evaluate and treat this problem. AIDS wasting syndrome (AWS) refers to weight loss that is not attributable to opportunistic infections (OIs), malignancies, or problems with swallowing. In 1987 the Centers for Disease Control and Prevention (CDC) revised the surveillance case definition of the acquired immunodeficiency syndrome (AIDS) to include AWS. Specifically AWS was defined as the involuntary weight loss of more than 10% baseline body weight plus either chronic diarrhea (at least two loose stools per day for more than 30 days) or chronic weakness and documented fever (for more than 30 days) in the absence of an explanatory concurrent illness or condition. The rather unwieldy definition has been somewhat simplified in general practice by the recognition that even a 5% weight loss is an independent risk factor for increased mortality, is a marker of HIV disease progression, and is associated with impaired physical functioning. In addition, people can and do lose weight without having diarrhea, and can likewise have diarrhea without losing weight. The same is also true of both fever and weakness.

AIDS Wasting Syndrome

In the post–*Pneumocystis carinii* pneumonia (PCP) prophylaxis era, AWS remains a commonly reported AIDS-defining illness. According to the CDC, over 27% of persons dying of AIDS had AWS at some time in the course of their HIV disease. It is the first AIDS-defining event for 8% of patients in the United States. Although precise figures are not available for the developing world, AWS or "slim disease" may complicate up to 50% of HIV/AIDS cases in Africa. Early studies demonstrated disproportionate loss of lean body mass (LBM) with relative sparing of body fat, even in asymptomatic patients. However, more recent data have suggested that patients tend to lose muscle and fat in proportion to their baseline body composition, similar to what is seen in simple starvation. Unlike starvation, AWS is not easily reversed by increased caloric intake. Kotler et al first reported on the direct impact of HIV-associated weight loss on mortality in 1989. Both total body weight and, more profoundly, LBM were linearly correlated with time to death. Their data strongly implicated the patients' nutritional status as a primary factor in HIV-related mortality, and indeed LBM has been found to be a better predictor of survival than CD4+ count or HIV viral load. In addition to mortality, AWS contributes significantly to morbidity.

Documentation

Weight loss can be documented with a scale. Certainly a patient's weight should be recorded at each visit. Some practitioners have noted that nutritional deficiency can occur without actual weight loss, or it may be underestimated by attention to total body weight alone. They have suggested that routine measurement of body composition be included in the management of all persons with HIV infection. A number of methods have been developed to analyze body composition. The most commonly employed is bioelectrical impedance analysis (BIA), which capitalizes on the differential resistances to a low-intensity electric current of fat, lean, and cellular tissues. BIA provides a reproducible three-compartment estimate of these tissues. The BIA technique has been validated against the more impractical methods of measuring total body potassium or of water immersion. The equipment for BIA is portable and thus well suited for outpatient clinical use, but it does require knowledgeable interpretation. Also it is not helpful for evaluating changes in body fat distribution. Other techniques include anthropometry using waist to hip ratios and the measurement of skinfold. Both are well suited for outpatient practice but suffer from limited reproducibility, and age, sex, and genetic factors affect them. Dual energy x-ray absorptiometry (DEXA) offers more sensitive and accurate estimates of body composition, but is generally available only at research sites.

Etiology and Pathogenesis

AWS is probably multifactorial. Factors that appear to be significant include decreased caloric intake, malabsorption, alterations in metabolism, an anabolic block, hypogonadism, and cytokine abnormalities (Box 22-1).

Of all of the potential factors responsible for AWS, none is likely to be as important as a decreased calorie intake. Box 22-1 lists many possible reasons for this.

In addition to a decrease in energy intake, alterations in metabolism may contribute to AWS. Resting energy expenditure (REE) is the energy needed to carry out normal metabolic functions. Total energy expenditure includes REE plus energy expended in all activities. Numerous studies have shown the REE to be increased in HIV-infected patients and that this increases further with acute illness. If a patient is unable to consume enough calories to overcome this increased REE, weight loss will occur. There appear to be other metabolism

BOX 22-1
Possible Etiologies of AIDS Wasting Syndrome

- Decreased calorie intake
    Dysphagia or odynophagia
    "Pill fatigue"
    Anorexia
    Psychosocial/economic factors
    Substance abuse
    Fatigue
    Altered mental status
    Nausea
- Malabsorption
- Alterations in metabolism
- Endocrine abnormalities
    Hypogonadism
    Growth hormone resistance
- Cytokine abnormalities

alterations in HIV-infected patients. Much has been written about lipodystrophy and alterations in lipid and protein metabolism as a result of medications used to treat HIV infection. It should be noted, however, that these changes were seen long before the introduction of highly active antiretroviral therapy (HAART). Triglyceride levels are higher in asymptomatic HIV-infected patents and even higher in patients with AWS. This is due to both decreased clearance of triglycerides and an increased de novo synthesis of triglycerides. Similarly, protein metabolism may be altered with HIV infection and wasting. Several studies have shown altered protein turnover in patients with AWS. In addition, others have postulated that there may be a misuse of amino acids, preventing the normal production of proteins. This phenomenon is referred to as anabolic block. This may also contribute to the cachexia associated with AWS.

Much interest has been directed at the endocrine abnormalities associated with HIV-related wasting. The two areas that have been given the most attention are hypogonadism (testosterone deficiency) and growth hormone (GH) resistance. In addition to androgenic effects, testosterone has anabolic activity. Many studies have now demonstrated that HIV-infected men and women have decreased levels of total and free testosterone. The etiology of the decreased testosterone levels is most often secondary to hypothalamic-pituitary dysfunction rather than primary gonadal failure. It is not unusual for serum testosterone levels to be low in patients with chronic illnesses. This, in fact, may be more of an adaptive response rather than a pathologic change. Several studies done recently have demonstrated that the fall in testosterone precedes AWS, suggesting that the abnormal levels may be a cause of wasting and not just a consequence. The effects of testosterone are numerous including changes in sexual function, depression, low energy, decreased appetite, osteoporosis, decreased muscle mass, and decreased strength. Many of these changes can be subtle. Unlike testosterone deficiency, HIV-infected patients are not deficient in GH. Rather, there appears to be a resistance to the effects of this hormone. Specifically, GH has a positive effect on nitrogen balance and protein synthesis. Whether or not this resistance to GH plays a role in AWS is still a matter of debate.

Another area for consideration regarding the pathogenesis of AWS involves the abnormal triggering of cytokines. Various animal studies have shown that cytokines such as tumor necrosis factor (TNF), interferons (IFN), and interleukins (IL) are associated with anorexia and weight loss. Elevated levels of IFN-α and TNF have been identified in HIV-infected patients, particularly in those with advanced disease. Elevations in IL-1 are seen in response to opportunistic infections and are associated with cachexia. Although no single cytokine has been definitively associated with HIV wasting, it is likely that multiple cytokine abnormalities do contribute to the condition.

Treatment

The initial management of wasting in a person infected with HIV should concentrate on controlling HIV infection itself with an effective antiretroviral regimen. Identification and treatment of opportunistic infections and malignancy are essential as well. Diarrheal diseases and malabsorption syndromes should be controlled. On occasion weight loss reflects socioeconomic problems. Adequate access to food is essential. No therapy will succeed without food.

The pathophysiology of HIV-related wasting is multifactorial. As such, the treatment of this condition needs to be multifaceted, and ranges from implementing sound nutritional and exercise principles to utilizing the newer available pharmacologic agents. An important distinction needs to be made between weight gain (or loss) and changes in LBM. Fat tissue does not serve as important a metabolic function as LBM. Thus one of the goals of treatment of AWS is to maintain LBM, not just total body weight. Although many of the available treatments help people maintain or gain weight, not all are capable of improving LBM.

Nutrition. One of the major causes of HIV-related wasting is inadequate energy intake. Therefore, a cornerstone of treatment is ensuring sufficient caloric intake. Nutritional assessment by an individual qualified to define energy goals is important and has been retrospectively demonstrated to improve nutritional status and to lead to weight gain in HIV-infected patients. Education regarding proper diet, food safety, appropriate vitamin and mineral supplementation, and drug-nutrient interactions is essential. A registered dietitian can also assist in symptom management of diarrhea, mouth sores, nausea, and vomiting. At the very least, the patient's weight should be recorded at each visit so that trends are identified early. If available, measurement of body composition is useful at baseline and at regular 3- to 6-month follow-up intervals.

The route of delivery of the calories will depend on the individual. The oral route is preferred. Oral nutritional supplements, generally in the form of liquid shakes, are the most commonly prescribed. However, their benefit is quite limited. The weight gain seen is primarily fat, and it may only be a short-term gain. After a month or so, the body autoregulates to decrease food intake back to its set point, so that people who utilize supplements wind up eating less. Furthermore, many of these products are expensive. The utility of supplements is probably limited to situations in which oropharyngeal discomfort compromises food intake or to people who do not have access to sufficient food or who are unwilling or unable to prepare meals for themselves. If the gastrointestinal tract is functional but the patient is unable to consume food orally, consideration should be given to using a nasogastric feeding tube, gastrostomy, or jejunostomy. People with profound nausea, anorexia, chronic oroesophageal ulcers, or neurologic disorders have benefited from these modalities. Finally, in cases in which the gastrointestinal tract cannot be used, such as malabsorption or persistent diarrhea, total parenteral nutrition (TPN) may be of benefit. However, TPN has not been beneficial in patients with AWS who did not have malabsorption or gastrointestinal disease. In patients who have been losing weight because of an OI or a malignancy, no increase in weight or LBM occurs despite TPN.

KEY POINTS

NUTRITION OPTIONS
- Nutritional assessment
- Nutritional supplements
    - Primarily fat gain
    - Short-term benefit
    - Expensive
    - Best for persons with limited access to food
- Feeding tubes
- Total parenteral nutrition

Exercise. Inactivity is associated with significant loss of LBM and a decrease in functional capacity. For various reasons, many people with AWS are inactive. In HIV-infected patients who do not have AWS, participation in a supervised progressive resistance (strength) training program resulted in increases in both strength and LBM, with a decrease in fat tissue. These benefits were maintained for several months after stopping exercise. In people who experienced AWS, the same benefits were seen. The advantages of this nonpharmacologic approach include low cost and low risk. In addition, there is often a psychological benefit associated with exercise. Often exercise training requires significant motivation on the patient's part and coaching by the health care provider. A gradual, graded exercise program can be outlined for a patient, and with encouragement some patients will be able to maintain it.

Appetite Stimulants. Currently there are two appetite stimulants approved for the treatment of AWS, megestrol acetate and dronabinol.

Megestrol Acetate. Megestrol acetate is a progestational agent used extensively in oncologic patients for weight loss. Several double-blind randomized placebo-controlled trials in patients with AWS have demonstrated an improvement in appetite, increased caloric intake, weight gain, and overall improvement in sense of well-being. Of note, the majority of the weight gain is fat, not LBM. The dose is 800 mg daily. Although this dose is generally very well tolerated, several complications can occur. As a steroid with glucocorticoid activity, megestrol at this dose can precipitate hyperglycemia, frank diabetes, and Cushing's syndrome. A steroid withdrawal syndrome can also occur when the drug is stopped after prolonged use. In addition, it can decrease gonadotropin secretion, leading to impotence and low testosterone levels. Patients on this drug should have regular monitoring of blood glucose and testosterone values. Because only LBM and not fat has been correlated with survival, megestrol acetate is not an ideal drug for the treatment of AWS. It is, however, an important adjunct when anorexia and caloric intake are clinical issues.

Dronabinol. Dronabinol is an oral cannabinoid, which is an active ingredient of marijuana. It has well-known appetite-enhancing effects. It has been studied in patients with AWS and is associated with an increase in appetite, improvement in mood, and decrease in nausea. However, weight gain is only minimal. The dose is 2.5 mg bid. At this dose the side effects most commonly seen are euphoria, somnolence, and thought-processing abnormalities. Overall, dronabinol can be useful in treating nausea, but the weight gain benefits are rarely significant.

Anabolic Block

Testosterone. Testosterone and other anabolic agents have been prescribed because patients with AWS may experience anabolic block, an inability to gain LBM despite adequate caloric intake. Low or borderline testosterone levels are quite common in both men and women and correlate with fatigue and weight loss. In HIV-infected patients who were both hypogonadal and wasting, testosterone replacement was shown to increase LBM and improve quality of life. The form of testosterone used was testosterone enanthate, 300 mg intramuscularly every 3 weeks, although it is more commonly given as 200 mg every 2 weeks. Other forms of testosterone exist including a transdermal patch, transdermal gel, and oral preparations. The available oral testosterone is hepatotoxic and should not be used. The various available transdermal preparations do not appear to be as effective as intramuscular testosterone in men with AWS. The standard dose is 5 mg per day. In androgen-deficient HIV-infected women, a low-dose patch (150 to 300 μg/day) was effective in producing a slight weight gain. Testosterone in these low doses is well tolerated and does not cause virilization, hirsutism, or changes in lipids or liver functions. The higher doses given by the IM route to men are also well tolerated. Polycythemia, liver toxicity, accelerated growth of prostate tumors, an increased risk of sleep apnea, and unfavorable lipid abnormalities are all potential side effects. Patients need to be monitored for the development of these conditions.

Oxandrolone, Nandrolone, and Oxymetholone. The anabolic agents, oxandrolone, nandrolone, and oxymetholone, have higher anabolic:androgenic ratios than testosterone. Nandrolone decanoate is available only as an intramuscular injection. It is relatively inexpensive and has less androgenic activity than testosterone, thus making it a better choice in eugonadal men as well as in women. It is given at 100 mg per week. Oxandrolone is an oral agent. Its dose is 10 mg twice a day. In both placebo-controlled and open-labeled trials, its use has resulted in significant increases in both weight and LBM. This was particularly true when paired with resistance exercise. Another oral testosterone derivative, oxymetholone, is available, although its Food and Drug Administration (FDA) approval is based on the treatment of anemia. It has been studied in AWS and appears to have beneficial effects on weight and LBM, as well as on quality of life. The dose studied was 50 mg three times a day, although no dose has been officially recommended. Both oral agents have the potential to cause liver toxicity, and they should be used with particular caution in patients on other hepatotoxins or who have chronic hepatitis. Overall, the long-term safety of all of these agents is unknown. In addition, there are currently very little data available on the use of these agents in women with AWS.

Growth Hormone. GH has anticatabolic/anabolic effects. Several studies have been done looking at the effects of recombinant GH in people with AWS. At an average dose of 6 mg per day given subcutaneously, increases in weight and LBM were seen. The results were more modest than the gains seen with the anabolic steroids. However, there was also a significant increase in exercise capacity and a loss of fat tissue. The most commonly reported side effects of GH include arthralgias, edema, hyperglycemia, and carpal tunnel syndrome. Because of the loss of fat tissue, some have advocated using GH to reverse the effects of lipodystrophy. Finally, the extraordinary cost and inconvenience of daily subcutaneous injections limit the utility of this agent.

Cytokine Modulators. Cytokine modulators have been studied in AWS. The only agent that has shown some benefit has been thalidomide. Thalidomide gained notoriety in the 1960s due to its teratogenicity. Recently, however, the drug has been reevaluated for its anticytokine benefits in treating erythema nodosum leprosum, as well as severe aphthous ulcers, and thalidomide is believed to work by inhibiting TNF. Weight gain and significant increases in LBM have been seen in studies of patients with AWS. Adverse effects include somnolence and a skin rash, which can be severe. Thalidomide is a known teratogen and should not be used in women who are or who could become pregnant. Its use in AWS currently remains experimental. Table 22-1 is a summary of pharmacologic therapies.

Approach to the Patient with AIDS Wasting Syndrome

Physical Examination to Exclude Opportunistic Infections. When an HIV-infected patient presents to a physician's office for evaluation of weight loss, it is incumbent on the physician to exclude an OI or malignancy. An OI will most often present with signs and symptoms particular to the organ involved. With some OIs the cause of the weight loss is obvious. For example, patients with thrush frequently also have esophageal candidiasis, leading to dysphagia and odynophagia and a resultant decreased caloric intake. This is also true of esophageal ulcers due to herpes simplex virus. With other OIs the cause of the weight loss can be the anorexia that often accompanies chronic infections.

Historical Features. Once an OI or malignancy has been excluded, historical features may provide a clue to the etiology of the weight loss. One of the common complaints in HIV-infected patients presenting with weight loss is diarrhea. A specific etiology for diarrhea should be sought. Infections and HAART side effects are the most common causes. Consideration should be given to the adequacy of the control of the HIV infection. Poorly controlled HIV infection, itself, can be responsible for weight loss. The history should also be used to look for evidence of depression. Depression is very common in any chronic illness and can manifest as anorexia and weight loss. In many circumstances a detailed nutritional history should be obtained and analyzed with a nutritionist for total caloric intake, nutrient content (carbohydrates, proteins, lipids), and micronutrient content (vitamins/minerals). A patient's perception of these things can be quite different from reality.

Laboratory Evaluation. The initial laboratory evaluation should include studies to exclude relevant OIs and malignancies. A thyroid-stimulating hormone (TSH) level is useful in ruling out hyperthyroidism. Testosterone, both total and free, should be measured in both men and women. Total testosterone is composed of free and protein bound hormone. In patients with weight loss and protein depletion, total testosterone may not accurately reflect the level of functionally available testosterone. Free testosterone may be a better indicator of the true testosterone pool in those circumstances. Consideration should also be given to measurement of LBM. This is superior to weight in its usefulness for both diagnosing wasting and following response to therapy. There are a number of methods, as mentioned earlier.

Pharmacologic Treatment. Once the history, physical examination, and laboratory data are obtained and an identifiable cause for AWS has been excluded, consideration needs to be given to treating the AWS with pharmacologic agents. In general, weight loss despite a good caloric intake should lead to considerations of malabsorption or increased catabolism. This type of loss will not benefit from medications to increase appetite. On the other hand, weight loss associated with a decrease in appetite suggests chronic infection, malignancy, or depression and may benefit from appetite stimulants.

KEY POINTS

EVALUATION AND MANAGEMENT OF AWS
- Maximize antiretroviral therapy
- Evaluate for opportunistic infection or malignancy
- Get a good dietary history
- Consider depression
- Consider malabsorption
- Measure serum testosterone and thyroid-stimulating hormone
- Measure lean body mass
- Consider pharmacologic treatment
    Appetite stimulants
    Anabolic agents
    Antinausea agents
- Encourage progressive resistance exercise

Illustrative Cases

Case 1 Analysis. John is a 40-year-old man who lost 20 lbs during a recent infection with PCP. His appetite is poor. He has been using a nutritional supplement five times a day instead of eating. He also has diarrhea.

Patients often lose weight with an OI. In addition, it is not unusual for appetite to be poor when patients are ill. Patients will often try to compensate for decreased food intake by taking nutritional supplements. Although these supplements can be very useful in helping to achieve adequate caloric intake, they should not be used as a substitute for food in a patient who can eat. Studies have shown that in such situations, people may compensate by decreasing food intake. If used in excess, these supplements can cause diarrhea. This patient would likely benefit from an appetite stimulant.

Case 2 Analysis. Mark is a 30-year-old man recently diagnosed with HIV infection. His CD4+ count is 75 cells/mm³ and his HIV viral load is 150,000 copies. He has not been on antiretrovirals. His only complaint is a 15-lb weight loss.

Patients with uncontrolled HIV infection may lose weight until viral replication can be controlled with HAART. Clearly, this patient would benefit from combination antiretroviral therapy rather than dietary supplements or pharmacologic agents to increase appetite.

TABLE 22-1
Pharmacologic Therapies for AIDS Wasting Syndrome

Therapy	Dose	Side effects	Comments
APPETITE STIMULANTS			
Megestrol acetate	800 mg po qd	Hyperglycemia Diabetes mellitus Cushing's disease Impotence	Progestational agent Majority of the weight gain is fat, not LBM
Dronabinol	2.5 mg po bid	Euphoria Somnolence	Active ingredient of marijuana Minimally effective for weight gain, but useful for nausea
ANABOLIC BLOCK			
Testosterone enanthate	300 mg IM q3w or 200 mg IM q2w	Polycythemia Liver abnormalities Prostate growth Lipid abnormalities	
Testosterone patch/gel	5 mg qd for men 150-300 μg qd for women		More expensive than IM These doses do not have androgen side effects associated with the IM
Testosterone oral	Do not use	Hepatotoxic	
Oxandrolone	10 mg po bid	Liver abnormalities	Results in gains in LBM, not just fat; little data in women
Nandrolone	100 mg IM qw	Less androgenic so preferred for eugonadal men and women, inexpensive	Results in gains in LBM, not just fat; little data in women
Oxymetholone	50 mg IM tiw	Liver abnormalities	Results in gains in LBM, not just fat; little data in women
Growth hormone	6 mg SQ qd	Arthralgias Edema Hyperglycemia Carpal tunnel syndrome	Increase in LBM, loss of fat Very expensive
CYTOKINE MODULATORS			
Thalidomide	100-300 mg po qd	Somnolence Rash	Known teratogen, cannot give to woman with pregnancy potential

Case 3 Analysis. Allen is a 32-year-old man with HIV infection who recently underwent an extensive evaluation for weight loss. The work-up did not reveal OIs or a malignancy. His only specific complaint is mild nausea.

Nausea is a frequent complaint among HIV-infected persons with weight loss. Often it can be a side effect of one or more of the numerous HIV-related medications. A full drug history of prescribed, over-the-counter, and alternative/herbal remedies should be taken. In addition, this patient's appetite is poor and he might benefit from an appetite stimulant. Dronabinol is an appetite stimulant that has the added benefit of possessing antiemetic properties.

Case 4 Analysis. Tim is a 50-year-old man diagnosed with AWS. He is generally inactive, and has lost 25 lbs. Serum total and free testosterone levels are decreased.

Many HIV-infected patients (both men and women), especially those with wasting, have low testosterone levels. Tim would likely benefit from anabolic therapy. Although there are several anabolic steroids available including oxandrolone, nandrolone, and oxymetholone, which can help increase weight and LBM, none is more effective than testosterone in hypogonadal men. In men who are not hypogonadal, these other therapies should be considered. It was also mentioned that Tim is inactive. Studies have demonstrated that anabolic agents in combination with progressive resistance exercise increase LBM to a greater degree than either alone.

Case 5 Analysis. James is a 30-year-old HIV-infected man with alcohol-related liver disease. He has AWS and has lost 20 lbs. OIs and malignancy have been excluded. He is started on megestrol and gains 10 lb, mostly fat according to BIA analysis. He is depressed by this excess fat and asks if there is anything else that can be done.

As already stated, the weight gain due to appetite stimulants is mostly fat. In order to increase LBM, an anabolic agent and/or progressive resistance exercise is necessary. Because of his liver disease, the anabolic steroids and possibly even testosterone should only be used with caution. In this situation GH should be considered. Its use has resulted in weight gain, increased LBM, and loss of fat. There is no significant liver toxicity associated with GH. The need for daily subcutaneous dosing, the high cost, and the uncomfortable side effects can limit its usefulness.

SUGGESTED READINGS

Corcoran C, Grinspoon S: Treatments for wasting in patients with the acquired immunodeficiency syndrome, *N Engl J Med* 340: 1740-1750, 1999.

Grunfeld C, Kotler DP: Wasting in the acquired immunodeficiency syndrome, *Semin Liver Dis* 12:175-187, 1992.

Kotler DP et al: Magnitude of body-cell-mass depletion and the timing of death from wasting in AIDS, *Am J Clin Nutr* 50:444-447, 1989.

Mulligan K, Tai VW, Schambelan M: Cross-sectional and longitudinal evaluation of body composition in men with HIV infection, *J Acquir Immune Defic Syndr Hum Retrovirol* 15:43-48, 1998.

23 Fever of Unknown Origin

KEVIN J. CROSS, JANET M. HINES, STEPHEN J. GLUCKMAN

Introduction

Fever is a very common sign in patients with the human immunodeficiency virus (HIV). Suppression of the immune system allows for the development of infections and neoplasms, both of which may present as fever. Additionally, some medications used in HIV characteristically cause drug-associated fever.

In most cases, fever is associated with signs and symptoms that suggest its source. However, immunosuppression can blunt or alter the body's response to infection and neoplasms, and mask their typical presentation. In some patients with advanced HIV, the only early evidence of a pathologic process is fever. In rare cases, this may remain the only clinically apparent sign for many weeks.

It is important to document fever. If the fever has an undulating course, it may be necessary to document it in the home. If a patient does not have a thermometer, or does not know how to use one, a thermometer and instructions on its use should be provided.

Definition

The clinical definition for fever of unknown origin (FUO) in an HIV-infected individual varies from study to study. Durack and Street established a set of criteria often used (Box 23-1).

Such strict definitions are most useful for epidemiologic case criteria to better define the scope of the problem of FUO. A more practical definition is useful for the clinical setting, and therefore is the one used in this discussion (Box 23-2).

Prevalence

Between 3% and 21% of HIV-infected patients will present with FUO at some time during the course of their illness. Most will have already been diagnosed with the acquired immunodeficiency syndrome (AIDS) due to the fact that FUO most often presents at times of advanced immunosuppression. The majority of patients with an FUO present when the CD4+ count is below 200 cells/mm^3. In fact, more than three fourths of all patients who present with FUO will have a CD4+ count below 100 cells/mm^3. Some studies have shown that a diagnosis is made in 60% to 90% of cases, but mortality rates run as high as 22%. The average fever duration is between 60 and 70 days, and amazingly a majority of patients experience fever for over a month before admission to a hospital. These findings demonstrate the need for physicians to make a diagnosis efficiently but to use diagnostics judiciously. Fever on its own in an HIV-infected patient does not require emergent evaluation and treatment (as opposed to fever in the neutropenic host). Attention to signs of clinical deterioration, as well as a reasonable understanding of the most likely causes of fever in these patients, will adequately guide the clinician's work-up.

As with non–HIV-infected patients with an FUO, the etiologic agent is most often infectious, although neoplastic causes are not uncommon. Furthermore, more than 19% of patients with HIV-FUO may have multiple sources of their fever, whereas non–HIV-infected patients will usually have a single cause. Therefore the physician must keep in mind that persistence of a fever in a patient after adequate treatment of one entity should inspire the search for another, previously undiagnosed, source of fever.

When the clinician is considering the possible causes of FUO the geographic location and the travel history of the patient are relevant. Tuberculosis and leishmaniasis are more prevalent in the Mediterranean and developing countries, and subsequently are the two leading infectious causes of FUO in HIV-infected individuals in those regions. In the United States, where these diseases are less commonly found, disseminated *Mycobacterium avium* complex (MAC), *Pneumocystis carinii* pneumonia (PCP), and cytomegalovirus (CMV) infection are the most common causes of FUO. Furthermore, within a general geographic location there may exist smaller communities where certain causes are more likely. Patients living or working in the inner cities of the United States, or those who have been incarcerated, are at higher risk of presenting with *M. tuberculosis* as the cause of their FUO than those residing in a more rural setting. For this reason, it is of the utmost importance that a good history be taken, one that includes place of residence, location of employment, and past travel history.

Initial Work-Up

The initial work-up of any patient with HIV and an FUO should begin with a meticulous history and physical examination. It is important to emphasize that any localizing signs or symptoms found should be specifically pursued. For instance, if there are significant headaches or if there are respiratory symptoms, these should be evaluated before doing a more general FUO evaluation. In addition, the evaluation of an FUO in this setting should be guided by the CD4+ count of the patient. Looking for opportunistic infections (OIs) that occur with low counts, such as CMV, *Cryptococcus*, *Pneumocystis*, and MAC, is generally inappropriate when CD4+ counts

BOX 23-1
Fever of Unknown Origin in HIV-Infected Patients

- Temperature higher than 101° F
- Fever of more than 4 weeks' duration for outpatients or more than 3 days' duration for inpatients, including at least 2 days' incubation of microbiologic cultures
- A diagnosis that remains uncertain after 3 days despite appropriate investigation including blood cell counts, liver enzyme tests, urinalysis, chest radiography, performance of cultures of blood and urine, and initial identification of localizing symptoms or specific findings on examination

BOX 23-2
Alternative Definition

- Fever that has no specific signs or symptoms that point to a likely cause
- Fever that has been present long enough that it can safely be presumed not to be related to a self-limited infection (in most cases, this would be 3-5 days without improvement of localization)

are more than 200 cells/mm³. Provided the initial evaluation does not reveal any localizing findings, several general laboratory tests are usually appropriate, including a complete blood count (CBC), renal and hepatic panel, blood cultures, urinalysis, and urine culture. Chest x-ray (CXR) should usually be performed.

Although long-term incubation of the original cultures will not increase the likelihood of making a diagnosis, repeating the blood cultures has been shown to be useful. Two sets of blood cultures give a yield of 93%, and repeating them a third time will increase it to around 99%, after which further culturing becomes futile. Use of nonstandard blood culture systems is appropriate at counts below 100 cells/mm³, and is discussed below.

If the initial testing does not lead the clinician in a specific direction, before initiating a more extensive work-up a drug fever should be strongly considered.

▶ KEY POINTS

INITIAL WORK-UP
⊃ Complete blood count
⊃ Renal and hepatic panel
⊃ Urinalysis
⊃ Blood cultures
⊃ Chest x-ray

Drug Fever

Drug fever should be among the first considerations in a patient with HIV who has a fever without any focal signs. If the patient is generally well despite the fever, and if the timing of the onset of the fever parallels (or follows) the initiation of a drug, it is reasonable to try empiric discontinuation of that drug. It should be remembered that drug fever usually occurs within days to a few weeks after initiating the medication, although occasionally the duration of medication prior to the onset of the fever can be much longer. Despite the severe suppression of the immune system seen in advanced stages of the disease, many HIV-infected patients can have drug reactions, ranging from mild elevations in body temperature to the occasionally fatal Stevens-Johnson syndrome. Drug fevers are seen in 20% of hospitalized AIDS patients at some time. Drug fevers are most commonly seen in response to sulfa drugs; however, HIV-infected patients are often on many medications, virtually any of which may produce a drug fever. Antiretroviral medications that are particularly associated with fever include the non-nucleoside reverse transcriptase inhibitors (NNRTIs), including nevirapine (Viramune), delavirdine (Rescriptor), and efavirenz (Sustiva). Abacavir (Ziagen) also deserves special mention. About 3% to 10% of patients on abacavir have a hypersensitivity reaction that can include fever (in over 90% of those having the reaction), and also fatigue, myalgias, rash, sore throat, and gastrointestinal or respiratory symptoms. Patients with the hypersensitivity reaction who either continue on the abacavir or are rechallenged with the drug are at high risk of developing progressive multiorgan system failure. Deaths have occurred. Most reactions occur within the first 6 weeks of being on or restarting the drug. If such a reaction is suspected, the physician prescribing the drug should be notified immediately, and strong consideration must be given to stopping the drug.

Empiric Drug Discontinuation

After the initial investigation is performed, utilizing noninvasive techniques and any invasive procedures deemed appropriate, a worthwhile next step for the clinician faced with a clinically stable HIV-FUO patient can include the discontinuation of as many drugs as possible. These agents should include any nonprescription medication and nutritional supplements. Patients will not typically suffer long-term ill effects from a "drug holiday." When the antiretrovirals are discontinued, they should all be discontinued simultaneously to prevent the development of viral drug resistance. Typically, drug fevers will resolve within 1 to 2 weeks of stopping the inciting agent, making this a reasonable duration for a drug-free trial.

Empiric drug discontinuation as a diagnostic test should be done fairly early in the diagnostic evaluation of a patient with an FUO. How early depends in part on how critical the medications are and how ill the patient is. Box 23-3 shows other drugs that commonly cause fever in HIV.

Empiric Drug Initiation

The need for empiric treatment can be considered at any time during the investigation. A successful trial of empiric treatment for an infection can be a useful way of inferring a causative relationship between the fever and the agent to which the treatment is being given. Factors that encourage the employment of early treatment include the worsening of a patient's clinical condition, a patient's unwillingness to allow invasive studies, concern about a transmissible disease, and any prolonged delay in the acquisition of laboratory results. In general, empiric treatment for an FUO is directed at mycobacterial infections, both tuberculous and nontuberculous.

Evaluation by Consideration of CD4+ Cell Count

The CD4+ cell count is useful in predicting the degree of impairment of the immune system. Thus using the CD4+ count to focus one's differential diagnosis in the evaluation of an FUO in an HIV-infected person is a safe and practical tactic. Obviously, there is some variability in CD4+ cell levels, and therefore the relationship between CD4+ cell count and possible diseases should only be used as a guide. See Box 23-4 for likely causes of FUO by CD4+ count.

CD4+ Count Higher than 200 cells/mm³

Tuberculosis. Tuberculosis can present in an HIV-infected patient at any CD4+ count. At higher counts it generally appears as a pulmonary disease, most commonly a subacute cough with weight loss, fevers, and night sweats associated with an x-ray revealing apical disease. In patients with very low CD4+ cell counts, tuberculosis generally manifests itself as disseminated disease (see below). Patients who have had a known exposure to tuberculosis at some time in their life or who have been incarcerated are at an increased risk for tuberculosis.

Sinusitis. Sinusitis should be considered in an HIV-infected person with fever, no matter what the CD4+ count. However, the likelihood of acute sinusitis increases as the CD4+ cell count drops. Up to 20% of patients with sinusitis will present only with a fever, so the clinician should have a low threshold for obtaining a computed tomography (CT) scan dedicated to evaluation of the paranasal sinuses, especially in a patient who has a past history of sinus infections.

Community-acquired Pneumonia. Community-acquired pneumonia (CAP) is one of the most common infections in patients with HIV. Although it usually is associated with cough or other pulmonary symptoms, occasionally early in its course CAP can present as an isolated fever. As it evolves, focal symptoms suggestive of pneumonia will generally result, but chest radiographic examination before it is differentiated allows for earlier diagnosis and treatment.

Malignancy. In general, the malignancies that are especially associated with fever include primary hepatoma or cancer metastatic to the liver, atrial myxoma, renal cell carcinoma, and lymphoma. In HIV-infected persons, non-Hodgkin's lymphoma, Kaposi's sarcoma, anal cancer, and cervical cancer are seen with increased frequency. The latter three malignancies are not associated with fever unless they are producing an obstruction with related infection. Therefore, in general, only lymphomas need to be considered when evaluating an HIV-infected patient with an FUO. It should be noted that primary central nervous system (CNS) lymphoma presents almost exclusively at counts below 50 to 100 cells/mm³ and is not typically associated with fever.

CD4+ Counts of 100 to 200 cells/mm³

Pneumocystis carinii Pneumonia. PCP is notorious for presenting with a prolonged, undifferentiated fever prior to onset of specific respiratory symptoms. Previous or even current prophylaxis against PCP does not ensure protection from the disease, although careful adherence to a prophylaxis regimen markedly decreases the likelihood of PCP.

Tuberculosis. Tuberculosis should remain a consideration as the CD4+ count drops; however, the presentation tends to shift from the more expected upper lobe pulmonary disease to

---

BOX 23-3
Drugs Commonly Causing Fever in HIV

Sulfonamides
Dapsone
Isoniazid
Rifampin
Amphotericin B
Pentamidine
Penicillins
Antiepileptics

BOX 23-4
Likely Causes of Fever of Unknown Origin by CD4+ Count

HIGHER THAN 200 cells/mm³
Tuberculosis
Sinusitis
Community-acquired pneumonia
Lymphoma

100-200 cells/mm³
Pneumocystis
Salmonella bacteremia

LOWER THAN 100 cells/mm³
Cytomegalovirus
Mycobacterium avium complex
Cryptococcus

---

lower lobe infiltrates, hilar lymphadenopathy, or extrapulmonary disease.

Salmonellosis. *Salmonella* bacteremia or focal suppurative infection may occur at any time in HIV, although it occurs more often at lower CD4+ counts. It may present as FUO without a supportive exposure history and without any symptoms or signs of gastrointestinal distress. It can be diagnosed by routine blood culture.

Other Diagnoses. Again, the diagnoses considered at higher CD4+ counts should also be considered here. Specifically, sinusitis, community-acquired pneumonia, and lymphoma may present at these counts. Unlike tuberculosis, they generally resemble their presentation at a higher CD4+ count.

CD4+ Counts Below 100 cells/mm³

Cytomegalovirus. CMV can be a clinical problem in patients with CD4+ counts below 100 cells/mm³, and becomes particularly prevalent when counts are below 50 cells/mm³. CMV may present as colitis, retinitis, meningoencephalitis, or much more infrequently pneumonia, but quite often fever will exist in a patient for a long period of time before focal symptoms are reported. Retinal involvement may be so mild or subtle that a patient has no visual complaints. Evaluation for CMV should begin with an ophthalmologic examination to look for the characteristic changes of CMV retinitis. The examination lacks sensitivity, however, and if CMV is suspected in a patient with an FUO, other diagnostic modalities, such as a polymerase chain reaction (PCR) for CMV on the blood or

> **BOX 23-5**
> **Specific Testing for Fever of Unknown Origin in HIV-Infected Patients**
>
> **CD4+ COUNT HIGHER THAN 200 cells/mm³**
> Sinus CT scan
>
> **CD4+ COUNT 100-200 cells/mm³**
> A-a gradient at rest and with exercise, and if abnormal consider *Pneumocystis carinii* pneumonia evaluation
>
> **CD4+ COUNT LOWER THAN 100 cells/mm³**
> Isolator blood cultures for mycobacteria
> Serum cryptococcal antigen
> Bone marrow biopsy
> Cytomegalovirus PCR on blood

spinal fluid, or histologic evidence of CMV in potentially involved organs must be explored. Antibody testing for active CMV infection lacks the sensitivity and specificity to be of any use in this setting.

Mycobacterium avium Complex. Although *M. avium* is ubiquitous, infection with this organism is uncommon in patients with healthy immune systems. As the CD4+ cell level drops, MAC infection becomes more prevalent. By the time of death, at least half of all patients with HIV are infected. MAC typically presents as an FUO associated with wasting. Focal symptoms can develop, in particular, abdominal pain and diarrhea. When evaluating an FUO in a patient with a very low CD4+ count, special blood cultures using isolator tubes should be utilized to check for MAC. Occasionally, a bone marrow or lymph node biopsy will reveal the diagnosis.

Cryptococcosis. In persons with very low CD4+ cell counts, cryptococcal infection may present as an FUO before the appearance of the more characteristic CNS disease or occasionally pulmonary disease. In this setting, a serum cryptococcal antigen is a good screening test and should be part of the evaluation of an FUO, even in the absence of headache or focal CNS signs or symptoms.

Endemic Mycoses. Disseminated endemic mycoses of histoplasmosis and coccidioidomycosis can produce an FUO in patients with very low CD4+ counts. These fungi are particularly likely if the patient has had the proper geographic exposure history. Histoplasmosis is a primary consideration in the midwestern United States and coccidioidomycosis is limited to the southwestern region in this country. The presentation as an FUO of disseminated disease is indistinguishable from disease cause by disseminated mycobacterial infections or CMV. Finding the fungi in tissue specimens generally makes the diagnosis.

Toxoplasmosis. Toxoplasmosis may rarely present as FUO in HIV patients. More typically, it will present as a sudden neurologic deterioration in motor function (as in a stroke) or as a new-onset seizure disorder. *Toxoplasma* should not generally be considered the source of an undifferentiated FUO, but work-up should commence if either of these syndromes is present.

Miscellaneous. Leishmaniasis is a common cause of HIV-FUO in the Mediterranean, Africa, India, and some areas of Southeast Asia and South America, especially when the CD4+ count drops below 100 cells/mm³. As the CD4+ count continues to fall, visceral leishmaniasis becomes more likely. It is commonly associated with a reduction in the platelet count to below 100,000 cells/mm³ and is rarely seen in patients who do not have platelet counts below this level. There is also an association between this disease and patients with low total leukocyte counts, low neutrophil counts, and low hemoglobin levels. Hepatosplenomegaly, an almost universal finding in non–HIV-infected patients with leishmaniasis, is less commonly seen in the immunosuppressed HIV-infected patient.

Further Testing

In addition to the standard FUO evaluation, the following specific testing should be considered in HIV-infected persons with unexplained prolonged fevers. Box 23-5 lists specific tests to be performed.

Diagnostic Tests

Routine Blood Cultures. Two sets of blood cultures are a standard part of an FUO evaluation, and in particular will identify occult *Salmonella* infection.

Chest Radiography. CXR is a standard part of an FUO evaluation. However, a normal chest radiograph cannot rule out the presence of PCP or of tuberculosis. In fact, chest radiographs may be normal in 10% to 20% of cases of PCP. The greater likelihood of extrapulmonary tuberculosis in patients with lower CD4+ counts should caution the physician not to dismiss tuberculosis as a diagnosis in the face of a normal chest radiograph.

Tuberculin Skin Testing. Skin testing for tuberculosis has a relatively low sensitivity and specificity for tuberculosis *disease* (as opposed to infection). A positive tuberculin skin test may reflect unrelated, coexistent asymptomatic mycobacterial infection and should generally not halt an FUO work-up. A negative tuberculin skin test does not eliminate tuberculosis from consideration as the cause of an FUO. Although a useful epidemiologic tool, tuberculin skin testing is not reliable enough to be definitive in the evaluation of a person with an FUO.

Computed Tomography Scanning. As in patients not infected with HIV, CT scanning can play an important diagnostic role in the evaluation of an FUO in HIV-infected patients. Thoracic CT scans have a diagnostic yield of 50% when used in patients with HIV-FUO, and this percentage goes up when mycobacterial disease is suspected. It has a central role in the evaluation of FUO during HIV infection. Abdominal CT is less effective in terms of overall diagnostic results, but is also very effective in finding evidence suggesting mycobacteriosis and lymphoma. These appear as either enlarged, often necrotic lymph nodes or single or multiple abscesses distributed throughout abdominal structures. Other than as a way to evaluate the sinuses, cranial CT scans are less effective as a screening tool for evaluating an FUO. Sinus evaluating can be accomplished by a simpler, quicker, directed CT scan.

Biopsy and Lumbar Puncture. Lymph node, bone marrow, liver, intestinal, and lung biopsies all have potential utility in the evaluation of an FUO in an HIV-infected patient. A clearly enlarged lymph node should be biopsied early in the work-up before a lot of less directed tests are done. Fine-needle aspiration (FNA) is a safe, quick, and less painful alternative to standard biopsy, but if the results of the FNA are negative, an excisional biopsy should be performed. A bone marrow biopsy may be particularly useful for diagnosing mycobacterial infection, lymphoma, and disseminated endemic fungi. Although the sensitivity for making this diagnosis may not be as high as it is for liver biopsy, it is generally a safer procedure to perform. When a patient has an unexplained pancytopenia or evidence of myelophthisis on peripheral smear, a bone marrow biopsy should be done relatively early in the diagnostic evaluation. Liver biopsy, a well-studied invasive procedure in HIV-FUO, yields a diagnosis in approximately 50% of cases. It is done looking for the same diagnoses as the bone marrow biopsy. The yield in persons with absolutely normal liver testing is too low to recommend this procedure. When a patient has evidence of infiltrative liver disease, as manifested by an elevation in alkaline phosphatase and γ-glutamyl transpeptidase out of proportion to transaminases, it is a particularly useful test. Several studies report on the use of intestinal biopsy, especially when intestinal lymphoma or CMV colitis is suspected, but the yield has been shown to be less than 15%. Lumbar puncture should be used in patients with severe or persistent headache, neurologic symptoms, or serum positive for cryptococcal antigen, but even in these cases a diagnosis will be made less than 20% of the time, and only half of these will be treatable. For these reasons, it is recommended that neither intestinal biopsy nor lumbar puncture be used in the standard HIV-FUO work-up in a patient without some signs, laboratory tests, or symptoms that suggest some localization to those regions.

Diagnosis of Specific Organisms
Cytomegalovirus

All CMV testing suffers from the problem that CMV is a ubiquitous virus and infection is common. The difficulty is distinguishing past infection from presently active disease. This problem makes antibody testing particularly unhelpful. The most promising recent development in the diagnosis of CMV has been the CMV antigenemia assay on blood, but it has not been shown to be sufficiently specific to use in HIV-infected patients. Since many patients with very low CD4+ counts have evidence of CMV antigenemia, finding CMV antigenemia in a patient does not establish CMV as the etiology of the FUO. Similarly, a positive culture for CMV may reflect profound immunosuppression alone, and not the cause of an FUO. The most specific test today for CMV infection is a tissue biopsy. CMV-infected tissue displays characteristic CMV inclusions in its cells.

Unfortunately, even finding CMV inclusions does not definitively diagnose CMV as the cause of an FUO. These can be seen in low numbers in patients with very low CD4+ counts without producing symptoms. The greater the number of CMV inclusions in a specimen, the more likely that CMV is causing disease rather than being merely a background presence. Often clinical judgment must be used to determine when to treat for CMV. CMV PCR is performed at some centers on an experimental basis, although it is not available for commercial use. However, its performance characteristics are favorable, depending on the laboratory, and it should come into widespread use soon. It is most commonly used on cerebrospinal fluid (CSF) for the diagnosis of CMV meningoencephalitis.

Mycobacterium avium Complex

The most useful way of identifying systemic MAC infection is in culture of the blood. Such culture requires the use of lysis-centrifugation tubes (isolators), and plating onto media appropriate for growth of mycobacteria. Such a culture requires 2 to 4 weeks for finalization. MAC can often be found colonizing the respiratory tract or stool, so sputum or stool specimens growing MAC are of no diagnostic value in the work-up of an FUO. Biopsy of an organ (liver, spleen, intestinal wall, or bone marrow) may be necessary if suspicion is high but blood cultures are negative.

Cryptococcosis

Serum cryptococcal antigen is a useful screen for the patient who has FUO without enough suspicion for cryptococcal meningitis to perform a lumbar puncture. A positive result requires CSF examination, since early in the course asymptomatic CNS infection can occur, and if CNS infection is present, the management of the patient is likely to be different.

Other Considerations
Immune Reconstitution Syndrome

An average of 6 weeks after the initiation of antiretroviral therapy in patients with CD4+ counts of less than 100 cells/mm^3, a small percentage of patients will develop what is known as immune reconstitution syndrome. The vigorous return of CD4+ cells and the cascade of the immune response that they put into play are characteristic of initiation of effective combination highly active antiretroviral therapy (HAART). It is believed that when the patient has a low-grade, subclinical infection (such as MAC) prior to the initiation of HAART, the now vigorous response to this infection is manifested by the development of the immune reconstitution syndrome. Typical symptoms include fever, anorexia, abdominal pain, and markedly tender and enlarged lymphadenopathy. Sometimes such nodes will suppurate. When the areas involved are less clinically apparent (e.g., abdominal symptoms), the patient may present with an FUO. Although this syndrome may occur with virtually any infection seen in advanced AIDS, it is best described at this point in patients with MAC infection. The optimal treatment is not yet described, and may include steroids, specific antimicrobial therapy, both, or neither. Antiretroviral therapy should not be stopped. Generally, the severity of the symptoms guides the institution of treatment.

Patients on Prophylaxis

The United States Department of Health and Human Services (DHHS) and the Infectious Disease Society of America (IDSA) issued guidelines for prevention of opportunistic infections in persons infected with HIV in 1995. They were updated in January 2000. They include recommendations for primary prevention of PCP, *Toxoplasma gondii,* tuberculosis, MAC, *Streptococcus pneumoniae,* and varicella-zoster virus. They also made strong recommendations for the secondary prevention of PCP, *T. gondii,* MAC, CMV, *Salmonella* species, *Cryptococcus neoformans,* and the endemic fungi. Although prophylaxis against OIs in HIV-infected patients is variably effective, it does not ensure protection. Furthermore, failed prophylaxis may result in atypical presentations of OIs by attenuating the breakthrough disease. One possible result of this is the development of a prolonged, nonlocalizing fever as the only initial symptom. As a rule, the lower the CD4+ count drops in HIV-infected patients who are not virologically controlled with HAART, the more likely prophylaxis will fail in providing protection against infection.

Nonspecific Focal Signs

Headache. Headache is a common generally nonspecific symptom that accompanies most fevers, particularly when it is bifrontal. In the febrile HIV-infected patient who has a low CD4+ cell count, it can also reflect specific disease processes such as meningitis, sinusitis, cerebral toxoplasmosis, or primary CNS lymphoma. It is impractical to evaluate every headache in a febrile patient with specific testing. However, headaches that last more than several days, get inexorably worse, or are associated with neurologic findings should be evaluated with a CNS imaging study and, if negative, a lumbar puncture.

Cough. Although most coughs are due to minor problems, cough associated with an FUO may be an important clue. Even in the presence of a normal CXR, this should be pursued. Infectious diseases such as PCP, sinusitis, and tuberculosis should be considered, as should noninfectious diseases such as allergic rhinitis, asthma, and gastroesophageal reflux.

Lymphadenopathy. Lymphadenopathy is commonly seen in HIV. It is often not clinically worrisome and does not have to be pursued. However, in the presence of an FUO it must be evaluated. This is particularly true if the nodes are localized, tender, hard, fixed, and/or greater than 1 cm.

What Not to Do
Serology

Antibody testing is available for many of the causes of HIV-FUO. Unfortunately, results must be interpreted with caution and are often of limited sensitivity and specificity in establishing a diagnosis of active infection. Specifically, highly immunocompromised individuals may not make a good antibody response, lowering the sensitivity of antibody testing. Furthermore, many of the infectious agents one might consider are ubiquitous, and antibodies are often found in healthy persons. Their presence may establish that the patient has been infected with an organism, but they cannot determine that the organism is presently causing disease; the specificity for the diagnosis of disease is limited. For example, as mentioned above, the positive predictive value of CMV serology is very poor due to the fact that anti-CMV antibodies are found in more than 80% of HIV-infected patients. Similarly, *Toxoplasma* serology has a sensitivity of less than 40% in diagnosing ongoing CNS infection, and a negative serology cannot eliminate the possibility of CNS *Toxoplasma* infection.

Antigen Testing

In general, antigen tests for a pathogen have higher positive predictive values than serologic tests because they more directly represent the presence of the infectious agent. Cryptococcal antigen testing is widely used in HIV-infected patients and has relatively high positive and negative predictive values. *Histoplasma* urinary antigen also has a high predictive value when used in the right setting. CMV antigen testing, however, is less useful in the HIV-infected population, since subclinical antigenemia can be seen in persons with very low CD4+ counts. As such, finding CMV antigen in the blood does not prove there is a causal relationship between the virus and the fever.

Ultrasound of the Abdomen

Ultrasonography should not be the first test for use in HIV-FUO. Although there has been some success with its use in diagnosing mycobacteriosis in Europe, where infections from these entities are numerous, its utility in the United States has been limited. It is rarely used other than for echocardiography in an intravenous drug user suspected of having endocarditis, or in the HIV-infected woman who has signs referable to the lower abdomen.

Radionuclide Imaging

Radionuclide imaging employing gallium-67 (^{67}Ga) citrate scintigraphy or indium-labeled white blood cells has been used with some success in the diagnosis of classic non-HIV FUO. Proponents believe that such imaging tests can help to localize the source of a fever. Many clinicians believe that this testing lacks the sensitivity and specificity to be of clinical value. It is our opinion that at the present time this testing is rarely helpful and is not generally part of our FUO work-up. Perhaps exception can be made in suspected colitis, where a small number of reports suggest that technetium-99m–labeled antigranulocyte monoclonal antibody studies show good sensitivity in demonstrating colitis. This information can then be used to justify a biopsy of colonic tissue.

Algorithm

Finding the etiology of an FUO in an HIV-infected patient can be a challenging endeavor given the wide spectrum of possible etiologies, the large number of available tests and studies, and the necessity to work quickly but in a cost-effective way. However, fever in HIV-infected patients should not be a cause for anxiety or overtesting on the part of the clinician. Generally, consideration of the CD4+ cell count in the context of a thorough history and physical examination will narrow the differential diagnosis down to a few likely possibilities. As with all diagnostic challenges common things do occur more commonly. The exceptional patient will have an unusual cause or a stubborn diagnosis that may require the consultation of an infectious disease specialist. It must always be remembered that in addition to being predisposed to specific problems, HIV-infected patients can still get any of the common causes of fever that non–HIV-infected persons can have. Therefore, when evaluating fever in a person who is infected with HIV, the clinician should also consider non–HIV-related causes. The following should be done in conjunction with each other, keeping in mind the possibility of multiple causes of the fever should one result come back positive.

Step One

An appropriate start to the work-up of any patient with FUO should include a good history and physical examination for localizing symptoms and signs. CBC, chemistries including liver-associated enzymes and lactate dehydrogenase (LDH), CXR, urinalysis, and blood and urine cultures should generally be done on all patients. Blood cultures may be repeated up to two more times before the yield drops to a point where further culturing is unlikely to be of help. Any localizing signs or symptoms from the history, physical examination, or initial laboratory testing should be evaluated further before going on to other less focused testing.

Step Two

Drug fever should be considered early, especially if the patient is on one of the more typical antiretrovirals (NNRTIs) or an antiretroviral whose fever could have a serious impact (i.e., abacavir).

Step Three

Consider the CD4+ count. *If the count is more than 200 cells/mm^3*, evaluate as one would an FUO in a non–HIV-infected person, although with particular concern for pulmonary tuberculosis, sinusitis, or lymphoma. *If the count is 100 to 200 cells/mm^3, in addition to the above* consider early PCP and obtain a measure of oxygen saturation. *If the count is below 100 cells/mm^3, obtain in addition to the above* (1) lysis-centrifugation blood cultures for mycobacteria, (2) serum cryptococcal antigen, (3) ophthalmologic examination for CMV retinitis, (4) consider bone marrow biopsy, (5) consider empiric treatment for MAC, and (6) if geographically appropriate, blood culture and urine antigen for *Histoplasma* may be performed.

Summary

FUO is a common illness in HIV-infected patients and can lead to a protracted course with much morbidity. Occasionally it will end with devastating results. Attempts at making a diagnosis in HIV-FUO are complicated by the spectrum of likely causes, which range from infectious to neoplastic to pharmacologic, and by the uniqueness by which a patient's signs and symptoms can present. Clinicians must always remember that in addition to being predisposed to specific problems, HIV-infected patients can still get any of the common causes of fever that non–HIV-infected persons can have. Finally, the clinician should remember that the possibility of multiple causes of the fever can exist in severely immunosuppressed persons. If a patient does not respond to the treatment of a proven diagnosis, further evaluation is warranted.

SUGGESTED READINGS

Armstrong WS, Katz JT, Kazanjian PH: Human immunodeficiency virus–associated fever of unknown origin: a study of 70 patients in the United States and review, *Clin Infect Dis* 28(2):341-345, 1999.

Mayo J, Collazos J, Martinez E: Fever of unknown origin in the HIV-infected patient: new scenario for an old problem, *Scand J Infect Dis* 29(4):327-336, 1997.

Miller RF, Hingorami AD, Foley NM: Pyrexia of undetermined origin in patients with human immunodeficiency virus infection and AIDS, *Int J STD AIDS* 7(3):170-175, 1996.

Sullivan M, Feinberg J, Bartlett JG: Fever in patients with HIV infection, *Infect Dis Clin North Am* 10(1):149-165, 1996.

24 Malignancy in HIV-Infected Patients

DAVID H. HENRY

Introduction

Chronic human immunodeficiency virus (HIV) infection can lead to profound immunosuppression, with a predisposition to opportunistic infection. With chronic immunosuppression there is also a tendency to develop certain cancers. Kaposi's sarcoma (KS), non-Hodgkins lymphoma, cervical cancer, and anal cancer are all more prevalent in HIV-infected patients. This chapter will discuss the presentation, natural history, diagnosis, and treatment of these HIV-related neoplasms.

Kaposi's Sarcoma
Presentation and Progression

Cause. KS is a growth of the endothelial cells and perivascular stromal cells of blood vessels. KS is found in four different patient groups. Classical KS was first described in 1870 in older men from the Mediterranean region. KS also develops in organ transplant patients receiving chronic immunosuppression, and it is endemic to certain areas of central Africa. Finally, HIV-related KS can occur in any HIV-infected patient, but it is primarily found in men who have sex with men. Curiously enough, we believe KS is *not* a true malignancy, which, by definition, would have the ability to sustain itself and to metastasize to other sites. KS does not appear to be self-sustaining and requires nearby cellular and humoral factors for growth. However, in advanced stages it behaves like a true malignancy and is treated as such. The KS lesion has proliferative, inflammatory, and angiogenic components that give the lesion its characteristic red-brown color and its tendency to develop an ecchymotic-like base.

Although still strongly associated with HIV, the incidence of HIV-related KS has been decreasing over the last few years. During the early years of the HIV epidemic, the number of KS cases was initially quite high. Since then, the number of cases has steadily declined. This decline has been attributed to the advent of highly active antiretroviral therapy (HAART), especially the protease inhibitors; safer sex practice among homosexual men; and a fall off in case reporting (Fig. 24-1).

Not all HIV-infected patients are equally likely to develop KS. The highest risk group are men who have sex with men. Intravenous drug abusers and those infected via heterosexual contact are nowhere near as prone to develop KS (Fig. 24-2). This observation has long suggested that a cofactor or coinfection is somehow involved in men who have sex with men.

In 1995, a new virus in the herpes family was discovered in KS cells. DNA from this new virus was found in the genome of every KS cell and named KS herpesvirus (KSHV), or more recently, human herpesvirus 8 (HHV-8). Subsequent research has determined that HHV-8 is found in the genome of every form of KS, whether it is classical, immunosuppressive, endemic, or HIV-related.

HHV-8 is a fascinating virus in its own right. Its closest relative among all herpesviruses is the herpesvirus Saimiri (HVS), whose natural host is the new world squirrel monkey. Its closest relative among other *human* herpesviruses is the Epstein-Barr virus (EBV), a virus long studied for its possible relationship to human neoplasms. Perhaps the most interesting aspect of HHV-8 is that it is an "eclectic traveler." There are a number of eukaryotic cellular genes in the HHV-8 genome that have been preserved over time. These genes were probably acquired from viral passage through former host cells and presumably kept by the HHV-8 virus because of some survival advantage conferred on the new virus.

What is the special role of the HHV-8 virus in the pathogenesis of KS? The answer is not yet clear, but interesting observations and theories abound. Research to answer these questions has been slow to develop. Even determining how common this virus is in different populations has been difficult. The assay for the HHV-8 virus is difficult to perform and standardization is still evolving. We know that HHV-8 seroprevalence in HIV-negative normal blood donors in the United States is only 3% to 8%. However, this number increases to 21% in HIV-negative blood donors in Greece (an endemic area for KS), and to 60% in Uganda. In the United States, 40% of homosexual men are HHV-8–positive, while 0% of heterosexual men are positive. The percentage positive increases in those homosexual men with multiple partners. Although these numbers underscore the probable route of sexual transmission in this country, it does not explain the marked seropositivity in central Africa, where even infants are positive and the rate increases with age. Maternal-child transmission and/or oral/fecal transmission is postulated to play a role in the underdeveloped world, although this is not proven. Recently, HHV-8 has been found in high concentration in saliva. Mothers in this area of the world premasticate food in their own mouths and then place it in the infant's mouth. This may explain the high maternal-infant transmission in this area.

HHV-8 infection must be necessary to develop KS. It is detectable some 3 to 10 years in HIV-infected patients before the development of clinical KS, but not all HHV-8–positive patients develop KS. With the advent of protected anal intercourse in men who have sex with men, the incidence of HHV-8 positivity has decreased. This may also explain, in part, the large decline in HIV-related KS over the last few years.

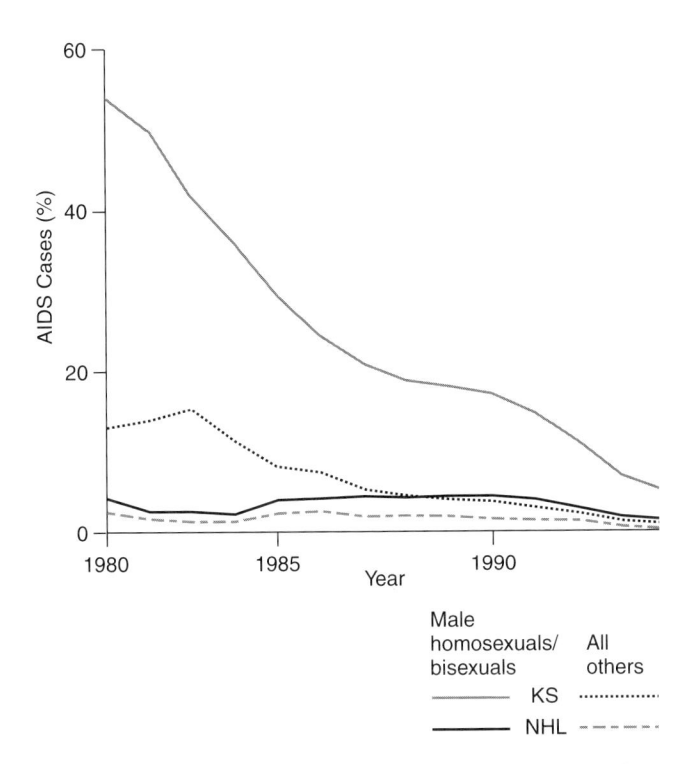

FIG. 24-1 Percent of U.S. AIDS cases presenting with Kaposi's sarcoma (KS) and with non–Hodgkin's lymphoma (NHL), male homosexual/bisexual AIDS cases versus all others, 1981-1994. (Data from AIDS Public Access Dataset, U.S. Centers for Disease Control and Prevention, 1996. Modified from Bigger RJ, Rabkin CS: The epidemiology of AIDS-related neoplasms, *Hematol Oncol Clin North Am* 10(5):999, 1996.)

In addition to HHV-8, other factors are necessary to provide the right environment for the development of a KS lesion. Inflammatory cytokines and angiogenesis growth factors are released from HIV-infected mononuclear cells that surround blood vessels and stromal tissues. These growth factors include interleukin (IL)-1, IL-6, fibroblast growth factor, GM-CSF, and the TAT protein gene product from the HIV itself.

Thus the development of a clinical KS lesion in any patient risk group involves multiple steps (Fig. 24-3) and may be summarized as follows. A genetic predisposition may be the necessary first step in some patients. This is followed by the development of an immunodeficiency state like an HIV infection or immunosuppressive therapy. Older age and chronic infection may account for the immunodeficiency "trigger" in classical and endemic KS, respectively. Then, HHV-8 activates or promotes growth somehow, transforming normal vascular endothelial cells into a malignant phenotype. Some of the genes acquired by the HHV-8 through its evolution could accomplish this transformation. Finally, the inflammatory cytokines and angiogenesis growth factors produced by HIV-infected mononuclear cells in the vicinity of the developing lesion continue the growth of the KS lesion in the HIV-infected patient.

Presentation. Most patients with HIV-related KS come to clinical attention because of one or more raised red-brown lesions on the skin. These lesions may occur anywhere. Areas of previous trauma, soles of the feet and toes, nose, and roof of the mouth are common sites for KS. Ten percent of patients will present with extracutaneous sites of KS first, such as lymph nodes or internal organs like the gastrointestinal (GI) or pulmonary regions.

Maculopapular Red-Brown Lesions. In the context of HIV, there is a very limited differential diagnosis for the raised red-brown pigmented lesion. First and foremost should be the consideration of KS. KS is most common in a white male who has sex with other men, but it can still occur in any other race or risk group. Rarely, bacillary angiomatosis can be confused with KS. This infectious lesion is caused by the cat scratch–like organism *Bartonella henselae*. It stains positive with the Warthin-Starry stain and is remarkably responsive to erythromycin.

Other causes of maculopapular red-brown lesions in the HIV-infected patient are given in Table 24-1.

Bilateral Pulmonary Infiltrates. Bilateral pulmonary infiltrates in the HIV-infected patient raise several infectious, neoplastic, and inflammatory possibilities. KS should always be considered in the differential diagnosis. Fully 50% of all patients with cutaneous KS will have internal organ involvement, usually GI or pulmonary. However, only 10% of patients will have symptomatic organ involvement. Bilateral pulmonary infiltrates are entirely consistent with pulmonary KS, which can also be either interstitial or nodular. In addition, pulmonary KS can present as hilar adenopathy or just as a pleural effusion. Lymphoma would be unlikely.

The most important infection to exclude with this presentation would be *Pneumocystis carinii* pneumonia (PCP). Sputum examination and/or bronchoalveolar lavage will usually confirm a diagnosis of PCP. A diagnosis of pulmonary KS would require a bronchoscopic examination of the lung and occasionally even an open lung biopsy. A useful noninvasive technique to differentiate these two possibilities is a thallium scan followed by a gallium scan. Pulmonary KS would be thallium-positive and gallium-negative, whereas PCP would be gallium-positive and thallium-negative.

Other infections to consider with bilateral pulmonary infiltrates would include *Mycobacterium tuberculosis, M. avium, Cryptococcus, Histoplasma, Coccidioides,* cytomegalovirus (CMV), and rarely herpesviruses such as simplex or zoster. Finally, the inflammatory entity of lymphocytic interstitial pneumonia (LIP) could cause bilateral pulmonary infiltrates.

Case. A 41-year-old male patient presents with a 1-week history of facial swelling. He is HIV-positive, with a recent CD4+ lymphocyte count of 220 cells/mm^3 and an HIV viral load of 30,000 copies/ml. He has taken zidovudine, lamivudine, and indinavir for the past year. For 3 months he has noticed a slight swelling of the lymph nodes in his neck and groin, and three new red, raised lesions have appeared on his back and chest, and under his right eyelid. He denies fever or night sweats, but he has lost 15 lb in the last 3 months.

On physical examination, he appears mildly ill, with a temperature of 99° F. His face is slightly swollen, with shotty bilateral cervical and inguinal lymphadenopathy. There is no jugular venous distention. Bibasilar rales are heard and a spleen tip is palpable.

Initial laboratory studies show hemoglobin of 10.5 g/dl, white blood cell count (WBC) 14.4 cells/ul, and normal creatinine, lactate dehydrogenase (LDH), and liver function tests. Chest x-ray reveals faint perihilar and lower lobe infiltrates, bilaterally. O$_2$ saturation is 92% on room air.

What are the diagnostic possibilities?
Would you biopsy his skin lesions?

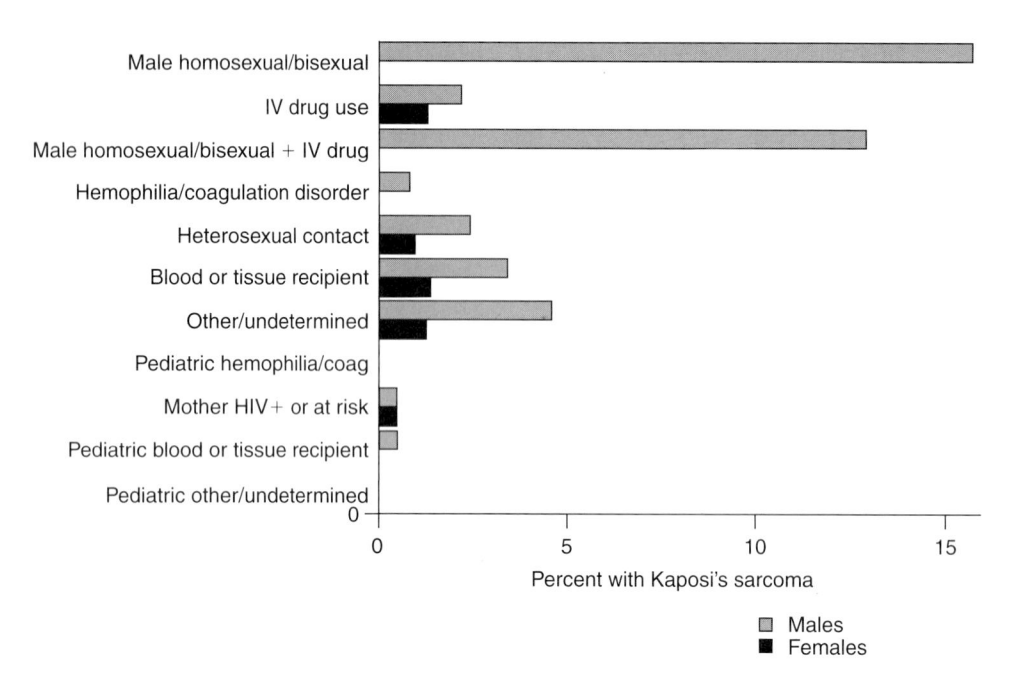

FIG. 24-2 Percent of U.S. AIDS cases presenting with Kaposi's sarcoma, by HIV exposure category and sex, 1981-1994. (Data from AIDS Public Access Dataset, U.S. Centers for Disease Control and Prevention, 1996. Redrawn from Bigger RJ, Rabkin CS: The epidemiology of AIDS-related neoplasms, *Hematol Oncol Clin North Am* 10(5):999, 1996.)

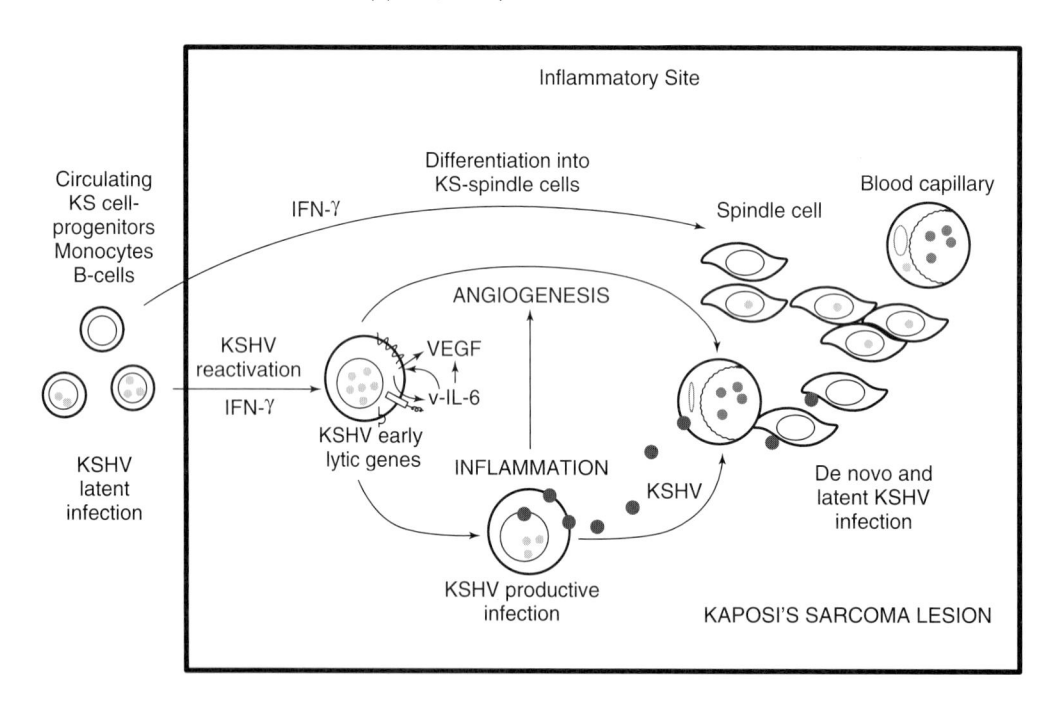

FIG. 24-3 Inflammatory reactivation and angiogenicity of KSHV/HHV-8. (Redrawn from *Blood* 93(12):4031-4032, 1999.)

Are the chest x-ray findings likely to be infectious or neoplastic?

Diagnosis

The HIV-infected patient described above clinically presents with a fairly typical case of skin KS, along with the more challenging finding of bilateral pulmonary infiltrates. This patient has fairly advanced HIV with a CD4+ lymphocyte count of 220 cells/mm^3. He is at risk for any neoplasm and most opportunistic infections.

The weight loss is worrisome, but nonspecific. Drug rash seems unlikely for two reasons. He only has three lesions, and

TABLE 24-1
Differential Diagnosis of Maculopapular Red-Brown Lesions

Cause	Appearance
Drug reaction	Usually pruritic and diffuse
Bacillary angiomatosis	Very similar to Kaposi's sarcoma
Cryptococcus	Nodular, ulcerating, or vesicular
Eosinophilic folliculitis	Pruritic papules and pustules
Histoplasma	Nodular, ulcerating, or vesicular
Herpes simplex	Grouped vesicles with erythematous base
Herpes zoster	Same rash as herpes simplex, except usually follow one dermatome
Insect bite	Erythematous, urticarial papule
Immune thrombocytopenic purpura	Tiny petechiae, ecchymoses, not raised
Kaposi's sarcoma	Firm red-brown
Molluscum	Usually flesh-colored
Seborrhea	Erythematous, scaling plaques
Staphylococcus aureus	May be erythematous papules or pustules
Syphilis	Chancre or diffuse rash, ± nodules

his medications (zidovudine, lamivudine, and indinavir) are not often associated with rash. The non-nucleoside reverse transcriptase inhibitors (efavirenz, nevirapine, delavirdine) are most often associated with rash.

The major infectious concern in this patient would be PCP, which can be very insidious in onset in an HIV-infected patient as opposed to a non–HIV-infected patient, in whom the pulmonary symptoms and findings are usually explosive. Community-acquired pneumonia would be a possibility. Pneumococcal pneumonia is common in HIV-infected patients, but would not likely be bilateral. Nonbacterial pneumonia due to *Legionella* or *Mycoplasma* would be a distant possibility.

The new raised red-brown lesions are very important in this case. The involvement of the right eyelid, facial swelling, and bilateral shotty cervical lymph nodes are typical of KS. The oropharynx should be carefully examined for red-brown lesions, especially the roof of the mouth, since this is a favorite site for KS. Likewise, stool for occult blood should be checked and may be positive with GI KS involvement.

The spleen tip most probably just represents advanced HIV and is nonspecific, but could indicate *M. avium* or lymphoma. KS only rarely involves the spleen.

The most efficient way to obtain a diagnosis in this patient would be to evaluate the skin and pulmonary findings. A skin biopsy should be performed to confirm suspected KS and to rule out the occasional case of bacillary angiomatosis, which can mimic KS.

The chest x-ray abnormalities and mild hypoxia also need evaluation. An arterial blood gas will determine the severity of the hypoxia. Sputum for PCP is easy enough to obtain if the patient has a productive cough. If negative, a bronchoscopy with lavage will rule out PCP and will also evaluate the patient for other infections and KS lesions.

In this patient, both a skin biopsy and bronchoscopic biopsy were positive for KS. The enlarged spleen was not involved with tumor, but was just a manifestation of systemic illness with visceral involvement with KS. This patient required systemic treatment with chemotherapy.

See Box 24-1 for a summary of the diagnosis.

BOX 24-1
Summary of Diagnosis of Kaposi's Sarcoma

Usually raised red-brown lesion
Always biopsy to establish diagnosis and rule out bacillary angiomatosis
Pulmonary and GI involvement common
HHV-8 *always* present
Most common in men who have sex with men

> **BOX 24-2**
> **Therapeutic Options for HIV-Related Kaposi's Sarcoma**
>
> **OBSERVATION**
>
> **LOCAL THERAPY**
> Topical altretinoin (Panretin gel)
> Cryotherapy
> Radiation therapy
> Intralesional chemotherapy
>   Vincristine
>   Vinblastine
>   Bleomycin
>   Interferon
>
> **SYSTEMIC THERAPY**
> Interferon
> Chemotherapy
>   Adriamycin, bleomycin, vincristine
>   Liposomal doxorubicin (Doxil)
>   Liposomal daunorubicin (Daunoxome)
>   Paclitaxel (Taxol)
> Angiogenesis inhibitors
>   TNP-470
>   Pentoxifylline
>   Thalidomide
>   Anti-VEGF
>   Interleukin-12

Natural History

HIV-related KS is a nonmalignant growth that can be totally benign, requiring no therapy, or widely spread and as deadly as any malignancy, even with therapy. Twenty percent of acquired immunodeficiency syndrome (AIDS) patients currently develop KS at some time during the course of their illness, but this number is decreasing. Although half of patients with skin KS have internal organ involvement, only 10% ever develop clinical symptoms.

Therefore the course of a patient with KS is quite variable, and many palliative therapies can improve the patient's quality of life. In general, the depth and duration of immunosuppression in the individual patient tend to correlate with a worse prognosis.

Treatment

When a diagnosis of KS is made, there are several therapeutic options (Box 24-2). For localized disease, observation only may be a reasonable option. In a patient with only a few lesions that are not cosmetically or medically a problem, no immediate therapy is necessary, since KS is not currently a curable disease. Careful attention to HAART with a regimen that increases CD4+ counts and lowers viral load may actually treat the KS by enhancing immune system function.

Several therapeutic options exist for the KS patient with localized skin lesions only. Alitretinoin (Panretin) is a 9-cis-retinoic acid that comes as a gel and is applied topically to KS lesions as often as four times a day. Response rates approach 50% with this new agent, which probably works via angiogenesis inhibition. Side effects are modest and include rash at the application site and pain/itching.

Intralesional therapy was popular in the 1980s before the advent of more effective and less toxic systemic therapy. Vincristine, vinblastine, bleomycin, and interferon have all achieved modest success, but their intralesional use has declined due to patient discomfort of injection and poor response.

Radiation therapy is an attractive option for localized KS. Painful and/or swollen lesions can be treated very effectively with a short course of radiation to areas like the soles of the feet, groin, rectum, face, or any other similar small field requiring palliation. Scarring or fibrosis of the skin can occur postradiation.

Interferon-α systemically has produced clinically significant responses in some patients with KS. Its mechanism of action is not fully understood, but probably includes angiogenesis inhibition. Its efficacy is usually confined to those patients with CD4+ counts over 200 cells/mm^3. Its principal toxicities of fever, chills, and myalgias are much worse and efficacy much less in those patients with CD4+ counts below 200 cells/mm^3.

Systemic chemotherapy for most any form of KS, localized or systemic, has enjoyed great success thanks to the novel liposomal technology used to deliver these drugs. Initially, regimens such as Adriamycin, bleomycin, and vincristine (ABV) were quite successful, but their side effects were a significant problem. Patients experienced nausea and vomiting, hair loss (Adriamycin), fevers (bleomycin), and myalgia/arthralgias/neuropathy (vincristine). In addition, myelosuppression was common and posed significant problems for the already immunocompromised patient. Finally, cumulative doses of Adriamycin had to be monitored to avoid cardiotoxicity.

Liposomal technology has eliminated many of the problems of systemic chemotherapy in the KS patient and is highly effective because of the particular growth characteristics of the tumor. Liposomal doxorubicin (Doxil) or liposomal daunorubicin (Daunoxome) encapsulates the active chemotherapy molecule in a tiny liposomal sphere. The liposomes are dissolved in aqueous solution and injected. The liposomes circulate systemically and stay within the circulation until they encounter a blood vessel wall that is "leaky." By their very nature, the blood vessels of KS are abnormal and more permeable than normal blood vessels. The liposomes "leak" through these vessels into the KS lesions. Soon thereafter, the liposomes are metabolized and release the chemotherapeutic agent into the lesion. Nuclear medicine studies have demonstrated this very mechanism in vivo using liposomes in animal tumor models. Studies in patients have demonstrated high concentrations of chemotherapy in KS skin 48 hours after injection with no active drug in adjacent normal skin using this liposomal delivery system. In addition, the side effect profile of Doxil and Daunoxome is remarkably low. Patients experience virtually no nausea and vomiting, hair loss, or cardiac toxicity. Care must still be taken to avoid clinically significant myelosuppression. Response rates to these liposomal drugs are quite high, with most patients achieving lesion flattening, decreased color, decreased swelling, and decreased size to some extent. Administration is likewise very convenient for the patient, consisting of a 30- to 60-minute infusion in the outpatient setting every 2 weeks. A maximum response is usually seen after 4 to 6 treatments, after which therapy may be stopped or continued at longer intervals. Time to initial lesion regression is usually 2 to 3 weeks, while time to regrowth of the KS lesion following cessation of treatment is usually 3 months.

Another active chemotherapy drug comes from the taxane family and is called paclitaxel (Taxol). It is also very effective, but its tendency to cause side effects has usually made it a second choice. Hair loss is the principal toxicity and is usually profound. Myelosuppression can also occur. Anaphylaxis can occur in 1% of patients receiving this drug.

A word about steroids in the treatment of KS is in order. Steroids can play a role in the management of the KS patient to relieve clinically significant swelling or pain. They are also effective antiemetics when given prior to chemotherapy. However, their general use should be discouraged, since they seem to enhance the growth of KS lesions and can further suppress the immune system of the HIV-infected patient.

Since abnormal angiogenesis plays such an important role in HIV-related KS, angiogenesis inhibitor therapy has been an active area of investigation. Several agents including TNP-470, pentoxifylline, thalidomide, vascular endothelial growth factor (VEGF) inhibitors, and IL-12 are currently under study. Likewise, since HHV-8 plays an instrumental role in the pathogenesis of KS, studies with antivirals to treat HHV-8 to prevent the development of KS or to treat KS if it is already present are underway.

When to Refer

Whenever possible, a biopsy diagnosis of KS should be made to rule out the occasional case of bacillary angiomatosis. Observation or topical therapy can be performed in the primary care setting, but the patient should be referred if more widespread skin disease develops and/or if internal organ involvement is suspected.

KEY POINTS

- About 50% of patients with skin Kaposi's sarcoma will have internal organ involvement
- Only 10% of internal organ involvement is symptomatic
- Steroids may exacerbate lesions if given too long
- Treatment with liposomal anthracyclines is very effective and has low toxicity

Lymphoma
Presentation and Progression

Cause. The principal type of lymphoma in HIV-infected patients is non-Hodgkin's lymphoma. Although the incidence of Hodgkin's disease is greater in HIV-infected patients, it is not as common as the non-Hodgkin's variety. HIV-related non-Hodgkin's lymphoma increased at an alarming rate throughout the 1980s and mid-1990s, growing by 21% each year. HAART did not decrease this trend according to data up through 1996, but recent observations suggest that the incidence is now decreasing with the advent of the protease inhibitors.

Approximately 3% to 4% of HIV-related lymphoma will be the patient's first AIDS-defining illness. However, it is more often a manifestation of previously diagnosed AIDS, accounting for 16% of AIDS deaths. Different from KS, no specific group is at increased risk for the development of lymphoma. Intravenous drug abusers, transfusion recipients, homosexual men, hemophiliacs, and heterosexual HIV-infected patients are all equally likely to develop lymphoma. For a brief time, it was believed that there was an association between zidovudine use and the appearance of lymphoma, but a case-control study dispelled this belief.

The best hypothesis currently to explain the occurrence of malignant lymphoma in the HIV-infected patient is that it occurs after prolonged, relentless B cell stimulation that finally goes awry. The probable sequence of events leading up to lymphoma begins early on after HIV infection when a polyclonal hypergammaglobulinemia develops as a consequence of T cell malfunction. Diffuse benign lymphadenopathy also occurs in some patients secondary to the chronic antigenic challenge of HIV. HIV-infected monocytes and T lymphocytes release cytokines IL-6 and IL-10, which enhance B cell proliferation. EBV infection may also play a role in some patients at this stage.

With so much polyclonal B cell stimulation going on, it is postulated that an error then occurs by random chance at the genetic level and a single clone of B cells is established. In fact, certain pathologic subtypes of lymphoma tend to correlate with different genetic errors. For example, immunoblastic lymphomas will usually have DNA from EBV in their genome. Small noncleaved lymphomas have a genetic malfunction from the c-myc oncogene, and diffuse large cell lymphoma overexpresses the gene product from the bcl-6 oncogene. HHV-8 plays very little role in this tumor compared with its role in KS, but there is one subtype of lymphoma that presents primarily in so-called body cavities. HHV-8 expression is commonly found in these body cavity lymphomas.

Presentation. HIV-related non-Hodgkin's lymphoma may be the patient's first AIDS-defining illness (3% to 4%), or more commonly it will present in a patient with already established AIDS. In contrast to non-HIV lymphomas that usually involve lymph nodes and occasionally spread to extralymphatic sites such as the liver and bone marrow, HIV lymphoma often involves non–lymph node sites and in some cases may not involve lymph nodes at all. Unusual extralymphatic sites of involvement include bone, buttocks, heart, head and neck structures, and GI or pulmonary sites. A central nervous system (CNS) mass lesion is a particularly bad site of initial presentation and usually occurs in a patient with far advanced AIDS who has no lymphoma elsewhere. However, cerebrospinal fluid (CSF)-positive leptomeningeal spread of lymphoma in a patient who already has lymphoma outside the brain does not confer such a grave prognosis.

In the general population non-Hodgkin's lymphoma histologies are categorized as low, intermediate, or high. HIV-related non-Hodgkin's lymphoma histology is typically intermediate to high grade. Consequently, the tumor is quite metabolically active so that the patient rarely presents with a long history of an asymptomatic lymph node or mass. There is usually a period of days to weeks when the patient experiences constitutional symptoms such as fever, night sweats, weight loss, or a symptom localizing to the area of greatest bulk disease. Since constitutional symptoms are nonspecific in HIV-infected patients, a diagnosis of lymphoma may not be suspected initially, but the evolution of symptoms and/or localizing signs within a few weeks usually leads to the early consideration of lymphoma as a diagnosis.

Some patients are quite metabolically active at the time of diagnosis. Because of the tendency of the tumor to grow rapidly, electrolyte and acid-base disturbances may be striking. Patients may be in an active tumor lysis syndrome at presentation, with elevated potassium, phosphate (with reciprocal calcium depression), uric acid, creatinine, and a metabolic lactic acidosis with respiratory compensation. Death is imminent at this stage without prompt diagnosis and treatment.

Case 1. A 28-year-old man tested positive for HIV 1 year ago. He had a history of thrush and shingles, but no other opportunistic infections or neoplasms. His CD4+ count was 10 cells/mm^3 and his viral load was 30,000 copies/ml. He was started on zidovudine, lamivudine, and efavirenz. He tolerated these medications well, but 1 year later his CD4+ count was only 40 cells/mm^3 and his viral load was 1,000 copies/ml.

He presented to the emergency room with a several-day history of abdominal pain and diarrhea. His temperature was 100° F orally and his examination was remarkable for no lymph node enlargement, but a right lower quadrant mass was palpated. CAT scan revealed a large right lower quadrant mass, possibly arising from the bowel, and hilar and mediastinal adenopathy with a large right pleural effusion. Percutaneous fine-needle aspirate and a core biopsy of the right lower quadrant mass were positive for an immunoblastic, B cell non-Hodgkin's lymphoma (high grade) with EBV in the tumor DNA. Pleural fluid was chylous and positive for lymphoma cells.

Laboratory values were quite remarkable, with a potassium of 6.0 mEq/l, phosphate of 8.0 mEq/l, uric acid of 12 mg/dl, LDH of 4,000 units, and a pH of 7.12 from lactic acidosis. Creatinine was 2.4 mg/dl and glucose was 30 mg/dl.

The patient was transferred to the intensive care unit for impending respiratory failure and intubated. Pressors were started to support a falling blood pressure. Electrolyte and acid-base disturbances were treated with volume and bicarbonate. Chemotherapy was initiated with cyclophosphamide, doxorubicin, vincristine, and prednisone (CHOP), and allopurinol was given to treat the elevated uric acid.

Within just a few days, the right lower quadrant mass was difficult to feel and the pleural effusion was markedly decreased. The patient was extubated and pressors were discontinued. G-CSF was given after chemotherapy to blunt the WBC nadir. A total of six courses of CHOP chemotherapy were required to achieve a complete remission and the patient remains free of relapse some 12 months after diagnosis. His antiretroviral regimen now includes a protease inhibitor, and his CD4+ count is 200 cells/mm^3 with an undetectable viral load.

Although this patient has achieved a complete remission, his median survival is still precarious because of his CD4+ count of less than 50 cells/mm^3 at the time of diagnosis and therapy. However, maintenance of his CD4+ count above 200 cells/mm^3 with protease inhibitor–based therapy may allow a prolonged remission.

Case 2. A 53-year-old man presents complaining of a right neck mass for 3 weeks and difficulty chewing. He denies fevers and nights sweats, but has a 15-lb weight loss. On his current antiretroviral regimen, the CD4+ lymphocyte count is 250 cells/mm^3 and viral load is undetectable. On examination his temperature is 99° F and there is a 4 × 4–cm right neck lymph node. There is a large pink ridge of tissue bulging from the gingiva at the base of his teeth on the lower right jaw. A spleen tip is palpable.

Laboratory reveals a mild anemia and normal renal function, but LDH is 450 units. CAT scans reveal a mass at the angle of the right jaw extending into the right cervical lymph nodes, normal chest, and enlarged spleen and several enlarged periaortic lymph nodes. Bone marrow and CSF are negative for lymphoma.

Biopsies of the right cervical lymph node and right buccal mucosal mass are positive for a diffuse, small noncleaved B cell lymphoma, with overexpression of the c-myc oncogene.

He was treated with cyclophosphamide, doxorubicin, and etoposide (CDE) infusional therapy for 4 days, repeated every 28 days. Antiretroviral therapy was continued during treatment. After six cycles, he is in complete remission and has remained so for 1 year of follow-up.

This patient stands an excellent chance of continuing in remission given his CD4+ count over 50 cells/mm^3 at the time of diagnosis and therapy.

Diagnosis

A diagnosis of lymphoma in an HIV-infected patient is a constant possibility. As patients live longer with HIV, they live longer with some degree of immunosuppression, which carries a constant risk of transformation from benign lymphoid hyperplasia to malignant lymphoma. The best way to make a diagnosis of lymphoma is to always suspect this possibility and to watch for its appearance.

Constitutional symptoms of fever, night sweats, and weight loss are usually indicative of infection; but if none is found, lymphoma should always be suspected. Likewise, unexplained lymphadenopathy *or* a mass in any location should be biopsied if other diagnoses are not made after a reasonable amount of time.

The diagnosis is ultimately made via biopsy of a lymph node or suspicious mass lesion. Aspirate cytology is usually not enough for the pathologist when lymphoma is being considered. Histologic architecture is most important along with immunophenotyping, and only a biopsy can provide enough material for these studies.

Once a diagnosis is made, complete work-up includes a CAT scan of the chest, abdomen, and pelvis. A bone marrow biopsy and CSF analysis are also needed to rule out involvement in these areas. Gallium or positron emission tomography (PET) scanning may also be helpful to evaluate response to therapy.

See a summary of the diagnosis in Box 24-3.

Natural History

The natural history of HIV-related non-Hodgkin's lymphoma depends on the response to therapy and the extent of immunosuppression. Untreated, this tumor will usually be fatal in a matter of weeks to months. Chemotherapy is always necessary to treat this tumor, since it behaves as a systemic, widespread disease, even when localized at presentation. With modern chemotherapy, complete remission rates of over 50% have been observed, but remission rates are very dependent on the patient's HIV status at the time of diagnosis. With a CD4+ count of less than 50 cells/mm^3, complete remission rates are only 35%, with a median survival of only 5 months. With a CD4+ count of over 50 cells/mm³, complete remission rates are 65%, with a median survival of 18 months, and many patients in this better prognostic category are alive and free of lymphoma over 5 years later. A list of several prognostic factors is given in Box 24-4.

Stage and location of lymphoma do not affect the chance for remission, except for the case of primary CNS lymphoma. A primary CNS presentation of HIV lymphoma without any other sites of disease confers a particularly bad prognosis. This presentation usually occurs in the patient with far advanced AIDS. Patients rarely survive beyond 6 months no matter what the therapy, which up to now has consisted of radiation therapy with or without chemotherapy.

Treatment

The mainstay of therapy in HIV-related lymphoma is multidrug chemotherapy. Even when a lymphoma appears to be localized, treatment with radiation alone has met with early relapse from distant unsuspected sites. Therefore HIV-related lymphoma is always treated as a systemic disease.

There are several chemotherapy regimens that have been successful and they include the CHOP regimen, mBACOD (methotrexate, bleomycin, doxorubicin, cyclophosphamide, dexamethasone), and CDE. All three chemotherapy regimens can produce durable complete remissions, but the chance for complete remission and the length of remission depend on the severity of the HIV-related immunosuppression at the time of diagnosis. Because of the tendency for HIV-related lymphoma to involve the CNS, all patients should have a spinal tap with CSF analysis for lymphoma cells. If positive, intrathecal therapy is added to the treatment regimen. If negative, patients may still receive intrathecal therapy if they are high risk to develop leptomeningeal disease. This would include patients with high-grade histology or bone marrow involvement.

Studies thus far indicate that patients with CD4+ lymphocyte counts less than 50 to 100 cells/mm³ have shorter survival, whereas those with CD4+ lymphocyte counts over 50 to 100 cells/mm³ can do very well from a lymphoma standpoint. However, in either risk category, if a patient should relapse, his or her chance for successful remission and survival again is quite poor. The treatment of patients with such relapses is currently an area of active investigation.

One of the most difficult areas for current and future therapy in HIV-related lymphoma is how to integrate HAART into the treatment regimen. Some of the antiretroviral drugs, especially the protease inhibitors, may significantly alter chemotherapy drug metabolism and vice versa, resulting in the potential for several scenarios in which either the HIV or the lymphoma may be undertreated or overtreated. Given this potential problem, some advocate withholding HAART entirely during the chemotherapy period. Others advocate continuing the antiretroviral regimen no matter what, so as not to lose ground against the HIV during chemotherapy. Results of studies are eagerly awaited to answer the questions of when and how to integrate HAART into the treatment process.

BOX 24-3
Summary of Diagnosis of Lymphoma

Commonly involves extralymphatic sites such as bone, bone marrow, and GI and pulmonary regions
Obtain tissue, not just cytology, for diagnosis
Send tissue for immunophenotyping and cytogenetics along with regular pathology studies
Complete staging should include CAT scans of chest, abdomen, and pelvis, bone marrow biopsy, and lumbar puncture
Systemic therapy should begin promptly after diagnosis

BOX 24-4
Factors Associated with Shorter Survival

CD4+ count less than 100 cells/mm³
Patient older than 35 years
History of injection drug use
Stage III or IV disease
Elevated lactate dehydrogenase

When to Refer

A patient with a biopsy diagnosis of HIV-related lymphoma should be referred to an oncology center familiar with such patient care. However, if a patient is suspected of having lymphoma and biopsy is contemplated, every effort should be made to obtain an actual biopsy and not just cytology. In addition, tissue should be held for special studies such as flow cytometry and gene rearrangement if the regular histology suggests lymphoma.

KEY POINTS

- Non-Hodgkin's lymphoma is most common type
- Histology usually intermediate to high grade
- Always treat as a systemic disease
- Primary CNS lymphoma occurs in advanced AIDS and carries poor prognosis
- About 3% to 4% present with lymphoma as initial manifestation of AIDS
- Certain viral (EBV) genes and oncogenes (c-myc and bcl-6) may be expressed in these lymphomas

---

Cervical Cancer
Presentation and Progression

Cause. Cervical cancer and its precursor lesion, cervical intraepithelial neoplasia (CIN), are closely linked to prior infection with human papillomavirus (HPV). In fact, certain HPV strains are associated with different degrees of CIN. HPV 6 and 11 are seen with condyloma and early dysplasia (CIN 1). CIN 1 usually does not progress to cervical cancer. HPV types 16, 18, 31, 32, 33, 35, and some of the 50s can lead to greater degrees of cervical dysplasia (CIN 2 + 3) and can be followed by frank neoplasia.

In the precursor lesion (CIN) cells, the HPV DNA travels as a plasmid and does not integrate into the host genome. However, in actual cervical cancer, the HPV DNA is found fully integrated into the host DNA. The HPV gene encodes for certain proteins, termed E6 and E7, which facilitate malignant transformation. The E6 protein inactivates the P53 tumor suppressor gene, and the E7 protein inactivates the retinoblastoma gene. Without normally functioning P53 or retinoblastoma genes, cell cycle activity is uncontrolled, and excessive cell growth can occur.

Presentation. Since HIV and HPV are both spread via sexual contact, HPV infection, with its tendency to CIN and cervical cancer, should always be suspected in any HIV-infected woman. Fifty-eight percent of HIV-infected women were HPV-positive in a National Institutes of Health (NIH) study versus only 26% of HIV-negative controls. The HPV infection rate is higher if the CD4+ count is lower. Seventy percent of HIV-infected women were HPV-positive if the CD4+ count was less than 200 cells/mm^3.

The presence or absence of gynecologic symptoms at presentation depends on the extent of the lesion. Precancerous lesions such as reactive, atypical, or CIN dysplasia are usually asymptomatic. However, patients with cervical cancer are usually symptomatic and most often present with irregular vaginal bleeding. Pelvic examination will usually reveal a mass, which may extend to adjacent structures.

If a routine Pap test suggests some degree of atypia, the patient must return for further evaluation. Invasive cervical cancer usually presents in the 40- to 50-year-old woman, but preinvasive changes can occur some 15 years earlier and will often be associated with an abnormal Pap test (CIN 1, 2, and 3). It may take as many as 7 years to progress from CIN 1 to 3 and another 5 to 7 years to progress from CIN 3 to invasive cancer. Conversely, CIN 1 lesions will regress spontaneously in 40% of patients. Risk factors for any dysplasia include multiple sex partners, early pregnancy, early sexual activity, sexually transmitted diseases (STDs), and cigarette smoking, in addition to HPV infection (Box 24-5).

Case 1. A 34-year-old HIV-infected woman presents for routine gynecologic examination. She has a history of condyloma, but denies any abnormal vaginal discharge or bleeding. She is sexually active with several partners. Her Pap test is positive for atypical cells only. Repeat Pap test 3 months later reveals CIN 1. HPV serology is positive for type 6. Since 40% of CIN 1 lesions regress spontaneously, no colposcopy or biopsy is performed. Repeat Pap test 3 months later shows improvement with atypical cells only. Continued periodic Pap testing every 3 months is recommended until at least two Pap tests are normal in a 6-month period.

Case 2. A 42-year-old HIV-infected woman presents for routine Pap testing. Previous Pap tests have been positive for atypia. She is asymptomatic. Her current CD4+ count is 120 cells/mm^3. Her Pap test is positive for CIN 2. HPV serology is positive for type 16. Loop evaluation and biopsy are performed to attempt to find and remove the entire lesion. The procedure is successful, and pathology reveals clear margins with complete excision of the CIN 2 lesion. Close follow-up every 3 to 6 months is recommended, since the relapse rate is 50% in HIV-infected patients, especially in those with lower CD4+ counts.

BOX 24-5
Risk Factors for Cervical Neoplasia

HIV
Human papillomavirus
CD4+ count less than 500 cells/mm^3
Early sexual intercourse, multiple partners
Smoking

BOX 24-6
Malignancies in HIV Infection

AIDS-DEFINING MALIGNANCIES
Kaposi's sarcoma
B cell lymphoma
Cervical carcinoma

NON–AIDS-DEFINING MALIGNANCIES
Hodgkin's disease
Squamous carcinoma
  Head and neck
  Anus
Melanoma
Plasmacytoma
Adenocarcinoma of the colon
Small-cell lung carcinoma
Germ cell (testicular) tumor
Basal cell tumor

BOX 24-7
Summary of Diagnosis of Cervical Cancer

Annual Pap test after two negative Pap tests, 6 months apart
CIN 1 spontaneously regresses in 40%
CIN 2 and 3 require complete, margin-free excision
About 50% of HIV CIN 2 and 3 patients relapse after 1 year

Diagnosis

In 1993, the Centers for Disease Control and Prevention (CDC) added cervical cancer to the list of AIDS-defining malignancies (Box 24-6). The CDC also recommended that HIV-infected women have an annual Pap smear, but only *after* two successive normal smears, performed 6 months apart. Even so, some clinicians favor testing every 6 months to be safe. The Pap test and its reliability have come under fire. Some studies of HIV-infected women have produced unacceptably high false-positive and false-negative results. However, this disparity has not been confirmed by others so that Pap testing still remains the best routine screening test in this patient population.

If the Pap test is abnormal, the degree of the abnormality dictates the next step in diagnosis and therapy. A reactive or atypical histology should be repeated in 3 to 4 months. If still abnormal, colposcopy with consideration for cervical biopsy should be performed. Since the degree of immunosuppression tends to correlate with the tendency to develop cervical dis-

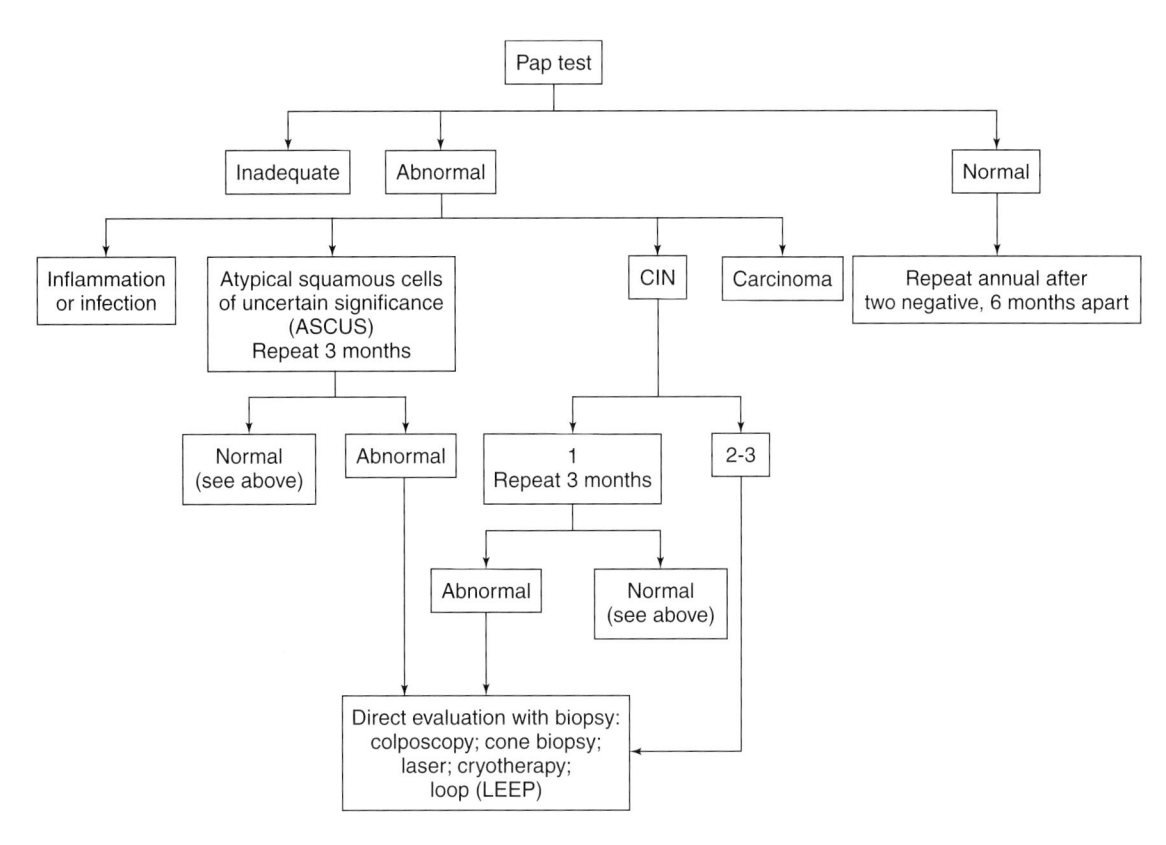

FIG. 24-4 Pap test algorithm.

ease, closer follow-up is especially important in the patient with lower CD4+ counts (less than 200 cells/mm^3).

See Box 24-7 for a summary of diagnosis.

Natural History

Once CIN is diagnosed, HIV-positive women tend to behave at first like their HIV-negative counterparts. CIN 1 changes may spontaneously regress in as many as 40% of patients. However, CIN 2 and 3 changes may have a different natural history in the HIV-infected patient. Properly treated, only 5% to 10% of HIV-negative women will experience recurrence 1 year later, whereas 50% of HIV-positive women will relapse after 1 year.

Invasive cervical cancer in HIV-positive women is usually more advanced at diagnosis than in HIV-negative women and may spread to unusual sites. It is more difficult to treat for cure because of the tendency to disseminate rapidly. Surgery and radiation therapy are employed the same as in the HIV-negative woman. Chemotherapy usually plays only a palliative role.

It is still unknown what change, if any, HAART will have on the natural history of cervical cancer and precancerous changes. Since cervical neoplasia is associated with lower CD4+ counts, it is anticipated that more effective antiretroviral therapy will decrease the frequency of these lesions.

Treatment

Treatment depends on the histologic grade and stage of the lesion diagnosed (Fig. 24-4). For reactive or atypical changes on the Pap test, a follow-up Pap test in 3 to 4 months is indicated. If an abnormality persists, direct cervical visualization via colposcopy with biopsy should be performed.

If a precancerous dysplastic lesion (CIN) is detected by Pap test, therapy depends on the grade of the lesion. For CIN 1, some 40% of women will regress spontaneously. No initial therapy is required, only repeat biopsy in 3 to 6 months. CIN 2 and 3 must be surgically removed, with the goal being to achieve negative margins. There are several techniques to accomplish this. They include cryosurgery, laser ablation, cone biopsy, or LEEP (loop electrosurgical excision procedure). The LEEP technique is very attractive because it allows direct visualization of the lesion and therapy at the same time. Lesions identified by prior colposcopy can then be biopsied and removed simultaneously with the LEEP technique. Complete excision rates with this procedure are quite high. In fact, the high relapse rate of CIN in HIV-infected patients probably reflects the fact that the premalignant changes in HIV are more widespread than usual, allowing a greater chance for incomplete resection.

Medical therapy with topical agents like 5-fluorouracil or the retinoids has met with some success in uncontrolled studies. An HPV vaccine to prevent infection with this virus is also under investigation.

If invasive cervical cancer is diagnosed, the stage dictates the treatment. An early stage I invasive cancer confined to the cervix can be treated with either cone biopsy or LEEP excision or simple hysterectomy. Radical hysterectomy is best reserved for larger stage I tumors. Radiation is given after primary surgery for either advanced stage I or stage II and greater.

The use of chemotherapy provides a dilemma for the locally advanced cervical cancer patient. Since patients with this stage often progress rapidly and often have advanced HIV disease, chemotherapy is best reserved for palliation. However, a recent National Cancer Institute alert documented a significantly improved outcome in all women with locally advanced cervical cancer who received cisplatin chemotherapy in addition to their radiation. Additional studies will be necessary to conclude if this also applies to HIV-infected women with cervical cancer.

When to Refer

Pap smears should be performed annually after two normal Pap tests, 6 months apart. Patients should be referred for colposcopy and/or biopsy if a reactive/dysplastic Pap test is not normal on repeat examination *or* if changes of CIN are detected of any grade.

▶ KEY POINTS

- Human papillomavirus infection tightly linked to pathogenesis of cervical dysplasia/cancer
- Cervical cancer and pre cancer more common when CD4+ count less than 200 cells/mm³
- Most CIN and cervix cancer relapse is due to incomplete resection
- Cervical cancer is preceded 7-15 years by CIN dysplasia

Anal Neoplasia
Presentation and Progression

Cause. There is a growing awareness that HIV infection and/or receptive anal intercourse is associated with anal neoplasia. Anal neoplasia can be either a noninvasive precancer or an invasive carcinoma. The noninvasive precancer is generally referred to as anal intraepithelial neoplasia (AIN). Synonyms would be dysplasia, squamous intraepithelial lesion, or carcinoma in situ.

Men who have sex with men are the highest risk group to develop a precancerous anal or AIN lesion. HIV infection and a falling CD4+ count were found to raise this risk even further early on in the HIV epidemic. There were 348 HIV-positive and 260 HIV-negative men evaluated for AIN 4 years after an initial normal evaluation. High-grade AIN developed in 19% of HIV-negative men and 30% of HIV-positive men with CD4+ counts over 500 cells/mm³. The incidence increased to 52% in HIV-positive men with CD4+ counts less than 200 cells/mm³. Positive smoking history is also significantly correlated with AIN risk.

Similar to the scenario of HPV infection and the risk of cervical cancer in women, HPV infection is strongly associated with anal neoplasia. The pathogenesis is very likely the same as it is in cervical cancer (see the section on Cervical Cancer). The oncogenes of HPV (HPV types 16, 18, 31, 33, and 35) infect the anal epithelial cells via sexual transmission. Viral gene products E6 and E7 bind to host P53 and retinoblastoma proteins, respectively. P53 and retinoblastoma proteins regulate cellular growth. If the function of these so-called tumor suppressor proteins is lost, malignant transformation can occur. The evidence thus far concerning HPV infection rates and HIV has documented the strong epidemiologic association between HPV and the development of anal neoplasia. HPV DNA probes have found HPV in anal precancer and invasive cancer.

TABLE 24-2
Relative Risk of Anal Cancer Among Never-Married Men Compared with Ever-Married Men in Urban Areas

Dates	Relative risk	95% confidence interval
1973-1978	5.8	0.9-8.7
1979-1984	6.7	4.7-9.5
1985-1989	10.3	7.5-14.1

P(trend)—0.02.
From Northfelt DW, Swift PS, Palefsky JM: Anal neoplasia, *Hematol Oncol Clin North Am* 10(5):1181, 1996.

There is also strong evidence to support the association of HIV and anal receptive intercourse with the development of anal neoplasia. Both New York City and San Francisco reported marked increases in anal cancers in never-married men during the first years of the HIV epidemic (Table 24-2), with the greatest increase in the HIV-infected man. Furthermore, the incidence of anal cancer in a homosexual man with recently diagnosed AIDS is now 40 times the general population.

Presentation. HIV-infected patients commonly have GI complaints as a consequence of their underlying disease or therapy. The protease inhibitors also can cause diarrhea and rectal irritation from frequent bowel movements, so symptoms specific to the anorectal area may be missed initially. Nevertheless, the clinician should be attuned to the symptoms of rectal bleeding, discharge, or pain. Most early lesions (AIN) will be asymptomatic, while invasive cancer will usually have symptoms of bleeding, pain, or constipation.

Case 1. A 34-year-old HIV-infected man is in for a routine follow-up. He takes a protease inhibitor combination regimen and feels well except for occasional diarrhea. His CD4+ count is 240 cells/mm³ and viral load is undetectable. Rectal examination is negative except for anal warts. Anal Pap test reveals an early dysplasia (AIN 1). Anoscopy is negative.

The patient is reassured that this is an early, precancerous lesion that often regresses spontaneously. Repeat anal Pap test in 6 months is normal, and routine anal Pap testing is scheduled for another 6 months.

Case 2. A 41-year-old HIV-infected man complains of occasional blood in stool. His CD4+ count is 80 cells/mm³ and viral load is 12,000 copies/ml. He is taking a protease inhibitor–containing regimen, which he tolerates poorly. Rectal examination is negative, but anal Pap test is positive for high-grade dysplasia (AIN 3). Anoscopy reveals a 1-cm raised, red lesion that is excised. Pathology reveals high-grade dysplasia (AIN 3) lesion, and cryoablation is performed to "sterilize" the area. Four quadrant biopsies are negative for any other lesion.

No further invasive procedures are performed, and follow-up resumes with every 3- to 6-month anal Pap testing.

Diagnosis

Assuming that a precancerous anal lesion is likely to progress to an invasive anal cancer, screening programs would offer a reasonable approach to intervene before this progression can occur. A screening program would be most appropriate for the high-risk patient. High-risk factors to develop anal neoplasia include HIV-positive, anal receptive intercourse, CD4+ count below 500 cells/mm^3, anal condyloma, and smoking (Box 24-8). Any symptoms such as anal discharge or bleeding, pruritus, or pain would make investigation even more important. The screening test could be an anal Pap test, anoscopy, or colposcopy. Although the best screening test is not known, the anal Pap test is fairly reliable and simple to perform. A wet Dacron swab is inserted at least 2 cm from the anal verge and withdrawn while rotating. Smears are prepared and fixed in the usual manner for a Pap test.

The appropriate frequency of screening is unknown. The asymptomatic, high-risk patient could be screened annually. The patient with any precancer AIN on examination should be followed up every 3 to 6 months. Such a screening program in HIV-infected men who have sex with men was judged cost-effective in a recent cost benefit analysis.

If screening detects no lesion or only an early dysplasia (AIN 1), a follow-up Pap test annually is reasonable. If a Pap test detects a high-grade dysplasia (AIN 2 or 3), direct visualization with anoscopy or colposcopy should be performed.

The symptomatic patient may have an invasive cancer. If Pap test and/or biopsy diagnoses an invasive cancer, then complete staging should be performed to evaluate the extent of disease. Testing should include a CAT scan of the abdomen and pelvis and a full colonoscopy.

See Box 24-9 for a summary of diagnosis.

Natural History

In the HIV-infected female, screening for cervical cancer in the precancer stage has offered patients the promise of earlier intervention in a cost-effective manner to diagnose and treat dysplastic lesions, before they can progress to invasive cancer. A similar strategy for HIV-infected patients and anal neoplasia may or may not be appropriate. Does AIN always progress to invasive cancer? The answer is not known. We know low-grade AIN can regress without therapy. High-grade AIN may progress to invasive cancer, but data to document this slowly progressive process, which takes years of follow-up, have been lacking. Perhaps the reason we are not yet sure is that patients have been dying of AIDS before they can develop invasive cancer. If so, the advent of HAART and longer life with HIV/AIDS may increase the incidence of anal cancer.

However, what if HAART lowers the frequency of anal neoplasia by restoring some degree of immune function? Patients with KS and CMV retinitis have decreased their need for disease-specific therapy just because of a rising CD4+ count. To date, follow-up studies to evaluate this issue in the protease inhibitor era do *not* demonstrate that HAART is decreasing the incidence of anal neoplasia.

Treatment

The safest approach is to assume that precancerous (AIN) lesions will presumably progress to invasive cancer. Therefore

---

BOX 24-8
Risk Factors for Anal Neoplasia

HIV
Human papillomavirus
Anal receptive intercourse
CD4+ count less than 500 cells/mm^3
Smoking

BOX 24-9
Summary of Diagnosis of Anal Neoplasia

Routine screening for anal neoplasia can be performed with Pap testing
Early dysplasia (AIN 1) usually regresses spontaneously
High-grade dysplasia (AIN 2 or 3) will likely progress to invasive cancer

---

such precancerous lesions should be treated aggressively and completely, depending on the degree of dysplasia.

Most early dysplastic lesions (AIN 1) will regress spontaneously, so anal Pap testing should be repeated in 3 to 6 months to document regression. A high-grade dysplastic anal Pap test (AIN 2 or 3) requires further investigation to completely ablate the lesion. Four-quadrant biopsy is performed in addition to detect an occult abnormality. The abnormal area viewed on anoscope or colposcopy is ablated with electrocautery, cryotherapy, or laser. High-grade dysplasia (AIN 2 or 3) can relapse, so careful follow-up testing should be employed on a regular 3- to 6-month basis.

Alternative therapies for dysplasia are under development. A very small lesion might be treated with topical cytotoxic therapy such as podophyllum resin or 5-fluorouracil. A vaccine against the HPV viral protein E7 is under development. Also, a novel adenovirus, type ONYX-015, has been cloned via recombinant gene technology. This adenovirus is toxic to cells that do not express the P53 tumor suppressor protein. Cells infected with HPV and expressing HPV protein E6 do not express P53 protein as a consequence of the HPV infection, so they would be targeted by this recombinant adenovirus.

Studies of HIV-infected patients with invasive anorectal cancer suggest that they tend to do worse when treated like the general population. This is because they have more advanced HIV and because they have more morbidity from the chemotherapy and radiation therapy employed. More recent information suggests that standard chemotherapy (5-fluorouracil and mitomycin or cisplatin) and radiation therapy for HIV-infected patients with invasive anorectal cancer are better tolerated with better results in the patient who is only mildly to moderately immunocompromised. Advanced AIDS patients still do poorly with aggressive treatment.

When to Refer

Routine screening for anal neoplasia with anal Pap testing is a procedure that can be practiced in the office after becoming familiar with the procedure. Patients with high-grade (AIN 2 or 3) anal Pap tests or those with palpable lesions should be referred for direct visualization procedures for biopsy and lesion ablation.

Any suspicious anal lesion, with or without an abnormal Pap test, should be referred to a medical or surgical oncologist or gastroenterologist for biopsy and treatment.

KEY POINTS

Anal neoplasia is more common in patients with:
⊃ HIV
⊃ Human papillomavirus
⊃ CD4+ count below 500 cells/mm^3
⊃ Anal receptive intercourse

SUGGESTED READINGS

Aoki Y et al: Angiogenesis and hematopoiesis induced by Kaposi's sarcoma–associated herpesvirus-encoded interleukin-6, *Blood* 93:4034, 1999.

Bigger RJ, Rabkin CS: The epidemiology of AIDS-related neoplasms, *Hematol Oncol Clin North Am* 10(5):999, 1996.

Monini P et al: Reactivation and persistence of human herpesvirus-8 infection in B cells and monocytes by Th-1 cytokines increased in Kaposi's sarcoma, *Blood* 93:4044, 1999.

Sande MA, Volberding PA, editors: *The medical management of AIDS,* Philadelphia, 1997, WB Saunders.

Straus DJ et al: Prognostic factors in the treatment of human immunodeficiency virus-associated non-Hodgkin's lymphoma: analysis of AIDS Clinical Trials Group protocol 142-low-dose versus standard-dose m-BACOD plus granulocyte-macrophage colony-stimulating factor, *J Clin Oncol* 16(11):3601-3606, 1998.

Tulpule A, Matheny SC: AIDS-related malignancies, *Prim Care* 25(2):473-482, 1998.

25 HIV Infection in Children and Adolescents

RICHARD M. RUTSTEIN, BRET J. RUDY

Introduction

Human immunodeficiency virus (HIV) infection was recognized in children soon after the first cases of the acquired immunodeficiency syndrome (AIDS) were reported in adults. As of the end of 1998, there were an estimated 1.2 million children less than 15 years old living with HIV/AIDS worldwide. Yearly, more than 500,000 infants are born with HIV infection. In addition, there are 8 million uninfected children who have lost one or both of their parents to HIV infection. In the United States, through 1998, there have been 8,500 cases of pediatric AIDS, with more than 90% occurring secondary to perinatal transmission.

Early reports on HIV-infected children stressed the rapid progression of immunodeficiency and early death. With the advent of antibody testing in 1985, and prospective longitudinal studies of HIV-infected neonates, it became clear that these "rapid progressers" only represented 25% to 40% of infected children. The majority of HIV-infected children follow a less rapid course, with symptoms developing in the middle of the first decade, and a median survival (prior to the use of highly active antiretroviral therapy [HAART]) of 8 to 12 years. In recent years, children have benefited from combination therapies, with decreased morbidity and increased survival.

The first part of this chapter is devoted to an overview of the epidemiology and clinical aspects of perinatally acquired HIV infection. In the second part we will cover aspects of HIV infection unique to adolescents.

Perinatally Acquired HIV Infection
Epidemiology

The vast majority of new pediatric infections are acquired perinatally. Transfusion-acquired infections are now rare in the United States and in most developed countries. Sexual abuse has been implicated in several cases, but the true extent of transmission via this route is unknown. Despite several well-publicized cases of pediatric HIV infection potentially transmitted within a home environment (over the nearly 20 years of the epidemic in this country), casual contact in the home has not been proven to be associated with transmission. Pooling data from two studies, there were no documented transmissions among families enrolled, covering more than 1,500 person-years. All of the cases of potential horizontal transmission described to date most likely involved exposure to the blood of an infected individual.

Perinatal transmission may occur in utero, intrapartum, or postpartum via breast-feeding. The actual timing and mechanisms underlying in utero and intrapartum transmission are still unknown. In utero infection is defined as having occurred when an infant is positive on viral testing (by blood co-culture or polymerase chain reaction [PCR] DNA assay) within the first 48 hours of life. Intrapartum infection is defined as having occurred in infants with negative viral tests in the initial 48 hours, but positive tests after 2 weeks of age. It is believed that in the absence of breast-feeding, approximately 25% of perinatally transmitted infections occur in utero, and the remaining 75% intrapartum. In areas where breast-feeding is common, the incidental risk of HIV infection from breast-feeding is in the range of 14% to 25%.

The prevalence of HIV infection among pregnant women varies widely worldwide. In the United States, the overall rate is believed to be between 0.15% and 0.2% (1 to 2/1,000 pregnant women), with an estimated 6,000 to 7,000 infants born each year to HIV-infected pregnant women. Prevalence rates as high as 6% to 8% have been reported from individual hospitals in urban areas in the United States; these rates pale in comparison with the prevalence rates of 10% and 35% reported from prenatal sites in the Caribbean and sub-Saharan Africa, respectively.

Worldwide, perinatal transmission rates range from 13% to 48%. In developing countries, a significant proportion of perinatal transmission occurs postnatally, secondary to breast-feeding. It has been estimated that the additional risk of transmission related to breast feeding is 0.5% per month of breast-feeding; another estimate is of an additional overall risk of 14% to 25% for breast-feeding. In the United States and Europe, where breast-feeding is discouraged for HIV-infected new mothers, reported transmission rates have ranged from 13% to 30%.

Women with high viral loads, low CD4+ counts, previous AIDS diagnosis, prolonged rupture of membranes (more than 4 to 8 hours), chorioamnionitis, and preterm delivery (prior to 34 weeks gestation) are at increased risk of having infected infants. When all factors are taken into account, maternal viral load is the main predictor of mother-infant transmission. In two perinatal studies no transmission was documented for women with undetectable viral loads (a total of 164 women with undetectable viral loads, many of whom were on antiretroviral therapy [ART], were included in the two studies). However, it must be kept in mind that there are reports of HIV transmission from mother to infant when the mother had an undetectable viral load, and there are women with very high viral loads who do not transmit the virus to their newborns.

Prevention of Perinatal Transmission

One of the major successes in the fight against HIV has been the remarkable decrease in perinatal transmission rates. The landmark National Institutes of Health (NIH)-sponsored multisite trial (ACTG 076) demonstrated the efficacy of perinatal zidovudine therapy in reducing transmission of HIV. Pregnant HIV-infected women with CD4+ counts higher than 200 cells/mm^3 were randomized to receive placebo or oral zidovudine from week 26 of gestation until the beginning of labor, intravenous placebo or drug during labor, and 6 weeks of placebo or oral zidovudine for the newborn. Transmission was decreased from 20% in the placebo group to 8% in the treatment group. In follow-up studies, transmission rates as low as 4% to 5% have been noted among women on the perinatal zidovudine regimen.

Decreased rates of mother-infant transmission have also been reported using modifications of the 076 treatment protocol. In studies in Africa and Asia, 1 month of prenatal oral zidovudine, followed by oral zidovudine during labor, with no infant therapy, decreased perinatal transmission by 50%. Transmission was also decreased with combined intrapartum and postnatal zidovudine therapy, although not to the extent seen in the original NIH 076 study. No effect was seen with intrapartum zidovudine therapy only.

In a study of an abbreviated course of dual drug therapy, intrapartum oral zidovudine and lamivudine, followed by 1 week of postnatal zidovudine/lamivudine therapy for the infant, reduced perinatal transmission by 37%. Lastly, one dose of oral nevirapine during labor, combined with a single infant dose by 72 hours of life, decreased infection by almost 40% when compared with short-course zidovudine therapy. Although these studies are not directly comparable because they were conducted in different areas of the world, with variations in maternal stage of illness, delivery practices, and allowances for breast-feeding, they do indicate that in resource-poor areas even short-course perinatal therapy has the potential to save lives.

Despite the success with these shorter courses of therapy, in developed countries the standard of care for therapy during pregnancy remains, at a minimum, zidovudine given as in the 076 treatment protocol (antenatal, intrapartum IV, and postnatally for 6 weeks). It should be stressed that perinatal zidovudine monotherapy would be the minimally acceptable therapy, applicable only to women with normal CD4+ counts and low viral loads. For all other women, combination therapy, as prescribed for nonpregnant women, would be the standard of care.

With increasing numbers of women infected with zidovudine-resistant virus, up to 10% in some areas, newer therapies to prevent perinatal transmission are desperately needed. Pharmacokinetic and safety data are needed on ART combination therapy for pregnant women and their neonates. There are small series of women treated with dual or triple ART (including protease inhibitor [PI]-containing combinations) during pregnancy; from these small studies, transmission rates appear to be well below 5%.

The risks of prenatal maternal HAART to the fetus have not been fully defined. In one study, the incidence of premature birth was increased in women on dual and triple therapy. This has not yet been confirmed with other studies, however. A large French study on the use of zidovudine/lamivudine for pregnant women reported two of the children developed a rare mitochondrial disease. Although these data have not been replicated, they underscore the importance of worldwide surveillance of women treated with ART during pregnancy and the need for long-term follow-up of children exposed in utero to ART.

The route of delivery also appears to impact on the risk of perinatal transmission. Combined United States and European data support the concept that prolonged rupture of membranes (more than 4 to 8 hours) increases the risk of HIV transmission to the infant, and elective cesarean section (defined as when the mother is not in active labor, and membranes are intact) decreases the risk. In a multicenter trial in Europe, women were randomized to elective cesarean section (E-CS) versus routine care. For the first 400 mothers/infants in the trial, those delivered by E-CS had a transmission rate of 1.8% versus 10.8% for those delivered vaginally. In addition, a large meta-analysis of perinatal treatment trials showed that when combined with perinatal zidovudine therapy, E-CS further decreased transmission (from 7.3% to 2.0%). The reduction in transmission was less marked in women taking perinatal zidovudine. HIV-infected pregnant women have a slightly higher rate of morbidity following surgical delivery, primarily postpartum fevers and infections.

There are no data available comparing outcomes of women on HAART delivered vaginally with women treated with zidovudine monotherapy and E-CS. For women already on HAART, with suppression of viral replication, the additional protective benefit of elective cesarean sections remains to be determined. Until these questions are answered, decisions on choice of perinatal therapy and mode of delivery must be made between individual women and their health care providers. In August of 1999, the American College of Obstetricians and Gynecologists (ACOG) issued a recommendation that HIV-infected women should be offered E-CS at 38 weeks of gestation.

In this fast-moving field, HIV-infected pregnant women must be informed of their therapeutic choices, and followed at centers with expertise in the field. Treatment of HIV-infected pregnant women should only be undertaken in consultation with HIV specialists.

It is imperative that all women receive counseling about, and be offered, HIV testing early in pregnancy. In addition, special efforts must be made to enroll and retain HIV-infected women in prenatal care. One of the barriers to the prevention of perinatal transmission has been the high rate of late/inadequate prenatal care among HIV-infected women. All centers must provide culturally sensitive, nonjudgmental care to HIV-infected/at-risk women, so as to remove as many barriers as possible that prevent women from remaining in care.

Testing

All infants born to HIV-infected women will be HIV enzyme-linked immunosorbent assay (ELISA)- and Western blot–positive at birth, by virtue of the transplacental transmission of immunoglobulin G (IgG) anti-HIV antibodies. These maternal antibodies are detectable in the infants' blood stream until 15 to 18 months of age. Therefore a positive HIV antibody test in an infant less than 18 months of age indicates HIV exposure, not infection. The antibody test is used to confirm an infant's exposure when the mother's serostatus is unknown.

The most reliable means of diagnosing HIV infection in infancy is by the use of the HIV blood co-culture or HIV PCR DNA assay. Both tests have a greater than 95% specificity and sensitivity for infants greater than 1 month of age. The culture appears to be slightly more sensitive and specific, but is technically more difficult and availability is limited. Only 30% of infected infants will be PCR-positive at one day of life, but more than 90% will be PCR-positive at ages greater than 21 days. Cord blood should not be used, since there are increased rates of false-positives.

Official recommendations are to perform the DNA PCR assay on day 1 of life, and repeat at 1 month of age and again at 3 to 5 months of age. A positive PCR should be repeated immediately. If the PCR assays at 1 month and 3 to 5 months of age are negative, the child is considered HIV-uninfected. Most centers suggest following the child at 3-month intervals until seroreversion (to HIV antibody negative status) is documented. The HIV RNA PCR test may prove to be an alternative test for HIV infection in infancy, but until further data are available, the qualitative DNA PCR should be used for diagnostic purposes.

For children over 18 months of age, the HIV ELISA (and Western blot, if positive) is usually sufficient. Two positive HIV ELISA/Western blot assays confirm HIV infection in children over 18 months of age. In rare cases, children may have negative antibody testing despite HIV infection. In children with parents at risk for infection, and illnesses compatible with HIV infection, further testing (HIV PCR DNA, CD4+ counts) may be considered. Consultation with a specialist is recommended.

For older infants and children, testing is indicated when family members are found to be positive (regardless of the health of the child). For neonates in whom the mother's HIV status is unknown, HIV antibody testing is recommended at the first well child visit. In addition, testing should be considered for the conditions noted in Box 25-1. The most common clinical presentations of HIV infection in children include failure to thrive (FTT), recurrent severe bacterial infections (pneumonia, bacteremia), idiopathic thrombocytopenic purpura (ITP), chronic parotitis, lymphocytic interstitial pneumonitis (LIP) noted on an incidental chest x-ray (a chronic reticulonodular infiltrate), and severe rapidly progressive pneumonia (indicative of *Pneumocystis carinii* pneumonia [PCP]).

Immunologic Evaluation

CD4+ counts are age specific. In infancy, absolute CD4+ counts range from 1,500 to 5,000 cells/mm^3, with mean values around 3,000 cells/mm^3. The absolute CD4+ counts then decrease slowly with age, reaching adult values (700 to 1,000 cells/mm^3) around age 7 (Box 25-2).

Immunoglobulin levels are elevated in more than 95% of HIV-infected children, and may be the first abnormal immunologic test noted, with IgG serum levels usually elevated to twice the normal values by 3 to 6 months of life.

Viral loads encountered in early childhood are much higher than seen in the adult population. Most infants have HIV RNA levels over 100,000 copies/ml. In the first year of life, viral loads average 185,000 copies/ml. They then decrease slowly, to levels more commonly seen in adults, by age 4. Although there is considerable overlap, higher levels in infancy are associated with increased risk of rapid progression of illness.

BOX 25-1
Indications for HIV Testing

Parents at risk for HIV infection, or known to be HIV-infected
Neonates when mothers' HIV status is unknown
Children/adolescents with documented sexually transmitted diseases and/or sexual abuse
Children with the following clinical conditions
   Failure to thrive
   Generalized adenopathy
   Hepatosplenomegaly
   Recurrent or chronic thrush, especially in children >2 yrs of age
   Chronic parotitis
   Chronic diarrhea
   Recurrent pneumonias/bacteremia
   Idiopathic thrombocytopenic purpura
   Severe pneumonia in an infant, or pneumonia unresponsive to initial antibiotics
   Progressive encephalopathy/loss of developmental milestones
   Lymphoid interstitial pneumonitis/reticulonodular infiltrate on chest radiograph

---

BOX 25-2
Revised Human Immunodeficiency Virus Pediatric Classification System

CLINICAL CATEGORIES

N = Asymptomatic
A = Mildly symptomatic (with two or more of the following chronic conditions: adenopathy, hepatomegaly, splenomegaly, dermatitis, parotitis, recurrent/chronic sinusitis/otitis media)
B = Moderately symptomatic (anemia, one episode of invasive bacterial infection, persistent thrush, cardiomyopathy, recurrent/chronic diarrhea, hepatitis, recurrent herpes simplex virus, more than one episode of zoster, lymphocytic interstitial pneumonitis [LIP], idiopathic thrombocytopenic purpura, disseminated varicella)
C = Severely symptomatic (any AIDS-defining condition with the exception of LIP)

IMMUNE STATUS

	CD4+ COUNT (% CD4+)		
Category	<12 months	1-5 years	6-12 years
1	>1,500 (>25)	>1,000 (>25)	>500 (>25)
2	750-1,499 (15-24)	500-999 (15-24)	200-499 (15-24)
3	<750 (<15)	<500 (<15)	<200 (<15)

In older children, viral loads are associated with prognosis and response to medication. For children over 1 year of age, risk of disease progression is associated with viral loads higher than 100,000 copies/ml and CD4+ % of less than 15%. As in adults, viral loads and CD4+ counts should be measured every 3 months in stable patients.

Clinical Presentation and Diagnosis

With the recommendation for routine testing of all pregnant women, many infected infants in urban areas are identified through testing in the neonatal period. For infants not diagnosed in early infancy, the clinical presentation may include FTT, generalized adenopathy, hepatosplenomegaly, recurrent thrush, frequent invasive bacterial infections, or most ominously, acute severe pneumonia refractory to standard antibiotic therapy (usually with PCP as the etiology). All infants admitted for FTT should have an evaluation for HIV infection. In addition, any child at any age should be HIV tested if his or her mother is found to be HIV-infected.

HIV-Related Infections. Table 25-1 lists the relative frequency of various AIDS-defining conditions in HIV-infected children. In general, LIP, although quite rare in HIV-infected adults, is the AIDS-defining illness for more than one third of HIV-infected children. Conversely, cytomegalovirus (CMV) retinitis and HIV-related lymphomas are unusual in children compared with the frequency in adults. Noted below are aspects of AIDS-defining conditions distinctive to the pediatric population.

Pneumocystis carinii Pneumonia. PCP remains one of the most common AIDS indicator illnesses in children. The majority of children with PCP present between 3 and 9 months of age, and are generally not known to be HIV-infected at the time of diagnosis of PCP. The presentation is that of a rapidly progressive pneumonia. Unlike the more varied, and at times indolent, clinical course seen in adults, the vast majority of infants with PCP present acutely ill and deteriorate rapidly, frequently requiring intubation within 24 hours of admission. The lactate dehydrogenase (LDH) is usually elevated at the time of diagnosis. Definitive diagnosis is made by histologic demonstration of the organism in lung fluid. Treatment is with high-dose trimethoprim-sulfamethoxazole, with adjunct steroid therapy.

In the first year of life, CD4+ counts are not predictive of risk of PCP in HIV-infected infants. Therefore all infected infants should receive PCP prophylaxis (150 mg/m2/day, in two divided doses, three days/week). After the age of 12 months, prophylaxis is offered to infected children with low (age-adjusted) CD4+ counts. In addition, all HIV-exposed infants, and at-risk older children/adolescents undergoing evaluation for HIV infection, should be placed on PCP prophylaxis until HIV infection is ruled out.

Lymphocytic Interstitial Pneumonitis. LIP is an AIDS-diagnosis illness distinct to pediatrics. Pathologically, there is an intense lymphocytic infiltration of the alveolar septa. Presumptive diagnosis may be made by chest radiographs revealing a reticulonodular pattern. Several studies have linked LIP to chronic immune stimulation, usually secondary to Epstein-Barr virus (EBV) infection. Many patients with LIP remain asymptomatic, and the chest x-ray findings improve as the children age and, paradoxically, as their immunodeficiency worsens. For patients with LIP who develop chronic lung disease, with resting hypoxemia, a definitive diagnosis is based on biopsy findings. Once confirmed, treatment with a prolonged course of steroids is indicated. Any HIV-infected patient on long-term steroids should also receive PCP prophylaxis.

Recurrent Bacterial Infections. Invasive recurrent bacterial infections (RBI) are more common in HIV-infected children than adults, and represent the AIDS diagnosis for 20%. The risk of pneumococcal bacteremia has been estimated at 10% per year for the first 3 years of life. There is a subgroup of children at risk for RBI. These children include those with two or more episodes of invasive bacterial disease, or one episode of invasive disease and B cell dysfunction as indicated by failure to mount an antibody response to childhood immunizations. Monthly immunoglobulin infusions, or chronic antibiotic therapy, may be indicated in these patients. The conjugate pneumococcal vaccine may afford some protection against pneumococcal disease in the first 2 years of life.

Disseminated Mycobacterium avium Complex. Disseminated *Mycobacterium avium* complex (DMAC) disease occurs in 5% to 10% of infected children, usually in children older than 6 years who are severely immunodeficient (CD4+ lower than 100 cells/mm^3). The presentation is generally that of an older school-aged child with prolonged high fevers, often accompanied by distinct gastrointestinal symptoms. Although no controlled studies have been performed on the efficacy of prophylaxis against DMAC in pediatric patients, based on adult data children with CD4+ counts lower than 100 cells/mm^3 should be offered either weekly azithromycin or daily therapy with either clarithromycin or rifabutin.

Cognitive Development and Encephalopathy. Secondary central nervous system (CNS) infections and complications (stroke, neoplasms, opportunistic infections [OIs]) are less common in pediatric patients than in adults. The most catastrophic CNS effect of pediatric HIV infection is a progressive encephalopathy (PE).

The diagnosis of PE is based on a loss of developmental milestones or a more than 15-point decrease in cognitive ability, and/or impaired head/brain growth associated with cerebral atrophy on neuroimaging, with or without basal ganglion calcifications, or acquired abnormalities in gross motor skills. In the pre-HAART era, the incidence of PE was 20%, with a peak age onset of symptoms of 12 to 24 months of age. The

TABLE 25-1
Pediatric AIDS-Defining Illnesses

Illness	Relative frequency (%)
Pneumocystis carinii pneumonia	24
Recurrent bacterial infections	20
Lymphoid interstitial pneumonitis	20
Progressive encephalopathy	17
Wasting syndrome	15
Disseminated *Mycobacterium avium* complex	6
Cytomegalovirus disease	6
HIV-related lymphoma	1

Modified from Centers for Disease Control and Prevention: *HIV/AIDS Surveillance Report* 8:1-40, 1996.

vast majority of cases of PE are diagnosed prior to age 3. The occurrence of PE is associated with increased risk of early mortality, generally within 24 months of diagnosis.

In addition to the PE, HIV-infected children are at an increased risk for a static encephalopathy. Up to 20% of infected children will be diagnosed with a static encephalopathy and/or specific learning disability, with or without attention deficit/hyperactivity disorder (ADHD).

Recent data suggest that in the absence of PE, children with HIV infection have stable developmental levels, without slow decrements of cognitive function as they age. It also appears that the incidence of PE has decreased in the era of HAART. Because of the frequency of neurocognitive deficits associated with perinatal HIV infection, all HIV-infected children should have neurodevelopmental testing at least yearly.

Management

Immunizations. Secondary viral and bacterial infections cause significant morbidity and mortality in HIV-infected children. Immunizations provide one means of protecting this population against common childhood pathogens. In general, the routine childhood immunization schedule is followed, with several modifications (Table 25-2). As with all immunocompromised children, poliovirus vaccine inactivated (IPV) should be substituted for all polio doses.

Although a live virus vaccine, the measles-mumps-rubella vaccine (MMR) is administered to infected children, except for those children with the most severely depressed CD4+ counts (class 3 immune status). Immunoglobulin should be given to unimmunized or nonresponding HIV-infected children during community measles outbreaks.

The results of a recent multisite NIH study support administration of the varicella vaccine to asymptomatic HIV-infected children. Safety studies of the varicella vaccine in children with advanced HIV disease are underway. It is recommended that exposed but uninfected children of HIV-infected adults should receive the varicella immunization, as transmission to susceptible persons following childhood immunization is a very rare event, and less likely to occur than following community-acquired infection.

HIV-infected children with varicella exposure should receive varicella-zoster immune globulin (VZIG) within 96 hours of exposure. There are also suggestive data that postexposure acyclovir treatment may prevent or ameliorate varicella in nonimmune contacts.

The conjugate pneumococcal vaccine is recommended for all infants. It is particularly important to immunize HIV-infected infants, since they are at such high risk for invasive disease. Yearly influenza immunizations are also recommended for HIV-infected children.

As would be expected for an immunocompromised population, HIV-infected infants and children have a significantly decreased response to childhood immunizations. The response rate, and titer of protective antibodies, is lower in infected children. Over one third of infected children will fail to produce protective antibody levels following immunization with measles (as a component of MMR) and hepatitis B. Although the response to the primary series of *Haemophilus influenzae* type B (HIB) vaccines is decreased (with 50% of children not developing antibody titers higher than 1.0 μg/ml,

TABLE 25-2
Immunizing the HIV-Infected Child

DTaP	Routine schedule
HIB	Routine schedule
Hepatitis B	Routine schedule
OPV/IPV	IPV only
MMR	Routine schedule, omit if immune class 3
Varicella	Administer to asymptomatic children and exposed, uninfected children. Safety and efficacy not established for symptomatic children
Influenza A/B	Yearly, once >6 months of age
Pneumococcal	Conjugated heptavalent vaccine at 2, 4, 6, and 12-15 months

considered adequate for long-term protection), following the booster dose a near normal response rate is seen.

Following completion of the primary series and, if needed, booster doses of vaccines (HIB; diphtheria, tetanus, and acellular pertussis [DTaP]; hepatitis B; and measles), postimmunization titers should be checked. If the response is inadequate, an additional booster is recommended, since a proportion of nonresponders will develop adequate titers following an additional dose of vaccine.

As with adults, mild increases in viral loads have been noted in children following immunizations. The increases are less in those on stable ART regimens; in general, the viral loads return to baseline values within 6 to 8 weeks of immunization. Most importantly, viral loads should not be checked within 2 months of an immunization to avoid finding a transient and misleading elevation.

Antiretroviral Treatment. As is the case for HIV-infected adults, recommended ART for infants and children dictates the use of three- or four-drug combinations (so-called HAART regimens), including at least one PI. State of the art guidelines have been published, and are readily available on the internet through the National Pediatric and Family HIV Resource Center. The guidelines are updated on line at regular intervals.

As an alternative to PI-containing combinations (PI-C), based on data from several small treatment studies, a non-nucleoside reverse transcriptase inhibitor (NNRTI) can be substituted for the PI. In addition, as another alternative to PI-C, triple nucleoside reverse transcriptase inhibitor (NRTI) therapy (zidovudine/lamivudine/abacavir) is under study in children. In some patients, the use of dual therapy, although suboptimal in terms of virologic response, may be an acceptable first-line therapy based on compliance issues or family preferences.

HAART in children has been associated with measures of virologic and immunologic improvement. As treatment protocols are now short-term studies of dosing, safety, and efficacy, large studies with clinical end points are not underway. However, anecdotal evidence indicates major gains in improved quality of life and decreased morbidity in children on HAART. Data from our center comparing the pre-HAART era with the present treatment regimens noted major clinical gains since the introduction of HAART (Table 25-3). These included decreased hospitalizations/100 patients, decreased hospital inpatient days/admission, decreased hospital inpatient days/patient, decreased occurrence of new OIs, and decreased mortality (from 5.8% 1-year mortality to no deaths in the first 12 months following the initiation of HAART in our clinic).

Although the use of HAART in a pediatric setting has resulted in the above noted clinical outcomes, the magnitude and duration of viral response to HAART in children have been less than found in adult studies. For treatment-naive patients, suppression of virus to less than 400 copies/ml is reported in 50% to 80% of children enrolled in clinical treatment protocols compared with the more than 75% to 85% response rate reported for triple-therapy regimens in naive adults. For previously treated children, suppression of viral load to less than 400 copies/ml is reported in 25% to 60% of patients. In one of the largest pediatric studies to date, NIH ACTG 338, stable HIV-infected children on NRTI therapy were randomized to dual- or triple-drug ritonavir-containing combinations; approximately 60% of patients had a drop in viral load to less than 400 copies/ml. In our review of experience from a clinical setting with the use of PI-C for older, ART-experienced children, only 32% of patients developed viral loads less than 400 copies/ml, although 85% of these patients (27% of the overall group) maintained viral suppression for at least 8 months.

The lower rate of virologic suppression in the pediatric setting compared with adults may be due to one of several factors, including children's higher baseline viral load, their immature immune system response to HIV, poor/inadequate drug exposure, and nonadherence. As noted earlier, children frequently enter therapy with higher baseline viral loads; several adult studies have found that baseline viral loads are inversely related to the chance of achieving viral suppression to levels below 400 or 50 copies/ml. In addition, perinatal HIV infection may disarm the immune system to a greater degree than adult-acquired infections (possibly accounting for the fact that in perinatal infection the time to reach a viral "set-point" is measured in years, not the months as seen in newly infected adults).

Pharmacokinetic monitoring indicates marked differences in overall systemic drug exposure in children. Oral absorption may be decreased or drug metabolism increased in infants and children. For instance, using the powdered formulation of nelfinavir, infants may require dosing that is near the total adult dose and may require three daily doses, in contrast to the well-accepted twice-daily dosing schedule employed for adults.

The problems of compliance/adherence found in treating adult patients are magnified in the pediatric population. In one study, more than 30% of families self-reported poor adherence to ART medication schedules (as indicated by omitting more than 20% of weekly doses). Of pediatric nonresponders to new treatment regimens, over 75% of families self-report poor adherence. It must be remembered that self-reports of compliance with medication schedules severely overestimate compliance.

TABLE 25-3
Impact of Combination Therapy on Pediatric HIV Infection

	1995-1996	1997-1998	p value
Infected patients	88	99	
Age (months)	65	81	<0.01
Patients on >2 ART medications	1%	67%	<0.01
Hospital admissions/patient/year	0.73	0.56	0.02
Inpatient days/patient/year	6.1	2.6	<0.05
New OIs or class C	12.5%	4%	<0.05
Mortality (12 month)	5.7%	0	<0.05

Data from the Children's Hospital of Philadelphia, Special Immunology Family Clinic.
ART, Antiretroviral therapy; *OIs*, opportunistic infections.

Central to the problem of poor compliance for pediatric patients is the lack of palatable liquid or suspension formulations for children too young to swallow capsules or pills. Of the currently available PIs, saquinavir and indinavir have no child-friendly formulation. The liquid preparations of ritonavir and amprenavir are refused by many children because of their distinctive bitter taste and high alcohol content. The nelfinavir powder is rejected for its grittiness and sweet taste. This makes the choice of, and compliance with, HAART regimens particularly difficult for infants. In contrast to the PIs, the NRTI and NNRTI agents are generally available in relatively child-friendly formulations.

The frequency of dosing is a major issue in choosing HAART regimens, as are food requirements/restrictions (such as the requirement that didanosine be administered on an empty stomach, and the extra fluid intake required with indinavir). Even with simplified dosing and palatable formulations, many children have behavioral issues around medicine-taking, adding further stress to the family. In some instances, where the main barrier to adherence has been the medicine-taking behavior of the child, pediatricians have resorted to the placement of gastrostomy tubes to facilitate medication administration. Many families also have other life stressors (inadequate housing, lack of adequate health insurance, lack of refrigeration) that make compliance with complex medication schedules difficult. Home visits have been extremely helpful to our team to get a true sense of the patient and his or her family in the home environment, and offer a visible sign of our support for the family. During a home visit, suggestions to simplify dosing schedules and improve administration of drug doses can be made and modeled.

For the future, there is hope that dosing regimens will be less complex; the NNRTI efavirenz is approved for once-daily dosing, and it appears that didanosine may also be dosed once daily. In the drug development process are at least two PIs that are touted as requiring only once-daily dosing. The hope is that within the next few years, there will be full HAART regimens active with only single daily dosing. As with adults, when faced with young patients who present with problems that place them at risk for poor adherence, clinicians may want to start with a simplified initial regimen, using the more palatable of the medicines, with less frequent dosing. PI-sparing therapy may also be considered, using three NRTIs (zidovudine/lamivudine/abacavir) or two NRTIs and one NNRTI. For instance, twice-daily stavudine with nighttime doses of didanosine (at least 2 hours after eating) and efavirenz would be a possible regimen with reasonable efficacy (and simplicity) in a treatment-naive population.

It is important to note that the long-term effects of HAART regimens on growing children are unknown. Up to 10% of children on PI-C regimens will develop changes in body fat reminiscent of the adult lipodystrophy syndrome. The incidence of increased cholesterol and triglyceride levels with PI-C regimens in children is not yet known, nor is the long-term effect of modestly elevated lipoprotein levels. As we begin to foresee the possibility of HIV-infected children and adults surviving for decades, not years, on HAART therapy, charting the long-term side effects of such therapies becomes increasingly important.

Prognosis. Before the advent of HAART for HIV infection, the median survival of perinatally infected children was in the range of 7 to 10 years. There was a subgroup (25% of the total group) who became symptomatic early in life, and usually succumbed to the illness by age 5. With HAART therapy, survival has been markedly improved. At our center, yearly mortality fell from more than 5% to 0 from 1996 to 1999 with the use of triple therapy. It is clear that many, if not most, perinatally infected children will now survive at least into their mid-late adolescence.

There is a cohort of older, treatment-experienced children and adolescents who, like their adult counterparts, have had treatment experience with most of the agents in each of the classes of antiretroviral agents. For these patients, new agents with retained potency for multiply resistant virus or that target novel viral sites are urgently needed.

Disclosure. One of the issues unique to pediatric HIV care is the issue of disclosure of the diagnosis to infected children. Unlike other pediatric chronic and/or fatal illnesses (e.g., cancer, cystic fibrosis), the diagnosis of HIV still carries with it the risk of significant social ostracism and discrimination. In addition, parents are understandably wary of discussing the diagnosis with children in fear that the children will then tell others (friends, teachers, relatives). For parents, disclosure requires that they face their own diagnosis and issues of denial of their disease, as well as their guilt and despair about transmission of the illness to their child.

Issues regarding disclosure are best dealt with in the context of a culturally sensitive, nonjudgmental team approach, with an appreciation that disclosing the diagnosis to the child is just one step in a long process of providing psychosocial support to the family.

Day Care and School Issues. The American Academy of Pediatrics (AAP) periodically releases policy statements on the care and management of HIV-infected and exposed infants and children. HIV-infected children should attend regular school programs. Nationwide, all school systems are instructed in universal precautions. The most recent AAP statement notes that gloves are not necessary in the general day-to-day care of HIV-infected infants (bathing, feeding, diaper changes). In general, infants and children should be encouraged to attend local preschool and school programs.

There are no cases of proven transmission of HIV infection within a school setting. Although two cases of potential spread of HIV via biting were reported early in the HIV epidemic, despite the frequency of biting behavior in preschool programs, this route has never been proven to result in HIV transmission between children.

Most states protect the confidentiality of the student in regards to HIV status, and do not require disclosure to school officials or on school health forms. Community providers unsure of local requirements should seek consultation with the nearest pediatric HIV specialty center prior to completing school health forms or disclosing a child's status to school officials. The treating physician and child's family need to be made aware of school outbreaks of certain infectious diseases (such as varicella and measles), since exposure to these agents requires prophylactic therapy for the child.

Prevention. With aggressive perinatal management, more than 90% of perinatal HIV infections can now be prevented (decreasing the transmission rate from 20% to 2%). Major barriers remain, including the failure to offer HIV testing to all pregnant women, and the high rate of inadequate or late prenatal care for many HIV-infected or at-risk women.

Despite the major advances in preventing perinatal HIV transmission and in the treatment of infected children, our primary goal must be the ultimate prevention of infection in susceptible adolescents and adults. Continued education and attempts at behavior change among adolescents and adults must remain a national priority.

Vaccine development holds out the only hope for true global control of HIV, but it remains a distant goal. In the meantime, primary prevention efforts in adolescents and adults, and targeted secondary prevention in HIV-infected women of childbearing age, must continue to be a major part of our national HIV treatment plan.

Adolescents and HIV

Adolescents pose unique issues for the practitioner caring for HIV-infected persons. Adolescents go through a series of both physical and psychosocial stages during puberty. These stages of development influence how adolescents deal with their changing body, peer relations, and stressors that confront them in everyday life. In addition, as their bodies change, the metabolism of some medications changes, thus influencing dosing in this age group. Thus it is essential that practitioners recognize these unique stages of adolescence and use this understanding as they approach HIV counseling and testing as well as care for the HIV-infected adolescent.

Epidemiology

It has been estimated, through adult studies based on new AIDS cases reported to the Centers for Disease Control and Prevention (CDC), that one in four new HIV infections occurs in persons under the age of 22. However, from surveys performed at centers providing care for HIV-infected children and adolescents, very few young people are engaged in care and are therefore underrepresented in reporting to the CDC. There are two possible reasons for this discrepancy in the numbers of adolescents suspected as infected compared with those engaged in care. First, adolescents may often be unaware of their infection, since they often do not seek HIV counseling and testing. Second, adolescents who are aware of their infection may not be adequately linked to HIV care in centers providing comprehensive HIV care services. Thus both of these issues may contribute to the low numbers of HIV-infected adolescents engaged in care.

The risk factors for those infected and reported to the CDC do give some insight into those youth most at risk. In young men ages 13 to 19, male to male sexual transmission accounts for 33% of reported AIDS cases. This percentage increases to 63% in those young men ages 20 to 24. Thus men who have sex with men are an important risk category in young men, including adolescents. As will be discussed, many of these young men do not yet self-identify as gay because they are still in earlier stages of sexual identity formation. Thus counseling of these young men requires special attention and understanding of sexual identity formation.

Young women continue to be at great risk for infection. In young women, the most important mode of transmission is heterosexual. This mode of transmission accounts for 54% of AIDS cases in 13- to 19-year-old females and for 53% of cases in 20- to 24-year-old females. It is quite apparent from CDC data that many young women with AIDS are unaware of the risk categories of their male partners. As will be discussed, offering counseling and testing only to those young people who identify themselves as at high risk will only identify a small number of those youth actually infected.

Adolescent Development

It is essential that the medical care provider who is either providing HIV counseling and testing to adolescents or providing care to HIV-infected adolescents understands the psychosocial development of adolescents. Adolescence can be divided into three stages: early, middle, and late. During early adolescence, young people are primarily family-oriented, although they begin to strive for some autonomy. Their thought processes are still fairly concrete, and they are mainly concerned with their physical development as opposed to romantic relationships. During middle adolescence, 15 to 17 years, they develop increasing independence and develop a strong alliance with their peer group. The focus of young people in this stage of development is about fitting in with a peer group. Although abstract thinking begins to emerge during this stage, concrete thought processes dominate under stressful circumstances. This is also the stage in which there is increasing sexual experimentation. During late adolescence, ages 18 to 19, young people develop a more adult relationship with their parents. Their relationships become more intimate, with both friends and romantic interests. It is during this late stage when young people really develop strong abstract thinking and a future orientation. It is important to realize that these stages are a continuum, and every adolescent goes through them in his or her own unique process. However, using these stages as a foundation for building discussion and counseling can markedly enhance the interaction with the young person.

For young people with issues concerning sexual orientation, there are also stages of sexual identity formation; these stages again can help to form the foundation for understanding the young person. As described by Troiden, these stages can be broken down into the following: sensitization, sexual identity confusion, sexual identity assumption, and finally integration and commitment. In the first stage, sensitization, the young person feels different from his or her peers and may begin to understand that this difference is based on sexual attractions. In the second stage, sexual identity confusion, the young person begins to understand his or her attractions to persons of the same sex; however, he or she is confused as to how to function in society with such feelings and attractions.

During sexual identity assumption, the young person begins to experiment and explore a life as a gay or lesbian person. In the final stage, integration and commitment, the young person has resolved many of the conflicts surrounding a gay identity and can be himself or herself as a functioning member of society. It is during this stage that the young person is ready to share these feelings with others; it is also during this stage that the young person will self-identify as gay or lesbian. Again, these are rough stages; some people never make it to the last stage and thus always have difficulty sharing their sexual orientation with others. In counseling young people, if a provider were to identify a young person in the sexual identity confusion stage as gay, then the provider would be labeling the young person before that young person had reached that stage of sexual identity formation, sometimes with very deleterious results. Again, understanding where the young person is in terms of these stages of development can help to guide counseling and ongoing care.

In assessing the psychosocial situation of an adolescent, the SHADSSS (*S*chool, *H*ome, *D*epression/self esteem, *S*ubstance use, *S*exuality, *S*afety) assessment can be a useful tool. The idea behind the SHADSSS assessment is to help the clinician gain better insight into the world of the adolescent. It can help identify areas of the adolescent's life that are especially troublesome, so that such issues can be discussed and addressed.

Treatment

Care for the HIV-infected adolescent follows the same principles as that for adults and for younger children. The medication dosing for adolescents is dependent on the sexual maturation scale of Tanner. For those adolescents who are Tanner stage 1 or 2, the pediatric dosing regimens should be followed. Those adolescents who are Tanner stage 3 or 4 should be monitored very closely using either pediatric or adult dosing guidelines, as deemed appropriate. Adolescents who are Tanner 5 should follow adult guidelines for dosing and regimens. The use of prophylactic medications should also follow the guidelines as established for adults and outlined elsewhere.

Probably of greatest concern for those treating HIV-infected adolescents is the issue of adherence. Recently, the Health Resource Services Administration published a monograph dealing with the treatment of HIV-infected adolescents that focuses heavily on the topic of adherence. As noted in this publication, it is essential that the clinician prescribing ART for adolescents has an in-depth understanding of the adolescent's lifestyle so that the regimen can be tailored to best fit that lifestyle. Issues surrounding school, work, disclosure, and nutrition can strongly influence which antiretrovirals may best fit into the life of the adolescent.

The frequency of monitoring CD4+ T lymphocyte counts and plasma RNA levels in adolescents is the same as that followed for younger children or adults. There are some important issues surrounding the care of the HIV-infected adolescent that must be considered. First, screening both adolescent males and females for other sexually transmitted diseases is essential to their care. In addition, Pap smears for adolescent females should be performed every 6 months to monitor for early dysplasia. Adolescents can also benefit from peer support, since living with HIV infection is often a very isolating experience. The use of peer educators as well as peer support groups can be a great help in keeping the HIV-infected adolescent engaged in care.

HIV Counseling and Testing

All sexually active young people should be made aware of the importance of HIV counseling and testing as part of good, comprehensive medical care. Several studies have noted that, if one were to rely only on risk factor assessment and to test only those adolescents with reported high-risk behavior, up to 60% of HIV-infected adolescents could be missed. Thus efforts are underway to make HIV counseling and testing more available and acceptable to adolescents. Although all sexually active young people are at risk for HIV, some groups are at particular risk. As based on preliminary REACH data (*R*eaching for *E*xcellence in *A*dolescent *C*are and *H*ealth), the only multicenter cohort study of HIV-infected young people infected through either sexual transmission or needle use, two groups appear most at risk. For the females, young African-American women make up 75% of the cohort. Many of these young women were identified through prenatal testing and many reported older male sexual partners. As would be expected, most of these young women reside in areas of high seroprevalence for HIV. For the males, 60% were African-American. For the HIV-positive males, 48% self-identified as homosexual, with 55% reporting that they are likely to have sex only with same-sex partners. Thus young women of color and young men who have sex with men, especially those residing in high seroprevalence areas of the country, are most at risk for HIV infection.

In most jurisdictions in the United States, adolescents can consent for HIV counseling and testing. It is important that the clinician has knowledge of both local and state laws governing HIV counseling and testing. It is also essential that counseling and testing be done in youth-sensitive environments. Adolescents are a group with one of the poorest return rates for posttest results and counseling. Thus it is imperative that the initial interaction that the adolescent has with the clinician or counselor be a positive one. Thus providing counseling in terms understood by adolescents and providing them with support through the process are key to successful HIV counseling and testing. Finally, HIV-infected adolescents require special efforts made to ensure that they are linked into comprehensive HIV care programs.

In addition, all young people who present for HIV care should have confirmation of their infection before considering beginning therapy. Although there may be several reasons that an uninfected youth may present for HIV care, such as a false-positive HIV ELISA not confirmed with a Western blot or a high-risk exposure to an infected person, infection should always be confirmed at the first visit.

SUGGESTED READINGS

American Academy of Pediatrics, Committee on Pediatric AIDS: Evaluation and medical treatment of the HIV-exposed infant, *Pediatrics* 99:909-917, 1997.

Centers for Disease Control and Prevention: Public Health Service Task Force recommendations for the use of antiretroviral drugs in pregnant women infected with HIV-1 for maternal health and for reducing perinatal HIV-1 transmission in the United States, *MMWR* 47(RR-02), 1998.

Centers for Disease Control and Prevention: *HIV/AIDS Surveillance Report*, 8:1-40, 1996.

Connor EM et al: Reduction of maternal-infant transmission of human immunodeficiency virus type 1 with zidovudine treatment, *N Engl J Med* 331:1173-1180, 1994.

D'Angelo LJ et al: Human immunodeficiency virus infection in urban adolescents: can we predict who is at risk? *Pediatrics* 88:982-986, 1991.

National Pediatric and Family HIV Resource Center: www.pedhivaids.org

Rosenberg PS, Biggar RJ, Goedert JJ: Declining age at HIV infection in the United States, *N Engl J Med* 330:789, 1994.

Slap GB: Normal physiologic and psychosocial growth in the adolescent, *J Adolesc Health Care* 7:3s-23s, 1986.

Troiden RR: Homosexual identity development, *J Adolesc Health Care* 9:105-113, 1988.

Working Group on Antiretroviral Therapy and Medical Management of HIV-Infected Children: Guidelines for the use of antiretroviral agents in pediatric HIV infection, *MMWR* 47(RR-04):1-48, 1988.

INDEX

A

Abacavir (ABC)
  acidosis and, 165
  as FDA-approved NRTI, 31
  characteristics of, 32t
  drug fever and, 230
  for children with AIDS, 253, 255
  for treatment intensification, 38
  gastrointestinal side effects from, 35-36
  rash/hypersensitivity reactions from, 36
  renal implications of, 162
  resistance to, 39
  rifabutin with, 47b
  rifamycin for TB and, 72
Abdomen
  cramps in
    Entamoeba histolytica and, 106
    Giardia lamblia and, 105
    primary HIV and, 119
  initial HIV assessment of, 26, 26b
  pain in, 190
    bacillary peliosis and, 115
    CMV colitis and, 86
    Cyclospora and, 104
    Entamoeba histolytica and, 106
    gastroenteritis and, 111
    immune reconstitution syndrome and, 233
    Isospora and, 103
    microsporidia and, 102
    ultrasound of, for fever of unknown origin diagnosis, 234
ABLC; see Amphotericin B lipid complex
Acanthamoeba, corneal ulcers and, 145
Acanthosis, Epstein-Barr virus and, 94
ACE; see Angiotensin converting enzyme inhibitors
Acetaminophen, and rash/hypersensitivity reactions from NNRTIs, 36
Acetylcysteine, for keratoconjunctivitis sicca, 141
Acid-fast bacilli (AFB) stains, 68
  for *Cryptosporidium parvum* diagnosis, 100, 100t, 218, 222
  for *Cyclospora cayetanensis* diagnosis, 104, 218, 222
  for *Isospora belli* diagnosis, 103, 218, 222
  for MAC diagnosis, 76
  for *Nocardia asteroides* diagnosis, 207
  for *Rhodococcus equi* diagnosis, 116
  for tuberculous diagnosis, 207, 213
  for tuberculous meningitis diagnosis, 172
Acidosis, 165
Acitretin, for psoriasis with HIV, 127
Activity level, mania and, 182

NOTE: Page numbers followed by b indicate boxes; f, figures; t, tables.

Acute retroviral syndrome (ARS), primary HIV and, 119
Acute tubular necrosis, in HIV
  causes of, 160, 160b
  diagnosis of, 161
Acyclovir
  atypical herpes zoster lesions and, 92
  CMV prophylaxis and, 89
  for CMV, 50
  for herpes simplex keratitis, 144
  for herpes zoster, 120, 174
  for herpes zoster encephalitis, 171
  for herpes zoster ophthalmicus, 144
  for HSV, 50, 54t, 90, 91, 119, 200
    with HIV, 133t, 136
  for HSV colitis, 220
  for HSV encephalitis, 171
  for oral hairy leukoplakia, 94, 121
    with HIV, 133t, 137
  for retinal necrosis, 150
  for varicella in children with AIDS, 253
  for varicella-zoster keratitis, 145
  for varicella-zoster retinitis, 150
  for VZV, 93, 93t
  intratubular crystallization and, 161, 161t
  neuropsychiatric side effects of, 181t
  PORN and, 150-151
  resistance to, 91, 93, 119, 120, 220
  TTP/HUS and, 159b
  ureteral obstruction from, 160b
Adenitis, cervical, in children, MAC and, 74
Adenocarcinoma, of lung, late HIV infection and, 211
Adenopathy, DMAC and, 75, 75t, 76
Adenovirus
  HIV-associated diarrhea and, 220
  pulmonary, late HIV infection and, 210
  recombinant, for anal neoplasia, 247
Adherence
  by adolescents with AIDS on HAART, 256-257
  by children with AIDS on HAART, 254
Adjustment disorders, 177
  severe, major depressive disorder *vs.,* 179
Adolescents
  HIV counseling and testing for, 257
  infectious mononucleosis and, 94
  with HIV infection, 249
    epidemiology of, 255-256
    treatment for, 256-257
Adrenal cortex insufficiency, hyponatremia and, 162
Adrenal glands
  cryptococcosis of, 81
  PCP and, 59
Adrenal insufficiency, hyperkalemia and, 164
β–Adrenergic blocking agents, for anxiety, 185
Adriamycin, for Kaposi's sarcoma, 240, 240b

Africa
  AIDS wasting syndrome in, 223
  HIV in, 6
  human herpesvirus 8 in, 236
  Isospora belli in, 103
  Kaposi's sarcoma in, 236
African Americans
  hepatitis C-associated immune complex glomerulonephritis and, 157, 158
  HIVAN and, 154, 155, 156
  Pneumocystis carinii pneumonia and, 58
Aging
  herpes zoster ophthalmicus and, 143
  keratoconjunctivitis sicca and, 141
Agitation
  major depressive disorder and, 179
  mania and, 183b
Agranulocytosis, from trimethoprim-dapsone for PCP, 63t
AIDS
  Cryptosporidium and, 100
  epidemiology of, international perspective, 6
  false-negative serologic tests for HIV and, 21
  surveillance case definition for, 6-7, 7b
  U.S. demographics overview of, 8-9
AIDS dementia complex, 167
AIDS retinopathy, 146, 146b
AIDS wasting syndrome (AWS)
  about, 223
  documentation of, 223
  etiology and pathogenesis of, 223-224
  evaluation and management of, 226, 226b
  exercise and, 225
  illustrative cases, 226-228
  nutrition options for, 224-225, 225b
  pharmacologic options for, 225-226, 226b
Albendazole
  cholestatic toxicity of, 195b
  for *Giardia lamblia,* 103t, 105
  for microsporidia, 101t, 102
    HIV-associated diarrhea and, 217
  for microsporidia keratitis, 145
Albenza; see Albendazole
Albumin; see also Hypoalbuminemia
  diarrhea diagnosis and, 216
Alcohol consumption habits
  hepatitis C and, 51
  HIV medical history and, 24
  sleep disturbances and, 191
Aldosteronism, 163
Alitretinoin, for Kaposi's sarcoma, 240, 240b
Alkaline phosphatase
  Bartonella and, 115
  biliary tract disease and, 198
  Cryptosporidia and, 100
  elevated, DMAC and, 75, 75t, 76
  fever of unknown origin and, 233

259

Alkaline phosphatase—cont'd
    in disseminated *Isospora,* 103
    microsporidia and, 102
Allergies, to penicillin, 114
Allopurinol
    for HIV-associated lymphoma, 242
    for renal failure and other renal abnormalities, 161
Alopecia, patchy, secondary syphilis and, 112
Alprazolam, for anxiety, 184
Alternative testing for HIV, 21-22
AmBisome, 83
American Academy of Pediatrics (AAP)
    on day care and school for children with AIDS, 255
Amikacin, for DMAC, 76, 77
    HIV-associated diarrhea and, 219
Amiloride, TMP structure and, 164
Aminoglycosides
    for corneal ulcers, 145
    for *Pseudomonas aeruginosa,* 207
    renal magnesium wasting and, 164
Amiodarone, contraindications for, 42t
Amitriptyline
    for neurologic adverse effects from antiretroviral therapy, 36
    potential antiretroviral interaction with, 182t
Amphetamines abuse, mania *vs.,* 183
Amphotericin B, 83-84, 84t
    acute renal failure and, 160
    for aspergillosis with HIV, 133t
    for blastomycosis, 83, 209
    for bloodstream candidiasis, 80
    for candidiasis with HIV, 124
        esophageal, 194
    for coccidioidomycosis, 54t, 82-83, 125
    for corneal infections, 145
    for cryptococcal meningitis, 171
    for cryptococcosis, 81, 125
        with HIV, 133t
        pulmonary, 208
    for *Cryptococcus neoformans,* 52t
    for fungal chorioretinitis, 153
    for geotrichosis with HIV, 133t
    for histoplasmosis, 53t, 82, 125
        pulmonary, advanced HIV and, 209
        with HIV, 133t
    for penicilliosis, 83
    for pregnant women with fungal infections, 49
    for sporotrichosis with HIV, 126
    for Zygomycetes, 83
    hypocalcemia and, 164
    hypokalemia and, 163
    neuropsychiatric side effects of, 181t
    renal magnesium wasting and, 164
    renal tubular acidosis and, 165
Amphotericin B cholesteryl complex, 84t
Amphotericin B lipid complex (ABLC), 83, 84t
Ampicillin
    for gastroenteritis, 111-112
    for HIV-associated diarrhea from *Salmonella,* 219

Ampicillin—cont'd
    for HIV-associated diarrhea from *Shigella,* 219
    for listeriosis, 112
    for *Salmonella* gastroenteritis in pregnant women, 49
Amprenavir, 31, 33
    characteristics of, 34t
    gastrointestinal side effects from, 35
    hepatic transaminases abnormalities from, 37
    liquid formulations for, children with AIDS and, 254
    neurologic adverse effects from, 36
    rash/hypersensitivity reactions from, 36
    resistance to, 40
    rifabutin for TB treatment and, 71
    rifabutin interactions with, 47b
    rifabutin treatment with, 72
Amyotrophic lateral sclerosis-like syndromes, HIV and, 168
Anabolic block
    AIDS wasting syndrome and, 223, 224
    treatment of, 225-226
Anal cancer
    high-grade squamous intraepithelial lesions (HSILs) and, 51
    relative risk for in urban areas, 246t
Anal intraepithelial neoplasia (AIN), 246, 247
Anal neoplasia, 246-248, 248b
    diagnosis of, 247b
    risk factors for, 247b
Analgesia, narcotic
    for neurologic adverse effects from antiretroviral therapy, 36
    xerostomia from, 132
Analgesics
    for aphthous ulcers, 139
    for pain, 191
    for pain in herpes zoster, 174
    opioid, for pain syndromes, 190
Anaphylaxis
    from paclitaxel for Kaposi's sarcoma, 241
    from pentamidine for PCP, 63t
    from TMP-SMX for PCP, 63t
Anemia
    DMAC and, 75
    from foscarnet, 87
    from ganciclovir, 87, 89
    from TMP-SMX for PCP prophylaxis, 65
    HIV-associated dementia and, 187
    MAC and, 76
    major depressive disorder and, 179
    microangiopathic hemolytic, HUS and, 159
    severe, AIDS retinopathy *vs.,* 146
    zidovudine and, 35, 37
Anergy testing, for inactive TB infection, 73-74, 211
Anesthetics, topical, for pain in herpes zoster, 174
Aneurysms, mycotic, *Salmonella* and, 111
Anger
    delirium and, 185
    release of, for reactive depression, 178

Angiogenesis inhibitors, for Kaposi's sarcoma, 240b, 241
Angiotensin converting enzyme (ACE) inhibitors
    for HIVAN, 156
    hyperkalemia and, 164
    renal failure or azotemia and, 160b
Angiotensin II receptor blockers, renal failure or azotemia and, 160b
Animals, domestic; *see* Pets
Anorectal lesions, 199-200, 200b
Anorexia
    AIDS wasting syndrome and, 226
    CMV colitis and, 86
    comprehensive history of, 25b
    Cryptosporidia and, 100
    Cyclospora and, 104
    from clindamycin-primaquine for PCP, 63t
    Giardia lamblia and, 105
    immune reconstitution syndrome and, 233
    in acute HIV-1 infection, 17b
    in *Rhodococcus equi,* 116
    Isospora and, 103
    MAC and, 76
    major depressive disorder and, 179
    megestrol acetate and, 225
    nasogastric feeding tube and, 225
    primary HIV and, 119
Anoscopy, for anal neoplasias, 247
Antacids, *Entamoeba histolytica* diagnosis and, 106
Anthracyclines, liposomal, for Kaposi's sarcoma, 130, 201
Anthropometry, for body fat measurement, 223
Antianxiety agents, xerostomia from, 132
Antibacterial mouth rinse, for linear gingival erythema, 134t
Antibiotics
    broad-spectrum, *Aspergillus* risk and, 211
    for aphthous ulcers, 139
    for corneal ulcers, 145
    for pyomyositis/lymphomatous infiltration of muscle, 175
    for *S. aureus,* 122
    for syphilis with HIV, 123
    macrolide, cholestatic toxicity of, 195b
    prolonged, bloodstream candidiasis and, 80
Antibody testing, for fever of unknown origin diagnosis, 234
Anticholinergics, xerostomia from, 132
Anticonvulsants
    drug-drug interactions and, 41, 184t
    for pain, 191
    for pain in herpes zoster, 174
Antidepressants
    anxiety disorders and, 184
    for HIV-associated dementia and, 188
    for pain, 191
    for pain syndromes, 190
    for reactive depression, 178, 179
    mania and, 183

Antidepressants—cont'd
  potential drug interactions with antiretrovirals, 182t
  tricyclic
    for anxiety, 185
    for bereavement, 179b
    for insomnia, 191
    for major depressive disorder, 180b, 181
    for mania, 183b
    for pain in herpes zoster, 174
    for sensory-motor axonal polyneuropathy, 169
    xerostomia from, 132
Antidiarrheal agents, for microsporidia, 102
Antidiuretic hormone (ADH), hypovolemia and, 162
Antidysrhythmics, drug-drug interactions and, 41
Antiepileptics, for toxoplasmic encephalitis, 98
Antifungal azoles, 84, 84t
  hepatocellular toxicity of, 195, 195b
Antifungals
  for angular cheilitis with HIV, 133t
  for aphthous ulcers, 139
  for candidiasis with HIV, 123-124, 133t
  for dermatophytosis with HIV, 124
  for esophageal candidiasis, 194
  for hyperplastic candidiasis, 138
  for linear gingival erythema, 138
  for necrotizing ulcerative gingivitis or periodontitis, 139
Antigen testing
  for cryptococcosis, 81, 171, 212
    with fever of unknown origin, 232, 233
  for fever of unknown origin diagnosis, 234
  for *Giardia lamblia,* 105
  for HSV diagnosis, 90
  for VZV diagnosis, 92
Antigenemia test, for CMV diagnosis, 86-87
Antigens, CD4, HIV-1 replication and, 3
Antihistamines
  antifungal azoles interactions with, 84
  for eosinophilic folliculitis in HIV, 129
  for insomnia, 192
  for pruritus in HIV, 126
  and rash/hypersensitivity reactions from NNRTIs, 36
  xerostomia from, 132
Antihypertensives, xerostomia from, 132
Antimicrobials
  bacterial pneumonia diagnosis and, 109
  for bacterial pneumonia, 110
  for *Bartonella,* 115
  for gastroenteritis, 111
  for immune reconstitution syndrome, 233
  for microsporidia, 217
  susceptibility testing, for *Rhodococcus equi,* 116
Antimotility agents, for HIV-associated diarrhea, 222
Antimucolytic therapy, for varicella-zoster keratitis, 145

Antimycobacterial agents, 42t
  drug-drug interactions and, 41
  for mycobacterial skin infections in HIV, 122
Antiplatelet agents, for TTP/HUS, 159
Antipsychotics, 183, 183b
  for HIV-associated delirium, 185-186
  for HIV-associated dementia, 188
  for HIV-associated psychosis, 189
Antiretroviral therapy (ART)
  about, 30
  adverse events from, 35-37
  clinical failure of, 38
  drug-drug interactions in, 40-41
  educational discussions on adherence to, 28
  for acute HIV-1 infection, 19
  for cytomegalovirus, with HIV, 136
  for HIV-associated dementia, 168
  for initial HIV management, 26-27
  for Kaposi's sarcoma, oral, 137
  for major depressive disorder, 180, 180b
  highly active
    anal neoplasia and, 247
    cervical cancer and, 245
    CMV retinitis and, 85, 88, 149
    drug-induced diarrhea and, 220
    for children with AIDS, 253-255, 254t
    for *Cryptosporidium parvum,* 100-101, 101t, 218
    for *E. bieneusi,* 217
    for HIVAN, 156
    for microsporidia, 101t, 102
    for primary HIV, 119
    herpes zoster and, 91
    HIV-related lymphoma and, 243
    HIV-related skin diseases and, 118
    human papillomavirus and, 133t
    Kaposi's sarcoma and, 201, 236, 240
    MAC treatment and, 198
    non-Hodgkin's lymphoma and, 241
    opportunistic infections and, 44
    prenatal maternal, 250
    T. gondii prophylaxis and, 98
  HIV epidemiology and, 12
  immunologic failure of, 37-38
  introduction of, 7, 30-31
  mania and, 183
  molluscum contagiosum and, 143
  monitoring patients on, 35
  PCP risk and, 64
  pharmacotherapy for major depressive disorder and, 180-181, 181t, 182t
  referrals for, 41
  renal implications of, 162
  resistance monitoring assays for, 39-40
  resistant virus and change in, 38-39
  skin reactions to, 129
  treatment intensification, 38
  viral rebound and, 31
  virologic failure of, 37
Antispasticity agents, for spasticity with vacuolar myelopathy, 168

Antiviral agents
  for HIV-associated delirium, 185
  for HIV-associated dementia, 187-188
  for human papilloma virus with HIV, 137
  for varicella-zoster keratitis, 145
Anxiety
  delirium and, 185
  pain syndromes and, 190
  sleep disturbances and, 191
Anxiety disorders, 183-185
  bereavement and, 179b
  Key Points, 185b
  reactive depression and, 177, 178
  SSRIs and, 180, 183
  T. gondii and, 96
  tricyclic antidepressants and, 180b, 183
Anxiolytics, 183b
  for pain, 191
Aortitis, tertiary syphilis and, 174
Apathy; *see also* Memory, impaired
  HIV-1–associated dementia complex and, 186
  HIV-associated dementia and, 167
Aphasia
  progressive multifocal leukoencephalopathy and, 170
  T. gondii and, 96
Aphthous ulcers
  as oral manifestation of HIV, 134t, 135t, 139
  CMV *vs.,* 136
  esophageal, 193
  esophageal candidiasis *vs.,* 80
  HSV-related ulcers *vs.,* 132
  necrotizing stomatitis *vs.,* 139
Appetite loss
  anxiety disorders and, 184
  biliary tract disease and, 198
  lithium carbonate and, 183
  major depressive disorder and, 179, 180b
  SSRIs and, 180
Appetite stimulants, AIDS wasting syndrome and, 225
Apprehension, anxiety disorders and, 183
Areflexia
  CMV polyradiculpathy and, 86
  Miller-Fisher syndrome and, 169
Argyll Robertson pupils, 152, 174
ARS; *see* Acute retroviral syndrome
ART; *see* Antiretroviral therapy
Arthralgias, 190
  aseptic meningitis and, 166
  coccidioidomycosis and, 82
  from vincristine for Kaposi's sarcoma, 240
  growth hormone for AWS and, 226, 227t
  mixed essentiual cryoglobulinemia and, 158
  primary HIV and, 119
Arthritis; *see also* Sjögren's syndrome
  coccidioidomycosis and, 82
  pain from, 190
  psoriatic, in HIV, 126, 127, 190
  reactive, *Giardia lamblia* and, 105
  Reiter's syndrome and, 127

Arthritis—cont'd
  septic
    bacterial pneumonia and, 109
    Salmonella and, 111
    sporotrichosis with HIV and, 126
Arthropathies, pain from, 190
Artificial tears
  for keratoconjunctivitis sicca, 141
  for microsporidia keratitis, 145
  for varicella-zoster keratitis, 145
Ascites, PCP and, 59
ASCUS; *see* Atypical squamous cells of undetermined significance
Asia
  HIV in, 6
    penicilliosis and, 83
  Isospora belli in, 103
  Southeast, infectious disease of, 211
Aspergillosis
  as oral manifestation of HIV, 133t, 135t
  fungal meningitis from, 171
  pulmonary, advanced HIV and, 209
Aspergillus fumigatus
  advanced HIV and, 209
  chorioretinitis and, 152-153
  focal CNS lesion and, 98t
  host defense to, 79
  Rhodococcus equi vs., 116
Aspergillus spp., 83
Aspirin, for membranoproliferative glomerulonephritis, 157
Astemizole
  alternatives to, 41
  antifungal azoles interactions with, 84
Astrovirus, HIV-associated diarrhea and, 220
Asymptomatic HIV
  antiretroviral therapy for, 30-31
  CBF examination for chronic meningitis in, 166-167
  chest radiographs and, 213
Atarax, for insomnia, 192
Ataxia
  CMV and, 86
  from TMP-SMX for PCP, 63t
  HIV-1–associated dementia complex and, 186
  Miller-Fisher syndrome and, 169
Atherosclerosis, from antiretroviral therapy, 36
Ativan; *see* Lorazepam
Atorvastatin
  for lipodystrophy from antiretroviral therapy, 37
  safety of, 41
Atovaquone
  for *Cryptosporidium*, 100, 101t
  for *E. bieneusi*, 217
  for microsporidia, 101t, 102
  for PCP, 52t, 60, 61, 63t, 206
    prophylaxis, 66, 206
  for *T. gondii*, 52t, 98, 99t
Attention deficit
  HIV-1–associated dementia complex and, 186
  MCMD and, 186
Atypical mycobacteria, 68

Atypical squamous cells of undetermined significance (ASCUS), human papillomavirus and, 51
AWS; *see* AIDS wasting syndrome
Axonal loss, Guillain-Barré syndrome and, 169
Azathioprine, for chronic inflammatory demyelinating polyneuropathy, 169
Azithromycin
  bacterial respiratory infections and, 48
  for bacterial pneumonia, 110
  for *Bartonella*, 115
  for *Cryptosporidium*, 100, 101t
  for DMAC, 48, 52t, 76, 76t
    HIV-associated diarrhea and, 219
    in children with AIDS, 252
  for DMAC prophylaxis, 76t, 77
  for *M. xenopi*, 78
  for MAC-induced choroiditis, 152
  for *Mycobacterium avium* complex, 198
  for *T. gondii*, 97, 98, 99t
  lactose-free, for *Cryptosporidium parvum*, 218
  rifabutin treatment and uveitis with, 72
  safety of, 41
  and standard PCP prophylaxis, 66
Azoles, antifungal, 84, 84t
  for *Pityrosporum ovale*, 124
AZT; *see* Zidovudine

B

B lymphocytes, HIV and, 108
  lymphoma development in, 241
Bacillary angiomatosis
  as skin manifestation of HIV, 122, 122b
  Bartonella and, 115
  initial HIV assessment for, 25, 26b
  Kaposi's sarcoma *vs.*, 129, 237
  maculopapular red-brown lesions and, 239t
  peliosis hepatis and, 196
Bacillary epithelioid angiomatosis, as oral manifestation of HIV, 134t
Bacillary peliosis, *Bartonella* and, 115
Bacille Calmette-Guérin (BCG), 68
  vaccine, 47
Baclofen, for spasticity with vacuolar myelopathy, 168
Bacteremia
  Bartonella and, 115
  HIV-associated diarrhea and, 219
  in *Rhodococcus equi*, 116
  pneumonia in late HIV infection and, 212
  Salmonella gastroenteritis and, 111, 112
Bacterial culture, for *S. aureus*, 122
Bacterial infections, recurrent, children with AIDS and, 251, 252, 252b
Bactrim; *see* Trimethoprim-sulfamethoxazole
Bactroban ointment, for *S. aureus*, 122
Barium studies
  Entamoeba histolytica diagnosis and, 106
  for esophagitis diagnosis, 193-194
  for *Giardia lamblia*, 105
  for HIV-associated diarrhea diagnosis, 216
Bartonella, 49, 115-116, 116b
  peliosis hepatis and, 196

Bartonella henselae, 115
  focal CNS lesion and, 98t
  Kaposi's sarcoma *vs.*, 237
Bartonella quintana, 115
  as skin manifestation of HIV, 122
Basal cell carcinoma, as skin manifestation of HIV, 130
Battey bacillus; *see Mycobacterium avium* complex
BCG (bacille Calmette-Guérin), 68
  vaccine, 47
Behavior disturbances
  delirium and, 185
  HIV-associated psychosis and, 189
  HSV encephalitis and, 170-171
Behavioral therapy, for pain, 191
Behçet's syndrome, ulcers from, HIV and, 135t
Benadryl, for insomnia, 192
Bengal solution, for varicella-zoster keratitis diagnosis, 144
Benzathine penicillin, for syphilis, 114
  with HIV, 123
Benzodiazepines
  drug-drug interactions and, 41
  for anxiety, 184-185
  for bereavement, 179b
  for insomnia, 191
  for reactive depression, 178
  safe choices of, 41
Bepridil, contraindications for, 42t
Bereavement, 179, 179b
  anxiety *vs.*, 185b
  major depressive disorder *vs.*, 179
Bethanechol, for salivary flow, 136
Bicarbonates
  for acidosis, 161
  for hyperkalemia, 164
Biliary tract disease, 198-199, 199b
  Cryptosporidium parvum and, 217
  I. belli and, 218
Bilirubin, elevation of, inidinavir and, 198
Bioelectrical impedance analysis (BIA), for body composition measurement, 223
Biofeedback, for pain, 191
Biopsy
  duodenal
    for *Giardia lamblia* diagnosis, 105
    for HIV-associated diarrhea diagnosis, 222
  excisional, for anogenital condylomata acuminata, 200
  for anal neoplasia, 247
  for anogenital warts diagnosis, 121
  for *Bartonella* diagnosis, 115, 122
  for biliary tract disease diagnosis, 198-199
  for blastomycosis diagnosis, 83
  for coccidioidomycosis diagnosis, 82, 125
  for esophageal ulcers diagnosis, 194
  for fever of unknown origin diagnosis, 232-233
  for HIVAN diagnosis, 155
  for HIV-associated lymphoma diagnosis, 242
  for Kaposi's sarcoma diagnosis, 129, 201

Biopsy—cont'd
  for MAC with very low CD4+ counts diagnosis, 232
  for molluscum contagiosum diagnosis, 120
  for *Rhodococcus equi* diagnosis, 116
  for zidovudine-related myopathy, 175
  of brain
    for CNS lymphoma diagnosis, 173
    for HSV encephalitis diagnosis, 171
    for progressive multifocal leukoencephalopathy diagnosis, 170
    for *T. gondii* diagnosis, 171
  of kidney
    for acute renal failure or other abnormalities, 160
    for hepatitis C-associated immune complex glomerulonephritis diagnosis, 158
    for mixed essential cryoglobulinemia, 158
  of liver, 196
  of lung
    for HIV-associated pneumonias diagnosis, 214
    for Kaposi's sarcoma diagnosis, 237
    for *T. gondii* diagnosis, 97
  of muscles
    for polymyositis, 170
    for pyomyositis/lymphomatous infiltration of, 174
  of nerves, for CMV radiculitis diagnosis, 173
  of oral lesions, for CMV diagnosis in HIV, 136
  of skin, for porphyria cutanea tarda diagnosis, 128
  percutaneous needle aspiration, for PCP diagnosis, 59-60
  transbronchial
    chest radiographs and, 212
    for CMV diagnosis, 86
    for coccidioidomycosis diagnosis, 209
    for HIV-associated pneumonias diagnosis, 213-214
    for Kaposi's sarcoma, 210
    for nonspecific interstitial pneumonitis diagnosis, 211
    for PCP diagnosis, 59, 206
    for tuberculosis diagnosis, 207
  vitreous, for uveitis diagnosis, 142
Bipolar disorder, 182-183, 183b
  HIV-associated psychosis *vs.*, 189
  major depressive disorder *vs.*, 180b
Bipolaris hawaiiensis, chorioretinitis and, 152-153
Birds
  Cryptosporidium and, 99
  T. gondii and, 96
Bisexual men
  CMV and, 85
  and condylomata acuminata in HIV, 121
  HIV screening for, 20
  natural history of HIV infection study among, 12
  U.S. HIV prevalence among, 9, 10f

Bismuth, *Entamoeba histolytica* diagnosis and, 106
Bismuth subsalicylate, for *Cryptosporidium*, 101
Bites, human, HIV transmission, 11
Bladder atony, sensory-motor neuropathy from vincristine and, 175
Bladder dysfunction, tertiary syphilis and, 174
Blastomyces dermatitidis, 83, 209
Blastomycosis, 83, 83b
  demographics of, 211
  pulmonary, advanced HIV and, 209
Bleeding; *see* Gastrointestinal bleeding; Rectal bleeding
Bleomycin
  for HIV-associated lymphoma, 243
  for Kaposi's sarcoma, 130, 240, 240b
  for warts, 121
  TTP/HUS and, 159b
Blepharitis, keratoconjunctivitis sicca and, 141
Blindness
  corneal ulcers and, 145
  herpes simplex keratitis and, 144
Blisters, porphyria cutanea tarda in HIV and, 128
Bloating, *Giardia lamblia* and, 105
Blood; *see also* Complete blood count
  blastomycosis in, 83
  candidiasis in, 80
  CMV in, 85
  cryptococcosis in, 81
  extrapulmonary TB in, 70
  for coccidioidomycosis diagnosis, 82
  histoplasmosis in, 209
  M. xenopi and, 78
  rapid plasma reagin test for syphilis and, 113
Blood count with differential
  initial HIV assessment of, 26b
  and TMP-SMX for PCP, 61
Blood culture/tests
  for bacterial pneumonia diagnosis, 109
  for *Bartonella* diagnosis, 115
  for fever of unknown origin diagnosis, 230, 232
  for gastroenteritis diagnosis, 111
  for HIV-associated delirium, 185
  for HIV-associated dementia, 187
  for MAC with very low CD4+ counts, 232, 233
  for mycobacteremia, 196
  for penicilliosis, 83
  for pneumococcal pneumonia diagnosis, 206
  for pulmonary disease in late HIV infection, 212
Blood products recipients
  HIV screening for, 20
  lymphoma and, 241
  U.S. HIV prevalence among, 11
Blood proteins, HIVAN and, 155
Blood urea nitrogen (BUN), renal failure and other renal abnormalities and, 162
Body composition, measurement of, 223, 224

Body fat
  distribution, measurement of, 223
  in children with AIDS, 255
Body piercing, hepatitis C and, 51
Bone marrow
  Bartonella and, 115
  biopsy of, for fever of unknown origin diagnosis, 232, 233
  M. xenopi and, 78
  PCP and, 59
  and trimetraxate for PCP, 63t
Bones
  Bartonella and, 115, 122
  lymphoma presentation in, 241
Bovine colostrum, for *Cryptosporidium parvum,* 218
Bowel, dysmotility, sensory-motor neuropathy from vincristine and, 175
Brachial neuritis, in acute HIV-1 infection, 17b
Brain, *Bartonella* and, 122
Brain abscess
  bacterial pneumonia and, 109
  Entamoeba histolytica and, 106
  in *Rhodococcus equi*, 116
  mybcobacterial infections and, 172
  Salmonella and, 111
Brain dysfunction
  from cryptococcal meningitis, 171
  HIV and, 166, 167b
  T. gondii and, 171
Brain imaging
  for HIV-associated delirium, 185
  for HIV-associated dementia, 187
Breast milk
  CMV in, 85
  perinatal transmission and, 249
Breasts, initial HIV assessment of, 26b
Breath, shortness of, *Cryptosporidia* and, 100
Brolene; *see* Propamidine isethionate
Bronchiectasis, late HIV infection and, 211
Bronchiolitis obliterans with organizing pneumonia (BOOP), late HIV infection and, 211
Bronchitis, *E. intestinalis* and, 217
Bronchoalveolar lavage (BAL)
  for bacterial pulmonary infections, 207
  for blastomycosis diagnosis, 83
  for CMV diagnosis, 86
  for coccidioidomycosis diagnosis, 82, 209
  for cryptococcosis diagnosis, 208
  for *Haemophilus influenzae* diagnosis, 206
  for HIV-associated pneumonias diagnosis, 213
  for *Nocardia asteroides* diagnosis, 207
  for PCP diagnosis, 59, 206
  for toxoplasmosis diagnosis, 97, 210
Bronchocospy, chest radiographs and, 212
Bronchoscopy
  fiberoptic
    for HIV-associated pneumonias diagnosis, 213-214
    for PCP diagnosis, 59
    PCP treatment and, 63
  for bacterial pneumonia diagnosis, 109, 110
  for *Rhodococcus equi* diagnosis, 116

Bronchospasm
  and aerosolized pentamidine for PCP prophylaxis, 66
  PCP and, 63
Bruises, Kaposi's sarcoma vs., 129
Brush fire border, in CMV retinitis, 148
Bupropion, potential antiretroviral interaction with, 182t
Buspirone, for anxiety, 185
Buttocks, lymphoma presentation in, 241

C

Caclium, depression of, HIV-associated lymphoma and, 242
Caffeine, sleep disturbances and, 191
Calcipotriene, for psoriasis with HIV, 127
Calcium, renal availability of, 164
Calcium glutonate, for hyperkalemia, 164
Calcivirus, HIV-associated diarrhea and, 220
Caloric intake
  decreased, AIDS wasting syndrome and, 223-224
  megestrol acetate and, 225
Campylobacter
  CMV colitis vs., 86
  gastroenteritis, *Shigella* gastroenteritis vs., 111
  HIV infection and, 111
  HIV-associated diarrhea and, 219, 219b
  Reiter's syndrome and, 127
Campylobacter cinaedi, 111
Campylobacter fennelliae, 111
Campylobacter fetus, 111
Campylobacter jejuni, 111
Candida albicans
  chorioretinitis and, 152-153
  CMV retinitis vs., 86
  corneal infections with, 145-146
  Epstein-Barr virus vs., 94
  focal CNS lesion and, 98t
  fungal meningitis from, 171
  host defense to, 79
  HSV esophagitis vs., 90
  oral hairy leukoplakia and, 136
  pulmonary, advanced HIV and, 209
Candidiasis, 80
  as cutaneous manifestation of HIV, 123-124
  atrophic, as oral manifestation of HIV, 135t, 137-138
  esophageal, 80, 138
    as AIDS-defining illness, 193
    CMV esophagitis vs., 86
    in acute HIV-1 infection, 18
  hyperplastic
    as oral manifestation of HIV, 133t, 135t, 138
    Epstein-Barr virus vs., 94
    oral hairy leukoplakia vs., 136
  Key Points, 124b
  oral
    as acute HIV-1 manifestation, 17b
    as HIV manifestation, 133t, 137-138
    HIV and, 118
    linear gingival erythema vs., 138
    oral hairy leukoplakia vs., 121
    Pneumocystis carinii pneumonia and, 12

Candidiasis—cont'd
  prophylaxis against, 49, 54t
  seborrheic dermatitis vs., 79
Candies, sugarless, for salivary flow, 135-136
Capnocytophaga spp., corneal infections with, 145
Capreomycin
  hypovolemic hyponatremia and, 162
  renal magnesium wasting and, 164
Capsaicin cream, for pain in herpes zoster, 174
Captopril, for IgA glomerulonephritis, 157
Carbamazepine
  contraindications for, 175
  for sensory-motor axonal polyneuropathy, 169
Carbon monoxide, diffusing capacity of, *Pneumocystis carinii* pneumonia and, 58, 212
Carcinoma, pulmonary, advanced HIV and, 205
Carcinoma in situ, anal, 246
Cardia dysrhythmias, Guillain-Barré syndrome and, 169
Cardiac tamponade, bacterial pneumonia and, 109
Cardiomegaly, *T. gondii* and, 97
Cardiopulmonary systems, initial HIV assessment of, 25-26, 26b
Cardiotoxicity, from vincristine for Kaposi's sarcoma, 240
Cardiovascular syphilis, 112
Carotid artery diseases, ocular hypotension and, 142
Carpal tunnel syndrome, growth hormone for AWS and, 226, 227t
CAT scan
  for anal neoplasia, 247
  for HIV-associated lymphoma diagnosis, 242
Cataracts
  from CMV treatment, 88
  from ganciclovir implants, 87
  herpes zoster ophthalmicus and, 144
  silicone oils for retinal detachment and, 148
Catheters
  central venous, bloodstream candidiasis and, 80
  line infections
    foscarnet administration and, 87
    fungal chorioretinitis and, 152-153
    ganciclovir administration and, 87
Cats
  Bartonella and, 115-116, 122
  gastroenteritis and, 111
  T. gondii and, 46, 96, 99, 210b
Cat-scratch disease; see *Bartonella henselae*
Cavitation
  bacterial pneumonia and, 109
  in *Rhodococcus equi*, 116
CC-CKR-5, HIV-1 replication and, 3
CC-CKR-S, 3
CCR5, macrophage-tropic HIV strains and, 15

CD4+ counts
  anal neoplasias and, 247
  aphthous ulcers and, 139
  Bartonella and, 115
  CMV encephalitis and, 170
  CMV radiculitis and, 173
  Cryptosporidium parvum and, 217
  cytomegalovirus and, 133t, 148
  eosinophilic folliculitis in HIV and, 128
  fever of unknown origin and, 229, 231-232, 231b
  for children with AIDS, 251, 251b
  for HIV-associated pneumonias diagnosis, 212
  for pregnant women, perinatal transmission and, 249
  herpes simplex disease and, 89-90
    chronic, 119
  herpes zoster complications and, 93, 120
  initial HIV assessment of, 44
  Isospora and, 103
  Kaposi's sarcoma and, 134t
  liver abnormalities and, 196
  lymphoma and, 243
  M. kansasii and, 208
  major oral aphthous ulcers and, 134t
  molluscum contagiosum and, 120
  necrotizing stomatitis and, 134t, 139
  necrotizing ulcerative peridontitis and, 139
  neurologic complication diagnosis and, 166
  NSIP and, 211
  ocular hypotension and, 142
  oral hairy leukoplakia and, 133t, 137
  PCP and, 57-58, 205
  PCP risk and, 64
  pulmonary disease likelihood based on, 212b, 214
  toxoplasmosis and, 94, 97
  tuberculosis and, 207
CD4+ T-lymphocyte counts
  CMV and, 85, 147
  CMV pneumonitis and, 86
  drug combinations and, 35
  educational discussions on, 27-28
  HIV infection and, 7, 12
  HIV staging and, 12
  immune system monitoring and, 28-29
  in acute HIV-1 infection, 16
  initial HIV assessment of, 26b, 44
  low, antiretroviral therapy for, 30-31
  Pneumocystis carinii choroiditis and, 152
  rise in response to antiretroviral therapy, 45
  skin diseases and, 118
  tuberculosis, HIV and, 68-69, 70
CD8+ T-lymphocyte counts, in acute HIV-1 infection, 16
CDE regimen, for HIV-associated lymphoma, 242, 243
Cefotaxime, for *Salmonella* gastroenteritis in pregnant women, 49
Ceftriaxone
  for bacterial pneumonia, 110
  for gastroenteritis, 112
  for pneumococcal pneumonia, 206

Ceftriaxone—cont'd
  for *Salmonella* gastroenteritis in pregnant women, 49
  for syphilis, 114
Celexa; *see* Citalopram
Celexa, for HIV-associated dementia, 188
Cellular cytotoxicity, antibody-dependent, ulcers from, 135t
Cellular immunity
  as host defense to fungi, 79
  mycobacterial infections and, 68
  Pneumocystis carinii pneumonia and, 57
  syphilis and HIV and, 112
Cellular potassium uptake, impaired; *see* Hyperkalemia
Cellulitis
  cryptococcosis and, 125
  from *S. aureus* in HIV, 121-122
Centers for Disease Control and Prevention (CDC), 6, 7
  on adolescents with HIV, 255-256
  on cervical cancer, 244
  on chronic mucocutaneous HSV lesions, 89
  on *Salmonella* septicemia, 111
  on syphilis, 114, 123
  on TB and HIV testing, 69
Central nervous system (CNS)
  abscesses, referral for, 176
  acyclovir and, 90
  Bartonella and, 115
  differential diagnosis of focal lesion of, 98t
  disseminated herpes zoster and, 92
  extrapulmonary TB in, 70
  for HIV-associated delirium and, 185
  HIV-1 manifestations of, 185t
  HIV-associated dementia and, 186-188
  HIV-related lymphoma in, 173, 241, 243
  immunosuppression and, 170-173, 173b
  MAC tuberculomas of, 76
  pediatric AIDS and, 252-253
  primary HIV complications in, 166-168, 167b
  T. gondii and, 96
  tumors of, AIDS-related papilledema *vs.*, 147
Central nervous system disease
  adverse reactions to tuberculosis treatment and, 71
  anxiety disorders and, 184
  CMV and, 86
    in HIV, 121
  major depressive disorder *vs.*, 180, 180b
  mania and, 182
  sleep disturbances and, 191
Central nervous system lymphoma, 172, 173
  T. gondii vs., 97, 171
Cephalosporins
  for corneal ulcers, 145
  for *S. aureus*, 122
Cerebellar tremor, *T. gondii* and, 96
Cerebral infarction, herpes zoster and, 120
Cerebrospinal fluid examination
  for aseptic meningitis diagnosis, 166
  for blastomycosis diagnosis, 83

Cerebrospinal fluid examination—cont'd
  for chronic inflammatory demyelinating polyneuropathy diagnosis, 169
  for chronic meningitis diagnosis, asymptomatic HIV and, 166-167
  for CMV radiculitis diagnosis, 173
  for CMV ventriculoencephalitis diagnosis, 86
  for cryptococcosal antigen diagnosis, 81, 171
  for gastroenteritis diagnosis, 111
  for Guillain-Barré syndrome diagnosis, 169
  for herpes zoster diagnosis, 174
  for HIV-associated delirium diagnosis, 185
  for HIV-associated dementia diagnosis, 167, 187
  for HIV-associated lymphoma diagnosis, 242
  for lymphomatous meningitis diagnosis, 175
  for motor neuropathy diagnosis, 168
  for neurologic complication diagnosis, 166
  for neurosyphilis diagnosis, 172
  for progressive multifocal leukoencephalopathy diagnosis, 170
  for subacute motor neuropathy from lymphoma diagnosis, 175
  for syphilis diagnosis, 114
    with HIV, 123
  for *T. gondii* diagnosis, 96, 171
  for tuberculous meningitis diagnosis, 172
  lymphoma presentation in, 241
  polymerase chain reaction and
    for CMV diagnosis, 170
    for CMV meningooencephalitis diagnosis, 233
    for HSV encephalitis diagnosis, 171
Cerebrovascular disease, as neurologic complication of HIV, 167b, 173
Cervical cancer
  diagnosis of, 244-245, 244b
  human papillomavirus and, 51, 199, 243-244
  Key Points, 246b
  natural history of, 245
  presentation of, 244
  risk factors in, 244b
  treatment of, 245-246
Cervical intraepithelial neoplasia (CIN)
  human papillomavirus and, 243-244
  natural history of, 245
  treatment of, 245
Cesarean section, elective, for delivery with HIV infection, 250
Cetirizine, safety of, 41
Chalazions, Kaposi's sarcoma *vs.*, 142-143
Chancre, syphilitic, 112
  rectal HSV *vs.*, 199
Charcot's joints, 174
Cheilitis, angular, as oral manifestation of HIV, 133t, 138
Chemofluorescent stain, for microsporidia diagnosis, 217
β-Chemokines, HIV-1 replication and, 3

Chemotherapy
  for cervical cancer, 246
  for HIV-associated lymphoma, 242
  for Kaposi's sarcoma, 129, 130, 201, 240b
    ocular, 143
    oral, 137
  for lymphoma, 175
  for non-Hodgkin's lymphoma, 134t, 242, 243
  for squamous cell carcinoma, 134t
Chest pain, 190
  anxiety disorders and, 184
  blastomycosis and, 83
  HSV esophagitis and, 90
  in *Rhodococcus equi*, 116
  M. kansasii and, 208
  Nocardia asteroides and, 207
  Rhodococcus equi and, 207
Chickenpox, 91
  HIV medical history and, 24
  prophylaxis against, 50, 93-94
  varicella-zoster antibody test and, 45
Children with AIDS; *see also* Perinatal transmission
  about, 249
  antiretroviral treatment for, 253-255, 254t
  classification of, 251b
  clinical presentation and diagnosis, 252-253
  and cyclosporine for HIVAN in, 156
  definition of, 7, 8t
  immunizations for, 253
  immunologic evaluation for, 251
  lymphoid interstitial pneumonitis and, 211
  opportunistic infections and, 44
  prognosis for, 255
  U.S. prevalence for, 11-12, 12f
  varicella-zoster virus and, 92
Children with immunodeficiency diseases, *Pneumocystis carinii* pneumonia and, 57
Chills
  from interferon for Kaposi's sarcoma, 240
  pneumococcal pneumonia and, 206
  pneumonia and, 108
  psoriasis and, 127
Chlamydia, initial HIV assessment for, 26b
Chlamydia pneumoniae, 108
Chlamydia trachomatis, Reiter's syndrome and, 127
Chlordiazepoxide, for anxiety, 184
Chlorhexidine gluconate
  for linear gingival erythema, 138
  for necrotizing stomatitis, 139
  for necrotizing ulcerative gingivitis or peridontitis, 139
Cholangiopancreatography, endoscopic retrograde (ERCP)
  for *Cryptosporidium*, 100
  for *Isospora*, 103
  for microsporidia diagnosis, 102

Cholangitis
    biliary tract disease and, 198
    gastrointestinal CMV and, 220
    microsporidia and, 217
    sclerosing
        Cryptosporidia and, 100
        microsporidia and, 102
Cholecystitis
    acalculous
        gastrointestinal CMV and, 220
        in disseminated *Isospora*, 103
        microsporidia and, 102, 217
    Cryptosporidia and, 100
    Giardia lamblia and, 105
Cholestasis, 198
Cholesterol, abnormalities of, from antiretroviral therapy, 36
Cholestyramine
    for *Cryptosporidium*, 101
    for HIV-associated diarrhea, 222
CHOP regimen, for HIV-related lymphoma, 242, 243
Choreiform movement disorder, toxomplasmosis and, 171
Choriamnioitis, perinatal transmission and, 249
Chorioretnal infiltrates, CMV retinitis *vs.*, 85
Chorioretinitis
    fungal, 152-153, 153b
    syphilitic, AIDS retinopathy *vs.*, 146
Choroid, ophthalmic lesions of
    AIDS retinopathy and, 146
    CMV retinitis and, 147
    MAC and, 152
    PCP and, 59
    Pneumocystis carinii and, 152
Cidofovir
    for CMV, 50, 53t
    for CMV esophagitis, 194
    for CMV pneumonitis, 209
    for CMV radiculitis, 173
    for CMV retinitis, 87, 88, 148, 149t
    for herpes simplex disease, 50, 91, 200
    for HIV-associated diarrhea from CMV, 220
    for molluscum contagiosum, 143
    for VZV, 93
    ocular hypotension and, 142
    renal failure and, 160, 161
    uveitis and, 142
Ciprofloxacin
    for bacterial enteric infections, 48-49
    for DMAC, 76, 77
        HIV-associated diarrhea and, 219
    for gastroenteritis, 111, 112
    for *M. xenopi*, 78
    for *Rhodococcus equi*, 207
    for *Salmonella*, 54t
    high-dose, intratubular crystallization and, 161t
Circinate exudate, AIDS retinopathy and, 146
Cisapride
    contraindications for, 42t
    drug-drug interactions and, 41
Cisplatin
    for anal neoplasia, 247
    for cervical cancer, 246

Citalopram, for major depressive disorder, 180b
Clarithromycin
    bacterial respiratory infections and, 48
    for *Bartonella*, 115
    for *Cryptosporidium parvum*, 218
    for DMAC, 48, 52t, 76, 76t
        HIV-associated diarrhea and, 219
        in children with AIDS, 252
    for DMAC prophylaxis, 76t, 77
    for *M. xenopi*, 78
    for MAC-induced choroiditis, 152
    for *Mycobacterium avium* complex, 198
    for *T. gondii*, 97, 98, 99t
    rifabutin treatment and uveitis with, 72
    safety of, 41
Clindamycin
    for *Pneumocystis carinii* pneumonia, 206
    for toxoplasmosis, 52t, 97, 98, 99t
        late HIV infection and, 210
    for toxoplasmosis retinochoroiditis, 151
    and primaquine for PCP prophylaxis, 66
    and pyrimethamine for PCP prophylaxis, 66
Clindamycin-primaquine, for *Pneumocystis carinii* pneumonia, 60, 62, 63t, 64
Clobetasol, for necrotizing stomatitis, 139
Clofazimine
    for DMAC, 76
    urine color changes with, 163t
Clomipramine, potential antiretroviral interaction with, 182t
Clonazepam
    for anxiety, 184
    for HIV-associated dementia with mania, 188
    for insomnia, 191
    for mania, 183
    for reactive depression, 178b
Clostridium difficile, HIV-associated diarrhea and, 219
Clotrimazole
    for angular cheilitis, 138
    for oral candidiasis, 138
    for oropharyngeal candidiasis, 80
    for vulvovaginal candidiasis, 80
Clozapine, contraindications for, 42t
CMV; *see* Cytomegalovirus
Coagulation, disseminated intravascular, histoplamosis and, 82
Coal tar shampoos, for seborrheic dermatitis, 127-128
Cocaine abuse, mania *vs.*, 183
Coccidioides immitis, 49-50, 82, 209
    as skin manifestation of HIV, 125, 125b
    Kaposi's sarcoma *vs.*, 237
    prophylaxis against, 54t
Coccidioidomycosis, 82-83, 83b
    demographics of, 211
    disseminated, fever of unknown origin and, 232
    fungal meningitis from, 171
    hepatitis in HIV and, 196
    molluscum contagiosum *vs.*, 120
    prophylaxis against, 49-50, 54t
    pulmonary, advanced HIV and, 209
Codeine, for *Cryptosporidium*, 101

Cognitive dysfunction
    absence of, motor neuropathy and, 168
    delirium and, 185
    HIV-associated psychosis and, 189
    in children with AIDS, 253
    referral for, 175
    sleep disturbances and, 191
Cognitive therapy
    for anxiety, 185
    for major depressive disorder, 180
Colitis
    cytomegalovirus, 86
        HSV colitis *vs.*, 220
        in acute HIV-1 infection, 18
    fulminant, *Entamoeba histolytica* and, 106
    HSV, 220
    pseudomembranous, *Clostridium difficile* and, 219
Collagen diseases, AIDS retinopathy *vs.*, 146
Colonic carcinoma, *Entamoeba histolytica* *vs.*, 106
Colonic mucosal polyps, condylomata acuminatum *vs.*, 199
Colonoscopy
    for CMV diagnosis, 86
    for HIV-associated diarrhea diagnosis, 222
Colposcopy
    for anal neoplasias, 247
    for cervical intraepithelial neoplasia, 245
Community-acquired pneumonia, 57; *see also* Pneumonia
    CD4+ counts and fever of unknown origin in, 231, 231b
    fluoroquinolone for, 63
Complementary therapies, 31
    educational discussions on, 28
Complete blood count (CBC), for fever of unknown origin diagnosis, 230
Computed tomography
    for biliary tract disease diagnosis, 198
    for *Entamoeba histolytica* diagnosis, 106
    for fever of unknown origin diagnosis, 232
    for hemorrhagic stroke diagnosis, 173
    for HIV-associated psychosis, 189
    for neurologic complication diagnosis, 166
    for progressive multifocal leukoencephalopathy diagnosis, 170
    for pyomyositis/lymphomatous infiltration of muscle, 174
    for sinusitis with low CD4+ count, 231
    for *T. gondii*, 96
    for tuberculous meningitis diagnosis, 172
    of brain, for cryptococcosis, 81
    of chest, for pulmonary diseases diagnosis, 213
Concentration deficits
    HIV-1–associated dementia complex and, 186
    HIV-associated dementia and, 167, 186
    major depressive disorder and, 179
    MCMD and, 186

Condylomata acuminata
  anal neoplasias and, 247
  anogenital, 199, 200
  as oral manifestation of HIV, 137
  in HIV, 121
Condylomata lata, secondary syphilis and, 112
Cone biopsy, for cervical intraepithelial neoplasia, 245
Confusion; *see also* Delirium
  anxiety disorders and, 184
  aseptic meningitis and, 166
  CMV ventriculoencephalitis and, 86
  CNS lymphoma and, 173
  from cryptococcal meningitis, 171
  in cryptococcosis, 81
  lymphomatous meningitis and, 175
  neurologic complications in HIV and, 166
  progressive multifocal leukoencephalopathy and, 170
  SSRIs and, 183
  T. gondii and, 96, 171
  tricyclic antidepressants and, 180b, 183
  tuberculous meningitis and, 172
Conjunctiva, herpes zoster ophthalmicus of, 143-144
Conjunctival tumors, Kaposi's sarcoma as, 142-143
Conjunctivitis
  chronic follicular, molluscum contagiosum and, 143
  papillary, syphilitic retinitis and, 152
  primary herpetic, herpes simplex keratitis *vs.*, 144
  Reiter's syndrome and, 127
Consciousness level
  delirium and, 185
  HSV encephalitis and, 170-171
Constipation
  anal neoplasias and, 246
  Giardia lamblia and, 105
  HSV proctitis and, 90
  SSRIs and, 183
  tricyclic antidepressants and, 180b, 183
Contraceptives, oral, drug-drug interactions and, 41
Control
  lack of
    anxiety disorders and, 184
    anxiety *vs.*, 185b
    pain and, 190
  out of, reactive depression and, 177
Cornea
  decompensation of, silicone oils for retinal detachment and, 148
  infections of
    herpes simplex keratitis and, 144
    herpes zoster ophthalmicus and, 143-144
    keratoconjunctivitis sicca and, 141
    microsporidia keratitis and, 145
  ulcers of, 145-146, 146b
Corticosteroids
  Aspergillis risk and, 211
  aspergillosis, advanced HIV and, 209
  CNS lymphoma and, 171

Corticosteroids—*cont'd*
  Entamoeba histolytica and, 105
  for aphthous ulcers, 134t
  for cerebral toxoplasmosis, 97-98
  for chronic inflammatory demyelinating polyneuropathy, 169
  for edema in tuberculous meningitis, 172
  for HIVAN, 156
  for intraocular inflammation with CMV treatment, 88
  for mononeuropathy multiplex, 169
  for necrotizing stomatitis, 134t
  for NSIP, 211
  for pain, 191
  for PCP, 206
  for polymyositis, 170
  for severe allergic interstitial nephritis, 161
  and rash/hypersensitivity reactions from NNRTIs, 36
Co-trimoxazole
  for bacterial pneumonia, 110
  for gastroenteritis, 111-112
  for PCP, *M. kansasii* and, 77
  neuropsychiatric side effects of, 181t
Cotton-wool spots
  AIDS retinopathy and, 146
  CMV retinitis *vs.*, 85, 148
Cough
  blastomycosis and, 83
  CMV pneumonitis and, 86
  comprehensive history of, 25b
  Cryptosporidia and, 100
  fever of unknown origin and, 234
  fungal pneumonias and, 208-209
  M. kansasii and, 208
  M. xenopi and, 78
  Nocardia asteroides and, 207
  nonproductive, PCP and, 205
  penicilliosis and, 83
  pneumococcal pneumonia and, 206
  pneumonia and, 108
  productive, in *Rhodococcus equi*, 116
  Rhodococcus equi and, 207
  T. gondii and, 96
  tuberculosis and, 207
Cox-2 inhibitors, renal failure or azotemia and, 160b
Cramps, abdominal
  Entamoeba histolytica and, 106
  Giardia lamblia and, 105
  primary HIV and, 119
Cranial nerve
  abnormalities of, syphilis and, 112
  CMV radiculitis and, 173
  palsies of, *T. gondii* and, 96
Cranial neuropathies
  aseptic meningitis and, 166
  CMV encephalitis and, 170
  CNS lymphoma and, 173
  from cryptococcal meningitis, 171
  lymphomatous meningitis and, 175
  neurosyphilis and, 172
  sensory-motor neuropathy from vincristine and, 175
  tuberculous meningitis and, 172

Creatinine
  for HIV-associated diarrhea diagnosis, 216
  HIV-associated lymphoma and, 242
  renal failure and other renal abnormalities and, 160, 162
  and TMP-SMX for PCP, 61
Creatinine kinase, *T. gondii* and, 97
Creatinine phosphokinase, polymyositis and, 170
Cresylecht violet staining, for PCP, 59
Crixivan; *see* Indinavir
Cross-resistance to drug combinations, 39, 149; *see also* Drug resistance
Cryoglobulinemia
  essential mixed, 158, 158b
  hepatitis C-associated immune complex glomerulonephritis and, 157-158
  membranoproliferative glomerulonephritis and, 157
Cryosurgery, for cervical intraepithelial neoplasia, 245
Cryotherapy
  for anogenital condylomata acuminata, 200
  for Kaposi's sarcoma, 129, 240b
  for molluscum contagiosum, 120, 143
  for oral hairy leukoplakia, 94
  for warts, 121
Cryptococcosis, 12, 81; *see also* Meningitis, cryptococcal
  as neurologic complication of HIV, 172
  as oral manifestation of HIV, 133t, 135t
  CD4+ counts, fever of unknown origin and, 232
  disseminated
    HSV *vs.*, 90
    in HIV-infected patients, 125
  hepatitis in HIV and, 196
  molluscum contagiosum *vs.*, 120
  pulmonary, advanced HIV and, 208
  diagnosis of, 212
  T. gondii vs., 97
Cryptococcus neoformans, 81
  as skin manifestation in HIV, 124-125, 125b
  chorioretinitis and, 152-153
  CMV retinitis *vs.*, 86
  cutaneous, 125f
  focal CNS lesion and, 98t
  Kaposi's sarcoma *vs.*, 237
  M. kansasii and, 77
  maculopapular red-brown lesions and, 239t
  optic nerve atrophy and, 147
  prophylaxis against, 49, 52t
  pyomyositis/lymphomatous infiltration of muscle and, 174-175
Cryptosporidiosis, 217-218
  exposure to, 46-47
  I. belli vs., 218
  TTP/HUS and, 159b
Cryptosporidium parvum, 46-47, 99-102
  CMV colitis *vs.*, 86
  Cyclospora vs., 104
  diarrhea and, 100t, 217-218

Cryptosporidium parvum—cont'd
   gastrointestinal CMV and, 86
   HIV-associated cholangiopathy and, 198, 199
   HSV esophagitis and, 90
   Isospora vs., 103
   Key Points, 102b, 218b
   treatment of, 101t
Crystalluria
   diagnosis of renal failure and renal abnormalities and, 161
   from indinavir, 161
   from TMP-SMX for PCP, 60
   from TMP-SMX for PCP prophylaxis, 65
Curettage
   for molluscum contagiosum, 120, 143
   for necrotizing stomatitis, 139
   for nonmelanoma skin cancer in HIV, 130
Cushing's syndrome, megestrol acetate and, 225, 227t
CXCR4, T cell–tropic HIV strains and, 15
Cyclophosphamide, for HIV-associated lymphoma, 242, 243
Cycloplegic drops, for photophobia from corneal ulcers, 145
Cycloserine, neuropsychiatric side effects of, 181t
Cyclospora cayetanensis, 99, 104, 104b
   CMV colitis *vs.,* 86
   Cryptosporidium vs., 100
   diarrhea and, 100t, 218
   treatment of, 101t
Cyclosporine
   antifungal azoles interactions with, 84
   for chronic inflammatory demyelinating polyneuropathy, 169
   for HIVAN, 156
   for psoriasis with HIV, 127
Cyclothymia, mania *vs.,* 182, 183b
Cystic calcification, visceral, PCP and, 59
Cysts, *T. gondii* and, 96
Cytokines
   AIDS wasting syndrome and, 223, 224, 226
   Kaposi's sarcoma and, 237
Cytomegalovirus (CMV), 12; *see also* Retinitis, cytomegalovirus
   antibody test (anti-CMV IgG), 45
      for fever of unknown origin diagnosis, 232
   as neurologic complication of HIV, 167b
   as oral manifestation of HIV, 133t, 135t, 136
   as skin manifestation of HIV, 121
   CD4+ counts and fever of unknown origin with, 231-232, 231b
   disseminated, hypercalcemia and, 164
   disseminated *Mycobacterium avium* complex and, 74
   encephalitis, 170
   esophageal candidiasis *vs.,* 80, 124
   esophagitis, 193, 194
   fever of unknown origin and, 229, 233
   focal CNS lesion and, 98t
   Guillain-Barré syndrome and, 168
   hepatitis in HIV and, 196

Cytomegalovirus (CMV)—*cont'd*
   HIV-associated
      anorectal lesions and, 199
      children with AIDS and, 252b
      cholangiopathy and, 198, 199
      diarrhea and, 220
   HSV esophagitis *vs.,* 90
   HSV *vs.,* 90
   hypuricemia and, 165
   Isospora vs., 103
   Kaposi's sarcoma *vs.,* 237
   Key Points, 89b, 121b, 220b
   M. kansasii and, 77
   optic nerve atrophy and, 147
   pneumonitis, late HIV infection and, 209-210, 210b
   prevention, 89t
   primary infection
      cause of, 85
      diagnosis of, 86-87
      guidelines for, 88-89
      in acute HIV-1 infection, 17, 17b
      natural history of, 87
      presentation of, 85-86
      referrals for, 88
      treatment of, 87-88
         complications in, 88
         expected response to, 88
   prophylaxis against, 50, 53t
   pulmonary cryptococcosis comborbidity with, 208
   pyomyositis/lymphomatous infiltration of muscle and, 174-175
   radiculitis, 170, 173, 174f
   refractory *vs.* relapse in, 87
   salivary gland dysfunction and, 132
   toxoplasmosis comborbidity with, 151
   toxoplasmosis retinochoroiditis *vs.,* 151
   TTP/HUS and, 159, 159b
Cytosine arabonside, for progressive multifocal leukoencephalopathy diagnosis, 170
Cytotoxic T lymphocytes, in acute HIV-1 infection, 16
Cytovene; *see* Ganciclovir

D

d4T; *see* Stavudine
Dapsone; *see also* Trimethoprim-dapsone
   didanosine interactions with, 41
   for PCP prophylaxis, 65, 65t, 66
   for *Pneumocystis carinii* pneumonia, 52t
   for toxoplasmosis, 52t, 97, 98, 99t
      late HIV infection and, 210
   motor-predominant polyneuropathy from, 175
   renal syndromes with, 163t
   skin reactions to, 129
Daunorubicin, liposomal, for Kaposi's sarcoma, 240, 240b
Daunoxome; *see* Daunorubicin, liposomal
Day care, children with AIDS and, 255
ddC; *see* Zalcitabine
ddI; *see* Didanosine
Decision making, ambivalence in, major depressive disorder and, 179
Decongestants, xerostomia from, 132

Dehydration, lithium carbonate and, 183, 183b
Delavirdine, 33
   characteristics of, 33t
   didanosine interactions with, 41
   drug fever and, 230
   drug-induced diarrhea from, 220
   headache from, 36
   rash/hypersensitivity reactions from, 36
   resistance to, 39-40
   rifabutin and uveitis with, 72
   rifabutin contraindications with, 47b, 74
Delirium, 185-186
   anxiety *vs.,* 185b
   etiologies in HIV/AIDS patients, 186b
   HIV-associated dementia and, 186
   HIV-associated psychosis *vs.,* 189
   Key Points, 186b
Delusions
   HIV-1–associated dementia complex and, 186
   HIV-associated dementia and, 186
   major depressive disorder and, 179
   mania and, 182
   somatic, HIV-associated psychosis and, 189
Dementia, 186
   anxiety *vs.,* 185b
   CMV and, 86
   delirium *vs.,* 185
   diagnosis of, 187
   HIV-associated, 166, 167-168, 167b
      brain imaging studies of, 167, 167f
      categories of, 186-187
      CMV encephalitis *vs.,* 170
      diagnosis of, 187
      Key Points, 188b
      major depressive disorder *vs.,* 179-180
      mania *vs.,* 182, 183b
      nomenclature and research case definitions for, 187b
      treatment of, 187-188
   neurosyphilis and, 172
   treatment of, 187-188
Demyelination
   Guillain-Barré syndrome and, 169
   HIV-associated dementia and, 167
   progressive multifocal leukoencephalopathy and, 170
   vacuolar myelopathy and, 168
Dental status, initial HIV assessment of, 26b
Depakote, for mania, 183
Depression; *see also* Major depressive disorder
   AIDS wasting syndrome and, 226
   anxiety disorders and, 184
   anxiety *vs.,* 185b
   comprehensive history of, 25b
   delirium and, 185
   from parenteral pegylated interferon, 197
   HIV-1–associated dementia complex and, 186
   HIV-associated dementia and, 167
   major depressive disorder and, 179
   pain syndromes and, 190
   reactive, 177-179, 178b
   sleep disturbances and, 191

Dermatitis
    atopic, pruritus vs., 126
    chronic actinic, photosensitivity in HIV and, 128
    seborrheic, 79
        as skin manifestation of HIV, 127-128, 128f
            Key Points, 128b
        dermatophytosis in HIV vs., 124
        HIV and, 118
        initial HIV assessment for, 25, 26b
        PCP and, 205
        Pityrosporum ovale vs., 124
Dermatographism, pruritus vs., 126
Dermatophytosis, as skin manifestation of HIV, 124, 124b
Dermatosis, pustular, HSV vs., 90
Desipramine
    for bereavement, 179b
    for HIV-associated dementia, 188
    potential antiretroviral interaction with, 182t
Despair, reactive depression and, 177
Developing countries, *Strongyloides stercoralis* and, 210
Dexamethasone
    for aphthous ulcers, 139
    for HIV-associated lymphoma, 243
    for necrotizing stomatitis, 139
Dexedrine, for HIV-associated dementia, 188
Dextroamphetamine, for HIV-associated dementia, 188
Diabetes mellitus, type II
    AIDS retinopathy vs., 146
    from antiretroviral therapy, 37
    megestrol acetate and, 225, 227t
    papillopathy, AIDS-related papilledema vs., 147
    and pentamidine for PCP, 61
Dialysis
    for HIVAN, 156
    for hyperkalemia, 164
    short-term, for severe hyperkalemia or renal fluid overload, 161
Diarrhea
    AIDS wasting syndrome and, 226
    anal neoplasia and, 246
    anxiety disorders and, 184
    chronic, AWS and, 223
    CMV colitis and, 86
    comprehensive history of, 25b
    Cryptosporidium and, 100
    Cyclospora and, 104
    DMAC and, 75t, 76
    Entamoeba histolytica and, 105, 106
    from acyclovir, 90
    from clindamycin-primaquine for PCP, 62, 63t
    from spore-forming organisms, 100t
        treatment of, 101t
    gastroenteritis and, 111
    Giardia lamblia and, 104-105, 105
    HIV-associated, 195, 216
        diagnosis and treatment of, 221-222
            algorithm for, 221f
        diagnosis of, 214

Diarrhea—cont'd
    HIV-associated—cont'd
        drug-induced, 220, 221
        from bacteria, 219
        from protozoa, 216-218
        from viruses, 220
        pathogens in, 217t
        unexplained, 220-221
    HUS and, 159
    hypokalemia and, 163
    hyponatremia and, 162
    in acute HIV-1 infection, 17b
    Isospora and, 103
    lithium carbonate and, 183, 183b
    microsporidia and, 102
    primary HIV and, 119
    renal magnesium wasting and, 164
    symptom management of, 224
    with antiretroviral therapy, 35-36
Diazepam, for anxiety, 184
Didanosine
    characteristics of, 32t
    drug-drug interactions with, 41
    drug-induced diarrhea from, 220
    for children with AIDS, 254, 255
    gastrointestinal side effects from, 36
    hepatocellular toxicity of, 195b
    hyperamylasemia from, 37
    hypocalcemia and, 164
    hypokalemia and, 163
    hypomagnesemia and, 164
    hypuricemia and, 165
    neurologic adverse effects from, 36
    neuropsychiatric side effects of, 181t
    nucleoside analogue-induced neuropathy and, 175
    pancreatitis from, 37
    and pentamidine for PCP, 61, 64
    renal implications of, 162
    resistance to, 39
    rifabutin with, 47b
    rifamycins for TB and, 72
    xerostomia from, 132
Dideoxycytidine, reaction to, as oral manifestation of HIV, 135t
Dideoxynucleoside reverse transcriptase inhibitors, neurologic adverse effects from, 36
Diff-Quick stain, for PCP, 59
Dihydroergotamine, contraindications for, 42t, 175
Dihydroxypropoxymethyl guanine; *see* Ganciclovir
Dilantin, antiretroviral drug interactions with, 41
Diphenoxylate
    for *Cryptosporidium*, 101
    for HIV-associated diarrhea, 222
Diphenylhydantoin, for sensory-motor axonal polyneuropathy, 169
Diptheria, tetanus, and acellular pertussis (DTaP) vaccine
    for children with AIDS, 253, 253b
Directly observed therapy (DOT), for tuberculosis treatment, 69, 70, 71, 74, 208
Disability, pain and, 190

Disclosure, of HIV infection to children, 255
Disorientation; *see also* Confusion
    delirium and, 185
    HIV-associated psychosis and, 189
    T. gondii and, 96
Disseminated disease, differential diagnosis of, fever of unknown origin and, 232
Disseminated *Mycobacterium avium* complex (DMAC)
    children with AIDS and, 252, 252b
    diagnosis of, 74
    epidemiology of, 74-75
    fever of unknown origin and, 229
    HIV-associated diarrhea and, 220b
    pathogenesis of, 75
    presentation and progression, 75-76
    prevention of, 77
    prophylaxis of, 76t
    symptoms, physical findings and laboratory abnormalities in, 75t
    treatment of, 76-77, 76t
Distractability, delirium and, 185
Diuretics
    for nephrosarca, 160
    with high-saline intravenous fluid for renal failure and other renal abnormalities, 161
    with saline for hyponatremia, 163
    xerostomia from, 132
DMAC; *see* Disseminated *Mycobacterium avium* complex
DNA polymerase chain reaction assay; *see* Polymerase chain reaction (PCR)
Dogs, gastroenteritis and, 111
Doxil; *see* Doxorubicin, liposomal
Doxorubicin
    for HIV-associated lymphoma, 242, 243
    for Kaposi's sarcoma, 130
    liposomal, for Kaposi's sarcoma, 201, 240, 240b
Doxycycline
    esophagitis and, 193
    for bacterial pneumonia, 110
    for *Bartonella*, 115, 122
    for syphilis, 114
        with HIV, 123
    for syphilitic retinitis, 152
Drinking water, contaminated
    Cryptosporidium and, 99, 101
    Cyclospora cayetanensis and, 104
    Giardia lamblia and, 104
Dronabinol, for appetite enhancement, 225, 227t
Drug abuse; *see also* Drug users, injecting
    acute psychosis vs., 189
    anxiety vs., 185b
    mania vs., 183, 183b
    pain control and, 191
    reactions to, major depressive disorder vs., 179
Drug allergies
    for HIV medical history, 24
    interstitial nephritis and, 160b

Drug combinations
    CDE, for HIV-associated lymphoma, 242, 243
    CHOP, for HIV-associated lymphoma, 242, 243
    for acute HIV-1 infection, 19
    for bacterial pneumonia, 110
    for children with AIDS, 253-255, 254t
    for cryptococcal meningitis, 171
    for cryptococcosis with HIV, 125
    for diarrhea from spore-forming protozoa, 101t
    for DMAC, 48, 52t, 76, 76t
        HIV-associated diarrhea and, 219
    for *Isospora*, 103
    for Kaposi's sarcoma, 130, 240b
    for MAC-induced choroiditis, 152
    for Mycobacetrial infections, 78
    for non-Hodgkin's lymphoma, 134t
    for PCP, 206
    for perinatal transmission reduction, 250
    for *Rhodococcus equi*, 116
    for squamous cell carcinoma, 134t
    for toxoplasmosis, 99t, 171
    for toxoplasmosis retinochoroiditis, 151
    for varicella-zoster keratitis, 145
    HIV cross-resistance to, 39
    hypuricemia and, 165
    initial selection of, 35
    mBACOD, for HIV-associated lymphoma, 243
    of three-NRTIs, 33, 35
    preferred, 31
    resistance testing and, 40
Drug fever, 230, 231b
Drug reactions
    acute tubular necrosis and, 160b
    as skin manifestation of HIV, 129, 129b
    linear gingival erythema *vs.*, 138
    maculopapular red-brown lesions and, 239t
    photoallergic, 128
    pruritus and, 126
    with antiretroviral drug combinations, 35
Drug resistance
    HSV and, 91
    in CMV treatment, 148-149
    Rhodococcus equi and, 116
    to acyclovir, 91, 93, 119, 120
        for HSV, 200, 220
        with severe immune deterioration and HSV-2, 133t
    to ampicillin, 111-112
    to antiretroviral therapy
        assays monitoring, 39-40
        testing before, 40
    to co-trimoxazole, 110, 111-112
    to famcyclovir, for HSV, 200
    to fluconazole for candidiasis, 80, 124
    to ganciclovir for CMV, 88
    to isoniazid, 208
    to itraconazole for candidiasis, 124
    to PCP prophylaxis, 65
    to penicillin in pneumococci, 110
    to quinolones for *Campylobacter*, 219
    to rifampin, 208
    to tuberculosis treatment, 69-70, 207-208

Drug resistance—cont'd
    to valacyclovir, for HSV, 200
    to zidovudine, 188
        perinatal transmission and, 250
    tuberculosis diagnosis and, 71
    tuberculosis prophylaxis and, 74
Drug toxicity, 195b
    anxiety *vs.*, 185b
    cholestatic, 195b
    hepatocellular, 195b, 196, 198
    major depressive disorder *vs.*, 180b
    mania and, 183, 183b
    pain and, 190
Drug users, injecting
    cytomegalovirus risk for, 45
    hepatitis C and, 51, 195
    HIV screening for, 20
    HIV-1 subtype B and, 6-7
    HIVAN and, 154, 155
    HIV-associated diarrhea and, 216
    HIV-associated nephropathy and, 154
    initial HIV management for, educational discussions on needles for, 28
    international HIV prevalence among, 6
    Kaposi's sarcoma and, 236
    lymphoma and, 241
    pulmonary sequelae, late HIV infection and, 211
    tuberculosis risk for, 211
    U.S. HIV prevalence among, 10-11, 10f
    with HIV
        M. fortuitum and, 122
        Staphylococcus aureus in, 207
        Streptococcus pneumoniae and, 108
        tuberculosis and, 207
Drug withdrawal syndromes
    anxiety disorders and, 184
    anxiety *vs.*, 185b
Drug-drug interactions, 47, 47b
    antifungal azoles and, 84
    in antiretroviral therapy, 40-41
        HIV-related lymphoma treatment and, 243
    neuropsychiatric side effects from, 180, 180b, 181t
    protease inhibitors and, 188
    TB treatment and, 71
Drugs
    contraindicated, 41, 42t
        neurologic complications from, 175
    recreational, *Aspergillis* risk and, 211
Dry eyes; *see* Keratoconjunctivitis sicca; Microsporidia keratitis
Dry mouth; *see* Xerostomia
Dual energy x-ray absorptiometry (DEXA), for body compositin, 223
Duodenal aspiration, for *Giardia lamblia*, 105
Duodenal sampling with string test, for *Giardia lamblia*, 105
Dysarthria
    Guillain-Barré syndrome and, 168
    T. gondii and, 96
Dyschromatopsia, optic nerve atrophy and, 147
Dysequilibrium
    HIV-associated dementia and, 167
    neurologic complications in HIV and, 166

Dysesthesia
    herpes zoster and, 173-174
    sensory-motor axonal polyneuropathy and, 169
Dysglycemia
    from pentamidine for PCP, 63t
    from trimetraxate for PCP, 63t
    and pentamidine for PCP, 61
Dyspepsia, with antiretroviral therapy, 35-36
Dysphagia
    comprehensive history of, 25b
    esophagitis and, 193
    gastrointestinal CMV and, 86
    Guillain-Barré syndrome and, 168
    HSV esophagitis and, 90
    in esophageal candidiasis, 80
    polymyositis and, 169
Dysphoria
    major depressive disorder and, 179
    reactive depression and, 177
Dysplasia, anal, 246
Dyspnea
    blastomycosis and, 83
    CMV pneumonitis and, 86
    comprehensive history of, 25b
    fungal pneumonias and, 208-209
    in *Rhodococcus equi*, 116
    M. kansasii and, 208
    M. xenopi and, 78
    Nocardia asteroides and, 207
    PCP and, 205
    penicilliosis and, 83
    pneumococcal pneumonia and, 206
    pneumonia and, 108
    T. gondii and, 96
Dysrhythmias, *T. gondii* and, 97
Dysruria, from indinavir, 161
Dysthymia, major depressive disorder *vs.*, 180b

E

Early HIV, diagnosis of, 22, 23
Ears
    assessment for initial HIV management, 25
    atypical presentations of PCP and, 58-59
Eastern Europe, HIV in, 6
Echinococcal cysts, *Entamoeba histolytica vs.*, 106
Economic concerns, educational discussions on, 28
Edema
    growth hormone for AWS and, 226, 227t
    hepatitis C-associated immune complex glomerulonephritis and, 157, 158
    macular
        AIDS retinopathy and, 146
        CMV retinitis and, 85
        cystoid, 88, 142
    of optic nerve, 146-147
    renal interstitial, acute renal failure and, 160
Education
    adolescent development of sexual identity, HIV and, 256
    for anxiety, 185
    for reactive depression, 178
    nutritional, 224

Educational discussions
  during primary care office visits, 44
  for initial HIV management, 27-28
Efavirenz, 33
  azithromycn and, 41
  birth defects from, 37
  characteristics of, 33t
  drug fever and, 230
  for children with AIDS, 254, 255
  neurologic adverse effects from, 36
  neuropsychiatric side effects of, 181t
  rash/hypersensitivity reactions from, 36
  resistance to, 39-40
  rifabutin interactions with, 47b
  rifabutin treatment for TB and, 72
Effexor; see Venlafaxine
Eflornithine, for *Pneumocystis carinii* pneumonia, 60, 62
Electroconvulsive therapy, for major depressive disorder, 181
Electrodesiccation
  for molluscum contagiosum, 143
  for nonmelanoma skin cancer in HIV, 130
Electroencephalogram, for HSV encephalitis diagnosis, 171
Electroencephalography, for HIV-associated delirium, 185
Electrolytes
  abnormalities of
    HIV-associated dementia and, 187
    HIV-associated lymphoma and, 242
    for HIV-associated diarrhea diagnosis, 216
  imbalance of
    hyponatremia and, 162-163
    potassium disorders and, 163-164
    psoriasis and, 127
    renal failure and other renal abnormalities and, 161
  and TMP-SMX for PCP, 61
Electromyography
  for chronic inflammatory demyelinating polyneuropathy, 169
  for CMV radiculitis diagnosis, 173
  for dapsone-induced motor-predominant polyneuropathy, 175
  for Guillain-Barré syndrome, 169
  for INH-related neuropathy, 175
  for mononeuropathy multiplex diagnosis, 169
  for motor neuropathy diagnosis, 168
  for nucleoside analogue-induced neuropathy, 175
  for polymyositis diagnosis, 170
  for pyomyositis/lymphomatous infiltration of muscle, 174
  for sensory-motor axonal polyneuropathy, 169
  for sensory-motor neuropathy from vincristine, 175
  for subacute motor neuropathy from lymphoma, 175
  for zidovudine-related myopathy, 175
Electron microscopy, for microsporidia diagnosis, 102
Eletroencephalograms, for HIV-associated psychosis, 189

Embarrassment, reactive depression and, 177, 178
Emotional distress, HIV-related skin diseases and, 118
Emptiness feeling, major depressive disorder and, 179
Encephalitis, 12
  diffuse, histoplamosis and, 82
  in acute HIV-1 infection, 17b
  post-varicella-zoster virus infectious, 92
  toxoplasmic
    diagnosis of, 97
    and *Pneumocystis carinii* pneumonia, 46
    T. gondii and, 96
    treatment for, 98
  viral, as neurologic complication of HIV, 167b
Encephalitozoon cuniculi, microsporidia keratitis and, 145
Encephalitozoon hellem, microsporidia keratitis and, 145
Encephalitozoon intestinalis, 102-103, 217; see also Microsporidia
  treatment for, 101t
Encephalopathy
  acyclovir and, 90
  HIV-associated, 17b, 167
    focal CNS lesion and, 98t
    in children, 252-253
  toxoplasma, TMP-SMX prophylaxis and, 64
Encoscopy, for *Entamoeba histolytica* diagnosis, 106
Endemic mycoses, 81-82
  blastomycosis, 83
  coccidioidomycosis, 82-83
  histoplamosis, 82
  penicilliosis, 83
Endocarditis
  bacterial and nonbacterial, cerbrovascular disease and, 173
  Bartonella and, 115
  Salmonella and, 111
  tricuspid valve, *Staphylococcus aureus* and, 108
Endophthalmitis, from ganciclovir implants, 87
Endoscopic retrograde cholangiopancreatography (ERCP), for biliary tract disease diagnosis, 198
Endoscopy
  for esophagitis diagnosis, 193, 194
  for HIV-associated diarrhea diagnosis, 216, 222
End-stage renal disease; see Renal failure, acute
Energy, loss of, major depressive disorder and, 179, 180b
Entamoeba histolytica, 105-106
  CMV colitis vs., 86
  diarrhea and, 218, 222
  Key Points, 106b, 218b
  treatment of, 103t
Enteric infections, bacterial, prophylaxis against, 48-49
Enterobacter cloacae, ulcers from, HIV and, 135t

Enterocytozoon bieneusi, 102-103, 217; see also Microsporidia
  treatment for, 101t
Env gene, HIV variants and, 3
Envelope genes, 3
Envelope glycoproteins, response to HIV infection by, 20
Enzyme immunoassay
  for *Clostridium difficile* diagnosis, 219, 222
  for *Cryptosporidium parvum* diagnosis, 218, 222
  for *Entamoeba histolytica* diagnosis, 218, 222
  for HIV screening, 20
  detuned for early diagnosis, 23
Enzyme-linked immunosorbent assays (ELISAs)
  for *Cryptosporidium* diagnosis, 100, 100t
  for *Giardia lamblia* diagnosis, 105
  for HSV diagnosis, 90
  for infants born to HIV-infected mothers, 250, 251
  for *T. gondii* diagnosis, 97
Eosinophilic folliculitis
  as skin manifestation of HIV, 128-129, 129b
  maculopapular red-brown lesions and, 239t
  pruritus vs., 126
Eosinophilic pustular dermatosis, 128
Epidemiology
  international perspective, 6
  of tuberculosis, 69-70
  U.S. background for, 6-8
Epidermal necrolysis, toxic, from drug hypersensitivity in HIV, 129
Epidermophyton, 80
Epiretinal membrane
  from CMV treatment, 88
  immune recovery vitritis and, 142
Epithelial herpes simplex keratitis, 144
Epivir; see Lamivudine
Epstein-Barr virus (EBV), 94
  herpesvirus Saimiri and, 236
  lymphocytic interstitial pneumonitis and, 252
  oral hairy leukoplakia and, 121, 136-137
Ergot alkaloids, 42t
  drug-drug interactions and, 41
Ergotamine, contraindications for, 42t, 175
Erythema multiforme
  coccidioidomycosis and, 82
  exudativum, necrotizing ulcerative gingivitis or peridontitis vs., 139
Erythema multiforme–like eruptions, from drug hypersensitivity in HIV, 129
Erythema nodosum, coccidioidomycosis and, 82
Erythematous candidiasis, as oral manifestation of HIV, 133t, 137-138
Erythroderma, with Sézary syndrome, as skin manifestation of HIV, 130
Erythrodermic psoriasis, as skin manifestation of HIV, 127

Erythromycin
  Entamoeba histolytica diagnosis and, 106
  for bacillary epithelioid angiomatosis, 134t, 237
  for *Bartonella*, 115, 122
  for *Entamoeba histolytica*, 103t, 106
  for *Rhodococcus equi*, 207
Escherichia coli
  hemolytic-uremic syndrome and, 159
  HIV-associated diarrhea and, 219
  pneumonia in late HIV infection and, 207
  TTP/HUS and, 159b
  ulcers from, HIV and, 135t
Esophageal candidiasis, 80, 138
  as AIDS-defining illness, 193
  in acute HIV-1 infection, 18
  treatment of, 194
Esophagitis, 193-194, 195b
  cytomegalovirus, diagnosis of, 86
  evaluation and treatment algorithm, 194f
  gastrointestinal CMV and, 86, 220
  HSV, 90
Esophagogastroduodenoscopy (EGD)
  for esophageal candidiasis diagnosis, 80
  for HIV-associated diarrhea diagnosis, 222
Essential mixed cryoglobulinemia, 158, 158b
Ethambutol
  dosage for initial treatment of TB, 72t
  for DMAC, HIV-associated diarrhea and, 219
  for *M. kansasii*, 77, 208
  for *M. xenopi*, 78
  for MAC-induced choroiditis, 152
  for *Mycobacterium avium* complex, 198
    disseminated, 48, 52t, 76, 76t
  for tuberculosis, 207
  for tuberculous meningitis, 172
  hypuricemia and, 165
  NRTIs or PIs and, 72
  safety of, 41
Etoposide
  for HIV-associated lymphoma, 242
  for Kaposi's sarcoma, 130
Euphoria, dronabinol and, 225, 227t
Euvolemic hyponatremia, AIDS and, 162
Excoriations, eosinophilic folliculitis in HIV and, 128
Exercise
  AIDS wasting syndrome and, 225
  capacity, growth hormone and, 226
  HIV medical history review of, 24
Extensor plantar responses, vacuolar myelopathy and, 168
Extrapulmonary tuberculosis, 70, 70t
  inactive infection and, 73
Eye hemorrhage
  AIDS retinopathy and, 146
  subconjunctival, Kaposi's sarcoma *vs.*, 142
Eyes; *see also* Retinal detachment; Retinal necrosis; Retinitis; Uveitis; Vitritis
  initial HIV assessment of, 25, 26b
  T. gondii and, 97

F

Failure to thrive
  blastomycosis and, 83
  children with AIDS and, 251

False-negative serologic tests for HIV, 20-21
False-positive serologic tests for HIV, 21
  with DNA polymerase chain reaction assay, 22
Famciclovir
  for herpes zoster, 120, 174
  for herpes zoster encephalitis, 171
  for herpes zoster ophthalmicus, 144
  for HSV, 50, 54t, 90, 91, 119, 200
  for varicella-zoster keratitis, 145
  for VZV, 93, 93t
  resistance to VZV, 93
Famvir; *see* Famciclovir
Fasciculations, motor neuropathy and, 168
Fat tissue
  growth hormone and, 226
  redistribution of, from antiretroviral therapy, 36-37
Fatigue; *see also* Lethargy; Malaise
  abacavir and, 230
  anxiety disorders and, 184
  comprehensive history of, 25b
  Cryptosporidia and, 100
  Cyclospora and, 104
  in acute HIV-1 infection, 17b
  PCP and, 205
  Rhodococcus equi and, 207
  sleep disturbances and, 191
  testosterone and, 225
Fearfulness
  anxiety disorders and, 183, 184
  delirium and, 185
Feces, CMV in, 85
Feline immunodeficiency virus, classification of, 3
Fetus, prenatal maternal HAART risks for, 250
Fever; *see also* Fever of unknown origin
  AIDS wasting syndrome and, 223
  aseptic meningitis and, 166
  bacillary peliosis and, 115
  biliary tract disease and, 198
  blastomycosis and, 83
  bronchoalveolar lavage for PCP diagnosis and, 59
  CMV colitis and, 86
  CMV pneumonitis and, 86
  CMV retinitis and, 85
  CMV ventriculoencephalitis and, 86
  comprehensive history of, 25b
  Cryptosporidia and, 100
  disseminated *Isospora* and, 103
  DMAC and, 75, 75t
  Entamoeba histolytica and, 106
  from atovaquone for PCP, 63t
  from bleomycin for Kaposi's sarcoma, 240
  from cryptococcal meningitis, 171
  from dapsone for PCP prophylaxis, 66
  from HSV encephalitis, 171
  from interferon for Kaposi's sarcoma, 240
  from pentamidine for PCP, 63t
  from TMP-SMX for PCP, 60, 63t
  from TMP-SMX for PCP prophylaxis, 65
  Giardia lamblia and, 105
  HIV-associated diarrhea and, 216
  HIV-associated lymphoma and, 242

Fever—*cont'd*
  HSV esophagitis and, 90
  immune reconstitution syndrome and, 233
  in acute HIV-1 infection, 16-17, 17b
  in gastroenteritis, 111
  in histoplamosis, 82
  in infectious mononucleosis, 94
  in penicilliosis, 83
  in pneumonia, 108
  in *Rhodococcus equi*, 116
  in secondary syphilis, 112
  Kaposi's sarcoma and, 201
  M. kansasii and, 208
  M. xenopi and, 78
  MAC and, 76
  microsporidia and, 102
  Nocardia asteroides and, 207
  PCP and, 205
  PCP prophylaxis and, 64
  pneumococcal pneumonia and, 206
  primary HIV and, 119
  psoriasis and, 127
  Rhodococcus equi and, 207
  T. gondii and, 96, 171
  TTP and, 159
  tuberculosis and, 207
  tuberculous meningitis and, 172
  varicella-zoster virus and, 92
Fever of unknown origin (FUO)
  algorithm for, 234-235
  CD4+ count and diagnosis of, 231-232, 231b
  definition of, 229, 230b
  drug fever and, 230, 231b
  immune reconstitution syndrome and, 233
  initial workup, 229-230, 230b
  nonspecific focal signs of, 234
  prophylaxis for opportunistic infections and, 233-234
  specific organism diagnosis and, 233
  specific testing for, 232-233, 232b
  what not to do for, 234
Fexofenadine, safety of, 41
Fiber supplements, for HIV-associated diarrhea, 222
Fibrates, for lipodystrophy from antiretroviral therapy, 37
Fibroblast growth factor, Kaposi's sarcoma and, 237
Fibromas, human papillomavirus *vs.*, 137
Fine needle aspiration, for fever of unknown origin diagnosis, 232-233
Fish, *Cryptosporidium* and, 99
Fish oil, for non-HIV IgA glomerulonephritis, 157
Flatulence
  Entamoeba histolytica and, 106
  Giardia lamblia and, 105
Flecainide, contraindications for, 42t
Floaters
  fungal chorioretinitis and, 153
  retinal necrosis and, 149
  toxoplasmosis and, 151
  uveitis and, 72, 142
Flourescein stain, for microsporidia keratitis diagnosis, 145

Flow cytometry, for lymphomatous meningitis, 175
Fluconazole, 84
   for candidiasis, 49, 54t, 80
      esophageal, 124, 194
      oral, 138
   for coccidioidomycosis, 50, 54t, 82-83
   for cryptococcal meningitis, 171
   for cryptococcosis, 81
   for cryptococcosis with HIV, 125
      pulmonary, advanced HIV and, 208
   for *Cryptococcus neoformans*, 49, 52t
   for fungal infections, 84t
   for histoplasmosis, 82, 125
   for penicilliosis, 83
   rifabutin treatment and uveitis with, 72
Flucytosine, 84t
   for cryptococcosis, 81, 125
      pulmonary, advanced HIV and, 208
Fluocinonide, for necrotizing stomatitis, 139
Fluorescent antibody tests, for HSV diagnosis, 119
Fluorescent stains, for tuberculosis diagnosis, 70-71
Fluorescent treponemal antibody-absorbed (FTA-abs) test
   for neurosyphilis, 172
   for syphilis, HIV and, 113
   for syphilitic retinitis, 152
Fluoride, nystatin with sucrose and, 138
Fluorochrome stain, for microsporidia diagnosis, 222
Fluoroquinolones
   for bacterial enteric infections, 48
   for bacterial pneumonia, 110
   for *Bartonella*, 115
   for community-acquired pneumonia, 63
   for gastroenteritis, 111, 112
   for *Rhodococcus equi*, 116
5-Fluorouracil
   for anal neoplasia, 247
   for cervical intraepithelial neoplasia, 245
   for warts, 121
Fluoxetine
   for bereavement, 179b
   for HIV-associated dementia, 188
   for major depressive disorder, 180b
   potential antiretroviral interaction with, 182t
Flurazepam
   contraindications for, 175
   for insomnia, 191
Flushing, anxiety disorders and, 184
Fluvastatin, safety of, 41
Fluvoxamine, potential antiretroviral interaction with, 182t
Focal epithelial hyperplasia, as oral manifestation of HIV, 137
Focal neurologic signs
   cerebrovascular disease and, 173
   cryptococcis and, 172
   lymphoma and, 173
   referral for, 175
   tuberculous meningitis and, 172
Folate
   deficiency of, ulcers from, 135t
   HIV-associated dementia and, 167, 187
Folliculitis, from *S. aureus* in HIV, 121-122

Follow-up visits, in initial HIV management, 29
Fomivirsen
   for CMV retinitis, 149, 149t
   for cytomegalovirus, 53t
Food contamination
   Cyclospora cayetanensis and, 104
   gastroenteritis and, 111
   Giardia lamblia and, 104
Foot drop, sensory-motor neuropathy from vincristine and, 175
Forgetfulness; *see* Memory, impaired
Former Soviet Union, HIV in, 6
Foscarnet
   acute renal failure and, 160
   for CMV, 50, 53t
      perianal ulcers in HIV, 121
   for CMV encephalitis, 170
   for CMV esophagitis, 194
   for CMV pneumonitis, 209
   for CMV radiculitis, 173
   for CMV retinitis, 87-88, 148, 149, 149t
   for herpes simplex disease, 50, 91, 119, 200
   for herpes zoster, 120
   for herpes zoster ophthalmicus, 144
   for HIV-associated diarrhea from CMV, 220
   for HSV colitis, 220
   for oral hairy leukoplakia, 94
   for varicella-zoster retinitis, 150
   for VZV, 93
   hypocalcemia and, 164
   hypokalemia and, 163
   hypomagnesemia and, 164
   neuropsychiatric side effects of, 181t
   reaction to, as oral manifestation of HIV, 135t
   skin reactions to, 129
   TTP/HUS and, 159b
   xerostomia from, 132
Foscavir; *see* Foscarnet
Frontal release signs, HIV-associated dementia and, 186
Fumagillin, for microsporidia keratitis, 145
Fumidil B; *see* Fumagillin
Funduscopy, for ocular VZV diagnosis, 92
Fungal infections
   about, 79
   candidiasis, 80
   cryptococcosis, 81
   endemic mycoses, 81-83
   host defense to, 79
   late HIV infection and, 208-209, 209b
   superficial, 79-80
Fungemia, pneumonia in late HIV infection and, 212
Fungizone; *see* Amphotericin B
Furuncles, from *S. aureus* in HIV, 121-122
Fusarum spp., chorioretinitis and, 152-153
Fusin, HIV-1 replication and, 3

G

Gabapentin
   for neurologic adverse effects from antiretroviral therapy, 36
   for sensory-motor axonal polyneuropathy, 169

Gag viral proteins, HIV-1 replication and, 3
Gag-pol viral proteins, HIV-1 replication and, 3
Gait
   instability of, tertiary syphilis and, 174
   slowing of, HIV-associated dementia and, 167
   unsteady, HIV-1–associated dementia complex and, 186
Gallbladder
   Cryptosporidia and, 100
   microsporidia and, 102
Gallium scanning
   for fever of unknown origin diagnosis, 234
   for HIV-associated lymphoma diagnosis, 242
   for Kaposi's sarcoma *vs.* PCP diagnosis, 237
   for pulmonary diseases diagnosis, 213
Gamma globulin, IV, for TTP/HUS, 159
Ganciclovir
   for CMV encephalitis, 170
   for CMV esophagitis, 194
   for CMV pneumonitis, 209
   for CMV radiculitis, 173
   for cytomegalovirus, 50, 53t
      prophylaxis of, 89t
      resistance to, 88
      retinitis, 87-88, 148, 149, 149t
      with HIV, 133t, 136
   for herpes simplex disease, 91, 200
   for HIV-associated diarrhea from CMV, 220
   for Kaposi's sarcoma-associated herpesvirus, 51
   for oral hairy leukoplakia, 94
   for perianal ulcers from CMV in HIV, 121
   for varicella-zoster retinitis, 150
   hepatocellular toxicity of, 195b
   reaction to, as oral manifestation of HIV, 135t
   resistance to VZV, 93
   TTP/HUS and, 159b
Gardening, *Cryptosporidium* and, 101
Gastric outlet obstruction, *Cryptosporidium parvum* and, 217
Gastritis, gastrointestinal CMV and, 220
Gastroduodenal ulcer disease, GI bleeding and, 200
Gastroenteritis, 111-112
Gastrointestinal bleeding, 200-201, 201b
Gastrointestinal disease, 193
   abacavir and, 230
   adverse reactions to tuberculosis treatment and, 71
   anorectal lesions, 199-200
   biliary tract disease, 198-199
   bleeding, 200-201
   diarrhea, 195
   esophagitis, 193-194, 195b
   from CMV with AIDS, 86, 87-88, 121, 220, 220b
   hepatitis, 195-198
   Reiter's syndrome and, 127

Gastrointestinal distress
  DMAC and, 75, 75t, 76
  from atovaquone for PCP, 63t
  from TMP-SMX for PCP, 63t
  from TMP-SMX for PCP prophylaxis, 65
  from trimethoprim-dapsone for PCP, 63t
  in acute HIV-1 infection, 16-17, 17b
  renal failure and, 160
Gastrointestinal pain, 190
Gastrointestinal reflux disease
  CMV esophagitis vs., 86
  HSV esophagitis vs., 90
Gastrointestinal system, lymphoma presentation in, 241
Gastrostomy, for nutrition, 225
General anxiety disorder, anxiety vs., 185b
Genetics
  HIVAN and, 154, 155
  oral ulcers, HIV and, 135t
Genital herpes simplex disease, 89-90, 199
Genital secretions, CMV in, 85
Genital warts
  HIV-associated anorectal lesions and, 199
  in HIV, 121
Genitourinary systems
  assessment for initial HIV management, 26
  extrapulmonary TB in, 70
  initial HIV assessment of, 26b
  Reiter's syndrome and, 127
Genotypic resistance, to antiretroviral therapy, 39
  assays of, 40
Geographic tongue, Epstein-Barr virus vs., 94
Geotrichosis, as oral manifestation of HIV, 133t
Geotrichum candidum, linear gingival erythema vs., 138
Giant cells, multinucleated
  HIV in, 167
  vacuolar myelopathy and, 168
Giardia lamblia, 104-105, 105b, 218, 222
  CMV colitis vs., 86
  Key Points, 218b
  treatment of, 103t
Giemsa staining
  for toxoplasmosis diagnosis, 210
  for VZV diagnosis, 92
Gingival erythema, linear, 138-139
  as oral manifestation of HIV, 134t
Gingival hemorrhage, from necrotizing ulcerative peridontitis, 139
Glaucoma
  silicone oils for retinal detachment and, 148
  syphilitic retinitis and, 152
  varicella-zoster keratitis and, 144
Gliomas, central nervous system, as neurologic complications of HIV, 172
Gliosis, HIV-associated dementia and, 167
Glomerulonephritis (GN)
  acute, renal failure or azotemia and, 160b
  immune complex, 156-157, 157b
    hepatitis C-associated, 157-158
    renal potassium excretion and, 164

Glomerulosclerosis, focal segmental (FSGS), HIV-associated nephropathy and, 154, 156
Glucocorticoids, for *Pneumocystis carinii* pneumonia, 62, 63-64, 63t
Glucocorticosteroids
  for aphthous ulcers, 139
  for necrotizing stomatitis, 139
Glucose, megestrol acetate and, 225
Glucose intolerance, from antiretroviral therapy, 37
Glucose-6-phosphate dehydrogenase (G6PD)
  and clindamycin-primaquine for PCP, 62
  and trimethoprim-dapsone for PCP, 61
γ-Glutamyl transpeptidase, fever of unknown origin and, 233
Gonadotropins, megestrol acetate and, 225
Gonorrhea, rectal HSV vs., 199
gp 41
  in HIV envelope, 3
  response to HIV infection by, 20
gp 120
  in HIV envelope, 3
  response to HIV infection by, 20
gp 160, response to HIV infection by, 20
Gram's stain
  for bacterial pulmonary infections, 207
  for hyperplastic candidiasis diagnosis, 138
  for microsporidia keratitis diagnosis, 145
  for pneumococcal pneumonia diagnosis, 206
  for *Pseudomonas aeruginosa* diagnosis, 207
  for pulmonary diseases diagnosis, 213
Grandiosity, mania and, 182
Granulocyte/macrophage-colony stimulating factor (GM-CSF), Kaposi's sarcoma and, 237
Granulocytopenia, advanced HIV and, 108
Granulomas
  chorioidal or retinal, MAC and, 152
  syphilitic, 172
Granulomatosis, Wegener's, syphilitic retinitis vs., 152
Granulomatous diseases, hypercalcemia and, 164
Grief
  pathologic, major depressive disorder vs., 180b
  reactive depression and, 178
Group M, HIV subtypes in, 3
Group O, divergent HIV subtypes in, 3
Growth hormone (GH), AIDS wasting syndrome and, 224, 226, 227t
Guidelines
  adherence to
    antiretroviral therapy educational discussions for, 28
    treatment failure and, 40
  for CMV, 88-89
  for community-acquired pneumonia, 110
  for HSV, 91
  for syphilis, 114
  for VZV, 93-94

Guillain-Barré syndrome
  Campylobacter and, 111, 219
  HIV and, 168-169, 169b
  in acute HIV-1 infection, 17b
Guilt
  major depressive disorder and, 179
  reactive depression and, 177, 178
Gum, chewing sugarless, for salivary flow, 135
Gummatous syphilis, 112, 172
Guttate psoriasis, as skin manifestation of HIV, 127
Gynecologic history, for HIV medical history, 24

H
H-2 blockers, contraindications for, 42t
HAART, see Antiretroviral therapy, highly active
HAD; see HIV-1–associated dementia complex
Haemophilus influenzae, 206
  pneumonia from, 108
  prophylaxis against, 48
  sputum culture and, 109
  TMP-SMX prophylaxis against, 65
Hair, seborrheic dermatitis and, 127
Hair loss
  from paclitaxel for Kaposi's sarcoma, 241
  from systemic chemotherapy, 240
Haldol; see Haloperidol
Halitosis, from necrotizing ulcerative peridontitis, 139
Hallucinations
  delirium and, 185
  HIV-1–associated dementia complex and, 186
  HIV-associated dementia and, 186
  HIV-associated psychosis and, 189
  major depressive disorder and, 179
  mania and, 182
Haloperidol
  for HIV-associated delirium, 186
  for HIV-associated dementia, 188
  for HIV-associated psychosis, 190b
  for mania, 183
Hand-washing
  Cryptosporidium and, 46, 47
  for *Cryptosporidium*, 101
  Toxoplasma gondii and, 46
Head
  assessment for initial HIV management, 25
  lymphoma presentation in, 241
Head drop, polymyositis and, 169
Headaches
  anxiety disorders and, 184
  aseptic meningitis and, 166
  CNS lymphoma and, 173
  comprehensive history of, 25b
  fever of unknown origin and, 234
  from cryptococcal meningitis, 171
  from HSV encephalitis, 171
  from progressive multifocal leukoencephalopathy, 170
  from *T. gondii*, 96
  from trimethoprim-dapsone for PCP, 63t
  from varicella-zoster virus, 92
  in acute HIV-1 infection, 16-17, 17b

Headaches—cont'd
  lymphomatous meningitis and, 175
  meningovascular syphilis and, 112
  neurologic complications in HIV and, 166
  neurosyphilis and, 172
  pain and, 190
  primary HIV and, 119
  tuberculous meningitis and, 172
"Headlight in the fog" sign, toxoplasmosis retinochoroiditis and, 151
Health care workers, U.S. HIV prevalence among, 11
Heart
  abnormalities, and pentamidine for PCP, 61, 63t
  lymphoma presentation in, 241
  PCP and, 59, 63
  T. gondii and, 97
Heart failure, congestive, late HIV infection and, 211
Heck's disease, as oral manifestation of HIV, 137
Helplessness
  anxiety disorders and, 184
  reactive depression and, 177
Hemangioma, cavernous, Kaposi's sarcoma vs., 142
Hematochezia, from HSV, 220
Hematologic disease
  adverse reactions to tuberculosis treatment and, 71
  malignancies, aspergillosis, advanced HIV and, 209
Hematuria
  hepatitis C-associated immune complex glomerulonephritis and, 157, 158
  membranoproliferative glomerulonephritis and, 157
Hemiparesis
  from cryptococcal meningitis, 171
  progressive multifocal leukoencephalopathy and, 170
  T. gondii and, 96, 171
Hemiplegia, T. gondii and, 96
Hemodialysis; see also Dialysis
  patient-to-patient HIV infection and, 156
Hemoglobin, fever of unknown origin and, 232
Hemolysis
  from ribavirin plus interferon for HCV, 197-198
  G6PD deficiency-related
    from clindamycin-primaquine for PCP, 63t
    from dapsone for PCP prophylaxis, 66
    from trimethoprim-dapsone for PCP, 63t
  and trimethoprim-dapsone for PCP, 61
Hemolytic-uremic syndrome (HUS), 158-159, 159b
  valacyclovir and, 91
Hemophiliacs
  HIV screening for, 20
  lymphoma and, 241
  U.S. HIV prevalence among, 11

Hemoptysis
  in *Rhodococcus equi,* 116
  M. kansasii and, 208
  Nocardia asteroides and, 207
Hemorrhage
  acute tubular necrosis and, 160b
  bronchoalveolar lavage for PCP diagnosis and, 59
  from Kaposi's sarcoma in HIV, 129
  pulmonary, late HIV infection and, 211
  retinal, AIDS retinopathy and, 146
  subconjunctival, Kaposi's sarcoma vs., 142
Hemorrhagic strokes, 173
Hemorrhoids, anal squamous cell carcinoma vs., 199
Heparin, hyperkalemia and, 164
Hepatitis
  CMV encephalitis and, 170
  from TMP-SMX for PCP, 61, 63t, 206
  from TMP-SMX for PCP prophylaxis, 65
  from trimethoprim-dapsone for PCP, 63t
  HIV-associated, 195-198
  and rifamycin for TB, 74
  secondary syphilis and, 112
Hepatitis A
  acute, acute HIV-1 infection vs., 17
  exposure or infection history of, 24
  prophylaxis against, 53t
  vaccine for, 45
Hepatitis B
  acute, acute HIV-1 infection vs., 17, 17b
  exposure or infection history of, 24
  hepatitis C-associated immune complex glomerulonephritis and, 157
  HIV-associated, 195-197
  initial HIV assessment for, 26b
  membranoproliferative glomerulonephritis comorbidity with, 157
  prophylaxis against, 53t
  protease inhibitors and, 35
  vaccine for, 45
    children with AIDS and, 253, 253b
  viral hepatitis antibody tests with, 45
Hepatitis C
  antiretroviral therapy and, 37
  HIV-associated, 195, 196
  initial HIV assessment for, 26b
  membranoproliferative glomerulonephritis comorbidity with, 157
  mixed essential cryoglobulinemia and, 158
  porphyria cutanea tarda in HIV and, 128
  prophylaxis against, 51
  protease inhibitors and, 35
  treatment for, 197-198
  viral hepatitis antibody tests with, 45
Hepatitis C-associated immune complex glomerulonephritis, 157-158, 157b, 158b
Hepatocellular carcinoma
  Entamoeba histolytica vs., 106
  HCV treatment and, 198
Hepatoma, CD4+ counts and fever of unknown origin with, 231

Hepatosplenomegaly
  disseminated histoplasmosis and, 125
  DMAC and, 75, 75t
  leishmaniasis and, 232
  penicilliosis and, 83
  pulmonary histoplasmosis and, 209
Herbal medicines, drug-drug interactions and, 41
Herpes simplex keratitis
  as ocular complication of AIDS, 144, 144b
  varicella-zoster keratitis vs., 144
Herpes simplex virus (HSV), 12, 50
  as oral manifestation of HIV, 133t
  as skin manifestation of HIV, 119
  cause of, 89
  chronic, 120f
  diagnosis of, 90
  esophageal candidiasis vs., 80
  focal CNS lesion and, 98t
  gastrointestinal CMV vs., 86
  guidelines for, 91
  hepatitis in HIV and, 196
  HIV-associated anorectal lesions and, 199-200
  HIV-associated diarrhea and, 220
  HIV-associated encephalitis and, 170-171, 171b
  Kaposi's sarcoma vs., 237
  Key Points, 91b, 119b
  maculopapular red-brown lesions and, 239t
  mania vs., 183
  natural history of, 90
  optic nerve atrophy and, 147
  oral lesions, 136
    aphthous ulcers vs., 132
    CMV vs., 136
  presentation of, 89-90
  prophylaxis against, 54t
  pulmonary, late HIV infection and, 210
  referral for, 91
  suggestive of HIV, 135t
  TTP/HUS and, 159b
Herpes zoster; see also Varicella-zoster virus
  as neurologic complication of HIV, 167b
  as skin manifestation of HIV, 120, 120b
  diagnosis of, 92-93
  famciclovir for, 90
  Kaposi's sarcoma vs., 237
  maculopapular red-brown lesions and, 239t
  presentation of, 92
  varicella-zoster virus and, 91
Herpes zoster encephalitis, 171
Herpes zoster ophthalmicus, 92, 120
  as ocular complication of AIDS, 143-144
    Key Points, 144b
  herpes zoster encephalitis and, 171
  VZV and, 93
Herpesvirus; see also Cytomegalovirus; Epstein-Barr virus
  Kaposi's sarcoma-associated, 51, 201
  retinitis and, 147
Herpesvirus 1, human
  herpes simplex keratitis and, 144
  herpes zoster ophthalmicus vs., 143

Herpesvirus 2, human, herpes zoster ophthalmicus vs., 143
Herpesvirus 8, human
 as oral manifestation of HIV, 137
 Kaposi's sarcoma and, 129, 201, 236, 238f, 241
Herpesvirus Saimiri (HVS), 236
Herpetic whitlow, chronic, in HIV, 119
Herpetiform ulcers, HIV and, 135t
Herplex; see Idoxuridine
Heterosexuals
 cytomegalovirus risk for, 45
 HIV-1 subtype E and, 6-7
 Kaposi's sarcoma and, 236
 lymphoma and, 241
 U.S. HIV prevalence among, 11
Hiccups, esophagitis and, 193
High-grade squamous intraepithelial lesions (HSILs), 51
Histoplasma capsulatum, 49, 82
 antigen testing, disseminated histoplasmosis in HIV and, 212
 as skin manifestation of HIV, 125
 chorioretinitis and, 152-153
 focal CNS lesion and, 98t
 HIV-associated diarrhea and, 220
 Kaposi's sarcoma vs., 237
 maculopapular red-brown lesions and, 239t
 prophylaxis against, 53t
Histoplasmosis, 82
 as oral manifestation of HIV, 133t, 135t
 demographics of, 211
 disseminated, fever of unknown origin and, 232
 fungal meningitis from, 171
 gastrointestinal CMV and, 86
 hepatitis in HIV and, 196
 HSV vs., 90
 Key Points, 82b, 125b
 late HIV infection and, 208-209
 molluscum contagiosum vs., 120
 prophylaxis against, 49
Hitzig zones, sensory loss in, 174
HIV; see also Early HIV; HIV-1; Late-stage HIV; Primary HIV
 acute
  antiretroviral therapy for, 30
  Key Points, 16b, 17b
  oral manifestations of, 136
 asymptomatic, antiretroviral therapy for, 30-31
 Cryptosporidium and, 99-100
 Cyclospora and, 104
 Entamoeba histolytica and, 105
 Epstein-Barr virus and, 94
 fitness, mutations and, 39
 Giardia lamblia and, 104-105
 HSV and replication of, 90
 initial management of
  antiretroviral therapy, 26-27
  baseline laboratory testing, 26, 26b
  basics of, 25b
  comprehensive history, 24-25, 25b
  educational discussions, 27-28
  follow-up visits, 29
  immune system monitoring, 28-29

HIV—cont'd
 initial management of—cont'd
  immunizations, 26
  opportunistic infection prophylaxis, 26-27
  physical examination, 25-26, 26b
  possible referrals, 27
 Isospora and, 103
 microsporidia and, 102
 natural history of, 12-13
 neurotropic nature of, 166
 psoriasis vulgaris and, 126
 serologic test for, 7
 symptomatic, antiretroviral therapy for, 30
 syphilis and, 112, 113-114
 T. gondii and, 96
 testing for, 20-23
  sexually transmitted infections and, 113
 tuberculosis and, 68-69
 varicella-zoster virus of central nervous system and, 92
HIV antibodies
 false-negative serologic tests and, 21
 in acute HIV-1 infection, 16, 16b, 20
 in infants born to HIV-infected mothers, 250
HIV blood co-culture, for HIV in infants born to HIV-infected mothers, 250
HIV encephalopathy, focal CNS lesion and, 98t
HIV RNA copy number, disease staging and, 13
HIV-1
 acute
  case presentation of, 14
  clinical manifestations of, 16-17, 17b
  diagnosis of, 17-18, 18b
  differential diagnosis of, 17b
  immune response to, 15-16, 16b
  natural history of, 18-19
  presentation and progression of, 14-15, 15f
  referral for, 19
  treatment of, 19, 19b
 Group M, clade B tests, false-negative serologic tests and, 21
 Key Points, 14b
 nomenclature and research case definitions for, 187b
 phylogenetic tree of, 5t
 regulatory proteins, 3, 5t
 replication cycle of, 3, 4f
  disease staging and, 13
HIV-1 antibodies, negative, in acute HIV-1 infection, 18
HIV-1 structural proteins, 3, 4t
HIV-1–associated dementia (HAD) complex, 186
HIV-1–associated minor cognitive/motor disorder (MCMD), 186-187
HIV-2
 false-negative serologic tests and, 21
 replication cycle of, 3
HIVAN, 154-156, 156b
 case, 155, 155b
 renal potassium excretion and, 164

HIV-associated cholangiopathy, 198-199, 199b
HIV-associated major congitive/motor disorder, 167
HIVID; see Zalcitabine
Hoarseness, *Cryptosporidia* and, 100
Hodgkin's disease, GI bleeding and, 201
Home HIV tests, 21
Homeless people
 Bartonella quintana and, 115
 M. kansasii and, 77
 tuberculosis risk for, 211
Homosexual men
 CMV and, 85
 and condylomata acuminata in HIV, 121
 Entamoeba histolytica and, 218
 Giardia lamblia and, 218
 HIV screening for, 20
 HIV-1 subtype B and, 6-7
 HIV-associated anal cancer and, 246
 HIV-associated diarrhea and, 216
  from HSV, 220
 HIV-associated nephropathy and, 154
 human herpesvirus 8 and, 236
 Kaposi's sarcoma risk for, 211
 lymphoma and, 241
 natural history of HIV infection study among, 12
 oral Kaposi's sarcoma and, 137
 U.S. HIV prevalence among, 9, 10f
Hopelessness
 pain and, 190
 reactive depression and, 177
Horses
 Pneumocystis carinii pneumonia and, 57
 Rhodococcus equi and, 116
Hospitalization
 for bacterial pneumonia, 110
 for Guillain-Barré syndrome, 169
 for major depressive disorder, 180
HSV; see Herpes simplex virus
Human T cell lymphotropic virus (HTLV-I), vacuolar myelopathy vs., 168
Humiliation, bereavement and, 179
Hutchinson's sign, herpes zoster ophthalmicus and, 143
Hydrocephalus, tuberculous meningitis and, 172
Hydroxymethylglutaryl-CoA reductase inhibitors
 for lipodystrophy from antiretroviral therapy, 37
 protease inhibitors and, 162
Hydroxyphosphonomethoxypropyl cytosine; see Cidofovir
Hyperaldosteronism, 163
 hyperkalemia and, 164
Hyperamylasemia, didanosine and, 37
Hyperbilirubinemia, indinavir and, 37
Hypercalcemia, from foscarnet, 87
Hypercholesterolemia, HIVAN and, 155
Hyperesthesia, and HSV-related anorectal ulcers, 199
Hypergammaglobulinemia
 HIVAN and, 155
 polyclonal, lymphoma and, 241

Hyperglycemia
    growth hormone for AWS and, 226, 227t
    megestrol acetate and, 225, 227t
Hyperkalemia
    from TMP-SMX for PCP, 61, 63t
    in HIV, 163-164, 164b
        drugs associated with, 161, 161t
Hyperkeratosis, HSV and, 90
Hyperlipidemia, from antiretroviral therapy, 36
Hyperparakeratosis, Epstein-Barr virus and, 94
Hyperphosphatemia, from foscarnet, 87, 165
Hyperpigmentation
    as oral manifestation of HIV, 134t, 140
    porphyria cutanea tarda in HIV and, 128
    toxoplasmosis retinochoroiditis and, 151
Hyperplasia, epithelial, Epstein-Barr virus and, 94
Hyperreflexia, vacuolar myelopathy and, 168
Hypersensitivity reactions
    from abacavir, 165
    from antiretroviral therapy, 36
    ulcers from, 135t
Hypersomnia, 191
    major depressive disorder and, 179
Hypertension
    AIDS retinopathy vs., 146
    Guillain-Barré syndrome and, 169
    hepatitis C-associated immune complex glomerulonephritis and, 157, 158
    HIVAN and, 155
    intercranial, papilledema and, 146-147
    membranoproliferative glomerulonephritis and, 157
    portal, GI bleeding and, 200
    pulmonary, late HIV infection and, 211
Hypertonia, HIV-associated dementia and, 186
Hypertrichosis, porphyria cutanea tarda in HIV and, 128
Hyperventilation, anxiety disorders and, 184
Hypervolemic hypernatremia, 162
Hypnotics, for reactive depression, 178
Hypoalbuminemia
    HIVAN and, 155
    renal failure and, 160
Hypocalcemia, 164
    from foscarnet, 87
Hypocomplementemia
    hepatitis C-associated immune complex glomerulonephritis and, 157-158
    membranoproliferative glomerulonephritis and, 157
Hypoglycemia, and pentamidine for PCP, 61
Hypoglycemics, antifungal azoles interactions with, 84
Hypogonadism, AIDS wasting syndrome and, 223, 224
Hypokalemia
    from foscarnet, 87
    in HIV, 163, 164
Hypomagnesemia
    from foscarnet, 87
    with hypocalcemia, 164

Hyponatremia, in HIV, 162-163, 163b
    CMV encephalitis and, 170
Hypophosphatemia, from foscarnet, 87, 165
Hypotension
    abacavir and, 165
    from pentamidine for PCP, 63t
    from trimetraxate for PCP, 63t
    Guillain-Barré syndrome and, 169
    ocular, 142, 142b
    postural, sensory-motor neuropathy from vincristine and, 175
    prerenal azotemia and, 160b
Hypothalamic-pituitary dysfunction, AIDS wasting syndrome and, 224
Hypothyoidism, 162
Hypotony
    from cidofovir, 87
    from ganciclovir implants, 87
Hypovitaminosis A, keratoconjunctivitis sicca and, 141
Hypovolemia
    acute tubular necrosis and, 160b
    diagnosis of renal failure and other renal abnormalities and, 161
    hyponatremia and, 162
    lactic acidosis and, 165
    prerenal azotemia and, 160b
    renal failure and, 160
Hypoxemia
    fungal pneumonias and, 208-209
    PCP and, 205
Hypoxia, lactic acidosis and, 165
Hypuricemia, uric acid transport abnormalities and, 165
Hysterectomy, for cervical cancer, 245

I

Ichthyosis, as skin manifestation of HIV, 126
Ideas, flight of, mania and, 182, 183b
Idoxuridine, for herpes simplex keratitis, 144
Ileus retention, Guillain-Barré syndrome and, 169
Illusions, delirium and, 185
Imipenem, for *Rhodococcus equi*, 116, 207
Imipramine, potential antiretroviral interaction with, 182t
Imiquimod
    for anogenital condylomata acuminata, 200
    for molluscum contagiosum, 121
    for warts, 121
Immune complex diseases, glomerulonephritis, 156-157
Immune complex glomerulonephritis; see Glomerulonephritis, immune complex
Immune reconstitution syndrome, fever of unknown origin and, 233
Immune recovery, vitritis, 142
Immune system
    and antiretroviral therapy failure, 37-38
    cell-mediated, 68
    monitoring, 28-29
Immunizations
    during primary office visit, 45
    for initial HIV management, 26

Immunofluorescent antibody testing
    for *Bartonella* diagnosis, 115
    for *Cryptosporidium parvum* diagnosis, 100, 100t, 218, 222
    for *Giardia lamblia* diagnosis, 105, 218, 222
    for HSV diagnosis, 90
    for PCP diagnosis, 59
    for toxoplasmosis diagnosis, 97, 210
    for VZV diagnosis, 92
Immunoglobulin, intravenous
    for chronic inflammatory demyelinating polyneuropathy, 169
    for Guillain-Barré syndrome, 169
Immunoglobulin A (IgA) glomerulonephritis, 157
Immunoglobulin G antibody, as *Toxoplasma gondii* test, 45
Immunoglobulin G anti-HIV antibodies, in infants born to HIV-infected mothers, 250
Immunoperosidase stain, for HSV diagnosis, 90
Immunosuppression
    aggressive anal neoplasia treatment and, 247
    anorectal disease and, 199
    assessment of, 211
    cytomegalovirus radiculitis and, 173
    herpes zoster and, 173-174
    microsporidiosis and, 217
    nervous system illness and neoplasms and, 166
    oral lesions in, 132
    pain and, 190
    pulmonary disease and, 205
    pyomyositis/lymphomatous infiltration of muscle and, 174-175
    tabes dorsalis and, 174
    tuberculosis and, 174, 207
Immunosuppressive therapy, *Pneumocystis carinii* pneumonia and, 57
Impetigo, from *S. aureus* in HIV, 121-122
Impotence
    megestrol acetate and, 225, 227t
    tertiary syphilis and, 174
In utero transmission, 249
Incontinence, vacuolar myelopathy and, 168
Indinavir, 31, 33
    biliary tract disease and, 198
    characteristics of, 34t
    children with AIDS and, 254
    cholestatic toxicity of, 195b
    didanosine interactions with, 41
    gastrointestinal side efects from, 35
    hyperbilirubinemia from, 37
    intratubular crystallization and, 161, 161t
    nephrolithiasis from, 37
    rash/hypersensitivity reactions from, 36
    renal implications of, 162
    resistance to, 39, 40
    rifabutin for TB treatment and, 71
    rifabutin interactions with, 47b
    rifabutin treatment with, 72
    skin reactions to, 129
    ureteral obstruction from, 160b

Infarcts, cerebral, varicella-zoster virus and, 92
Infectious Diseases Society of America (IDSA) guidelines
   for community-acquired pneumonia, 110
   for opportunistic infections, 88-89, 233-234
   for VZV, 93-94
Inflammatory demyelinating polyneuropathy
   acute (see also Guillain-Barré syndrome)
      as neurologic complication of HIV, 167b, 168-169
   chronic, as neurologic complication of HIV, 167b, 169
Influenza
   prophylaxis against, 53t
   pulmonary, late HIV infection and, 210
Influenza vaccine, 45
   for children with AIDS, 253, 253b
Informed consent, for HIV screening, 20
Injecting drug users; see Drug users, injecting
Insect bites, Kaposi's sarcoma vs., 129
Insight-oriented psychotherapy
   for anxiety, 185
   for major depressive disorder, 180
Insomnia; see also Sleep disturbances
   from atovaquone for PCP, 63t
Inspiration, tightness with, PCP and, 205
Insulin resistance, from antiretroviral therapy, 37
Insulin/D50W, for hyperkalemia, 164
Intensive care, for Guillain-Barré syndrome, 169
Interferon
   acute HIV-1 increases in, 16, 16b
   depressive side effects from, 180
   for hepatitis B, 198
   for hepatitis C, 197
   for human papilloma virus with HIV, 133t
   for Kaposi's sarcoma, 240b
   for mixed essential cryoglobulinemia, 158
   for warts, 121
   reaction to, as oral manifestation of HIV, 135t
Interferon footprints, of HIVAN, 155
Interferon-α
   AIDS wasting syndrome and, 224
   for anogenital condylomata acuminata, 200
   for hepatitis C-associated immune complex glomerulonephritis, 158
   for human papilloma virus with HIV, 137
   for Kaposi's sarcoma, 130, 240
   for progressive multifocal leukoencephalopathy diagnosis, 170
   neuropsychiatric side effects of, 181t
Interferon-α-2a, for Kaposi's sarcoma, ocular, 143
Interferon-γ
   MAC and, 75
   tuberculosis and, 68
Interleukin-1 (IL-1)
   Kaposi's sarcoma and, 237
   opportunistic infections and, 224
Interleukin-2 (IL-2)
   MAC and, 75
   tuberculosis and, 68

Interleukin-2 receptor, soluble, acute HIV-1 increases in, 16, 16b
Interleukin-6 (IL-6), Kaposi's sarcoma and, 237
Interleukin-10, acute HIV-1 increases in, 16, 16b
Interleukin-12 (IL-12)
   for Kaposi's sarcoma, 240b, 241
   MAC and, 75
International Aids Society, CMV treatment recommendations of, 87
Intertrigo, candidal, 124
Intestinal biopsy, for fever of unknown origin diagnosis, 232, 233
Intestinal obstruction, PCP and, 59
Intracerebral gumma, neurosyphilis and, 172
Intracranial pressure
   CNS lymphoma and, 173
   cryptococcosis and, 81
   in tuberculous meningitis, corticosteroids for, 172
Intrapartum transmission, 249
   decreases in, 250
Inverse psoriasis, as skin manifestation of HIV, 127
Involuntary movements, absence of, motor neuropathy and, 168
Iodinated contrast agents, acute tubular necrosis and, 160b
   acute tubular necrosis and, 161
Iodoquinol, for Entamoeba histolytica, 103t, 106
IPV; see Poliovirus vaccine inactivated
Iridocyclitis; see Uveitis
Iritis
   herpes zoster ophthalmicus and, 144
   ocular hypotension and, 142
Iron deficiency, ulcers from, 135t
Irritability
   delirium and, 185
   from glucocorticoids for PCP, 63t
   and glucocorticoids for PCP, 62
   MCMD and, 186
Ischemics strokes, 173
Isoniazid (INH)
   depressive side effects from, 180
   drug resistant TB and, 69-70, 208
   for M. kansasii, 77, 208
   for M. xenopi, 78
   for tuberculosis, 207
   for tuberculosis prophylaxis, 47, 53t, 74
   for tuberculosis treatment, 71, 174, 207
      initial dosage for, 72t
   for tuberculous meningitis, 172
   hepatocellular toxicity of, 195b
   mania and, 183
   neuropsychiatric side effects of, 181t
   NRTIs or PIs and, 72
   sensory-motor neuropathy from, 175
Isospora belli, 99, 103-104
   Cryptosporidium vs., 100
   Cyclospora vs., 104
   diarrhea and, 100t, 218
   Key Points, 104b, 218b
   TMP-SMX prophylaxis against, 65
   treatment of, 101t

Isotretinoin, for eosinophilic folliculitis in HIV, 129
Itraconazole, 84
   didanosine interactions with, 41
   for blastomycosis, 83, 209
   for candidiasis, 49, 54t
      esophageal, 124, 194
      oral, 138
   for coccidioidomycosis, 50, 54t, 82, 83
   for cryptococcosis with HIV, 125
   for Cryptococcus neoformans, 52t
   for dermatologic mycoses, 80
   for eosinophilic folliculitis in HIV, 129
   for fungal infections, 84t
   for histoplasmosis, 49, 53t, 82, 125
      pulmonary, advanced HIV and, 209
   for microsporidia keratitis, 145
   for onychomycosis with HIV, 124
   for oropharyngeal candidiasis, 80
   for penicilliosis, 83
   for seborrheic dermatitis, 79
   for sporotrichosis with HIV, 126
   for Zygomycetes, 83
   hypokalemia and, 163
   renal syndromes with, 163t
Ivermectin, for scabies in HIV, 126

J

Jarisch-Herxheimer reaction, from Bartonella treatment, 115
Jaundice, biliary tract disease and, 198
JC virus, progressive multifocal leukoencephalopathy and, 170
Jejunostomy, for nutrition, 225
Joint complaints
   Charcot's joints and, 174
   comprehensive history of, 25b
Judgment impairment, mania and, 182, 183b

K

Kaletra; see Lopinavir/ritonavir fixed-dose combination
Kaolin-pectin
   for Cryptosporidium, 101
   for HIV-associated diarrhea, 222
Kaposi's sarcoma, 6, 12
   as ocular complication of AIDS, 142-143
   as oral manifestation of HIV, 134t, 135t
   as skin manifestation of HIV, 129-130, 130f
   Bartonella vs., 115, 122
   brain metastasis of, 173
   focal CNS lesion and, 98t
   gastrointestinal CMV vs., 86
   GI bleeding and, 200-201
   herpesvirus associated with, 51
   HIV and, 118
      cause of, 236-237, 238f
      diagnosis of, 238-239, 239b
      initial assessment for, 25, 26b
      natural history of, 240
      presentation of, 237-238
      treatment of, 240-241, 240b
   HIV-associated diarrhea and, 220
   HSV esophagitis vs., 90
   Key Points, 130b, 143b, 211b, 241b

Kaposi's sarcoma—cont'd
  liver abnormalities and, 196
  maculopapular red-brown lesions and, 239t
  oral, human herpes virus 8 and, 137
  pain from, 190
  pulmonary
    late HIV infection and, 205, 210, 211b
      diagnosis of, 212
    transbronchial biopsy for diagnosis of, 59
  TTP/HUS and, 159b
  ureteral obstruction from, 160b
  U.S. AIDS cases with, 237b
    by HIV exposure category and sex, 238f
Kayexalate, for hyperkalemia, 161, 164
Keratinolytic agents, for human papilloma virus with HIV, 137
Keratitis
  herpes simplex, 144
  herpes zoster, 143
Keratoconjunctivitis sicca, 141, 141b
Keratoderma blennorrhagicum, as skin manifestation of HIV, 127
Keratolytics, for xerosis/ichthyosis in HIV, 126
Keratosis, frictional, Epstein-Barr virus *vs.*, 94
Ketoacidosis, diabetic, pentamidine-associated pancreatitis and, 165
Ketoconazole
  didanosine interactions with, 41
  for angular cheilitis, 138
  for candidiasis, 54t
    oral, 138
  for eosinophilic folliculitis in HIV, 129
  for fungal infections, 84t
  for *Pityrosporum ovale*, with HIV, 124
  for seborrheic dermatitis, 79, 127
  hyperkalemia in HIV and, 161t, 164
  hyponatremia and, 162
Kidney; *see also* Renal failure; Renal failure, acute
  antiretroviral drugs and, 162
  blastomycosis and, 83
  HIV-associated dementia and, 167
  HIV-associated diseases of, 154-156
    acidosis and, 165
    divalant cations and, 164-165
    electrolyte abnormalities and, 162-163
    hepatitis C-associated immune complex glomerulonephritis, 157-158, 157b
    immune complex glomerulonephritis, 156-157, 157b
    immunoglubulin A (IgA) glomerulonephritis, 157
    lupus-like nephritis, 157
    membranoproliferative glomerulonephritis (MPGN), 157
    mixed essential cryoglobulinemia, 158
    potassium disorders, 163-164
    renal failure and other abnormalities, 160-162
    thrombotic microangiopathy syndromes, 158-159

Kidney—cont'd
    intratubular crystallization, drugs associated with, 161t
    microsporidia and, 102
    PCP and, 59
    trimetraxate for PCP and, 63t
Kidney transplantation, 156
Klebsiella pneumoniae
  pneumonia in late HIV infection and, 207
  ulcers from, HIV and, 135t
Klonopin, for mania, 183, 183b

L

Labia, primary syphilis and, 112
Laboratory tests
  baseline assessment for initial HIV management, 26, 26b
  for AIDS wasting syndrome, 226
  for diarrhea in HIV, 216
  for pulmonary diseases in HIV, 212
  HIV medications and, 35
β–Lactam, extended spectrum; *see also* Ceftriaxone
  for *Pseudomonas aeruginosa*, 207
  neuropsychiatric side effects of, 181t
Lactate dehydrogenase (LDH), PCP and, 205, 211
Lactic acidosis, 165
  from antiretroviral therapy, 37, 162
  HIV-associated lymphoma and, 242
Lamivudine, 198
  as FDA-approved NRTI, 31
  characteristics of, 32t
  drug-induced diarrhea from, 220
  for children with AIDS, 253, 255
  for perinatal transmission reduction, 250
  neuropsychiatric side effects of, 181t
  renal implications of, 162
  resistance to, 39
  rifabutin with, 47b
  rifamycins for TB and, 72
  skin reactions to, 129
  treatment intensification and, 38
Lamotrigine
  for neurologic adverse effects from antiretroviral therapy, 36
  for sensory-motor axonal polyneuropathy, 169
Langerhans cells, HIV-1 subtype E replication and, 6
Laser ablation
  for cervical intraepithelial neoplasia, 245
  for human papilloma virus with HIV, 137
Laser photocoagulation, for retinal detachment, 88, 148
Late-stage HIV, false-negative serologic tests and, 21
Latin America, HIV in, 6
Laxatives, *Entamoeba histolytica* diagnosis and, 106
Lean body mass
  AIDS wasting syndrome and, 223, 226
  growth hormone and, 226, 227t
  oxandrolone and, 225, 227t
  testosterone and, 225
  weight gain or loss *vs.*, 224

Learning disabilities
  in children with AIDS, 253
Legionella
  pneumonia from, 108
  TMP-SMX prophylaxis against, 65
Legionella pneumophila, 207
Legs
  CMV polyradiculpathy and, 86
  sensory-motor axonal polyneuropathy and, 169
Leishmania, HIV-associated diarrhea and, 220
Leishmaniasis, fever of unknown origin and, 229, 232
Lentiviruses, about, 3
Leprosy, lepromatous, *Mycobacterium avium* complex *vs.*, 75
Lethargy; *see also* Fatigue; Malaise
  aseptic meningitis and, 166
  CMV ventriculoencephalitis and, 86
  Cryptosporidia and, 100
  Giardia lamblia and, 105
  HIV-1–associated dementia complex and, 186
  in acute HIV-1 infection, 16-17, 17b
  in cryptococcosis, 81
  Isospora and, 103
  primary HIV and, 119
  T. gondii and, 96, 171
Leucovorin
  and dapsone for PCP prophylaxis, 66
  for *Isospora*, 101t
  for *Pneumocystis carinii* pneumonia, 52t, 60
  for *T. gondii*, 52t, 97, 99t
  and trimetrexate for PCP, 61-62, 64
Leukemia, necrotizing ulcerative gingivitis or peridontitis *vs.*, 139
Leukemia/lymphoma, T cell, HTLV-I-associated, hypercalcemia and, 164
Leukocyte counts, fever of unknown origin and, 232
Leukocytosis with bandemia, bacterial pneumonia diagnosis and, 212
Leukoencephalitis, varicella-zoster virus and, 92
Leukoencephalopathy, progressive multifocal
  as neurologic complication of HIV, 167b, 170, 170f
  focal CNS lesion and, 98t
  T. gondii vs., 97
Leukopenia, from TMP-SMX for PCP, 206
Leukoplakia
  oral hairy (*see* Oral hairy leukoplakia)
  smoker's, Epstein-Barr virus *vs.*, 94
Librium; *see* Chlordiazepoxide
Lichen planus
  Epstein-Barr virus *vs.*, 94
  oral, linear gingival erythema *vs.*, 138
Lichenification, eosinophilic folliculitis in HIV and, 128
Lidocaine, for aphthous ulcers, 139
Lifestyle issues, educational discussions on, 28
Lightning pain, tertiary syphilis and, 174
Lindane, for scabies in HIV, 126

Lipids
    abnormalities of, testosterone and, 225, 227t
    testing, initial HIV assessment and, 26b
Lipodystrophy
    AIDS wasting syndrome and, 224
    from antiretroviral therapy, 36-37
    growth hormone for AWS and, 226
Liposomal amphotericin B, 83, 84t
Liposomal daunorubicin, for Kaposi's sarcoma, 240-241, 240b
Liposomal doxorubicin, for Kaposi's sarcoma, 201, 240-241, 240b
Listeria, TMP-SMX prophylaxis against, 65
Listeria monocytogenes, 111
Listerosis, 48, 111
Lithium carbonate, for mania, 183, 183b
    and HAD, 188
Liver; *see also* Hepatitis
    Bartonella and, 122
    biopsy of, for fever of unknown origin diagnosis, 232, 233
    blastomycosis and, 83
    cryptococcosis of, 81
    Entamoeba histolytica and, 106
    microsporidia and, 102
    PCP and, 59
Liver function
    adverse reactions to tuberculosis treatment and, 71
    algorithm for evaluation of, 197f
    antiretroviral therapy and, 37
    and clindamycin-primaquine for PCP, 62, 63t
    HIV-associated dementia and, 167
    initial HIV assessment of, 26b
    nevirapine and, 35
    testing, for fever of unknown origin diagnosis, 230
    and TMP-SMX for PCP, 61
    valproic acid and, 183
Liver toxicity
    anabolic agents and, 225, 227t
    from testosterone, 225, 227t
    from trimetraxate for PCP, 63t
Loop electrosurgical excision procedure (LEEP), for cervical intraepithelial neoplasia, 245
Loperamide
    for *Cryptosporidium*, 101
    for HIV-associated diarrhea, 222
Lopinavir/ritonavir fixed-dose combination, 31
    characteristics of, 34t
    gastrointestinal side efects from, 35
    PI-associated mutations and, 40
Loratadine, safety of, 41
Lorazepam
    for anxiety, 184, 185
    for insomnia, 191
    for reactive depression, 178b
    safety of, 41, 175
Los Angeles County Medical Center, pulmonary and extrapulmonary TB study, 70, 70t
Lovastatin
    alternatives to, 41
    protease inhibitors and, 162

Low-grade squamous intraepithelial lesions (LSILs), 51
Lumbar puncture, for fever of unknown origin diagnosis, 233
Lungs; *see also Pneumocystis carinii* pneumonia; Pneumonia; Pneumonitis; Pulmonary diseases
    abscess/empyema
        Entamoeba histolytica and, 106
        Salmonella and, 111
    bilateral infiltrates of, Kaposi's sarcoma and, 237-238
    biopsy of
        for fever of unknown origin diagnosis, 232
        procedures for, 214
    blastomycosis in, 83
    cryptococcosis and, 81
    functional testing of, 212
    histoplamosis and, 82
    lymphoma presentation in, 241
    M. xenopi and, 78
    MAC and, 76
    microsporidia and, 102
    necrosis of, bacterial pneumonia and, 109
    T. gondii and, 96-97
Lupus erythematosus, systemic, AIDS retinopathy *vs.*, 146
Lupus vulgaris, tuberculosis and, 122
Lupus-like nephritis, 157
Lymph nodes
    biopsy of, for fever of unknown origin diagnosis, 232
    blastomycosis and, 83
    cryptococcosis of, 81
    extrapulmonary TB in, 70
    initial HIV assessment of, 25, 26b
    Kaposi's sarcoma and, 201
    M. xenopi and, 78
    microsporidia keratitis and, 145
    swollen, comprehensive history of, 25b
Lymphadenitis
    Bartonella and, 115
    tuberculosis and, 122
Lymphadenopathy
    aseptic meningitis and, 166
    diffuse benign, lymphoma and, 241
    disseminated histoplasmosis and, 125
    fever of unknown origin and, 234
    HIV-associated lymphoma and, 242
    immune reconstitution syndrome and, 233
    in acute HIV-1 infection, 16-17, 17b
    infectious mononucleosis and, 94
    inguinal, HSV proctitis and, 90
    mediastinal, disseminated MAC and, 208
    PCP and, 59
    penicilliosis and, 83
Lymphatic obstruction, from Kaposi's sarcoma in HIV, 129
Lymphocytic interstitial pneumonitis (LIP), children with AIDS and, 251, 252, 252b
Lymphocytosis, atypical, infectious mononucleosis and, 94
Lymphocytosis syndrome, infiltrative
    corticosteroids for, 161
    interstitial nephritis and, 160

Lymphoid interstitial pneumonitis, late HIV infection and, 211
Lymphomas; *see also* Non-Hodgkin's lymphoma
    AIDS-related papilledema *vs.*, 146-147
    as neurologic complication of HIV, 167b
    bulky, acute uric acid nephropathy from chemotherapy for, 161
    cause of, 241
    CD4+ counts and fever of unknown origin with, 231, 231b
    central nervous system
        as neurologic complications of HIV, 172, 173
        T. gondii vs., 97, 171
    clinical failure of antiretroviral therapy and, 38
    CMV colitis *vs.*, 86
    CMV esophagitis *vs.*, 86
    Epstein-Barr virus and, 94
    focal CNS lesion and, 98t
    GI bleeding and, 200, 201
    HIV-associated
        cause of, 241
        children with AIDS and, 252, 252b
        diagnosis of, 242, 243b
        jaundice and, 198
        Key Points, 243b
        presentation of, 241-242
        treatment for, 243
    HSV esophagitis *vs.*, 90
    hypercalcemia and, 164
    intraocular, CMV retinitis *vs.*, 85
    liver abnormalities and, 196
    pulmonary, advanced HIV and, 205
        CD4+ counts in, 211
    small bowel, HIV-associated diarrhea and, 220
    subacute motor neuropathy from, 175
    T. gondii vs., 97
    T cell, as skin manifestation of HIV, 130
    treatment of, 175
    ureteral obstruction from, 160b
Lymphomatous meningitis, 175
Lysis-centrifugation, for tuberculosis diagnosis, 71

M

MAC; *see Mycobacterium avium* complex
Macrolides
    cholestatic toxicity of, 195b
    for bacterial pneumonia, 110
    for *Bartonella*, 115
    for *Campylobacter*, 112
    for HIV-associated diarrhea from *Campylobacter*, 219
    for *Rhodococcus equi*, 116
Maculopapular rash, in acute HIV-1 infection, 16-17, 17b, 18f
Magnesium salts
    for hypomagnesemia, 164
    for stroke, 173
Magnetic resonance imaging
    for CMV radiculitis diagnosis, 173, 174f
    for CMV ventriculoencephalitis, 86
    for *Entamoeba histolytica* diagnosis, 106
    for HIV-associated dementia, 167, 167f

Magnetic resonance imaging—*cont'd*
  for HIV-associated psychosis, 189
  for lymphomatous meningitis, 175
  for neurologic complication diagnosis, 166
  for progressive multifocal leukoencephalopathy diagnosis, 170, 170f
  for pyomyositis/lymphomatous infiltration of muscle, 174
  for spinal cord for progressive myelopathy, 168
  for subacute motor neuropathy from lymphoma, 175
  for *T. gondii* diagnosis, 96, 171, 171f
  for tuberculous meningitis diagnosis, 172
Major depressive disorder, 179, 180b
  diagnosis of, 179-180
  treatment of, 180-181
Malabsorption, AIDS wasting syndrome and, 223
Malaise; *see also* Fatigue; Lethargy
  biliary tract disease and, 198
  from parenteral pegylated interferon, 197
  tuberculous meningitis and, 172
Malassezia furfur, 79
Malignancies
  CD4+ counts and fever of unknown origin with, 231
  immunosuppression and, 236
  in HIV infection, 244b
Malnutrition
  Entamoeba histolytica and, 105
  in AIDS patients, hypophosphatemia and, 165
  keratoconjunctivitis sicca and, 141
Mania, 182-183
  sleep disturbances and, 191
Mantoux skin test, for inactive TB, 73
mBACOD regimen, for HIV-associated lymphoma, 243
MCMD; *see* HIV-1–associated minor cognitive/motor disorder (MCMD)
Measles
  acute HIV-1 infection *vs.*, 17, 17b
  pulmonary, late HIV infection and, 210
Measles-mumps-rubella vaccine
  for children with AIDS, 253, 253b
Mediastinitis, bacterial pneumonia and, 109
Medical history taking
  for AIDS wasting syndrome, 226
  for fever of unknown origin, 229-230
  for HIV, 24
    comprehensive, 25b
    of medications, 41
  for HIV-associated diarrhea diagnosis, 216
  for initial primary care office visit, 44
  for neurologic complications in HIV, 166
  for pulmonary disease in HIV, 211
Medications
  child behavior and, 254
  current
    for HIV medical history, 24, 211
    for HIV-associated diarrhea diagnosis, 216
Megestrol acetate, for appetite stimulation, 225, 227t

Melanoma
  Kaposi's sarcoma *vs.*, 143
  malignant, HIV and, 130
Membranoproliferative glomerulonephritis (MPGN), 157
Membranous glomerulopathy, atypical, 157
Memory, impaired
  CMV and, 86
  delirium and, 185
  HIV-1–associated dementia complex and, 186
  HIV-associated dementia and, 167, 186
  HSV encephalitis and, 170-171
  sleep disturbances and, 191
Memory disturbance, MCMD and, 186
Men who have sex with men
  anal neoplasia and, 246
  Entamoeba histolytica and, 218
  Giardia lamblia and, 218
  Kaposi's sarcoma and, 200, 236
    U.S. AIDS cases with, 237b
  precancerous anal neoplasia and, 246
  pulmonary Kaposi's sarcoma and, 210
Meningitis
  aseptic
    as neurologic complication of HIV, 166, 167b
    from TMP-SMX for PCP, 61, 63t
    from TMP-SMX for PCP prophylaxis, 65
    in acute HIV-1 infection, 16-17, 17b
    secondary syphilis and, 112
    varicella-zoster virus and, 92
  chronic, as neurologic complication of HIV, 166-167, 167b
  cryptococcal, 81, 81b
    as neurological complication of AIDS, 171
    fungal chorioretinitis and, 153
    mania *vs.*, 183
    papilledema *vs.*, 146
    pulmonary cryptococcosis and, 208
  gastroenteritis and, 111
  lymphocytic
    blastomycosis and, 83
    histoplasmosis and, 82
  lymphomatous, 175
  mycobacterial infections and, 172
  referral for, 176
  Salmonella and, 111
  tuberculous, 70, 208
    hypovolemic hyponatremia in, 162
    in acute HIV-1 infection, 18
Meningoencephalitis
  as neurologic complication of HIV, 166
  coccidioidomycosis and, 82
Meningomyeloardiculitis, varicella-zoster virus and, 92
Meningovascular syphilis, 112, 172
  cerbrovascular disease and, 172
Menses, ulcers from, 135t
Menstrual problems, comprehensive history of, 25b
Mental status
  changes in, 177
    delirium and, 189

Mental status—*cont'd*
  changes in—*cont'd*
    neurologic complications in HIV and, 166
    histoplamosis and, 82
    in cryptococcosis, 81
    major depressive disorder and, 180
Menthol lotions, for pruritus in HIV, 126
Meperidine, xerostomia from, 132
Mepron; *see* Atovaquone
Mesangioproliferative glomerulonephritis, 157
Metabolic disorders
  AIDS wasting syndrome and, 223
  neurologic symptoms of HIV and, 166
Metadone, antiretroviral drug interactions with, 41
Metastasis
  AIDS-related papilledema *vs.*, 147
  Kaposi's sarcoma *vs.*, 143
  of CNS lymphoma to brain, 173
Metformin, for insulin resistance from antiretroviral therapy, 37
Methadone
  PI or NNRTI and, 35
  rifampin and pyrazinamide for TB and, 74
Methemoglobinemia
  from dapsone for PCP prophylaxis, 66
  from trimethoprim-dapsone for PCP, 63t
  and trimethoprim-dapsone for PCP, 61
Methenamine silver staining, for PCP, 59
Methotrexate
  for chronic inflammatory demyelinating polyneuropathy, 169
  for CNS lymphoma, 173
  for HIV-associated lymphoma, 243
  for psoriasis with HIV, 127
  neuropsychiatric side effects of, 181t
  tubular precipitate of, 161
Methylpheindate, for HIV-associated dementia, 188
Methylprednisone
  for *Pneumocystis carinii* pneumonia, 63t
  PCP treatment and, 62
Metronidazole
  for *Clostridium difficile*, 219
  for *E. bieneusi*, 217
  for *Entamoeba histolytica*, 103t, 106, 218
  for eosinophilic folliculitis in HIV, 129
  for *Giardia lamblia*, 103t, 105, 218
  for linear gingival erythema, 134t
  for microsporidia, 101t, 102
  for necrotizing stomatitis, 134t, 139
  for necrotizing ulcerative gingivitis or peridontitis, 139
  hepatocellular toxicity of, 195b
Miconazole
  for angular cheilitis, 138
  for vulvovaginal candidiasis, 80
Microaneurysms, AIDS retinopathy and, 146
Microglia
  HIV in, 167
  vacuolar myelopathy and, 168
β_2-Microglobulin, HIV-associated dementia and, 167

β-Microglobulin, acute HIV-1 increases in, 16, 16b
Microhemagglutination-*T. pallidum* (MHA-TP), 113
  for neurosyphilis, 172
  for syphilitic retinitis, 152
Microscopy
  darkfield, for syphilis, 113
  light, for liver abnormalities, 196
Microsporidia, 47, 99, 102-103, 103b
  Cryptosporidium parvum and, 217-218
  Cryptosporidium vs., 100
  Cyclospora vs., 104
  diarrhea and, 100t
  HIV-associated cholangiopathy and, 198, 199
  HIV-associated diarrhea and, 216, 217
    Key Points, 217b
  Isospora vs., 103
  treatment of, 101t
Microsporidia keratitis, as ocular complication of AIDS, 145, 145b
Microsporidiosis, 47
  TTP/HUS and, 159b
Microsporidium, CMV colitis vs., 86
Microsporum, 80
Midazolam, contraindications for, 42t, 175
Milia, porphyria cutanea tarda in HIV and, 128
Miller-Fisher syndrome, 168-169
Mirtazapine, potential antiretroviral interaction with, 182t
Misperceptions, delirium and, 185
Mitochondrial dysfunction
  lactic acidosis and, 165
  prenatal maternal HAART risks for, 250
Mitomycin
  for anal neoplasia, 247
  TTP/HUS and, 159b
Mixed essential cryoglobulinemia, 158, 158b
Mohs' micrographic surgery, for non-melanoma skin cancer in HIV, 130
Molluscum contagiosum (MC)
  as ocular complication of AIDS, 143
  as skin manifestation of HIV, 120-121
  cryptococcosis vs., 125
  Key Points, 121b, 143b
  maculopapular red-brown lesions and, 239t
Monoclonal antibody testing
  for *Entamoeba histolytica* diagnosis, 218
  for HSV diagnosis, 90
  for VZV diagnosis, 92
Mononeuritis multiplex, mixed essentiual cryoglobulinemia and, 158
Mononeuropathy multiplex
  as neurologic complication of HIV, 167b, 169, 169b
  progressive vascular, CMV radiculitis and, 173
Mononucleosis, infectious
  acute HIV-1 infection vs., 17, 17b
  adolescents with Epstein-Barr virus and, 94

Mood disorders
  bereavement, 179
  case report, 178b
  in HIV/AIDS, 180
  major depressive disorder, 179-181
  mania, 182-183
  reactive depression, 177-179
Morbilliform eruptions, from drug hypersensitivity in HIV, 129
Mother-child transmission; *see also* Perinatal transmission
  of HHV-8, 236
  U.S. HIV prevalence of, 11-12
Motor nerve conduction studies
  for Guillain-Barré syndrome, 169
  for motor neuropathy diagnosis, 168
Motor neuropathy
  as neurologic complication of HIV, 167b, 168
  referral for, 175
  vertebral tubercular process and, 174
Mouth mucosa, ulcer of
  in acute HIV-1 infection, 16-17, 17b, 18f
  nasogastric feeding tube and, 225
Mouth sores
  comprehensive history of, 25b
  symptom management of, 224
Mucocutaneous candidiasis, 80, 81b
  pulmonary pathogens and, 211-212
Mucocutaneous disorders, HIV serotesting indications and, 119b
Mucocutaneous herpes simplex, 89-90
Mucocutaneous neoplasms, aphthous ulcers vs., 132
Mucormycosis, fungal meningitis from, 171
Multiple organ failure, histoplasmosis and, 82
Muscle dysfunction
  Guillain-Barré syndrome and, 168
  HIV and, 167b
  motor neuropathy and, 168
  polymyositis and, 170
Muscle mass, low, TTP/HUS and, 159
Muscles
  microsporidia and, 102
  pyomyositis/lymphomatous infiltration of, 174-175
Mutism, HIV-1–associated dementia complex and, 186
Myalgias, 190
  abacavir and, 230
  CMV retinitis and, 85
  from interferon for Kaposi's sarcoma, 240
  from parenteral pegylated interferon, 197
  from vincristine for Kaposi's sarcoma, 240
  in acute HIV-1 infection, 16-17, 17b
  polymyositis and, 169-170
  primary HIV and, 119
  T. gondii and, 97
  varicella-zoster virus and, 92
  zidovudine-related, 175
Mycobacteremia, pneumonia in late HIV infection and, 212
Mycobacteria other than tuberculosis (MOTT), 68

Mycobacterial infections
  about, 68
  as skin manifestation of HIV, 122, 122b
  pulmonary, advanced HIV and, 208, 208b
Mycobacterium avium, Kaposi's sarcoma vs., 237
Mycobacterium avium complex (MAC), 12, 68; *see also* Disseminated *Mycobacterium avium* complex
  antiretroviral therapy and, 198
  as ocular complication of AIDS, 152, 152b
  as skin manifestation of HIV, 122
  diagnosis of, 71, 76
  disseminated, HIV-associated diarrhea and, 219
  epidemiology of, 74-75
  fever of unknown origin diagnosis and, 232, 233
  gastrointestinal CMV and, 86
  HSV esophagitis and, 90
  hypuricemia and, 165
  incidence by CD4 count without prophylaxis, 75t
  Kaposi's sarcoma vs., 201
  late HIV infection and, 208
  liver abnormalities and, 195
  M. kansasii and, 77
  microbiology of, 74
  pathogenesis of, 75
  prophylaxis against disseminated infection with, 48, 52t, 76t
  treatment of, 76-77, 76t
  TTP/HUS and, 159b
Mycobacterium avium intracellulare (MAI)
  as neurologic complication of HIV, 172
  pyomyositis/lymphomatous infiltration of muscle and, 174-175
Mycobacterium bovis, 68
Mycobacterium celatum, 78
Mycobacterium chelonei, 78
Mycobacterium fortuitum, 78
  as skin manifestation of HIV, 122
Mycobacterium genavense, 78
Mycobacterium gordonae, 78
  diagnosis of, 71
Mycobacterium haemophilum, 78, 208
  as skin manifestation of HIV, 122
Mycobacterium intracellulare, 68, 74
  suggestive of HIV, 135t
Mycobacterium kansasii, 77
  advanced HIV and, 208
  diagnosis of, 71
  Rhodococcus equi vs., 116
Mycobacterium leprae, 68
Mycobacterium malmoense, 78
Mycobacterium marinum, 78
Mycobacterium microti, 68
Mycobacterium scrofulaceum, 78, 208
Mycobacterium simiae, 208
Mycobacterium tuberculosis, 68; *see also* Tuberculosis
  as neurologic complication of HIV, 172
  CMV retinitis vs., 86
  cultures for diagnosis of, 70-71
  gastrointestinal CMV and, 86
  HSV esophagitis and, 90

Mycobacterium tuberculosis—cont'd
  injecting drug users and, 205
  Kaposi's sarcoma *vs.*, 237
  late HIV infection and, 207-208, 208b
    CD4+ counts in, 212
  suggestive of HIV, 135t
Mycobacterium xenopi, 77-78, 208
Mycoplasma pneumoniae, 108
Myelitis
  CMV and, 170
  from herpes simplex or herpes zoster, 171
  varicella-zoster virus and, 92
  VZV and, 93
Myelopathy
  CNS lymphoma metastsis and, 173
  HIV-related, 166
  vacuolar, as neurologic complication of HIV, 167b, 168, 168b
Myelophthisis, fever of unknown origin and, 233
Myelosuppression, from paclitaxel for Kaposi's sarcoma, 241
Myocardial infarction, acute, acute tubular necrosis and, 160b
Myoclonus, syphilitic dementia and, 172
Myopathy
  HIV-related, 166, 169-170, 170b
  pain from, 190
  zidovudine and, 37
Myositis, pain from, 190
Myxoma, atrial, CD4+ counts and fever of unknown origin with, 231

N

Nails
  psoriasis as manifestation of HIV in, 127
  pyogenic granuloma from indinavir and, 129, 129f
Nandrolone decanoate, for anabolic block, 225, 227t
Nasogastric feeding tubes, 225
Natacyn; *see* Natamycin
Natamycin, for corneal infections, 145
National Pediatric and Family HIV Resource Center
  HAART guidelines from, 253
Nausea
  aseptic meningitis and, 166
  Cryptosporidia and, 100
  Cyclospora and, 104
  DMAC and, 75t, 76
  from acyclovir, 90
  from antiretroviral therapy, 35-36
  from clindamycin-primaquine for PCP, 63t
  from cryptococcal meningitis, 171
  from systemic chemotherapy, 240
  from TMP-SMX for PCP, 60, 63t, 206
  from TMP-SMX for PCP prophylaxis, 65
  Giardia lamblia and, 105
  in acute HIV-1 infection, 17b
  lithium carbonate and, 183b
  microsporidia and, 102
  nasogastric feeding tube and, 225
  primary HIV and, 119
  SSRIs and, 180
  symptom management of, 224
  T. gondii and, 96

Navane; *see* Thiothixene
Neck
  lymphoma presentation in, 241
  stiff, primary HIV and, 119
Necrotizing folliculitis, HSV and, 90
Necrotizing retinitis, varicella-zoster virus and, 92
Necrotizing stomatitis, as oral manifestation of HIV, 134t, 135t, 139
Necrotizing ulcerative gingivitis (NUG), as oral manifestation of HIV, 135t, 138, 139
Necrotizing ulcerative periodontitis (NUP), as oral manifestation of HIV, 134t, 135t, 138, 139
Necrotizing vasculitis
  Buerger's disease–like, PCP and, 59
  of peripheral nerve, 169
Needles, educational discussions on, 28
Nefazodone, potential antiretroviral interaction with, 182t
Nelfinavir, 31, 33
  characteristics of, 34t
  drug-induced diarrhea from, 220
  for children with AIDS, 254
  gastrointestinal side efects from, 35
  hepatocellular toxicity of, 195b
  resistance to, 40
  rifabutin for TB treatment and, 71
  rifabutin interactions with, 47b
  rifabutin treatment with, 72
Nemaline rod myopathy
  as neurologic complication of HIV, 167b
  polymyositis *vs.*, 170
Neoplasms
  as neurologic complication of HIV, 166, 167b, 172-173
  as skin manifestation of HIV, 129-130
    Key Points, 130b
  referral for, 176
Neopterin, acute HIV-1 increases in, 16, 16b
Nephritis
  E. intestinalis and, 217
  interstitial
    acute
      diagnosis of, 161
      drug interactions and, 160
    from indinavir, 161
    from TMP-SMX for PCP, 61
    from TMP-SMX for PCP prophylaxis, 65
    hypovolemic hyponatremia in, 162
    renal failure and, 160b
    Sjögren's syndrome, renal failure and, 160
Nephrolithiasis, indinavir and, 37
Nephropathy, HIV-associated, 154-156
  case, 155
    diagnostic points, 155b
Nephrosarca, 160
Nephrotoxicty
  acute tubular necrosis and, 160
  from cidofovir, 87, 148, 220
  from foscarnet, 87
  from pentamidine for PCP, 63t
  and pentamidine for PCP, 61

Nerve conduction studies
  for chronic inflammatory demyelinating polyneuropathy, 169
  for CMV radiculitis diagnosis, 173
  for dapsone-induced motor-predominant polyneuropathy, 175
  for Guillain-Barré syndrome, 169
  for INH-related neuropathy, 175
  for mononeuropathy multiplex diagnosis, 169
  for nucleoside analogue-induced neuropathy, 175
  for sensory-motor axonal polyneuropathy, 169
  for sensory-motor neuropathy from vincristine, 175
  for subacute motor neuropathy from lymphoma, 175
Nerve palsy, facial, in acute HIV-1 infection, 17b
Nerve root dysfunction, HIV and, 167b
Neuralgia
  post-herpetic, herpes zoster ophthalmicus and, 143
  VZV and, 93
Neuritis
  anterior ischemic, AIDS-related papilledema *vs.*, 147
  optic, etiologies of, 147
  prednisone for herpes zoster and, 93
Neuroimaging, for motor neuropathy diagnosis, 168
Neuroleptics
  for anxiety, 185
  for HIV-associated psychosis, 189
  for pain, 191
Neurologic systems
  abnormalities of, TTP/HUS syndrome and, 159
  adverse effects from antiretroviral therapy, 36
  disorders of, as HIV complications and, 166, 167b
  initial HIV assessment of, 26, 26b
Neuropathy
  from vincristine for Kaposi's sarcoma, 240
  HIV-related, 166
  medication-induced, 175
  VZV and, 93
Neuropsychiatric complications, 177
  anxiety disorders, 183-185
  case report, 178b
  classification of, 189f
  mood disorders, 177-183
  organic manifestations of, 185-188
  pain syndromes, 190-191
  psychotic disorders, 188-190
  sleep disturbances, 191-192
  suicide, 190
Neuropsychiatric testing, for HIV-associated dementia, 187
Neuropsychologic testing, for HIV-associated dementia, 187
Neurosyphilis, 112-113, 114
  as neurologic complication of HIV, 172
  immune status and, 151

Neurosyphilis—cont'd
  mania vs., 183
  with HIV, 123
Neutrexing; see Trimetrexate
Neutropenia
  advanced HIV and, 108
  Aspergillus spp. and, 83, 212
  bloodstream candidiasis and, 80
  from ganciclovir, 87, 89, 220
  from TMP-SMX for PCP prophylaxis, 65
  ulcers from
    aphthous ulcers vs., 132
    HIV and, 135t
    zidovudine and, 37
Neutrophil counts, fever of unknown origin and, 232
Nevi, benign, Kaposi's sarcoma vs., 129
Nevirapine, 33
  characteristics of, 33t
  drug fever and, 230
  for perinatal transmission reduction, 250
  hepatic transaminases abnormalities from, 37
  rash/hypersensitivity reactions from, 36
  resistance to, 39-40
  rifabutin treatment for TB and, 72
  rifabutin with, 47b
Night sweats
  DMAC and, 75, 75t
  HIV-associated lymphoma and, 242
  in acute HIV-1 infection, 16-17, 17b
Nikolsky's sign, toxic epidermal nerolysis and, 129
Nitazoxanide, for *Cryptosporidium parvum*, 218
Nitrogen balance, growth hormone and, 224
Nocardia
  focal CNS lesion and, 98t
  pulmonary, advanced HIV and, CD4+ counts in, 211
  Rhodococcus equi vs., 116
  TMP-SMX prophylaxis against, 65
Nocardia asteroides, 207
Nonadherance
  by adolescents with AIDS on HAART, 256-257
  by children with AIDS on HAART, 254
Non-Hodgkin's lymphoma
  as oral manifestation of HIV, 134t, 135t, 140
  as skin manifestation of HIV, 130
  DMAC vs., 75
  GI bleeding and, 201
  HIV-related (see also Lymphomas, HIV-associated)
    cause of, 241
    natural history of, 242-243
    presentation of, 241-242
    prognostic factors for, 243b
  late HIV infection and, 210-211
Non-nucleoside reverse transcriptase inhibitors (NNRTIs), 31
  characteristics of, 33t
  clinical failure of antiretroviral therapy and, 38
  drug fever and, 230
  drug-drug interactions and, 40-41

Non-nucleoside reverse transcriptase inhibitors (NNRTIs)—cont'd
  for children with AIDS, 253, 254
  lipodystrophy and, 36-37
  and NRTI combination, 33
  rash/hypersensitivity reactions from, 36
  renal implications of, 162
  resistance to, 39-40
  rifampin or rifabutin interactions with, 47
  TB drug treatment interactions with, 71
Nonspecific interstitial pneumonitis (NSIP), 211, 211b
  CD4+ counts in, 211
Nonsteroidal antiinflammatory drugs
  for pain, 191
  hyperkalemia and, 164
  photosensitivity in HIV and, 128
  renal failure and, 160
  renal failure or azotemia and, 160b
Nontuberculous mycobacteria (NTM), 68
  pulmonary, late HIV infection and, 208, 208b
Norpramin; see Desipramine
Nortriptyline
  for bereavement, 179b
  for HIV-associated dementia, 188
  for neurologic adverse effects from antiretroviral therapy, 36
  potential antiretroviral interaction with, 182t
Norwegian scabies, in HIV, 126
Nose
  assessment for initial HIV management, 25
  histoplasmosis of, 125
NSIP; see Nonspecific interstitial pneumonitis
Nuchal rigidity
  aseptic meningitis and, 166
  from cryptococcal meningitis, 171
Nucleoside analogue-induced neuropathy, 167b, 169b, 175
  sensory-motor axonal polyneuropathy and, 169
Nucleoside reverse transcriptase inhibitors (NRTIs)
  characteristics of, 32t
  combination of three, 33, 35
  for acute HIV-1 infection, 19
  for children with AIDS, 253, 254, 255
  gastrointestinal side effects from, 35-36
  lactic acidosis from, 37
  lipodystrophy and, 37
  and PI combinations, 31, 33
  preferred combinations of, 31
  renal excretion and, 162
  resistance to, 39
  triple, for children with AIDS, 253
  tuberculosis prophylaxis and, 47b
Nutritional deficiency, body composition measursments and, 223
Nutritional disorders, neurologic symptoms of HIV and, 166
Nutritional status
  assessment for initial HIV management, 25, 26b, 226
  HIV-related mortality and, 223

Nutritional supplementation
  for AIDS wasting syndrome, 224-225
  for *Cryptosporidium*, 101
Nystatin
  for angular cheilitis, 138
  for candidiasis with HIV, 124
  for oral candidiasis, 138
  for oropharyngeal candidiasis, 80

O

Obtundation, in cryptococcosis, 81
Occupational exposure to HIV, HIV screening for, 20
Octreotide
  for *Cryptosporidium parvum*, 100, 101t, 218
  for *E. bieneusi*, 217
  for HIV-associated diarrhea, 222
Ocular complications of AIDS, 141
Ocular hypotension, 142, 142b
Odynophagia
  comprehensive history of, 25b
  esophageal candidiasis and, 80, 193
  gastrointestinal CMV and, 86
  HSV esophagitis and, 90
Olanzapine
  for HIV-associated dementia, 188
  for HIV-associated psychosis, 190b
  for mania, 183
Onychomycosis
  as nail manifestation of HIV, 124
  sex differences in HIV-related incidence of, 118
Ophthalmic zoster; see Herpes zoster ophthalmicus
Ophthalamologic examinations, for CMV retinitis, 89, 136
  CMV pneumonitis and, 209-210
  fever of unknown origin and, 231
  monitoring of, 87, 148, 149
Ophthalmoplegia, Miller-Fisher syndrome and, 169
Opiates
  for HIV-associated diarrhea, 222
  for pain, 191
  for pain relief in sensory-motor axonal polyneuropathy, 169
  for pain syndromes, 190
Opium, tincture of, for *Cryptosporidium*, 101
Opportunistic infections (OIs), 7, 12; see also *Pneumocystis carinii* pneumonia
  AIDS wasting syndrome and, 226
  clinical failure of antiretroviral therapy and, 38
  cytomegalovirus, 85-89
  HAART and, 118
  hypuricemia and, 165
  low CD4+ counts, fever of unknown origin and, 229-230
  major depressive disorder and, 179
  mania vs., 183, 183b
  neurologic complications of, 166
  prophylaxis for, 44
    educational discussions on adherence to, 28

Opportunistic infections (OIs)—cont'd
  prophylaxis for—cont'd
    fever of unknown origin and, 233-234
    for bacterial infections, 48-49
    for fungi, 49
    for initial HIV management, 26-27
    for protozoan infections, 45-48
    for viruses, 50-51
    guidelines for, 51
  total parenteral nutrition and, 225
  tuberculosis, 69
Optic disc drusen, AIDS-related papilledema *vs.*, 147
Optic nerve
  atrophy of, 147, 147b
    silicone oils for retinal detachment and, 148
    tertiary syphilis and, 174
  CNS lymphoma and, 173
  edema of, 146-147
  herpes zoster ophthalmicus and, 144
  hyperemia of, immune recovery vitritis and, 142
  PORN and, 150
  syphilitic retinitis and, 152
  T. gondii and, 97
  varicella-zoster retinitis and, 150
Optic neuritis, syphilitic retinitis and, 151
Optic neuropathy
  from cryptococcal meningitis, 171
  inflammatory, AIDS-related papilledema *vs.*, 147
Oral hairy leukoplakia
  as oral manifestation of HIV, 121, 133t, 136-137
  Key Points, 121b
  Epstein-Barr virus and, 94
  hyperplastic candidiasis *vs.*, 138
  initial HIV assessment for, 26b
  Key Points, 94b
  sex differences in HIV-related incidence of, 118
Oral manifestations
  about, 132
  examination for, 132
  guide to, 133-134t
Oral pain, 190
OraSure, HIV test, 21-22
Organ donations
  HIV screening for, 20
  U.S. HIV prevalence among, 11
Oroesophageal ulcers, nasogastric feeding tube and, 225
Orolabial herpes simplex disease, 89
Oropharyngeal candidiasis, 80, 193
  as cutaneous manifestation of HIV, 123-124
  PCP prophylaxis and, 64
Osteomyelitis
  coccidioidomycosis and, 82
  Salmonella and, 111
  vertebral, tuberculosis and, 174
Osteopenia, from antiretroviral therapy, 37
Oxandrolone, for anabolic block, 225, 227t
Oxazepam
  for anxiety, 185
  for insomnia, 191
  for reactive depression, 178b

Oxymetholone, for anabolic block, 225
Oysters, *Cryptosporidium* and, 99-100, 101

P

p7, response to HIV infection by, 20
p18, response to HIV infection by, 20
p24 antigen
  acute HIV testing with, 22-23
  in acute HIV-1 infection, 18
  response to HIV infection by, 20
p31, response to HIV infection by, 20
p53, anal neoplasia and, 246
p55, response to HIV infection by, 20
p66, response to HIV infection by, 20
P450 enzyme system
  antidepressants and, 180
  protease inhibitors and, 175
Paclitaxel, for Kaposi's sarcoma, 130, 201, 240b, 241
Pain
  abdominal
    bacillary peliosis and, 115
    CMV colitis and, 86
    Cyclospora and, 104
    Entamoeba histolytica and, 106
    gastroenteritis and, 111
    immune reconstitution syndrome and, 233
    Isospora and, 103
    microsporidia and, 102
  anorectal
    anal neoplasias and, 246, 247
    HSV proctitis and, 90, 220
  as neuropsychiatric complication of HIV/AIDS, 190-191, 191b
  back, tuberculosis and, 174
  chest
    anxiety disorders and, 184
    blastomycosis and, 83
    HSV esophagitis and, 90
    in *Rhodococcus equi,* 116
    Nocardia asteroides and, 207
    Rhodococcus equi and, 207
  CMV radiculitis and, 173
  dermatomal, herpes zoster and, 173, 174
  esophageal, 194
  from alitretinoin, 240
  HIV-associated diarrhea and, 216
  jaw, from necrotizing ulcerative peridontitis, 139
  ocular
    corneal ulcers and, 145
    herpes zoster ophthalmicus and, 143
    retinal necrosis and, 149
    retro-orbital, in acute HIV-1 infection, 16-17, 17b
    retrosternal chest, in esophageal candidiasis, 80
    shooting, syphilis and, 112
    syphilitic retinitis and, 151
    T. gondii and, 97
    varicella-zoster keratitis and, 144
  of peripheral nerve, mononeuropathy multiplex and, 169
  pleuritic chest, pneumonia and, 108
  right upper quadrant, biliary tract disease and, 198

Pain—cont'd
  sensory loss in tertiary syphilis and, 174
  sensory-motor axonal polyneuropathy and, 169
  sleep disturbances and, 191
Palpitations, anxiety disorders and, 184
Pamelor; *see* Nortriptyline
Pancreas, PCP and, 59
Pancreatitis
  and aerosolized pentamidine for PCP prophylaxis, 66
  from didanosine, 37
  from pentamidine for PCP, 63t
  from TMP-SMX for PCP, 61, 63t
  from TMP-SMX for PCP prophylaxis, 65
  from trimetraxate for PCP, 63t
  gastrointestinal CMV and, 220
  Giardia lamblia and, 105
  and pentamidine for PCP, 61, 64
  pentamidine-associated, diabetic ketoacidosis and, 165
Pancytopenia
  Bartonella and, 115
  from TMP-SMX for PCP, 61, 63t
  unexplained, fever of unknown origin and, 233
Panic disorder, anxiety *vs.*, 185b
Panophthalmitis, uveitis and, 142
Panretin; *see* Alitretinoin
Pap smear
  abnormal, 244-245
  algorithm of, 245f
  anal, 247-248
  for adolescent females, 257
  for human papillomavirus, 51
  initial HIV assessment and, 26b
Papilledema, 146-147, 147b
  CNS lymphoma and, 173
Papillomavirus, human (HPV), 51
  anal neoplasia and, 246
  as oral manifestation of HIV, 133t, 137
  as skin manifestation of HIV, 121, 121b
  cervical intraepithelial neoplasia, cervical cancer and, 243-244
  HIV and, 244
  HIV-associated anorectal lesions and, 199
  Key Points, 246b
Paracentesis, for uveitis diagnosis, 142
Paracoccidioides brasiliensis, 83
Paralysis, areflexic, Guillain-Barré syndrome and, 169
Paranoia
  delirium and, 185
  HIV-associated psychosis and, 189
Paraplegia
  CMV polyradiculpathy and, 86
  CMV radiculitis and, 173
Parasthesia
  and HSV-related anorectal ulcers, 199
  perioroal, from neurologic effects of antiretroviral therapy, 36
Parenchymatous neurosyphilis, 112
Parenteral nutrition, total, AIDS wasting syndrome and, 225
Paresis, general, syphilis and, 112

Paresthesias
  comprehensive history of, 25b
  Guillain-Barré syndrome and, 168
  sacral, HSV proctitis and, 90, 220
  sensory-motor neuropathy from vincristine and, 175
Parkinsonian symptoms, antipsychotics and, 183b
Paromomycin
  for *Cryptosporidium,* 100, 101t
    HIV-associated diarrhea and, 218
  for *Entamoeba histolytica,* 103t, 106
Parotitis, chronic, children with AIDS and, 251
Paroxetine
  for bereavement, 179b
  for HIV-associated dementia, 188
  for major depressive disorder, 180b
  potential antiretroviral interaction with, 182t
Paxil; *see* Paroxetine
PCP; *see Pneumocystis carinii* pneumonia
Peer support
  for adolescents with HIV, 257
Peliosis hepatis, *Bartonella* and, 196
Pelvic abscess, in *Rhodococcus equi,* 116
Pemphigoid, benign mucous membrane
  linear gingival erythema *vs.,* 138
  necrotizing ulcerative gingivitis or periodontitis *vs.,* 139
Penicillins
  for neurosyphilis, 172
  for syphilis, 114, 134t
    tertiary, 174
    with HIV, 123
  for syphilitic retinitis, 152
  penicillinase-resistant, for *S. aureus,* 122
  resistance in pneumococci to, 110, 206
Penicilliosis, 83
  molluscum contagiosum *vs.,* 120
Penicillium marneffei, 83, 211
  advanced HIV and, 209
Penis
  primary syphilis and, 112
  ulcer of, in acute HIV-1 infection, 18f
Pentam; *see* Pentamidine
Pentamidine
  acute renal failure and, 160
  aerosolized
    atypical presentations of PCP and, 58
    for PCP prophylaxis, 66, 206
      Pneumocystis carinii choroiditis and, 152
      TMP-SMX *vs.,* 65
  for *Pneumocystis carinii* pneumonia, 52t
  for PCP, 60, 63t, 64, 206
  hepatocellular toxicity of, 195b
  hyperkalemia in HIV and, 161t, 164
  hypocalcemia and, 164
  intravenous, for PCP prophylaxis, 66
  neuropsychiatric side effects of, 181t
  renal magnesium wasting and, 164
  renal tubular acidosis and, 165
Pentamidine isethionate
  for PCP, 61
  intravenous, for ocular PCP, 152

Pentoxifylline, for Kaposi's sarcoma, 240b, 241
Percutaneous transthoracic needle aspiration, 214
Perianal area
  HIV and human papillomavirus of, 121
  HSV-related ulcers and, 199
  primary syphilis and, 112
Pericardial tamponade, *T. gondii* and, 97
Pericarditis
  Entamoeba histolytica and, 106
  penicilliosis and, 83
  T. gondii and, 97
Pericardium
  extrapulmonary TB in, 70
  PCP and, 59
Perinatal transmission
  epidemiology of, 249
  immune system and, 254
  of HHV-8, 236
  prevention of, 250, 255
  testing for, 250-251, 251b
  U.S. HIV prevalence of, 11-12
Periodontal status, initial HIV assessment of, 26b
Periodontitis, necrotizing ulcerative, as oral manifestation of HIV, 134t, 138-139
Peripheral nervous system, HIV and, 166, 167b
  Guillain-Barré syndrome, 168-169
  immunosuppresion and, 173-175
  motor neurons disorders, 168
Peripheral neuropathy
  drug combinations and, 35
  from antiretroviral therapy, 36
  from thalidomide, 139
  from trimethoprim-dapsone for PCP, 63t
  in acute HIV-1 infection, 17b
  pain from, 190
Peritoneal dialysis; *see also* Dialysis
  patient-to-patient HIV infection and, 156
Peritonitis
  E. intestinalis and, 217
  penicilliosis and, 83
  Salmonella and, 111
Perlèche; *see* Cheilitis
Permethrin
  for eosinophilic folliculitis in HIV, 129
  for scabies in HIV, 126
Persantine, for membranoproliferative glomerulonephritis, 157
Persecutory fantasies, HIV-associated psychosis and, 189
Personality changes
  HIV-1–associated dementia complex and, 186
  T. gondii and, 96
Personality disorders, major depressive disorder *vs.,* 179
Petechiae, initial HIV assessment for, 25, 26b
Pets
  Bartonella infections and, 49, 115-116
  Cryptosporidium and, 47, 101
  gastroenteritis and, 111
  T. gondii and, 96

Pharmacotherapy, for major depressive disorder, 180-181
Pharyngeal muscles, polymyositis and, 169
Pharyngeal pain, 190
Pharyngitis, in acute HIV-1 infection, 16-17, 17b
Phenobarbital, antiretroviral drug interactions with, 41
Phenotypic resistance, to antiretroviral therapy, 39
  assays of, 40
Phenytoin
  acute insterstitial nephritis and, 160
  antifungal azoles interactions with, 84
Phosphate, elevated, HIV-associated lymphoma and, 242
Phosphorus, abnormalities in, 165
Photophobia
  aseptic meningitis and, 166
  corneal ulcers and, 145
  from cryptoccocal meningitis, 171
  fungal chorioretinitis and, 153
  primary HIV and, 119
  retinal necrosis and, 149
  syphilitic retinitis and, 151
  toxoplasmosis and, 151
  uveitis and, 72, 141, 142
Photosensitivity; *see also* Porphyria cutanea tarda
  as skin manifestation of HIV, 128
Physical examination
  for AIDS wasting syndrome, 226
  for fever of unknown origin, 229-230
  for HIV-associated diarrhea diagnosis, 216
  for initial HIV management, 25-26, 26b
  for neurologic complications in HIV, 166
  for pulmonary diseases in HIV, 211-212
Physical health, loss of, bereavement and, 179
Picornavirus, HIV-associated diarrhea and, 220
Pigment epithelium, retinal, CMV retinitis and, 147
Pill esophagitis, 193
Pilocarpine, for salivary flow, 136
Pimozide, contraindications for, 42t
Pinworm infection, anal squamous cell carcinoma *vs.,* 199
Pityrosporum ovale
  as skin manifestation of HIV, 124, 124b
  seborrheic dermatitis and, 127
Plaques, vegetating, cryptococcosis and, 125
Plasmacytic interstitial nephritis, acute, renal failure and, 160, 160b
Plasmaphersis
  for chronic inflammatory demyelinating polyneuropathy, 169
  for Guillain-Barré syndrome, 169
  for TTP/HUS, 159
Platelet counts, fever of unknown origin and, 232
Pleocytosis, CMV polyradiculpathy and, 86
Pleura, extrapulmonary TB in, 70
Pleural fluid, for *Rhodococcus equi* diagnosis, 116

Pneumatosis intestinalis, *Cryptosporidium parvum* and, 217
Pneumococcal vaccine
 23-valent, against *Streptococcus pneumoniae*, 45, 48, 54t
 for children with AIDS, 252, 253, 253b
Pneumocystis carinii, HIV-associated diarrhea and, 220
Pneumocystis carinii chorioretinitis
 CMV retinitis *vs.*, 86
 Haemophilus influenzae vs., 206
Pneumocystis carinii choroiditis, 152, 152b
Pneumocystis carinii pneumonia (PCP), 6, 12
 atypical presentations of, 58-59
 bacterial pneumonia *vs.*, 108
 cause of, 57-58
 CD4+ counts and fever of unknown origin with, 231, 231b
 children with AIDS and, 251, 252, 252b
 clinical presentation of, 58
 diagnosis of, 59-60
  sputum examination for, 213
 empirical treatment for, 214b, 215
 exposure to, 45
 fever of unknown origin and, 229
 fiberoptic bronchoscopy for diagnosis of, 213
 in acute HIV-1 infection, 18
 Kaposi's sarcoma *vs.*, 237
 Key Points, 67b, 206b
 laboratory presentation of, 58
 late HIV infection and, 205-206
  CD4+ counts in, 211
 M. kansasii and, 77
 natural history of, 60
 NSIP *vs.*, 211
 prophylaxis against, 52t, 64-66
  duration of, 46
  for HIV-infected infants, 252
  initiation of, 45
  with TMP-SMX, 46
 pulmonary cryptococcosis comborbidity with, 208
 radiographic presentation of, 58
 T. gondii vs., 96
 treatment of, 60-64
Pneumonia; *see also Pneumocystis carinii* pneumonia
 bacterial, 108-110, 110b
  diagnosis and treatment of, 109f
  diagnostic tests for, 110t
  late HIV infections and, 206-207
 histoplasmosis and, 82
 late HIV infection and, 205
 and MAC in AIDS, 208
 severely rapid, children with AIDS and, 251
 subacute, coccidioidomycosis and, 82
 and TMP-SMX three times a week, 66
 varicella, 92
Pneumonitis
 CMV encephalitis and, 170
 cytomegalovirus, 86, 87-88
  in acute HIV-1 infection, 18
  late HIV infection and, 209-210, 210b
 interstitial, 205

Pneumonitis—cont'd
 lymphocytic interstitial, children with AIDS and, 251
 M. kansasii and, 77
 MAC and, 76
 nonspecific interstitial, 211
Pneumothorax
 and aerosolized pentamidine for PCP prophylaxis, 66
 bronchoalveolar lavage for PCP diagnosis and, 59
 lung biopsy and, 213, 214
 with PCP
  smoking and, 205
  treatment for, 206
Pneumovax, vaccine for *Streptococcus pneumoniae*, 45
Podophyllin, topical, for oral hairy leukoplakia, 94
Podophyllin resin, for anogenital condylomata acuminata, 200
Podophyllotoxin, for anogenital condylomata acuminata, 200
Podophyllum resin
 for anal neoplasia, 247
 for human papilloma virus with HIV, 137
 for molluscum contagiosum, 120
 for oral hairy leukoplakia, 121, 137
 for warts, 121
Poliovirus vaccine inactivated (IPV)
 for children with AIDS, 253, 253b
Polycythemia
 testosterone and, 225
 testosterone enthate and, 227t
Polymerase chain reaction (PCR)
 for *Bartonella* diagnosis, 115
 for CMV diagnosis, 86-87
  fever of unknown origin and, 233
 for *Cryptosporidium*, 100, 100t
 for *Cryptosporidium parvum* diagnosis, 218
 for *Cyclospora*, 104
 for direct detection of HIV, 22
 for *Entamoeba histolytica* diagnosis, 106
 for fever of unknown origin diagnosis with CMV diagnosis, 231-232
 for *Giardia lamblia*, 105
 for HIV in infants born to HIV-infected mothers, 251
 for HSV diagnosis, 90
 for microsporidia diagnosis, 217
 for PCP diagnosis, 60
 for *T. gondii* DNA, 97
 for tuberculous meningitis diagnosis, 172
 for VZV diagnosis, 92
 of CSF for CMV diagnosis, 170
Polymerase proteins, response to HIV infection by, 20
Polymyositis, as neurologic complication of HIV, 167b, 169-170
Polyradiculopathy, CMV and, 86
Porphyria cutanea tarda (PCT), as skin manifestation of HIV, 128, 128b
Positron emission tomography (PET) scanning, for HIV-associated lymphoma diagnosis, 242
Potassium disorders, 163-164
 HIV-associated lymphoma and, 242

Potassium hydroxide
 for hyperplastic candidiasis diagnosis, 138
 for *Pityrosporum ovale* diagnosis, 124
Poverty
 M. kansasii and, 77
 Shigella and, 219
 tuberculosis and, 69
Pravastatin, safety of, 41
Prednisone
 for aphthous ulcers, 139, 194
 for eosinophilic folliculitis in HIV, 129
 for herpes zoster, 93
 for HIV-associated lymphoma, 242, 243
 for necrotizing stomatitis, 139
 for paradoxical ("reversal") reactions in TB, 73
Pregnant women
 ciprofloxacin contradindications for, 49
 Cryptococcus neoformans and, 49
 efavirenz contraindications for, 37
 Entamoeba histolytica and, 105
 HIV screening for, 20, 250
 HIV-infected
  antiretroviral therapy for, 31
  prevalence of, 249
  sulfur ointment for scabies of, 126
  with syphilis, 123
 Mycobacterium avium disease prophylaxis against, 48
 pneumococcal vaccine for, 48
 thalidomide and, 139
 TMP-SMX and, 46
 with candidiasis, 49
 with cytomegalovirus, 50
 with herpes simplex disease, 50
 with tuberculosis, 47-48
Preterm delivery, perinatal transmission and, 249
Primaquine, for *Pneumocystis carinii* pneumonia, 206
Primary care office visits
 disease specific recommendations, for protozoan infections, 45-48
 initial
  blood texts, 44-45
  immunizations, 45
  medical history taking, 44
  patient education, 44
  tuberculosis testing, 45
Primary HIV, 119
 diagnosis of, 22
Primates, nonhuman, *Pneumocystis carinii* pneumonia and, 57
Probenecid, for nephrotoxicty from cidofovir, 53t, 148
Procaine penicillin, for syphilis, 114
Procarbazine, neuropsychiatric side effects of, 181t
Proctitis
 from HSV, 90, 220
 treatment of, 200
Prognosis, educational discussions of, 27
Progressive encephalopathy
 in children with AIDS, 252-253
Progressive multifocal leukoencephalopathy; *see* Leukoencephalopathy, progressive multifocal

Progressive outer retinal necrosis (PORN), 150-151
  herpes zoster ophthalmicus and, 144
  toxoplasmosis retinochoroiditis vs., 151
Progressive vascular mononeuropathy multiplex syndrome, CMV radiculitis and, 173
Propafenone, contraindications for, 42t
Propamidine isethionate, for microsporidia keratitis, 145
Prostacyclin, for TTP/HUS, 159
Prostate, cryptococcosis and, 81
Prostate tumors, testosterone and, 225, 227t
Protease inhibitors (PI)
  characteristics of, 34t
  contraindicated drugs with, 41
  diarrhea and, 246
  drug-drug interactions and, 40-41
  for acute HIV-1 infection, 19
  for children with AIDS, 253, 254
    once daily, 254-255
  for treatment intensification, 38
  gastrointestinal side efects from, 35
  HIV-associated dementia and, 168
  HPV infections and, 137
  Kaposi's sarcoma and, 236
  lipodystrophy and, 36-37
  liver disease from, 195, 198
  and NRTI combinations, 31, 33
  osteopenia from, 37
  P450 enzyme system and, 175
  rash/hypersensitivity reactions from, 36
  reaction to, as oral manifestation of HIV, 135t
  renal implications of, 162
  resistance to, 39, 40
  rifampin or rifabutin interactions with, 47, 47b
  TB drug treatment interactions with, 71
  xerostomia from, 132
Protein metabolism, AIDS wasting syndrome and, 224
Proteinuria
  diagnosis of renal failure and other renal abnormalities and, 161
  hepatitis C-associated immune complex glomerulonephritis and, 158
  HIVAN and, 155
    ACE-inhibitors for, 156
  in IgA glomerulonephritis, 157
  membranoproliferative glomerulonephritis and, 157
  renal failure and, 160
Proton pump inhibitors, contraindications for, 42t
Protozoa, HIV-associated diarrhea and, 216-218
Proviral DNA polymerase chain reaction assay, for acute HIV-1 infection, 18
Prozac; see Fluoxetine
Pruritus
  anal neoplasias and, 247
  as skin manifestation of HIV, 126, 126b
  eosinophilic folliculitis in HIV and, 128
  from alitretinoin, 240
  from TMP-SMX for PCP, 60, 63t
  from TMP-SMX for PCP prophylaxis, 65

Pruritus—cont'd
  from trimethoprim-dapsone for PCP, 63t
  HSV proctitis and, 90
  in vulvovaginal candidiasis, 80
  Norwegian scabies in HIV vs., 126
  seborrheic dermatitis and, 127
Pseudomembranous candidiasis; see Thrush
Pseudomonas aeruginosa
  corneal infections with, 145
  pneumonia from, 108
    late HIV infection and, 207
  Rhodococcus equi vs., 116
Psoriasis vulgaris
  as skin manifestation of HIV, 126-127, 127b, 127f
  pain from, 190
  Reiter's syndrome comorbidity with, 127
Psychiatric illness and psychological reactions
  anxiety disorders, 183-185
  case report, 178b
  mood disorders, 177-183
  organic manifestations of, 185-188
Psychomotor retardation
  HIV-associated dementia and, 167, 186
  major depressive disorder and, 179, 180b
Psychopharmacologic therapy, for reactive depression, 178
Psychosis, 188-189
  HIV-1–associated dementia complex and, 186
  Key Points, 190b
  major depressive disorder vs., 179
  mania and, 182, 183b
  T. gondii and, 96
Psychostimulants, for major depressive disorder, 181
Psychotherapy
  for anxiety, 185
  for bereavement, 179b
  for HIV-associated dementia, 188
  for major depressive disorder, 180
  for pain, 191
  for reactive depression, 177-178
Psychotic disorders, 188-190
Psyllium, for Cryptosporidium, 101
Pulmonary diseases
  bilateral infiltrates, Kaposi's sarcoma and, 237-238
  diagnosis with HIV disease of, 214b
    algorithm for, 215f
    chest computed tomography for, 212-213
    chest radiograph for, 212-213
    fiberoptic bronchoscopy for, 213-214
    Gallium scanning for, 213
    issues to consider, 214b
    laboratory studies for, 212
    medical history taking and, 211
    physical examination for, 211-212
    sputum examination for, 213
    when PCP not confirmed, 214b
  late HIV infection and, 205, 206b
    from bacterial infections, 206-207, 207b
    from fungal disease, 208-209
    from mycobacterial infections, 207-208, 208b

Pulmonary diseases—cont'd
  late HIV infection and—cont'd
    from nontuberculous mycobacteria, 208, 208b
    from PCP, 205-206, 206b
    from viral diseases, 209-210, 210b
    noninfectious, 210-211, 211b
    treatment with HIV disease of, algorithm for, 215f
Pulmonary embolism
  late HIV infection and, 211
  PCP and, 63
Pulse oximetry, and TMP-SMX for PCP, 61
Pupils
  abnormal responses of, neurosyphilis and, 172
  Argyll Robertson, 174
  syphilitic retinitis and, 152
Purpura
  histoplamosis and, 82
  mixed essentiual cryoglobulinemia and, 158
Pustular psoriasis, as skin manifestation of HIV, 127
Pustules, cryptococcosis and, 125
PUVA therapy, for psoriasis with HIV, 127
Pyogenic abscess, Entamoeba histolytica vs., 106
Pyogenic granuloma
  from indinavir, 129, 129f
  Kaposi's sarcoma vs., 143
Pyomyositis, 174
Pyrazinamide
  dosage for initial treatment of TB, 72t
  for M. kansasii, 77
  for M. xenopi, 78
  for tuberculosis, 174, 207
  for tuberculosis prophylaxis, 47, 53t
  for tuberculous meningitis, 172
  hepatocellular toxicity of, 195b
  hypuricemia and, 165
  NRTIs or PIs and, 72
  with rifampin for TB prophylaxis, 74
Pyridoxine
  for tuberculous, 174
  for tuberculous meningitis, 172
  sensory-motor neuropathy from isoniazid and, 175
  tuberculosis prophylaxis and, 47, 53t, 74
Pyrimethamine
  and dapsone for PCP prophylaxis, 66
  for Cyclospora, 104
  for E. bieneusi, 217
  for Isospora, 101t, 103
  for Pneumocystis carinii pneumonia, 46, 52t
  for toxoplasmosis, 52t, 97, 98, 99t, 171-172
    late HIV infection and, 210
  for toxoplasmosis retinochoroiditis, 151
  renal failure and, 160, 160b
  and sulfadiazine for PCP prophylaxis, 66
Pyuria, diagnosis of renal failure and renal abnormalities and, 161

Q

Quality of life
  for children with AIDS on HAART, 253-254
  testosterone and, 225

Quality of life—cont'd
    treatment of HIV-related skin diseases
        and, 118
Quinacrine, for *Giardia lamblia*, 103t,
    105
Quinidine, contraindications for, 42t
Quinolone antibiotics
    didanosine interactions with, 41
    for HIV-associated diarrhea from *Campylobacter*, 219
    for HIV-associated diarrhea from *Salmonella*, 219
    for HIV-associated diarrhea from *Shigella*, 219
    neuropsychiatric side effects of, 181t

R
R5 viruses, 15
Radiation exposure, of lacrimal gland, keratoconjunctivitis sicca and, 141
Radiation therapy
    for anal neoplasia, 247
    for cervical cancer, 245
    for CNS lymphoma, 173
    for Kaposi's sarcoma, 129, 130, 134t,
        240, 240b
        ocular, 143
        oral, 137
    for non-Hodgkin's lymphoma, 134t
    for pyomyositis/lymphomatous infiltration of muscle, 175
    for squamous cell carcinoma, 134t
    xerostomia from, 132
Radiculitis, CMV, 169b, 170, 173, 174f
Radiculopathy
    in acute HIV-1 infection, 17b
    tuberculosis and, 174
Radiographs
    chest
        bronchoalveolar lavage for PCP
            diagnosis and, 59
        for bacterial pneumonia diagnosis, 109,
            206
        for blastomycosis diagnosis, 83
        for CMV pneumonitis diagnosis, 86
        for cryptococcosis diagnosis, 81
        for fever of unknown origin diagnosis,
            230, 232
        for histoplamosis diagnosis, 82
        for Kaposi's sarcoma, 210
        for *M. kansasii* diagnosis, 208
        for *M. xenopi* diagnosis, 78
        for *Nocardia asteroides* diagnosis,
            207
        for PCP diagnosis, 205
        for pulmonary diseases diagnosis,
            212-213
        for *Rhodococcus equi* diagnosis, 207
        for tuberculosis diagnosis, 45, 47, 70,
            207
        PCP treatment and, 62-63
        and TMP-SMX for PCP, 61
    of brain, for CNS lymphoma diagnosis,
        173
Radionuclide imaging, for fever of unknown
    origin diagnosis, 234
Ramsay Hunt syndrome, 174

Rapid plasma reagin (RPR) test
    for neurosyphilis, 172
    for syphilis, 152
    HIV and, 113
Rashes; *see also* Varicella-zoster virus
    abacavir and, 230
    and clindamycin-primaquine for PCP, 62
    coccidioidomycosis and, 82
    comprehensive history of, 25b
    dermatomal, herpes zoster and, 174
    diagnosis of renal failure and renal abnormalities and, 161
    from acyclovir, 90
    from alitretinoin, 240
    from antiretroviral therapy, 36
    from atovaquone for PCP, 63t
    from clindamycin-primaquine for PCP,
        63t
    from dapsone for PCP prophylaxis, 66
    from pentamidine for PCP, 63t
    from thalidomide, 139, 226, 227t
    from TMP-SMX for PCP, 60, 63t, 206
    from TMP-SMX for PCP prophylaxis, 65
    from trimethoprim-dapsone for PCP, 63t
    in secondary syphilis, 112
    maculopapular, aseptic meningitis and,
        166
    papular, pulmonary histoplasmosis and,
        209
    unremitting or recurrent, referrals for,
        118-119
Reactive depression, 177-179, 178b
    major depressive disorder *vs.*, 180b
Recombinant immunoblot agency (RIBA),
    for HCV RNA, 45
Rectal bleeding
    anal neoplasia and, 246
    anal neoplasias and, 247
Rectal herpes simplex disease, 89-90
Red eye
    herpes simplex keratitis and, 144
    molluscum contagiosum and, 143
    toxoplasmosis and, 151
    uveitis and, 72, 142
Red-brown lesions, maculopapular
    differential diagnosis of, 239t
    Kaposi's sarcoma and, 237
Reference standards, for drugs, on-line, 41
Referrals
    for abnormal Pap smears, 246
    for acute HIV-1, 19
    for AIDS retinopathy, 146
    for anal neoplasia, 247-248
    for anogenital condylomata acuminata,
        200
    for bacterial pneumonia, 110
    for bacterial pulmonary infections, 207
    for CMV pneumonitis, 209
    for CMV retinitis, 88, 149
    for *Cryptosporidium*, 101-102
    for *Cyclospora*, 104
    for *Entamoeba histolytica*, 106
    for esophagitis, 194
    for fungal pulmonary infections, 209
    for GI bleeding, 201
    for *Giardia lamblia*, 105
    for hepatitis B and C, 198

Referrals—cont'd
    for hepatitis C-associated immune complex glomerulonephritis, 158
    for herpes simplex keratitis, 144
    for HIVAN, 156
    for HIV-associated diarrhea, 222
    for HIV-associated lymphoma, 243
    for HIV-associated skin diseases, 118-119
    for HSV, 91
    for hyperkalemia, 164
    for initial HIV management, 27
    for *Isospora*, 103
    for Kaposi's sarcoma, 211, 241
        ocular, 143
    for keratoconjunctivitis sicca, 141
    for microsporidia, 102-103
    for microsporidia keratitis, 145
    for mixed essential cryoglobulinemia,
        158
    for neurologic complications, 175-176
    for nontuberculous mycobacterial infections, 208
    for ocular molluscum contagiosum,
        143
    for PCP, 67, 206
    for pulmonary malignancy, 211
    for renal failure and other renal abnormalities, 162
    for retinal necrosis, 150
    for sleep disturbances, 192
    for syphilis, 114
    for *T. gondii*, 99
    for toxoplasmosis retinochoroiditis,
        151
    for TTP/HUS, 159
    for tuberculosis, 208
    for uveitis, 142
    for varicella-zoster keratitis, 145
    for VZV, 93
Reflexes
    chronic inflammatory demyelinating
        polyneuropathy and, 169
    segmental, herpes zoster and, 174
Rehydration, for *Cryptosporidium*, 101
Reiter's syndrome
    as skin manifestation of HIV, 127, 127b
    ulcers from, HIV and, 135t
Relaxation techniques, for anxiety, 185
Relaxation therapy, for pain, 191
Remeron, for insomnia, 192
Renal abscess, in *Rhodococcus equi*, 116
Renal cell carcinoma, CD4+ counts and
    fever of unknown origin with, 231
Renal failure
    acute
        hepatitis C-associated immune complex glomerulonephritis and, 157
        HIVAN and, 154
            among African Americans, 155, 156
        in HIV, 160-162
            causes of, 160b
        renal potassium excretion and, 164
    acyclovir and, 90
    from foscarnet, 220
    from TMP-SMX for PCP, 61, 63t
    HIVAN and, 155
    Key Points, 162b

Renal failure—cont'd
  obstructive
    causes of, 160b, 161
      drugs associated with intratubular crystallization and, 161t
    pentamidine and, 164
    TTP/HUS and, 159
Renal tubular acidosis, hyperkalemia and, 164
Repetitive movements, impairment with, HIV-associated dementia and, 186
Reporting, confidential name-based HIV infection, 7-8
Reptiles
  Cryptosporidium and, 99
  gastroenteritis and, 111
Rescriptor; see Delavirdine
Respiration, artificial, for *Pneumocystis carinii* pneumonia, 64
Respiratory distress, abacavir and, 230
Respiratory distress syndrome, adult
  PCP and, 63
  toxoplasmosis and, 210
Respiratory isolation, PCP treatment and, 62
Respiratory muscles, Guillain-Barré syndrome and, 168
Respiratory syncytial virus, late HIV infection and, 210
Respiratory tract infections, bacterial
  prophylaxis against, 48
  TMP-SMX prophylaxis against, 65
Respirgard II nebulizer, *Pneumocystis carinii* pneumonia and, 52t
Resting energy expenditure (REE), AIDS wasting syndrome and, 223
Restlessness
  major depressive disorder and, 179
  mania and, 182
Restriction fragment length polymorphism (RFLP), for tuberculosis diagnosis, 71
Retardation, psychomotor, CMV and, 86
Retinal artery occlusion
  central, varicella-zoster retinitis *vs.*, 150
  toxoplasmosis retinochoroiditis *vs.*, 151
Retinal detachment
  from ganciclovir implants, 87
  retinal necrosis and, 150
  rhegmatogenous
    CMV retinitis and, 87
    ocular hypotension and, 142
  surgical considerations for, 88
  varicella-zoster retinitis and, 150
  varicella-zoster virus and, 92
Retinal hemorrhage
  AIDS retinopathy and, 146
  CMV retinitis and, 148
Retinal necrosis; *see also* Progressive outer retinal necrosis; Syphilitic retinitis
  acute
    as AIDS complication, 149-150, 150b
    toxoplasmosis retinochoroiditis *vs.*, 151
  herpes zoster ophthalmicus and, 144
  varicella-zoster virus and, 92

Retinitis
  cytomegalovirus, 12, 50, 85-86
    AIDS retinopathy *vs.*, 146
    children with AIDS and, 252
    CMV encephalitis and, 170
    diagnosis of, 86, 148
    foscarnet for, 53t
    in contralateral eye, ganciclovir implants and, 87, 148
    in HIV, 121
    Key Points, 149b
    ocular hypotension and, 142
    PORN *vs.*, 150
    presentation and progression of, 147-148
    pulmonary CMV and, 212
    toxoplasmosis retinochoroiditis *vs.*, 151
    treatment for, 87, 148-149, 149t
    valganciclovir for, 87
  disseminated varicella-zoster virus and, 93
  herpersvirus-associated, 147
  PCP and, 59
  syphilitic retinitis and, 151
  varicella-zoster, 150
    herpes zoster ophthalmicus and, 144
Retinoblastoma proteins, anal neoplasia and, 246
Retinochoroiditis, toxoplasmosis, 151
Retinoids, topical
  for cervical intraepithelial neoplasia, 245
  for oral hairy leukoplakia, 94
  for psoriasis with HIV, 127
Retinopathy, AIDS, 146, 146b
Retrosternal discomfort, PCP and, 205
Retrovir; see Zidovudine
Retroviruses, about, 3
Reverse transcriptase
  HIV-1 replication and, 3
  p66, response to HIV infection by, 20
Reverse transcriptase polymerase chain reaction, for HCV RNA, 45
Rhabdomyolysis, acute tubular necrosis and, 160, 160b
  diagnosis of, 161
Rheumatologic pain, 190
Rhodococcus equi, 116, 116b, 211
  focal CNS lesion and, 98t
  late HIV infection and, 207
Rhomboencephalitis, meningitis with gastroenteritis *vs.*, 111
Ribavirin
  for hepatitis C, 197
  for mixed essential cryoglobulinemia, 158
Rifabutin
  alternatives to, 41
  contraindications for, 42t
  for DMAC, 48, 52t, 76, 76t
    HIV-associated diarrhea and, 219
    in children with AIDS, 252
  for DMAC prophylaxis, 76t, 77
  for *M. kansasii,* 77
  for tuberculosis, 207
  for tuberculosis prophylaxis, 53t
  for tuberculosis treatment, 71, 74
  potential interactions with, 47b
  protease inhibitors and, 74

Rifabutin—cont'd
  urine color changes with, 163t
  uveitis and, 141, 142
Rifampin
  contraindications for, 42t
  drug resistant TB and, 69-70
  for *Bartonella* with endocarditis, 115
  for DMAC, 76
  for *M. kansasii,* 208
  for *M. xenopi,* 78
  for *Rhodococcus equi,* 116, 207
  for tuberculosis prophylaxis, 47, 53t
  for tuberculosis treatment, 71, 174, 207
    initial dosage for, 72t
  for tuberculous meningitis, 172
  hyperkalemia in HIV and, 161t, 164
  hypokalemia and, 163
  potential interactions with, 47b
  renal syndromes with, 163t
  uric acid excretion and, 165
  urine color changes with, 163t
  with pyrazinamide for TB prophylaxis, 74
Rifamycins
  hepatocellular toxicity of, 195b
  PI and NNRTI interactions, 71
Rigors, primary HIV and, 119
Riluzole, motor neuropathy response to, 168
Risperidone (Risperdal)
  for HIV-associated dementia, 188
  for HIV-associated psychosis, 190b
  for mania, 183
Ritalin, for HIV-associated dementia, 188
Ritonavir, 31
  characteristics of, 34t
  creatine kinase increases from, 37
  didanosine interactions with, 41
  drug-induced diarrhea from, 220
  for children with AIDS, 254
  for treatment intensification, 38
  gastrointestinal side efects from, 35
  hepatic transaminases abnormalities from, 37
  hepatocellular toxicity of, 195b
  hypuricemia and, 165
  liquid formulations for, children with AIDS and, 254
  morphine metabolism and, 41
  neurologic adverse effects from, 36
  renal implications of, 162
  resistance to, 40
  rifabutin interactions with, 47b, 74
  and tuberculosis treatment, 72
RNA
  acute HIV testing with, 22-23
  messenger, HIV-1 replication and, 3
Rochalimaea; see *Bartonella*
Rodents, *Pneumocystis carinii* pneumonia and, 57
Rotavirus, HIV-associated diarrhea and, 220
Roth's spots, AIDS retinopathy and, 146
Roxithromycin, for *Cryptosporidium parvum,* 218
Rubella, acute HIV-1 infection *vs.*, 17, 17b

S

Sabin-Feldman dye test, for *T. gondii*, 97
Sadness
    major depressive disorder and, 179, 180b
    reactive depression and, 177, 178
Salicyclic acid shampoos, for seborrheic dermatitis, 128
Saline, for hyponatremia, 163
Saliva, CMV in, 85
Salivary flow, reduced; *see also* Xerostomia
    treatment of, 136t
Salivary gland disease, in HIV, 132
Salmonella
    CD4+ counts and fever of unknown origin with, 231, 231b
    CMV colitis vs., 86
    gastroenteritis and, 111
    HIV-associated diarrhea and, 219
    Key Points, 112b, 219b
    prophylaxis against, 54t
    Reiter's syndrome and, 127
    TMP-SMX prophylaxis against, 65
    TTP/HUS and, 159b
Salmonella enteritidis, 111
Salmonella typhimurium, 111
Salmonellosis, 48
Salvage therapy, PCP treatment and, 62-64
Saquinavir, 31
    bioavailability of hard-gel, 33
    characteristics of, 34t
    children with AIDS and, 254
    contraindications for, 175
    gastrointestinal side efects from, 35
    hepatic transaminases abnormalities from, 37
    hepatocellular toxicity of, 195b
    rifabutin interactions with, 47b
Sarcoidosis, syphilitic retinitis vs., 152
Sarcoptes scabiei (scabies)
    as skin manifestation of HIV, 126, 126b
    pruritus vs., 126
Scarring, porphyria cutanea tarda in HIV and, 128
Schizoaffective disorder
    major depressive disorder vs., 180b
    mania vs., 183b
Schizoaffective schizophrenia, mania vs., 182
Schizophrenia
    delirium vs., 185
    HIV-associated psychosis vs., 189
School
    for children with AIDS, 255
Scotomas
    CMV retinitis and, 85
    fungal chorioretinitis and, 153
Scrofuloderma, tuberculosis and, 122
Seborrheic dermatitis, 79
    as skin manifestation of HIV, 127-128, 128f
        Key Points, 128b
    dermatophytosis in HIV vs., 124
    HIV and, 118
    initial HIV assessment for, 25, 26b
    maculopapular red-brown lesions and, 239t

Seborrheic dermatitis—cont'd
    PCP and, 205
    Pityrosporum ovale vs., 124
Sedation
    clonazepam and, 183b
    for insomnia, 191
    SSRIs and, 183
    tricyclic antidepressants and, 180b, 183
Seizures
    acyclovir and, 90
    aseptic meningitis and, 166
    CNS lymphoma and, 173
    HIV-associated dementia and, 167
    lymphomatous meningitis and, 175
    neurosyphilis and, 172
    T. gondii and, 96
    tuberculous meningitis and, 172
Selective serotonin receptor inhibitors (SSRIs)
    drug-drug interactions and, 41
    for anxiety, 185
    for bereavement, 179b
    for HIV-associated dementia, 188
    for major depressive disorder, 180, 180b
    for reactive depression, 179
    tricyclic, 183b
Self-esteem
    major depressive disorder and, 179
    mania and, 182
Self-recriminatory thoughts, major depressive disorder and, 179
Semen donors, HIV screening for, 20
Sensory conduction studies, for subacute motor neuropathy from lymphoma, 175
Sensory loss
    absence of, motor neuropathy and, 168
    chronic inflammatory demyelinating polyneuropathy and, 169
    CMV radiculitis and, 173
    delirium and, 185
    herpes zoster and, 174
    mononeuropathy multiplex and, 169
    neurologic complications in HIV and, 166
    referral for, 175
    tertiary syphilis and, 174
    vacuolar myelopathy and, 168
    vertebral osteomyelitis from tuberculosis and, 174
Sensory nerve conduction studies, for Guillain-Barré syndrome, 169
Sensory-motor axonal polyneuropathy, as neurologic complication of HIV, 167b, 169
Sepsis
    acute tubular necrosis and, 160, 160b
    Clostridium difficile and, 219
    lactic acidosis and, 165
    pulmonary histoplasmosis and, 209
Sepsis-like reaction, from TMP-SMX for PCP, 61
Septata intestinalis; see Encephalitozoon intestinalis
Septic shock
    bacterial pneumonia vs., 109
    histoplamosis and, 82

Septic syndrome, gastroenteritis and, 111
Serax; *see* Oxazepam
Serosurveys, HIV, 7-8
Sertraline
    for bereavement, 179b
    for HIV-associated dementia, 188
    for major depressive disorder, 180b
    potential antiretroviral interaction with, 182t
Serum creatinine, initial HIV assessment of, 26b
Sexual abuse, perinatal transmission and, 249
Sexual activity
    educational discussions on, 28
    Kaposi's sarcoma and, 236
    mania and, 182
Sexual dysfunction, SSRIs and, 180
Sexual function, anxiety disorders and, 184
Sexual history, for HIV medical history, 24
Sexual identity, adolescent development of, HIV and, 256
Sexually transmitted diseases
    adolescent screening for, 257
    exposure or infection history of, 24
    genital molluscum contagiosum as, 120
    hepatitis C and, 195
    HIV screening and, 20
    oral Kaposi's sarcoma and, 137
Sexually-abused children, U.S. HIV prevalence for, 11
SHADSSS (School, Home, Depression/self-esteem, Substance use, Sexuality, Safety) assessment, 256
Shame
    anxiety disorders and, 184
    reactive depression and, 177, 178
Shigella
    CMV colitis vs., 86
    HIV infection and, 111
    HIV-associated diarrhea and, 219
    Reiter's syndrome and, 127
    type 1, TTP/HUS and, 159b
Shigella flexneri, 111
Shigella sonnei, 111
Shigellosis, 48, 111, 112
Shingles; *see also* Herpes zoster
    prophylaxis against, 50, 93-94
    with HIV, 137
Shock syndrome, abacavir and, 165
Shopping sprees, mania and, 182
Sigmoidoscopy
    flexible
        for condylomata acuminatum diagnosis, 199
        for HIV-associated diarrhea diagnosis, 216, 222
        for rectal lesions diagnosis, 200
        for CMV diagnosis, 86, 220
Sildenafil, drug-drug interactions and, 41
Silicone gels, for retinal detachment, 88
Silicone oils, for retinal detachment, 148
Simian immunodeficiency virus
    classification of, 3
    intravaginal model, presentation and progression of, 14-15

Simvastatin
  alternatives to, 41
  contraindications for, 42t
  protease inhibitors and, 162
Single use diagnostic system (SUDS) test for HIV, 22
Singultus, esophagitis and, 193
Sinuses
  CT scan for fever of unknown origin diagnosis, 232b
  microsporidia and, 102
Sinusitis
  E. intestinalis and, 217
  fever of unknown origin and, CD4+ count and, 231, 231b
  and TMP-SMX three times a week, 66
Sjögren's syndrome, 141
  interstitial nephritis and, 160
Skin
  assessment for initial HIV management, 25
  Bartonella and, 115
  coccidioidomycosis and, 82
  cryptococcosis of, 81
  disseminated varicella-zoster virus and, 92
  extrapulmonary TB in, 70
  fragility of, porphyria cutanea tarda in HIV and, 128
  histoplamosis and, 82
  HIV manifestations in, 118-119, 119b
    drug reactions, 129
    infections, 119-126
    infestations, 126
    inflammatory conditions, 126-129
    neoplasms, 129-130
  MAC and, 76
  painful conditions of, 190
  penicilliosis and, 83
Skin cancer; *see also* Neoplasms
  as skin manifestation of HIV, 130
Skinfold measurement, of body fat, 223
Sleep apnea, testosterone and, 225
Sleep disturbances
  anxiety disorders and, 184
  as neuropsychiatric complication of HIV/AIDS, 191-192
  bereavement and, 179b
  major depressive disorder and, 179, 180b
  mania and, 182, 183b
  reactive depression and, 177
Sleep medications, for reactive depression, 178
Slim disease, 223; *see also* AIDS wasting syndrome
Slowed rapid movements, motor neuropathy and, 168
Smoking
  anal neoplasias and, 247
  pneumothorax with PCP and, 205
Smoking cessation, ulcers from, 135t
Social disorganization, tuberculosis and, 69
Social interaction, anxiety disorders and, 184
Social withdrawal
  HIV-1–associated dementia complex and, 186
  HIV-associated dementia and, 186

Sodium, for hyperkalemia, 164
Sodium polystyrene sulfonate, for hyperkalemia, 161
Sodium tetradecyl sulfate, for Kaposi's sarcoma, 134t
  oral, 137
Soil, *Rhodococcus equi* and, 116
Somnolence
  from dronabinol, 225, 227t
  from thalidomide, 139, 226, 227t
South America, *Isospora belli* in, 103
Spasticity with hyperreflexia
  motor neuropathy and, 168
  vacuolar myelopathy and, 168
Speech, disorganized, HIV-associated psychosis and, 189
Sphincter dysfunction, lymphomatous meningitis and, 175
Sphincter incompetence, absence of, motor neuropathy and, 168
Spinal cord abscess, mybcobacterial infections and, 172
Spinal cord dysfunction
  HIV and, 166, 167b, 168
  toxomplasmosis and, 171-172
Spleen
  Bartonella and, 122
  blastomycosis and, 83
  PCP and, 59
Splenomegaly, Kaposi's sarcoma and, 201
Sporanox; *see* Itraconazole
Sporothrix schenckii, 83
  chorioretinitis and, 152-153
Sporotrichosis, as skin manifestation of HIV, 126, 126b
Sputum examination
  for bacterial pneumonia diagnosis, 109, 110
  for coccidioidomycosis diagnosis, 82, 209
  for *M. kansasii* diagnosis, 77
  for *M. xenopi* diagnosis, 77
  for MAC diagnosis, 208
  for *Nocardia asteroides* diagnosis, 207
  for PCP diagnosis, 59
  for pneumococcal pneumonia diagnosis, 206
  for pulmonary diseases diagnosis, 213
  for *Rhodococcus equi* diagnosis, 116
Squamous cell carcinoma, 51
  anal
    diagnosis of, 200
    human papillomavirus and, 199
  as oral manifestation of HIV, 134t, 140
  as skin manifestation of HIV, 130
  Epstein-Barr virus *vs.*, 94
  HSV *vs.*, 90
  in HIV, 121
  ulcers from, HIV and, 135t
Squamous intraepithelial lesion, anal, 246
St. John's wort, antiretroviral drug interactions with, 41
Staphylococcus aureus, 108
  as skin manifestation of HIV, 121-122
    Key Points, 122b
  corneal infections with, 145
  eosinophilic folliculitis in HIV and, 128

Staphylococcus aureus—cont'd
  maculopapular red-brown lesions and, 239t
  photosensitivity in HIV and, 128
  pneumonia in late HIV infection and, 207
  and pruritus in HIV, 126
  and scabies in HIV, 126
  TMP-SMX prophylaxis against, 65
  with HSV in HIV, 119
Staphylococcus epidermidis, corneal infections with, 145
Stavudine
  as FDA-approved NRTI, 31
  characteristics of, 32t
  for children with AIDS, 255
  hepatic transaminases abnormalities from, 37
  lactic acidosis from, 37
  neurologic adverse effects from, 36
  neuropsychiatric side effects of, 181t
  nucleoside analogue-induced neuropathy and, 175
  and pentamidine for PCP, 61, 64
  renal implications of, 162
  resistance to, 39
  rifabutin with, 47b
  rifamycins for TB and, 72
Steroid withdrawal syndrome, from megestrol acetate, 225
Steroids
  acute interstitial nephritis and, 161
  anxiety disorders and, 184
  depressive side effects from, 180
  for CNS lymphoma, 173
  for herpes zoster, 93
  for immune reconstitution syndrome, 233
  for Kaposi's sarcoma, 241
  for lymphocytic interstitial pneumonitis, 252
  for non-HIV IgA glomerulonephritis, 157
  for optic nerve atrophy, 147
  for photosensitivity in HIV, 128
  for toxoplasmosis retinochoroiditis, 151
  for TTP/HUS, 159
  for uveitis, 142
  for varicella-zoster keratitis, 145
  for varicella-zoster retinitis, 150
  mania and, 183
  topical
    for eosinophilic folliculitis in HIV, 129
    for pruritus in HIV, 126
    for psoriasis with HIV, 127
    for seborrheic dermatitis, 127
Stevens-Johnson syndrome
  drug fever and, 230
  drug hypersensitivity in HIV and, 129
  from TMP-SMX for PCP, 61
  nevirapine and, 36
Stimulants, for pain, 191
Stool, microscopic examination of
  for diarrhea diagnosis, 216, 218, 221-222
  for microsporidia diagnosis, 217
Stool cultures
  for gastroenteritis diagnosis, 111
  for porphyria cutanea tarda in HIV, 128
Street drugs, HIV medical history and, 24

Streptococci, α-hemolytic, corneal infections with, 145
Streptococcus, psoriasis vulgaris and, 126
Streptococcus pneumoniae
  pneumonia from, 108, 206
  prophylaxis against, 48, 54t
  TMP-SMX prophylaxis against, 65
  TTP/HUS and, 159b
  vaccine for, 45
Streptomycin, dosage for initial treatment of TB, 72t
Stress
  herpes zoster ophthalmicus and, 143
  ulcers from, 135t
Stroke
  as neurologic complication of HIV, 173
  tuberculous meningitis and, 172
Stromal herpes simplex keratitis, 144
Strongyloides stercoralis, 211
  hyperinfection syndrome with pulmonary involvement, late HIV infection and, 210
Subcutaneous abscesses
  cryptococcosis and, 125
  M. xenopi and, 78
Substance abuse, mania *vs.*, 182
Subtype distribution, HIV-1, 5-6, 5t
Suicide, 190
  major depressive disorder and, 179, 180
  risk of, from parenteral pegylated interferon, 197
Sulfa drugs
  drug fever and, 230
  skin reactions to, 129
Sulfadiazine
  acute renal failure from, 161
  for *Pneumocystis carinii* pneumonia, 46
  for toxoplasmosis, 52t, 97, 98, 99t, 171-172
    late HIV infection and, 210
    retinochoroiditis, 151
  intratubular crystallization and, 161, 161t
  ureteral obstruction from, 160b
Sulfadoxine, for *Isospora*, 101t, 103
Sulfamethoxazole, intratubular crystallization and, 161, 161t
Sulfonamides
  neuropsychiatric side effects of, 181t
  photosensitivity in HIV and, 128
Sulfur ointment, for scabies in HIV, 126
Sunburn, photosensitivity in HIV and, 128
Sunlight, herpes zoster ophthalmicus and, 143
Support systems
  educational discussions on, 28
  HIV medical history and, 24
Supportive care
  for anxiety, 185
  for bereavement, 179, 179b
  for HIV-associated delirium, 186
  for major depressive disorder, 180
  for motor neuropathy, 168
Surgery
  blood loss from, renal failure and, 160
  for tuberculomas, 172

Surgical excision
  for anogenital condylomata acuminata, 200
  for cervical intraepithelial neoplasia, 245
  for human papilloma virus with HIV, 133t, 137
  for Kaposi's sarcoma
    ocular, 143
    oral, 137
  for molluscum contagiosum, 143
  for non-Hodgkin's lymphoma, 134t
  for nonmelanoma skin cancer in HIV, 130
  for oral hairy leukoplakia, 94
  for *Rhodococcus equi*, 116
Surgical history, for HIV medical history, 24
Survivor guilt, 179b
Sustiva; *see* Efavirenz
Sweats, comprehensive history of, 25b
Sympathomimetics, mania and, 183
Syphilis
  anorectal HSV *vs.*, 199
  as neurologic complication of HIV, 167b, 172
  as oral manifestation of HIV, 134t
  cause of, 112
  chorioretinitis and, AIDS retinopathy *vs.*, 146
  CMV retinitis *vs.*, 86
  diagnosis of, 113-114
  HIV-associated dementia diagnosis and, 167
  in HIV-infected individuals, 113f
  Key Points, 114b, 123b
  maculopapular red-brown lesions and, 239t
  natural history of, 114
  optic nerve atrophy and, 147
  presentation of, 112-113
  secondary
    acute HIV-1 infection *vs.*, 17, 17b
    as skin manifestation of HIV, 118, 123f
    syphilitic retinitis and, 152
  tertiary, HIV and, 174
  testing, initial HIV assessment and, 26b
  vacuolar myelopathy *vs.*, 168
  with HIV, 122-123
Syphilitic retinitis, 151-152, 152b
  toxoplasmosis retinochoroiditis *vs.*, 151

T
T cell dysfunction, ulcers from, 135t
Tabes dorsalis
  HIV and, 174
  neurosyphilis and, 172
  syphilis and, 112
Tachycardia, anxiety disorders and, 184
Tachypnea, PCP and, 205
Tarsorrhaphy, for keratoconjunctivitis sicca, 141
TAT protein gene product, Kaposi's sarcoma and, 237
Tatoos, hepatitis C and, 51
Taxol; *see* Paclitaxel
Tearfulness, major depressive disorder and, 179
Tearing, corneal ulcers and, 145

Temazepam
  for insomnia, 191
  safety of, 41
Tenesmus, HSV proctitis and, 90, 220
Tension, anxiety disorders and, 184
Terbinafine
  for dermatologic mycoses, 80
  for onychomycosis with HIV, 124
Terfenadine
  alternatives to, 41
  antifungal azoles interactions with, 84
Testing for HIV, 20-23
  history of, 24
Testosterone
  AIDS wasting syndrome and, 224, 226
  anabolic block and, 225
  megestrol acetate and, 225
Testosterone enthate, 225
  for anabolic block, 227t
Testosterone patch/gell, for anabolic block, 225, 227t
Tetanus booster, 45
Tetracyclines
  didanosine interactions with, 41
  Entamoeba histolytica diagnosis and, 106
  for *Entamoeba histolytica*, 103t, 106
  for linear gingival erythema, 134t
  for necrotizing stomatitis, 134t, 139
  for necrotizing ulcerative gingivitis or peridontitis, 139
  for toxoplasmosis retinochoroiditis, 151
  hepatocellular toxicity of, 195b
  resistance in pneumococci to, 206
Thalidomide
  for AIDS wasting syndrome, 226, 227t
  for aphthous ulcers, 139, 194
  for *E. bieneusi*, 217
  for Kaposi's sarcoma, 240b, 241
Thallium-201 SPECT
  for CNS lymphoma diagnosis, 173
  for Kaposi's sarcoma *vs.* PCP diagnosis, 237
Thiabendazole
  for *Strongyloides stercoralis*, 210
  neuropsychiatric side effects of, 181t
Thiamine deficiency, lactic acidosis and, 165
Thinking problems, comprehensive history of, 25b
Thioglitazone derivatives, for insulin resistance from antiretroviral therapy, 37
Thiothixene
  for HIV-associated psychosis, 190b
  for mania, 183
Thoracentesis, chest radiographs and, 212
Thought insertions, HIV-associated psychosis and, 189
Thoughts, racing, mania and, 182
3TC; *see* Lamivudine
Throat
  assessment for initial HIV management, 25
  sore
    abacavir and, 230
    infectious mononucleosis and, 94
    primary HIV and, 119

Thrombocytopenia
  Bartonella and, 115
  from ganciclovir, 87, 220
  from pentamidine for PCP, 63t
  from TMP-SMX for PCP prophylaxis, 65
  linear gingival erythema *vs.*, 138
  MAC and, 76
  and pentamidine for PCP, 61
  TTP and, 159
Thrombocytopenic purpura
  idiopathic, children with AIDS and, 251
  immune, maculopapular red-brown lesions and, 239t
Thrombotic microangiopathy (TMA) syndromes, 158-159
  renal failure or azotemia and, 160b
Thrombotic thrombocytopenic purpura (TTP) and hemolytic-uremic syndrome (HUS), 158-159, 159b
  valacyclovir and, 90-91
Thrush
  as cutaneous manifestation of HIV, 123-124
  from glucocorticoids for PCP, 63t
  initial HIV assessment for, 26b
  oral
    as HIV manifestation, 133t, 137-138
    and glucocorticoids for PCP, 62
    PCP and, 205
    with HIV, 123-124
  oropharyngeal, PCP prophylaxis and, 64
  Pneumocystis carinii pneumonia and, 12
Thyroid
  HIV-associated dementia and, 167
  medications for, anxiety disorders and, 184
Thyroid dysfunction, HIV-associated dementia and, 187
Thyroiditis, PCP and, 59
Thyroid-stimulating hormone (TSH) level, AIDS wasting syndrome and, 226
Tinea capitis, AIDS and, 79-80
Tinea corporis, AIDS and, 79-80
Tinea cruris, AIDS and, 79-80
Tinea faciei, dermatophytosis in HIV *vs.*, 124
Tinea pedis, AIDS and, 79-80
Tinea versicolor
  AIDS and, 79-80
  as skin manifestation of HIV, 124
Tinidazole
  for *Entamoeba histolytica*, 103t, 106
  for *Giardia lamblia*, 103t, 105
Tissue donations, U.S. HIV prevalence among, 11
TMP-SMX; *see* Trimethoprim-sulfamethoxazole
TNP-470, for Kaposi's sarcoma, 240b, 241
Tobacco habits, HIV medical history and, 24
Toluidine blue staining, for PCP, 59
Tooth mobility, necrotizing ulcerative gingivitis or peridontitis and, 139
Torsades de pointes, and pentamidine for PCP, 61
Total parenteral nutrition, AIDS wasting syndrome and, 225

Toxic disorders, neurologic symptoms of HIV and, 166
Toxic megacolon
  Clostridium difficile and, 219
  Cryptosporidium parvum and, 217
Toxoplasma gondii
  cause of, 96
  diagnosis of, 97
  exposure prevention from, 46
  HIV-associated diarrhea and, 220
  IgG test for, 45
  presentation of, 96-97
  prophylaxis against, 46, 52t, 98-99, 99t
  pulmonary, late HIV infection and, 210
  referral for, 99
  toxoplasmosis retinochoroiditis and, 151
  treatment for, 97-99, 99t
Toxoplasmosis, 12
  acute HIV-1 infection *vs.*, 17, 17b
  as neurologic complication of HIV, 167b, 171-172
  as ocular complication of AIDS, 151
  atovaquone for prophylaxis of, 66
  cerebral, in acute HIV-1 infection, 18
  CMV retinitis *vs.*, 85
  CNS lymphoma *vs.*, 173
  fever of unknown origin and, 232
  focal CNS lesion and, 98t
  intercranial, papilledema *vs.*, 146
  Key Points, 99b, 151b
  mania *vs.*, 183
  pulmonary, late HIV infection and, 210
  TMP-SMX prophylaxis against, 65
Tranquilizers
  for pain syndromes, 190
  for reactive depression, 178
Transforming growth factor (TGF)-β, MAC and, 75
Transfusion recipients; *see* Blood products recipients
Transgenic mice, HIVAN pathogenesis studies in, 154
Transmembrane glycoprotein, response to HIV infection by, 20
Transminases, elevation of
  Bartonella and, 115
  from ganciclovir, 87
Transmission, HIV, educational discussions of, 27
Transplantation
  Kaposi's sarcoma and, 236
  of kidneys, end-stage renal disease and, 156
Trauma, oral ulcers and, 132
Traums, ulcers from, 135t
Travel, international
  fever of unknown origin and, 229
  Giardia lamblia and, 104
  HIV medical history and, 24, 211
  Strongyloides stercoralis and, 210
Trazodone
  for insomnia, 191
  potential antiretroviral interaction with, 182t
Treatment; *see* Antiretroviral therapy; Drug combinations; Drug resistance; Drugs, contraindicated

Treatment intensification, 38
Tremors
  from TMP-SMX for PCP, 63t
  HIV-1–associated dementia complex and, 186
  HIV-associated dementia and, 186
  syphilitic dementia and, 172
Trench fever; *see Bartonella henselae*
Treponema pallidum, 112; *see also* Syphilis
  suggestive of HIV, 135t
  syphilitic retinitis and, 151-152
Tretinoin
  for molluscum contagiosum, 121
  for oral hairy leukoplakia, 121
  for warts, 121
Triamterene, TMP structure and, 164
Triazolam, contraindications for, 42t, 175
Trichloracetic acid
  for molluscum contagiosum, 120
  for warts, 121
Trichome stains, for microsporidia diagnosis, 102, 217, 222
Trichophyton, 80
Trichophyton rubrum, as skin manifestation of HIV, 124
Trifluridine
  for herpes simplex keratitis, 144
  for varicella-zoster keratitis, 145
Triglycerides, AIDS wasting syndrome and, 224
Trimethoprim
  hyperkalemia in HIV and, 161t, 164
  renal failure and, 160, 160b
Trimethoprim-dapsone
  for ocular PCP, 152
  for *Pneumocystis carinii* pneumonia, 60, 61, 63t, 206
  vs. TMP-SMX, hyperkalemia and, 164
Trimethoprim-sulfamethoxazole (TMP-SMX)
  acute insterstitial nephritis and, 160
  acute renal failure and, 160
  bacterial respiratory infections and, 48
  for bacterial enteric infections, 48
  for *Cyclospora*, 101t, 104
  for *E. bieneusi*, 217
  for HIV-associated diarrhea from *Salmonella*, 219
  for HIV-associated diarrhea from *Shigella*, 219
  for *Isospora belli*, 101t, 103, 218
  for *Nocardia asteroides*, 207
  for NSIP, 211
  for ocular PCP, 152
  for PCP, 46, 52t, 60-61, 63t, 64, 206
    prophylaxis, 65-66, 65t
  for *Salmonella* gastroenteritis in pregnant women, 49
  for *T. gondii*, 46, 52t, 98, 99t
    maintenance, 171
  for toxoplasmosis retinochoroiditis, 151
  hepatocellular toxicity of, 195, 195b
  hypovolemic hyponatremia and, 162
  renal tubular acidosis and, 165
  resistance in pneumococci to, 206
  skin reactions to, 129

Trimetrexate, for *Pneumocystis carinii* pneumonia, 60, 61-62, 63t, 64, 206
Trisodium phosphonoformate hexahydrate; *see* Foscarnet
TTP/HUS; *see* Thrombotic thrombocytopenic purpura (TTP) and hemolytic-uremic syndrome (HUS)
Tuberculin skin test, 26b, 45, 71, 207
   for fever of unknown origin diagnosis, 232
   for tuberculosis diagnosis, HIV-infection and, 211
   for tuberculous meningitis diagnosis, 172
Tuberculoma, mybcobacterial infections and, 172
Tuberculosis; *see also Mycobacterium tuberculosis*
   and aerosolized pentamidine for PCP prophylaxis, 66
   as neurologic complication of HIV, 167b
   blastomycosis *vs.*, 83
   clinical course of, 72-73
   clinical presentation of, 70, 70t
   cutaneous, as skin manifestation of HIV, 122
   demographics of, 211
   diagnosis of, 70-71
   epidemiology of, 69-70
   exposure or infection history of, 24
   fever of unknown origin and, 229
      CD4+ count and, 231, 231b
   fiberoptic bronchoscopy for diagnosis of, 213
   focal CNS lesion and, 98t
   inactive infection screening and treatment for, 73-74
   oral lesions without pain of, 132
   paradoxical ("reversal") reactions, 73
   pathogenesis of, 68-69
   prophylaxis against, 47-48, 53t
   Rhodococcus equi vs., 116
   rifamycin for, drug combinations for HIV and, 35
   sputum examination cautions and, 213
   syphilitic retinitis *vs.*, 152
   T. gondii vs., 97
   treatment for, 71-72
      initial dosage for, 72t
   vacuolar myelopathy *vs.*, 168
   vertebral osteomyelitis and associated radiculopathy from, 174
Tuberculous meningitis, 172
Tubulointerstitial disease, renal potatssium excretion and, 164
Tumor lysis syndrome
   alkali-forced and saline diuresis for, 161
   uric acid and ureteral obstruction from, 160b
Tumor necrosis factor
   AIDS wasting syndrome and, 224
   tuberculosis and, 68
Tumor necrosis factor α, acute HIV-1 increases in, 16, 16b
Tumor suppressor proteins, anal neoplasia and, 246
Typhoid fever, *Salmonella* gastroenteritis *vs.*, 111

Tzank smear
   for HSV diagnosis, 90, 119, 120f
      varicella-zoster virus *vs.*, 200
   for VZV diagnosis, 92

U

UL97 gene, drug resistance to ganciclovir and, 88
Ulcers; *see also* Herpes simplex virus
   anorectal, herpes simplex virus and, 199
   corneal, 145-146, 146b
   cryptococcosis and, 125
   cutaneous
      blastomycosis and, 83
      histoplamosis and, 82
      penicilliosis and, 83
   esophageal, HIV-associated, 193, 194
   from MAC as skin manifestation of HIV, 122
   gastrointestinal, from trimetraxate for PCP, 63t
   genital, in acute HIV-1 infection, 16-17, 17b, 18f
   herpetiform, HIV and, 135t
   initial HIV assessment for, 26b
   oral
      conditions and etiologies associated with, 135t
      differentiation of, 132
      from trimetraxate for PCP, 63t
      in acute HIV-1 infection, 16-17, 17b, 18f
   perianal
      from CMV in HIV, 121
      from HSV, 220
Ultrasound
   abdominal, for fever of unknown origin diagnosis, 234
   for biliary tract disease diagnosis, 198
   for *Cryptosporidium*, 100
   for *Entamoeba histolytica* diagnosis, 106
   for HIVAN, 155
Ultraviolet B (UVB) light, for pruritus in HIV, 126
Ultraviolet B (UVB) radiation, for psoriasis with HIV, 127
Ultraviolet radiation, for eosinophilic folliculitis in HIV, 129
United States
   AIDS cases overview for, 8-9
   estimated number of person living with AIDS in, 8f
      by race and ethnicity, 9f
      by region, 9f
   heterosexual HIV transmission in, 11
   HIV epidemiology in, 6-8
   homosexual and bisexual HIV transmission in, 9, 10f
   injecting drug users HIV transmission in, 10-11, 10f
   mortality from AIDS in, 12
   perinatal HIV transmission in, 11-12
United States Department of Health and Human Services guidelines, for opportunistic infections, 233-234

United States Public Health Service
   opportunistic infections guidelines of, 88-89
   VZV guidelines of, 93-94
Urethritis, Reiter's syndrome and, 127
Uric acid, abnormalities in, 165
   HIV-associated lymphoma and, 242
Urinalysis
   for CMV diagnosis, 85
   for diagnosis of renal failure and other renal abnormalities, 161
   for fever of unknown origin diagnosis, 230
   for histoplasmosis diagnosis, 82, 209, 212
   for HIVAN diagnosis, 155
   for *Legionella* pneumonia diagnosis, 109-110
   for membranoproliferative glomerulonephritis diagnosis, 157
   for porphyria cutanea tarda diagnosis, 128
   initial HIV assessment of, 26b
Urinary retention
   CMV polyradiculpathy and, 86
   Guillain-Barré syndrome and, 169
Urinary symptoms, of CMV radiculitis, 173
Urine culture, for fever of unknown origin diagnosis, 230
Urticaria, *Giardia lamblia* and, 105
Uveitis; *see also* Syphilitic retinitis
   acute
      rifabutin treatment with antiretroviral therapy and, 71-72
      and rifamycin for TB, 74
   anterior
      retinal necrosis and, 149
      secondary syphilis and, 112
      syphilitic retinitis and, 151
      toxoplasmosis retinochoroiditis and, 151
   as ocular complication of AIDs, 141-142, 142b
   from cidofovir, 87
   from CMV treatment, 88
   granulomatous
      herpes zoster ophthalmicus and, 144
      hypercalcemia and, 164
      retinal necrosis and, 149
      varicella-zoster keratitis and, 144
      varicella-zoster virus and, 92

V

Vaccinations
   for children with AIDS, 253
   for influenza, 210
   HIV medical history and, 24
   pneumococcal, 206
Vaccines
   for human papillomavirus, 245
   for human papillomavirus viral protein E7, 247
Vacuolar myelopathy, as neurologic complication of HIV, 167b, 168, 168b
Vaginal candidiasis, 193
Vaginal discharge, in vulvovaginal candidiasis, 80
Vaginitis, comprehensive history of, 25b

Valacyclovir
    CMV prophylaxis and, 89
    for cytomegalovirus, 50
    for herpes zoster, 120, 174
    for herpes zoster encephalitis, 171
    for herpes zoster ophthalmicus, 144
    for HSV, 50, 54t, 90-91, 119, 200
        with HIV, 136
    for VZV, 93, 93t
    resistance to VZV, 93
Valganciclovir
    for CMV esophagitis, 194
    for CMV retinitis, 148
    for cytomegalovirus, 50, 87
Valium; see Diazepam
Valproic acid, for mania, 183, 183b
Valtrex; see Valacyclovir
Vancomycin
    for *Clostridium difficile,* 219
    for pneumococcal pneumonia, 206
    for *Rhodococcus equi,* 116, 207
Varicella vaccine
    for children with AIDS, 253, 253b
Varicella zoster immunoglubulin, 53t, 94
    for children with AIDS, 253
Varicella-zoster keratitis, 144-145, 145b
Varicella-zoster retinitis, 92, 93, 150-151, 151b
Varicella-zoster virus (VZV), 50, 53t; *see also* Herpes zoster; Herpes zoster ophthalmicus
    anorectal HSV *vs.,* 199
    cause of, 91
    diagnosis of, 92-93
    encephalitis from, 171
    focal CNS lesion and, 98t
    guidelines for, 93-94
    HIV-associated anorectal lesions and, 199
    HSV *vs.,* 90
    natural history of, 93
    optic nerve atrophy and, 147
    presentation of, 92
    pulmonary, late HIV infection and, 210
    referrals for, 93
    retinal necrosis and, 85, 150
    suggestive of HIV, 135t
    treatment for, 93, 93t
    with HIV, 137
Vascular disorders, neurologic symptoms of HIV and, 166
Vascular endothelial growth factor inhibitors, for Kaposi's sarcoma, 240b, 241
Vascular lesions, *Bartonella* and, 115
Vasculitis
    cerbrovascular disease and, 173
    mixed essential cryoglobulinemia and, 158
    parenchymal lesions with, 171
    tuberculous meningitis and, 172
Venereal Disease Research Laboratory (VDRL) tests
    for neurosyphilis, 172
    for syphilis, HIV and, 113, 114
Venlafaxine
    for HIV-associated dementia, 188
    for major depressive disorder, 180b
    potential antiretroviral interaction with, 182t

Ventriculitis, varicella-zoster virus and, 92
Ventriculoencephalitis, CMV and, 86
Verruca vulgaris, as oral manifestation of HIV, 137
Verrucae, in HIV, 121
Verrucous carcinoma, anal, diagnosis of, 200
Vibrio spp., HIV-associated diarrhea and, 219
Vidarabine monohydrate, for herpes simplex keratitis, 144
Video-assisted thoracoscopic surgery (VATS), 214
Videx; *see* Didanosine
Videx EC; *see* Didanosine
Vinblastine
    for Kaposi's sarcoma, 134t, 240, 240b
    neuropsychiatric side effects of, 181t
Vinblastine sulfate, for Kaposi's sarcoma, oral, 137
Vincalkaloids, for Kaposi's sarcoma, 130
Vincristine
    for HIV-associated lymphoma, 242, 243
    for Kaposi's sarcoma, 130, 240, 240b
    for TTP/HUS, 159
    sensory-motor neuropathy and, 175
Vinorelbine, for Kaposi's sarcoma, 130
Vira-A; *see* Vidarabine monohydrate
Viral culture, for HSV diagnosis, 119
    varicella-zoster virus *vs.,* 200
Viral genotype, 13
Viral load, 13
    acute HIV-1 infection and, 15
    antiretroviral therapy and, 31
    drug combinations and, 35
    for children with AIDS, 251, 251b
        after immunizations, 253
    for pregnant women, perinatal transmission and, 249
    high, antiretroviral therapy for, 30-31
    initial HIV assessment of, 26b
    measurements
        educational discussions on, 27-28
        for antiretroviral therapy monitoring, 35
    PCP risk and, 64
    viral RNA assay for, 18
    virologic failure of antiretroviral therapy and, 37
        genotypic resistance and, 39
Viral phenotype, 13
Viral RNA, in acute HIV-1 infection, 18
Viramune; *see* Nevirapine
Virologic failure, of antiretroviral therapy, 37
    genotypic resistance and, 39
    resistance testing and, 40
Viroptic; *see* Trifluridine
Vision; *see also* Blindness
    AIDS-related papilledema and, 147
    blurred
        fungal chorioretinitis and, 153
        retinal necrosis and, 149
    changes in, comprehensive history of, 25b
    CMV and, 85, 147, 148
    optic nerve atrophy and, 147

Vision—cont'd
    PORN and, 150
    syphilitic retinitis and, 151
    toxoplasmosis and, 151
    varicella-zoster retinitis and, 150
Visual disturbances
    neurologic complications in HIV and, 166
    progressive multifocal leukoencephalopathy and, 170
Visual field defects, *T. gondii* and, 96
Vital signs, assessment for initial HIV management, 25, 26b
Vitality, loss of, HIV-1–associated dementia complex and, 186
Vitamin A, for keratoconjunctivitis sicca, 141
Vitamin B_{12} deficiency
    as neurologic complication of HIV, 167, 167b
    HIV-associated dementia and, 187
    mania *vs.,* 183
    ulcers from, 135t
    vacuolar myelopathy *vs.,* 168
Vitrasert (intracolular depot device), 148
Vitrectomy
    for fungal chorioretinitis, 153
    with intravitreal gas, for retinal detachment, 88
Vitreous hemorrhage
    from ganciclovir implants, 87
    intravitreal injections and, 148
Vitritis
    from CMV treatment, 88
    fungal chorioretinitis and, 153
    immune recovery, 142
    retinal necrosis and, 150
    syphilitic retinitis and, 151
    toxoplasmosis retinochoroiditis and, 151
    varicella-zoster virus and, 92
Vomiting
    Cryptosporidia and, 100
    Cyclospora and, 104
    DMAC and, 76
    from acyclovir, 90
    from clindamycin-primaquine for PCP, 63t
    from cryptococcal meningitis, 171
    from systemic chemotherapy, 240
    from TMP-SMX for PCP, 206
    hyponatremia and, 162
    in acute HIV-1 infection, 17b
    microsporidia and, 102
    symptom management of, 224
    T. gondii and, 96
    with antiretroviral therapy, 35-36
von Zumbusch's psoriasis, as skin manifestation of HIV, 127
Vulvovaginal candidiasis, 80
VZV; *see* Varicella-zoster virus

W

Warfarin, antifungal azoles interactions with, 84
Warthin-Starry stain, for *Bartonella* diagnosis, 115, 237

Warts
    as oral manifestation of HIV, 137
    as skin manifestation of HIV, 121, 121b
    in HIV, 121
Wasting
    disseminated *Mycobacterium avium* complex and, 74, 77
    MAC and fever of unknown origin with, 232
    of muscles, zidovudine-related, 175
    renal magnesium, 164
    T. gondii and, 97
    tuberculosis and, 70
    without fever, *E. bieneusi* and, 217
Wasting syndrome
    as neurologic complication of HIV, 167b
    polymyositis *vs.*, 170
Water purification, *Cryptosporidium* and, 47, 101
Weakness
    chronic, AWS and, 223
    chronic inflammatory demyelinating polyneuropathy and, 169
    CMV radiculitis and, 173
    comprehensive history of, 25b
    Guillain-Barré syndrome and, 168
    lymphoma, motor neuropathy and, 175
    lymphomatous meningitis and, 175
    mononeuropathy multiplex and, 169
    motor neuropathy and, 168
    neurologic complications in HIV and, 166
    of legs
        HIV-1–associated dementia complex and, 186
        vacuolar myelopathy and, 168
    polymyositis and, 169-170
    sensory-motor neuropathy from vincristine and, 175
    T. gondii and, 96, 97
    zidovudine-related, 175
Weight, assessment for initial HIV management, 25
Weight gain
    growth hormone and, 226
    lean body mass and, 224
    oxandrolone and, 225
Weight loss; *see also* Wasting
    blastomycosis and, 83
    CMV colitis and, 86
    CMV retinitis and, 85
    comprehensive history of, 25b
    Cryptosporidia and, 100
    Cyclospora and, 104
    DMAC and, 75, 75t, 76
    documentation of, 223
    Entamoeba histolytica and, 106
    fungal pneumonias and, 208-209
    Giardia lamblia and, 105
    histoplamosis and, 82
    HIV-associated diarrhea and, 216

Weight loss—*cont'd*
    HIV-associated lymphoma and, 242
    in *Rhodococcus equi*, 116
    Isospora and, 103
    Kaposi's sarcoma and, 201
    lean body mass and, 224
    M. kansasii and, 208
    M. xenopi and, 78
    MAC and, 76
    microsporidia and, 102
    Nocardia asteroides and, 207
    PCP and, 205
    penicilliosis and, 83
    Rhodococcus equi and, 207
    testosterone and, 225
    tuberculosis and, 207
Wellness, loss of, bereavement and, 179
Western blot tests
    for HIV in infants born to HIV-infected mothers, 250, 251
    for HIV screening, 20
    indeterminate, 21
Wheezing, *Cryptosporidia* and, 100
Whipple's disease, Kaposi's sarcoma *vs.*, 201
White blood cells, biliary tract disease and, 198
White matter
    for HIV-associated dementia and, 167, 186
    subcortical, progressive multifocal leukoencephalopathy and, 170
Women
    anabolic agents effects for, 225
    androgen-deficient, transdermal testosterone for, 225, 227t
    cytomegalovirus risk for, 45
    nandrolone decanoate for anabolic block in, 225
    of reproductive age, acitretin and, 127
    pain undertreatment and, 190
Worry, anxiety disorders and, 183
Worthlessness, bereavement and, 179
Wright-Giemsa stain, for PCP, 59
Wrist drop, sensory-motor neuropathy from vincristine and, 175

X
X4 viruses, 15
Xanax; *see* Alprazolam
Xerosis, as skin manifestation of HIV, 126
Xerostomia; *see also* Sjögren's syndrome
    angular cheilitis and, 138
    as oral manifestation of HIV, 132, 135-136
    treatment of, 136t

Y
Yeast cells, fungal chorioretinitis and, 153
Yersinia
    HIV-associated diarrhea and, 219
    Reiter's syndrome and, 127

Z
Zalcitabine
    as FDA-approved NRTI, 31
    characteristics of, 32t
    esophagitis and, 193
    neurologic adverse effects from, 36
    neuropsychiatric side effects of, 181t
    nucleoside analogue-induced neuropathy and, 175
    and pentamidine for PCP, 61, 64
    rifabutin with, 47b
ZDV; *see* Zidovudine
Zerit; *see* Stavudine
Ziagen; *see* Abacavir
Zidovudine
    as FDA-approved NRTI, 31
    characteristics of, 32t
    creatine kinase increases from, 37
    depressive side effects from, 180
    drug-induced diarrhea from, 220
    esophagitis and, 193
    for children with AIDS, 253, 255
    for HIVAN, 156
    for HIV-associated dementia, 187, 188
    for oral hairy leukoplakia, 121
    for perinatal transmission prevention, 250
    for uveitis, 142
    gastrointestinal side effects from, 35-36
    headache from, 36
    hepatocellular toxicity of, 195b
    lactic acidosis and, 165
    monotherapy, for acute HIV-1 infection, 19
    neuropsychiatric side effects of, 181t
    other adverse effects from, 37
    reaction to, as oral manifestation of HIV, 135t
    renal syndromes with, 163t
    resistance to, 39
    rifabutin with, 47b
    rifamycins for TB and, 72
    skin reactions to, 129
    and TMP-SMX for PCP, 61
    valproic acid and, 183
    xerostomia from, 132
Zidovudine-related myopathy, 175
    as neurologic complication of HIV, 167b
    polymyositis *vs.*, 170
Zinc pyrithione shampoos, for seborrheic dermatitis, 128
Zoloft; *see* Sertraline
Zoster, HIV medical history and, 24
Zygomycetes, late-stage AIDS and, 83
Zyprexa; *see* Olanzapine